Orthopaedic Knowledge Update

Shoulder and Elbow

American Academy of Orthopaedic Surgeons

Orthopaedic Knowledge Update
Shoulder and Elbow

Edited by
Tom R. Norris, MD

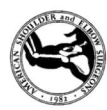
Developed by the
American Shoulder and Elbow Surgeons

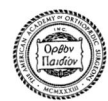
Published by the
American Academy of Orthopaedic Surgeons
6300 North River Road   Rosemont, IL 60018

Orthopaedic Knowledge Update: Shoulder and Elbow

American Academy of Orthopaedic Surgeons

The material presented in *Orthopaedic Knowledge Update: Shoulder and Elbow* has been made available by the American Academy of Orthopaedic Surgeons for educational purposes only. This material is not intended to present the only, or necessarily best, methods or procedures for the medical situations discussed, but rather is intended to represent an approach, view, statement, or opinion of the author(s) or producer(s), which may be helpful to others who face similar situations.

Some drugs or medical devices demonstrated in Academy education programs or materials have not been cleared by the FDA or have been cleared by the FDA for specific uses only. The FDA has stated that it is the responsibility of the physician to determine the FDA clearance status of each drug or device he or she wishes to use in clinical practice.

Furthermore, any statements about commercial products are solely the opinion(s) of the author(s) and do not represent an Academy endorsement or evaluation of these products. These statements may not be used in advertising or for any commercial purpose.

The material contained in this volume was submitted as previously unpublished material, except in the instances in which credit has been given to the source from which some of the illustrative material was derived.

Materials appearing in this book prepared by individuals as part of their official duties as U.S. Government employees are not covered by the above-mentioned copyright.

All rights reserved. No part of this publication may be reproduced, stored in a retrieval system, or transmitted, in any form, or by any means, electronic, mechanical, photocopying, recording, or otherwise, without prior written permission from the publisher.

First Edition
Copyright © 1997 by the
American Academy of Orthopaedic Surgeons

ISBN 0-89203-170-0

Acknowledgments

Editorial Board, OKU: Shoulder and Elbow
Tom R. Norris, MD
Ralph B. Blasier, MD
John J. Brems, MD
Evan L. Flatow, MD
Gary M. Gartsman, MD
Joseph P. Iannotti, MD, PhD
Shawn W. O'Driscoll, MD, PhD, FRCSC
Louis J. Soslowsky, PhD
Michael Watson, MA, MRCP, FRCS
Joseph D. Zuckerman, MD

**American Academy of Orthopaedic Surgeons
Board of Directors, 1997**
Douglas W. Jackson, MD, *President*
John A. Bergfeld, MD
John J. Callaghan, MD
S. Terry Canale, MD
Richard D. Coutts, MD
Alvin H. Crawford, MD
Robert D. D'Ambrosia, MD
Kenneth E. DeHaven, MD
James D. Heckman, MD
Stuart A. Hirsch, MD
George L. Lucas, MD
Edward A. Rankin, MD
Aaron G. Rosenberg, MD
Scott B. Scutchfield, MD
James W. Strickland, MD
Edward A. Toriello, MD
William W. Tipton, Jr, MD *(ex officio)*

**American Shoulder and Elbow Surgeons
Board of Directors, 1997**
Robert D. Leffert, MD, *President*
Louis U. Bigliani, MD
Edward V. Craig, MD
Harvard Ellman, MD
Gary M. Gartsman, MD
Thomas J. Neviaser, MD
Robin R. Richards, MD, FRCSC

Staff
Marilyn L. Fox, PhD, *Director, Department of Publications*
Bruce Davis, *Senior Editor*
Joan Abern, *Associate Senior Editor*
Lisa Claxton Moore, *Associate Senior Editor*
Loraine Edwalds, *Production Manager*
Sophie Tosta, *Production Coordinator*
Jana Ronayne, *Production Assistant*
Geraldine Dubberke, *Production Assistant*

Contributors

David W. Altchek, MD
Assistant Attending Orthopaedic Surgeon
Sports Medicine and Shoulder Service
The Hospital for Special Surgery
New York, New York

Kai-Nan An, PhD
Director, Biomechanics Laboratory
Division of Orthopedic Research
Mayo Clinic
Professor of Bioengineering
Mayo Medical School
Rochester, Minnesota

James R. Andrews, MD
Clinical Professor of Surgery
Division of Orthopaedic Surgery
University of Alabama at Birmingham
Birmingham, Alabama

LTC Robert A. Arciero, MD
Orthopaedic Surgery Department
Keller Army Community Hospital
United States Military Academy
West Point, New York

Christopher T. Behr, MD
Fellow, Sports Medicine and Shoulder Service
The Hospital for Special Surgery
New York, New York

Bruce D. Beynnon, PhD
Director of Research
McClure Musculoskeletal Research Center
Department of Orthopaedics and Rehabilitation
The University of Vermont
Burlington, Vermont

Ralph B. Blasier, MD
Chief of Orthopaedic Surgery
Grace Hospital
Detroit, Michigan

Erin Boynton, MD, FRCSC
Assistant Professor
Division of Orthopaedics
University of Toronto
Toronto, Ontario, Canada

John J. Brems, MD
Head-Section of Upper Extremity
Department of Orthopaedic Surgery
Cleveland Clinic Foundation
Cleveland, Ohio

Professor Timothy D. Bunker, FRCS
Consultant Orthopaedic Surgeon
Hunterian Professor
Princess Elizabeth Orthopaedic Hospital
Exeter, England

James E. Carpenter, MD
Assistant Professor of Surgery
Section of Orthopaedic Surgery
University of Michigan Shoulder Group
Ann Arbor, Michigan

Patrick M. Connor, MD
The Shoulder and Elbow Center
Miller Orthopaedic Clinic
Charlotte, North Carolina

Frances Cuomo, MD
Associate Chief, Shoulder Service
Orthopaedic Surgery
Hospital for Joint Diseases
New York, New York

Donald F. D'Alessandro, MD
Associate
The Shoulder and Elbow Center
Miller Orthopaedic Clinic
Charlotte, North Carolina

James D. Dalton, Jr, MD
Clinical Fellow, Shoulder and Sports Medicine
Department of Orthopaedic Surgery
Center for Sports Medicine
University of Pittsburgh
Pittsburgh, Pennsylvania

Maj Thomas M. Deberardino, MD
Orthopaedic Surgery Department
Keller Army Community Hospital
United States Military Academy
West Point, New York

David T. Dellaero, MD
The Hughston Clinic
Columbus, Georgia

David G. Duckworth, MD
Acting Instructor
Department of Orthopaedics
University of Washington
Seattle, Washington

Larry D. Field, MD
Co-Director, Upper Extremity Service
Mississippi Sports Medicine and Orthopaedic Center
Clinical Instructor, Department of Orthopaedic Surgery
University of Mississippi School of Medicine
Jackson, Mississippi

Evan L. Flatow, MD
Professor of Orthopaedic Surgery
Associate Chief, The Shoulder Service
New York Orthopaedic Hospital
Columbia-Presbyterian Medical Center
New York, New York

Eileen Fowler, PhD, PT
Assistant Professor
Orthopaedic Surgery
UCLA
Los Angeles, California

Gary M. Gartsman, MD
Fondren Orthopedic Group
Texas Orthopedic Hospital
Houston, Texas

Andrew Green, MD
Assistant Professor of Orthopaedic Surgery
Brown University School of Medicine
Providence, Rhode Island

Patrick E. Greis, MD
Assistant Professor, Orthopaedic Surgery
The University of Pittsburgh
Pittsburgh, Pennsylvania

S. Wendell Holmes, Jr, MD
Orthopaedic Sports Medicine Fellow
American Sports Medicine Institute
Birmingham, Alabama

Robert N. Hotchkiss, MD
Chief of Hand Service
Hospital for Special Surgery
New York, New York

Joseph P. Iannotti, MD, PhD
Associate Professor, Orthopaedic Surgery
Director, Shoulder and Elbow Service
University of Pennsylvania
Department of Orthopaedics
Philadelphia, Pennsylvania

Jesse B. Jupiter, MD
Associate Professor of Orthopaedic Surgery
Harvard Medical School
Chief, Hand Surgery Service
Massachusetts General Hospital
Department of Orthopaedic Surgery
Boston, Massachusetts

W. Ben Kibler, MD
Medical Director
Lexington Clinic
Sports Medicine Center
Lexington, Kentucky

Graham J.W. King, MD, MSc, FRCSC
Assistant Professor, Department of Surgery
University of Western Ontario
London, Ontario, Canada

Kenneth J. Koval, MD
Chief, Fracture Service
Hospital for Joint Diseases
New York, New York

John E. Kuhn, MD
Assistant Professor
The University of Michigan Shoulder Group
Division of Sports Medicine
Section of Orthopaedic Surgery
The University of Michigan
Ann Arbor, Michigan

Scott A. Lintner, MD
Orthopaedics Indianapolis, Inc.
Indianapolis, Indiana

Joachim F. Loehr, MD, FRCSC
Department of Orthopaedics
Clinic Lilthelm Schulthess
Zurich, Switzerland

George M. McCluskey III, MD
Orthopaedic Surgeon
The Hughston Clinic
Columbus, Georgia

Anthony Miniaci, MD, FRCSC
Head, Sports Medicine Program
Associate Professor
Department of Surgery
University of Toronto
Toronto, Ontario, Canada

Gary W. Misamore, MD
Methodist Sports Medicine Center
Indianapolis, Indiana

Bernard F. Morrey, MD
Chairman, Department of Orthopaedic Surgery
Department of Orthopaedic Surgery
Mayo Clinic
Rochester, Minnesota

R. John Naranja, Jr, MD
Chief Resident
University of Pennsylvania
Department of Orthopaedics
Philadelphia, Pennsylvania

Claude E. Nichols, MD
Associate Professor
McClure Musculoskeletal Research Center
Department of Orthopaedics and Rehabilitation
The University of Vermont
Burlington, Vermont

Gregory P. Nicholson, MD
Clinical Assistant Professor
Department of Orthopaedic Surgery
Indiana University
Indianapolis, Indiana

Tom R. Norris, MD
California-Pacific Medical Center
San Francisco, California

John E. Novotny, MS
Senior Biomedical Engineer
McClure Musculoskeletal Research Center
Department of Orthopaedics and Rehabilitation
The University of Vermont
Burlington, Vermont

Shawn W. O'Driscoll, MD, PhD, FRCSC
Mayo Clinic
Rochester, Minnesota

Kevin D. Plancher, MD, MS
Assistant Professor
Albert Einstein College of Medicine
Bronx, New York

Gary G. Poehling, MD
Professor and Chairman
Department of Orthopaedics
Wake Forest University Medical Center
Winston-Salem, North Carolina

Roger G. Pollock, MD
Assistant Professor of Orthopaedic Surgery
Columbia University
New York Orthopaedic Hospital
Columbia-Presbyterian Medical Center
New York, New York

David Ring, MD
Resident
Harvard Combined Orthopedic Residency
Massachusetts General Hospital
Boston, Massachusetts

Anthony A. Romeo, MD
Assistant Professor
Department of Orthopaedic Surgery
Rush-Presbyterian-St. Luke's Medical Center
Chicago, Illinois

Hirotaka Sano, MD
Research Fellow
Bone and Joint Research Laboratory
University of Ottawa
Ottawa, Ontario, Canada

C. Craig Satterlee, MD
Clinical Assistant Professor of Orthopaedic Surgery
University of Missouri, Kansas City
Kansas City, Missouri

Felix H. Savoie, MD
Mississippi Sportsmedicine
Jackson, Mississippi

Jerry S. Sher, MD
Clinical Assistant Professor
University of Miami School of Medicine
Shoulder and Knee Institute of Florida
Miami Beach, Florida

Kevin L. Smith, MD
Assistant Professor
Department of Orthopaedics
University of Washington
Seattle, Washington

Louis J. Soslowsky, PhD
Associate Professor of Surgery and Bioengineering
Director of Orthopaedic Research
Orthopaedic Research Laboratory
University of Pennsylvania
Philadelphia, Pennsylvania

A. Marc Tetro, MD, FRCSC
Department of Orthopaedic Surgery
Washington University School of Medicine
St. Louis, Missouri

Craig D. Tifford, MD
Senior Orthopaedic Resident
Department of Orthopaedic Surgery
Albert Einstein College of Medicine
Bronx, New York

Hans K. Uhthoff, MD, FRCSC
Professor Emeritus
Division of Orthopaedic Surgery
University of Ottawa
Ottawa, Ontario, Canada

Martti Vastamäki, MD, PhD
Associate Professor
Orton Orthopaedic Hospital of the Invalid Foundation
Helsinki, Finland

Jon J.P. Warner, MD
Director, Shoulder Service
Assistant Professor of Orthopaedic Surgery
Assistant Director of the Center for Sports Medicine
The University of Pittsburgh
Pittsburgh, Pennsylvania

Michael Watson, MA, MRCP, FRCS
Orthopaedic Surgeon
Suy's Hospital
Correron, United Kingdom

Thomas W. Wright, MD
Associate Professor of Orthopaedics
University of Florida
Department of Orthopaedics
Gainesville, Florida

Ken Yamaguchi, MD
Assistant Professor
Shoulder and Elbow Service
Department of Orthopaedic Surgery
Washington University School of Medicine
St. Louis, Missouri

Joseph D. Zuckerman, MD
Chief, Shoulder Service
Chairman, Department of Orthopaedic Surgery
Hospital for Joint Disease
New York, New York

Table of Contents

	Acknowledgments		v
	Contributors		vii
	Preface		xv

Section I: Basic Science

Section Editors — **Ralph B. Blasier, MD**
Louis J. Soslowsky, PhD

1	Tissues and Their Structure	Gregory P. Nicholson, MD Scott A. Lintner, MD	3
2	Biomechanics of Glenohumeral Stability	John E. Kuhn, MD	11
3	Basic Science of the Rotator Cuff	James E. Carpenter, MD	19
4	Shoulder Kinematics and Kinesiology	Bruce D. Beynnon, PhD Claude E. Nichols, MD John E. Novotny, MS	31
5	Basic Science Considerations in Glenohumeral Arthroplasty and Proximal Humeral Fractures	A. Marc Tetro, MD, FRCSC Ken Yamaguchi, MD	37
6	Evaluating Outcomes in the Treatment of Shoulder Disorders	John E. Kuhn, MD Ralph B. Blasier, MD	47

Section II: Instability and Athletic Injuries

Section Editor — **Evan L. Flatow, MD**

7	Clinical Assessment, Imaging, and Classification	Erin Boynton, MD, FRCSC Anthony Miniaci, MD, FRCSC	59
8	Acute and Chronic Dislocations of the Shoulder	LTC Robert A. Arciero, MD Maj Thomas M. Deberardino, MD	67
9	Recurrent Anterior Instability	Jon J.P. Warner, MD Patrick E. Greis, MD	77
10	Multidirectional and Posterior Instability of the Shoulder	Roger G. Pollock, MD	85
11	Arthroscopic Anterior Glenohumeral Reconstruction	Gary M. Gartsman, MD	95

12	Special Issues in Athletes	George M. McCluskey III, MD David T. Dellaero, MD		**101**
13	Complications, Failed Repairs, and Revision Surgery	Christopher T. Behr, MD David W. Altchek, MD		**111**

Section III: Rotator Cuff Impingement

Section Editor — **Joseph P. Iannotti, MD**

14	Anatomy, Function, Pathogenesis, and Natural History of Rotator Cuff Disorders	Jerry S. Sher, MD	**123**
15	Nonsurgical Treatment of Rotator Cuff Tears	Craig D. Tifford, MD Kevin D. Plancher, MD, MS	**135**
16	Surgical Treatment of the Intact Cuff and Repairable Cuff Defect: Arthroscopic and Open Techniques	Joseph P. Iannotti, MD, PhD R. John Naranja, Jr, MD Gary M. Gartsman, MD	**151**
17	Complications of Rotator Cuff Surgery	R. John Naranja, Jr, MD Joseph P. Iannotti, MD, PhD Gary M. Gartsman, MD	**157**
18	Massive Rotator Cuff Tears	Anthony Miniaci, MD, FRCSC	**167**
19	Cuff Tear Arthropathy	David G. Duckworth, MD Kevin L. Smith, MD	**173**

Section IV: Trauma/Fracture

Section Editor — **Joseph D. Zuckerman, MD**

20	Proximal Humerus Fractures	Frances Cuomo, MD	**181**
21	Clavicle Fractures	Anthony A. Romeo, MD	**191**
22	Scapular Fractures	Andrew Green, MD	**199**
23	Humeral Shaft Fractures	Kenneth J. Koval, MD	**205**

Section V: Arthritis/Arthroplasty

Section Editor — **John J. Brems, MD**

24	Inflammatory Arthritis of the Shoulder	Patrick M. Connor, MD Donald F. D'Alessandro, MD	**215**
25	Management of Osteoarthritis of the Shoulder	Gary W. Misamore, MD	**227**
26	Osteonecrosis and Other Noninflammatory Degenerative Diseases of the Glenohumeral Joint Including Gaucher's Disease, Sickle Cell Disease, Hemochromatosis, and Synovial Osteochondromatosis	C. Craig Satterlee, MD	**233**

Section VI: Miscellaneous Shoulder Problems

Section Editor — **Michael Watson, MA, MRCP, FRCS**

27	Brachial Plexus Injuries	James D. Dalton, Jr, MD Jon J.P. Warner, MD	**243**
28	Frozen Shoulder	Timothy D. Bunker, FRCS	**255**
29	Suprascapular Nerve Entrapment	Martti Vastamäki, MD, PhD	**265**
30	Lesions of the Superior Aspect of the Shoulder	Felix H. Savoie, MD Larry D. Field, MD	**269**
31	Calcifying Tendinitis, Chondrocalcinosis, Heterotopic Ossification, and Pigmented Villonodular Synovitis	Hans K. Uhthoff, MD, FRCSC Hirotaka Sano, MD Joachim F. Loehr, MD, FRCSC	**277**
32	Rehabilitation of the Shoulder	W. Ben Kibler, MD	**289**

Section VII: Elbow Trauma/Fracture/Reconstruction

Section Editor — **Shawn W. O'Driscoll, MD, PhD, FRCSC**

33	Biomechanics and Functional Anatomy of the Elbow	Graham J.W. King, MD, MSc, FRCSC Kai-Nan An, PhD	**301**
34	Athletic Injuries of the Elbow	James R. Andrews, MD S. Wendell Holmes, Jr, MD	**311**
35	Stiffness and Ankylosis of the Elbow	Graham J.W. King, MD, MSc, FRCSC	**325**
36	Tendon Injuries and Tendinopathies About the Elbow	Bernard F. Morrey, MD	**337**
37	Elbow Instability	Shawn W. O'Driscoll, MD, PhD, FRCSC	**345**
38	Loose Bodies of the Elbow	Shawn W. O'Driscoll, MD, PhD, FRCSC	**355**
39	Osteochondritis Dissecans of the Elbow	Gary G. Poehling, MD	**363**
40	Nerve Injuries and Neuropathies About the Elbow	Thomas W. Wright, MD	**369**
41	Elbow Arthritis	Bernard F. Morrey, MD Shawn W. O'Driscoll, MD, PhD, FRCSC	**379**
42	Fractures of the Radial Head	Robert N. Hotchkiss, MD	**387**
43	Fractures of the Distal Humerus	Jesse B. Jupiter, MD David Ring, MD	**397**
44	Olecranon and Coronoid Fractures	Shawn W. O'Driscoll, MD, PhD, FRCSC	**405**
	Index		**414**

Preface

Orthopaedic Knowledge Update: Shoulder and Elbow, the newest addition to the *OKU* Specialty Series, was developed in response to the explosion of knowledge and interest in the field of shoulder and elbow disorders. While a dream of many, this labor of love was championed by the late Harvard Ellman, MD. It was his vision that has enabled earlier chapters on shoulder and elbow topics in *OKU* to be expanded into this book to address many of the exciting advances in our field.

Codman published the first book on the shoulder in 1934. The field advanced with the anatomic investigations of DePalma and Moseley. McLaughlin, Rowe, Bateman, and Neviaser contributed clinical advances. It was Neer who made clinically useful the Codman four-part proximal humerus fracture classification system and developed a prosthetic replacement for the shoulder. He led the way in the study of many of the topics presented here, including new concepts in impingement and cuff pathology, instability, fractures, and prosthetic arthroplasty.

Of equal importance, Neer and Rockwood responded to the expansion of knowledge with the development of fellowship training for the many orthopaedic surgeons who now lead the field in research and clinical advances. In addition to our section editors, these include Bigliani, Cofield, Matsen, Hawkins, Warren, Craig, Kessel, and Gerber who have published and organized courses in the shoulder, and Coonrad, Morrey, and Ewald in the elbow.

This up-to-date book summarizing the current status of the shoulder and elbow is only made possible by the generous donation of time and expertise of the chapter contributors, and of the section editors: Blasier and Soslowsky for basic science; Flatow for shoulder instability and athletic injuries; Iannotti for impingement and rotator cuff pathology; Zuckerman for trauma, including fractures of the proximal humerus and clavicle; Brems for shoulder arthroplasty; Watson, who truly made this an international collaboration with the European authors to address the many additional shoulder topics; and O'Driscoll for coordinating all the elbow topics. Gartsman acted as consultant, helping develop and coordinate the arthroscopy topics. In this book, each author is identified with each chapter; thus, their efforts can be directly acknowledged.

This *OKU: Shoulder and Elbow* would not have been possible without the strong support of the publications staff at the American Academy of Orthopaedic Surgeons: Marilyn Fox, PhD, Director of Publications; Lisa Claxton Moore, Associate Senior Editor; and the entire publications staff for their coordinated efforts in the editing, production, and overall management of this project. Their frequent communications kept us on track.

All of us who have contributed to the completion of this book know that this update will be a valuable resource in the study of the shoulder and elbow.

Tom R. Norris, MD
Editor

I
Basic Science

Ralph B. Blasier, MD
Louis J. Soslowsky, PhD
Section Editors

1
Tissues and Their Structure
Gregory P. Nicholson, MD and Scott A. Lintner, MD

The functional abilities of the shoulder are made possible by the unique structural characteristics of the osseous, ligamentous, cartilaginous, tendinous, and muscle tissues of the shoulder girdle. The shoulder girdle consists of three joints: glenohumeral, acromioclavicular, sternoclavicular; and two main spaces, subacromial and scapulothoracic. Many recent advances in our knowledge of the structure of the tissues of the shoulder girdle have led to a better understanding of the function of the shoulder as a whole. This chapter will focus on these recent advances.

The Glenohumeral Joint

Osseous Structures

Most studies on glenohumeral joint geometry have been performed in conjunction with shoulder arthroplasty system design. Different measurement techniques (direct specimen measurement, radiographs, stereophotogrammetry), and diagnostic methods (radiographs, magnetic resonance imaging (MRI), gross specimen examination) have provided somewhat contradictory data on the congruency of the glenohumeral joint surfaces. Using measurements from gross specimens, a difference between the radius of curvature of the joint surface of the humerus and the glenoid has been shown. The average radius of curvature of the humeral head in the coronal plane is 24 mm ± 1.2 mm. The glenoid radius of curvature averaged 2.3 mm greater than that of the humeral head.

The articular geometry of the bone and cartilage surfaces of the glenohumeral joint was analyzed using stereophotogrammetry. The congruence of radii between the two joint surfaces was found to be within 2 mm in 88% of specimens. The articular cartilage of the humeral head was thickest at its center, and that of the glenoid was thickest at its periphery. This may partially explain why data from plain radiographic studies showed a larger radius of curvature to the glenoid compared to that of the humeral head. The articular surface geometry of the glenohumeral joint approaches congruency in the majority of specimens studied. Continuing study is needed in this area to clarify this issue.

The superior part of the articular surface of the humeral head averages 8 mm (range of 3 to 23 mm) above the level of the greater tuberosity. The center of the humeral head is offset approximately 9 mm posteriorly in relationship to the center of the humeral shaft. The retroversion of the humeral articular surface has been noted in the literature to be anywhere from 10° to 45°. Using the intramedullary canal as a reference point, the retroversion has been shown to widely vary from specimen to specimen, from 10° to 55°, with an average of 29.8° (±11°). Thus, with the posterior offset of the humeral head and the variability in retroversion angle, the position of a humeral prosthesis must be individualized. Glenoid position in relation to the scapula has not shown as much variability. The glenoid has an average of 5° of superior tilt in relationship to the scapula and a retroversion of 3° to 9° in relationship to the long axis of the scapula.

The main blood supply to the humeral head is provided by the anterolateral ascending branch of the anterior circumflex humeral artery. It is consistently located in the lateral aspect of the intertubercular groove. It enters the bone at the proximal end of the groove at the junction with the greater tuberosity. The interosseous continuation of the arcuate artery supplies the vast majority of the articular segment. There are, however, other sources of blood supply via anastomosis to the humeral head. The posterior circumflex artery sends multiple branches into the posterior humeral neck and greater tuberosity. Anastomosis from the rotator cuff tendon insertions have been thought to provide some vascular supply to limited portions of the proximal humerus. There are also anastomotic connections to supply the humeral head through the arcuate artery by way of the anterior circumflex, thoracoacromial, and suprascapular arteries.

Labrum

The labrum is a fibrous structure surrounding the periphery of the glenoid. The labrum consists of fibrous tissue that is attached to the glenoid cartilage through a fibrocartilaginous transition zone. Like the meniscus of the knee, the labrum contains proteoglycans and stains intermediate with saffron-O. Labrum specimens from young individuals contain very little elastin, but there does appear to be an increase in elastin composition with age.

The labrum is triangular in cross section in the superior portion of the joint and becomes more rounded and less elevated on the inferior glenoid. Branches of the suprascapular artery, the circumflex scapular artery, and the posterior humeral circumflex artery serve as the labrum's vascular supply. Vessels are more numerous peripherally, but unlike the knee meniscus, there are vessels found centrally with no areas identified as being avascular. There is less vascularity at the fibrocartilaginous junction between the glenoid rim and the labrum. There does not appear to be any vascular contribution to the labrum from the underlying glenoid rim.

The attachment of the labrum to the underlying glenoid is variable. The long head of the biceps inserts into the superior labrum, where the collagen fibers of each intermingle. There is usually a synovial reflection beneath the labrum superiorly, where the articular cartilage extends over the rim of the glenoid under the area of biceps attachment.

The anterior-superior labrum can be the site of origin for the middle glenohumeral ligament (MGHL) or the inferior glenohumeral ligament (IGHL) rather than the glenoid itself.

The anterior glenolabral attachments are variable at the equator, with a sublabral hole communicating with the subscapularis recess in some shoulders. The superior labrum is generally more mobile and loosely attached to the glenoid in comparison to the inferior labrum.

The mean depth of the labrum anteriorly is 3.1 mm (1.0 to 6.4 mm); posteriorly, 3.3 mm (1.1 to 6.6 mm); superiorly, 3.0 mm (1.3 to 5.2 mm); and inferiorly, 3.8 mm (1.6 to 7.7 mm). The elevation of the glenolabral socket when including the labrum is increased by approximately 50%. The labrum increases the contact surface area of the glenohumeral joint by 38% in the long axis and 36% in the short axis. The labrum also increases the humeral head coverage area by 72% in the long axis and 59% in the short axis when compared to the glenoid devoid of labrum. The labrum has been shown to contribute approximately 20% to glenohumeral stability when the humeral head is compressed onto the glenoid when the capsule and musculature are absent.

Capsule

The shoulder joint capsule is a complex structure reinforced with distinct thickenings or "ligaments." The posterior capsule is relatively thin with no obviously identifiable thickenings. In the posterior capsule there is a simple pattern of radial and circular collagen fibers. The anterior-inferior capsule has thickenings identifiable as the superior glenohumeral ligament (SGHL), MGHL, and the IGHL (Fig. 1).

The SGHL is visible only from the articular side of the capsule and is always detectable under polarized light, but the collagen orientation is quite variable. Almost 20% of the time the SGHL fibers cross under the biceps tendon and form a portion of a fibrous canal for the biceps tendon.

The MGHL is quite variable in orientation and presentation. It originates from the labrum approximately 86% of the time and from the glenoid rim approximately 14% of the time. In only 33% of shoulders does the MGHL represent a distinct band. In the remaining shoulders the MGHL is blended with the capsule.

The IGHL is the most consistent in orientation and presentation of the glenohumeral ligaments. The IGHL consists of a thicker anterior band and a thinner, inconsistent posterior band separated by an intervening pouch. The anterior and inferior capsule collagen fiber bundles are oriented so that they radiate spirally in three layers to attach into the glenolabral area. There are three layers to the inferior glenohumeral ligament complex. The thinner, middle layer is oriented 90° to the two thicker outer layers that run in the coronal plane from the glenoid to the humerus. The anterior band and the posterior band may consist of identifiable thickenings of the inner layer. These thickenings, when present, are distinct bundles of well-organized, coarse collagen fibers running coronally. The axillary pouch has a less organized pattern of collagen fibers.

Studies of the anatomy and tensile properties of the IGHL complex revealed that the superior band is thickest (mean, 2.23 mm) and that the complex becomes thinner more posteriorly (Fig. 2). The anterior pouch averaged 1.94 mm, and the posterior pouch thickness averaged 1.59 mm. This thickness calls into question the actual existence of the posterior band as a discrete structure. It was also noted that the thickness decreased in a proximal-to-distal fashion, thus being thicker near the glenoid insertions (mean, 2.30 mm) than near the humerus (mean, 1.61 mm). The length of all three regions was similar and consistent (mean, 43 mm).

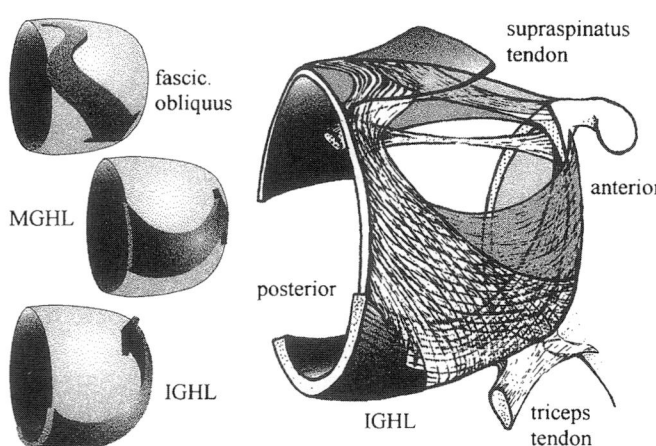

Fig. 1 Orientation of collagen fiber bundles in ligamentous reinforcements of anterior capsule. MGHL, middle glenohumeral ligament; IGHL, inferior glenohumeral ligament. (Reproduced with permission from Gohlke F, Essigkrug B, Schmitz F: The pattern of the collagen fiber bundles of the capsule of the glenohumeral joint. *J Shoulder Elbow Surg* 1994;3:111-128.)

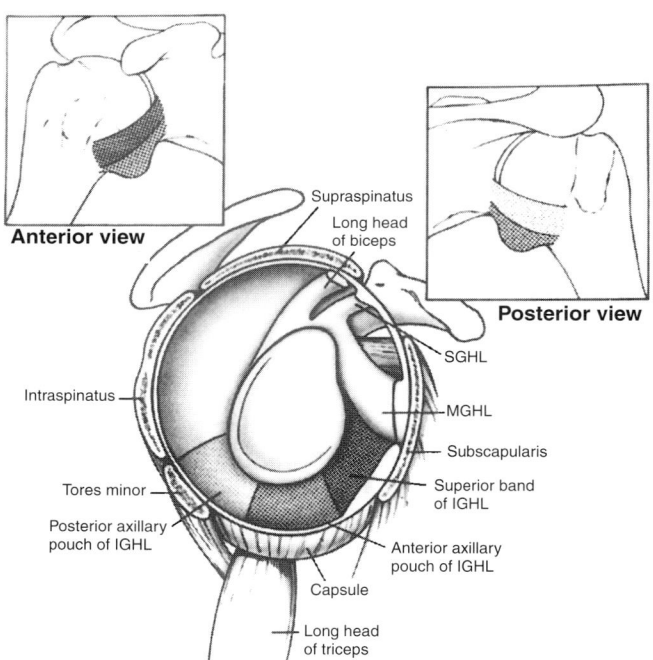

Fig. 2 Anatomic drawings of the three regions of the inferior glenohumeral ligament (IGHL) from intracapsular and extracapsular views. MGHL = middle glenohumeral ligament; SGHL = superior glenohumeral ligament. (Reproduced with permission from Bigliani LU, Kelkar R, Flatow EL, et al: Glenohumeral stability: Biomechanical properties of passive and active stabilizers. *Clin Orthop* 1996;330:13-30.)

Tensile studies, both at low strain rates and higher, near-physiologic strain rates, showed that the superior band of the IGHL had the greatest stiffness, and that the bone insertion site experiences greater strain than the midsubstance of the ligament. When subjected to force, the anterior axillary pouch, along with the anterior band, exhibited a viscoelastic stiffening effect. The anterior portion of the IGHL complex demonstrated increased stiffness and strength at higher, near-physiologic strain rates. This supports the concept that the anterior IGHL complex stabilizes the humeral head in the abducted, externally rotated position from excessive translation.

The SGHL appears to be a restraint to inferior translation and external rotation in the adducted shoulder position. The MGHL appears to contribute to anterior stability in the mid-abducted shoulder as well as limiting external rotation in this position. In the midranges of motion, capsular mechanisms of joint restraint seem to play a small role in glenohumeral joint stability.

Rotator Cuff Interval

The rotator cuff interval is the triangular space between the subscapularis and supraspinatus. The coracoid forms the base medially, and the apex is at the transverse humeral ligament over the bicipital groove laterally. The long head of the biceps tendon runs through the interval as does the superior glenohumeral ligament. The coracohumeral ligament, which covers the interval, has a constant insertion off the lateral border of the base of the coracoid. This insertion has been described as shaped as an inverted "V". The fibers of the coracohumeral ligament then run laterally, blending with the capsular fibers to insert into the deep and superficial layers of both the supraspinatus and subscapularis. Histologically, the coracohumeral ligament does not resemble a true ligament, most notably because of the absence of organized bundles of collagen fibers; it appears to be a fold of anterosuperior capsule. Tissue in the rotator cuff interval does limit inferior translation, and in some studies the release of the interval tissue leads to significant posterior and inferior translations. Imbrication of the interval leads to limitations of glenohumeral external rotation, extension, and inferior translation. The obligate anterior translation seen with flexion was also noted to increase with a tightened rotator interval capsule (coracohumeral ligament). These findings have clinical implications in surgical reconstruction procedures. Our knowledge in this area of the shoulder capsule is increasing, but more study is needed to continue to clarify the structure and function of the rotator cuff interval.

Long Head of the Biceps Tendon

In the rotator cuff interval between the supraspinatus and subscapularis, the long head of the biceps tendon passes from its intra-articular portion into the bicipital or intertubercular groove. A sling to support the tendon proximal to the groove is formed by fibers from the subscapularis and supraspinatus (Fig. 3). The subscapularis fibers branch off and form the floor of the sheath and fibers from the supraspinatus branch form the roof over the long biceps tendon. The coracohumeral ligament covers this sheath. The long head of the biceps tendon has a unique anatomic course. Its origin is from the supraglenoid tubercle, approximately 5 mm medial to the superior articular rim of the

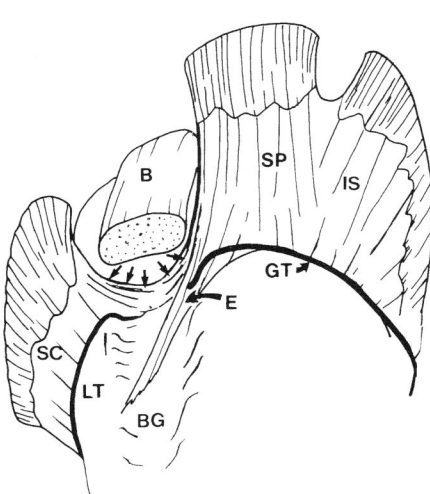

Fig. 3 The bed for the long head of biceps tendon is formed primarily by fibers from the subscapularis (small arrows). The lateral extension (E) of fibers from the supraspinatus normally forms the roof over the biceps groove. SC = subscapularis; B = biceps; SP = supraspinatus; IS = infraspinatus; LT = lesser tuberosities; BG = bicipital groove; GT = greater tuberosity. (Reproduced with permission from Clark JM, Harryman DT II: Tendons, ligaments, and capsule of the rotator cuff: Gross and microscopic anatomy. *J Bone Joint Surg* 1992;74A:713-725.)

glenoid. It also has a Y-shaped origin from the superior glenoid labrum. The tendon course is intra-articular through the previously described sheath/sling and turns sharply inferiorly into the intertubercle groove. The tendon length averages approximately 100 mm. The cross-sectional area of the tendon changes as the tendon courses distally. Proximally it is largest, averaging 8.4 mm by 3.4 mm. As it proceeds into the intertubercular groove (which anatomically gets narrower distally) the tendon size decreases to an average of 4.5 mm by 2.1 mm. Within the groove, the tendon is covered by a synovial sheath (a reflection of the glenohumeral joint synovium) and has been shown to be well vascularized throughout its course.

Tendon failure is most likely caused by mechanical stresses and friction related to its anatomic course and structure. Degenerative lesions have been shown to be most prevalent at the distal biceps groove (the most narrow anatomic enclosure) and near the origin superiorly.

The exact function of the long head of the biceps tendon is still under debate. Clinically and biomechanically it appears that this structure can act as a head depressor. However, its action does not aggravate inferior instability. Investigations have shown that it also contributes to anterior-posterior stability. In certain arm positions, the long head of the biceps tendon appears to act as a dynamic stabilizer of the humeral head. In other positions, its action does aggravate posterior instability. Further work is necessary to clarify its functional role.

Subacromial Space

The most prominent structure in the boundary of the subacromial space is the acromion. It is formed by the fusion of epiphyseal growth centers around the age of 21 to 24 years, and variations in size, shape, angle, and sagittal morphology have been noted. Acromion length, width, and anterior thickness have recently been reported, with a fundamental difference in size between men and women being noted. The average dimensions for males were: length, 48.5 mm; width, 19.5 mm; anterior thickness, 7.7 mm. For females, the average dimensions were 40.6 mm, 18.4 mm, and 6.7 mm, respectively.

Changes in sagittal morphology of the undersurface of the acromion have been associated with rotator cuff disease. Studies have shown that acromial morphology that protrudes into the subacromial space increases the contact force on the rotator cuff tendons and increases pressure readings in the subacromial space with simulated arm motion. There is debate over whether the acromion undergoes a change in its morphology. A recent longitudinal study of acromial morphology showed no significant alteration in the morphology with advancing age. According to outlet view radiographs, the morphology of the acromion was not affected by an age-dependent anterior acromial spur formation. Thus, morphology and spur formation are two independent factors that will impact the subacromial space.

Another structural component to the superior boundary of the subacromial space is the coracoacromial ligament, which connects two osseous processes of the scapula, the coracoid and the acromion. The origin from the coracoid is off the anterior and superior surface of the most distal aspect of the coracoid. Three main variants have been described: quadrangular, Y-shaped, and broad banded. The average length of the attachment on the coracoid is approximately 32 mm, whereas the narrower insertion on the undersurface of the acromion averages approximately 19 mm. There is usually a distinct lateral band and medial band structure separated by a small, less organized area near the coracoid. In specimens with intact rotator cuffs the average dimensions for the lateral band were: length, 34 mm; thickness, .96 mm; and width, 8.0 mm. For the medial band, average length was 32.4 mm; thickness, .99 mm; and width, 6.3 mm. In specimens with rotator cuff tears the lateral band showed increased thickness (average, 1.21 mm) and decreased length (average, 26.6 mm).

The insertion of the coracoacromial ligament under the anterolateral aspect of the acromion has been noted to be the site of spur formation. As the ligament itself comes under tension and the anterolateral acromion sees contact forces, the ligament insertion may undergo endochondral ossification. This scenario marks the beginning of age-dependent spur formation off the acromion.

The coracoid forms the superior or anterior boundary of the subacromial space. The coracoid process is quite variable in size, shape, and degree of inclination into the space above the subscapularis. Studies on the clinical significance of subcoracoid impingement are lacking. The role of the coracoid process on suprarotator cuff space pathologies is unclear.

The acromioclavicular joint does form the most medial superior roof of the subacromial space. The acromial facet and the distal clavicle are stoutly held by capsule and ligaments. Impingement on the rotator cuff can occur from the inferior aspect of the acromioclavicular joint. As the arm elevates, the contact force on the acromion moves from the anterolateral acromion to medial and somewhat posterior on the acromion and then to the inferior capsule of the acromioclavicular joint as elevation continues. On the supraspinatus, contact is initially proximal at 0° of elevation and moves distally to the insertion of the tendon as elevation continues.

Between the superior structural boundary of the subacromial space (acromion, coracoacromial ligament, coracoid, acromioclavicular joint) and the inferior structural boundary of the subacromial space (superficial surface of rotator cuff and interval tissue) is the anatomic structure of the subacromial bursa, which is normally synovium-lined and variable in size, but extends from approximately the midpoint of the acromion laterally (thus about the junction of the supraspinatus and infraspinatus) to the superior third of the subscapularis. From medial to lateral it extends from just lateral to the acromioclavicular joint and coracohumeral ligament origin to down over the greater tuberosity for a distance of approximately 3 to 5 cm from the lateral acromial border. Outside of the bursal confines the rest of the subdeltoid space is fibrofatty areolar tissue. Histologically, the subacromial space under the anterolateral border of the acromion has four layers: synovial (bursal wall), collagen fibers (coracoacromial ligament), fibrocartilage (coracoacromial ligament insertion), and then bone (acromion). In other areas without coracoacromial ligament insertion, it is a synovial layer (bursa), areolar tissue, and the bone of the acromion. The bursa itself has been shown to have neural elements that were in the form of diffuse, copious free nerve endings. The majority of neural elements were found on the roof of the bursa near the coracoacromial ligament. Pacinian corpuscles and Ruffini endings were also seen, but in smaller numbers than the diffuse free nerve endings. The presence of these structures may be evidence that the bursa does mediate pain perception in pathologic conditions. The bursa has also been shown to be a structure that can begin the repair process with vascular ingrowth and fibroblast migration into bursal-sided tendon tears.

Acromioclavicular Joint

The acromioclavicular joint is diarthrodial, with a shallow concave facet on the acromion that averages 17.3 mm in length and 9.1 mm in height. The convex surface of the distal clavicle is approximately twice this surface area. The joint is usually medially or vertically oriented, and very rarely is laterally tilted in relation to the frontal plane. A meniscus attached to the superior capsule is usually perforated or incomplete. The capsule itself is the primary restraint to anteroposterior translation of the joint. The capsule has been noted to be thickest superiorly and posteriorly. The capsular insertions on the distal clavicle have been shown to average 16.1 mm superiorly and 15.6 mm posteriorly from the joint line. Distal clavicle resection proximal to these capsular insertions may lead to excessive anteroposterior motion at the distal clavicle. The primary restraint to superior-inferior displacement of the acromioclavicular joint are the coracoclavicular ligaments: the trapezoid and the conoid ligaments. The conoid ligament provides restraint to superior-inferior displacement, whereas the trapezoid ligament resists compressive forces (lateral displacement of the clavicle) at the acromioclavicular joint. The amount of motion at the acromioclavicular articulation between scapula and clavicle appears to be slight. The joint does compress, translate, and rotate, but usually in concert with scapular motion. Most of the clavicular motion appears to occur at the sternoclavicular joint.

Sternoclavicular Joint

The medial end of the clavicle is concave in the anteroposterior plane and convex vertically. The much smaller sternal articular fossa is not congruent and thus allows free motion, limited only by the constraints of the ligamentous structures. The stability of the sternoclavicular joint is totally dependent on the ligamentous anatomy. The most important ligament is the capsular ligament, which covers the anterosuperior and posterior aspect of the joint. This structure prevents upward displacement of the medial clavicle caused by downward forces on the outer clavicle. The capsular ligament provides stability, but allows the clavicle to move approximately 30° upward, 30° in combined anteroposterior motion, and through 45° of rotation along the long axis. Biomechanical studies encompassing loads at the joint and stresses on the ligaments coupled with differing arm position have yet to be done.

Scapulothoracic Articulation

The scapula slides over the cone of the thoracic cage. Its stability and motion are controlled by the scapular rotator muscles, the most important of which seems to be the serratus anterior muscle. This muscle is responsible for holding the medial scapula to the chest wall, and it has been shown to have the highest muscle activity throughout the range of motion of all scapular muscles. It also assists in rotation and elevation of the scapula. Scapular rotation is necessary to place the glenohumeral joint in a position of maximum stability.

The scapulothoracic articulation can be divided into two triangular spaces. The serratus anterior space is surrounded by the rib cage anteriorly, the serratus anterior muscle posteriorly, and the rhomboid muscles medially. There is a well-defined bursa filling the area of this space. A smaller subscapularis space is surrounded by the subscapularis posteriorly, serratus anterior muscle anteriorly, and the axilla laterally. The serratus anterior obliquely separates these two spaces from one another as it traverses the scapulothoracic articulation from anterior laterally to posterior medially.

Selected Bibliography

Osseous Structures

Iannotti JP, Gabriel JP, Schneck SL, et al: The normal glenohumeral relationships: An anatomical study of 140 shoulders. *J Bone Joint Surg* 1992;74A:491-500.

Using both cadavers and magnetic resonance imaging, the authors measured the dimensions of the humeral and glenoid articular surfaces in 140 shoulders. The radius of curvature of the humeral head and glenoid were measured. The average thickness of the humeral head was measured and a strong correlation between the size of the humeral head and the lateral humeral offset measurement was noted. This study gives measurement parameters for reconstruction of the glenohumeral joint with prosthetic replacement.

Jobe CM, Iannotti JP: Limits imposed on glenohumeral motion by joint geometry. *J Shoulder Elbow Surg* 1995;4:281-285.

The authors studied 50 cadaveric shoulders and analyzed the arc of articular cartilage available off the humeral head and matching glenoid. The radius of curvature of the humeral head was measured. The surface area of the humeral head and matching glenoid were also calculated. The geometry of the articular surface of the glenohumeral joint limits the motion that is available in simple arcs.

Pearl ML, Volk AG: Retroversion of the proximal humerus in relationship to prosthetic replacement arthroplasty. *J Shoulder Elbow Surg* 1995;4:286-289.

The authors measured the retroversion of the humeral head in relationship to the surgically reamed humeral canal. They found that retroversion is highly variable, ranging from 10° to 55° with a mean of 30°.

Soslowsky LJ, Flatow EL, Bigliani LU, et al: Articular geometry of the glenohumeral joint. *Clin Orthop* 1992;285:181-190.

Using stereophotogrammetry, the authors were able to obtain accurate quantitative results for the three-dimensional geometry of the articular surfaces of the glenohumeral joint. The humeral head and glenoid articular surfaces were found to be congruent with radii within 2 mm in 88% of cases. The articular cartilage was found to be thickest at the center of the humeral head, and at the periphery of the glenoid. The articular surfaces of the humeral head and glenoid can be thought of as arcs of a sphere and do not significantly deviate from congruence. The relative areas of the articular surfaces, however, are markedly different. The average humeral head to glenoid surface area ratio was approximately 3:1.

Tillett E, Smith M, Fulcher M, et al: Anatomic determination of humeral head retroversion: The relationship of the central axis of the humeral head to the bicipital groove. *J Shoulder Elbow Surg* 1993;2:255-256.

The authors found the central axis of the humeral head was an average of 9 mm posterior to the posterior margin of the bicipital groove. This study was performed on 18 fresh cadaver specimens.

Capsule and Rotator Cuff Interval

Bigliani LU, Pollock RG, Soslowsky LJ, et al: Tensile properties of the inferior glenohumeral ligament. *J Orthop Res* 1992;10:187-197.

This biomechanical study of the inferior glenohumeral ligament complex evaluated the superior band, anterior axillary pouch, and posterior axillary pouch under uniaxial tensile load to failure. Under low strain rates, the anterior axillary pouch failed at a higher strain than the posterior pouch or superior band. Capsular stretching was noted to occur prior to failure in all specimens.

Cooper DE, Arnoczky SP, O'Brien SJ, et al: Anatomy, histology, and vascularity of the glenoid labrum: An anatomical study. *J Bone Joint Surg* 1992;74A:46-52.

The authors used 23 fresh frozen shoulders to explore the gross anatomy, histology, and vascularity of the glenoid labrum. The biceps tendon was found to insert consistently in the supraglenoid tubercle 5 mm medial to the superior rim of the glenoid, but also have a consistent insertion into the superior glenoid labrum. The inferior labrum was found to be smaller and more firmly attached to the glenoid rim as opposed to its more mobile superior portion. The arteries supplying the periphery of the glenoid labrum were described, and vascularity was noted to be limited to the periphery of the labrum.

Cooper DE, O'Brien SJ, Arnoczky SP, et al: The structure and function of the coracohumeral ligament: An anatomic and microscopic study. *J Shoulder Elbow Surg* 1993;2:70-77.

The authors studied the coracohumeral ligament in 12 fresh frozen cadavers by gross dissection and histologic section. The study revealed that the coracohumeral ligament is lined by synovium on its undersurface, but that it contains no discretely organized collagen bundles as would be seen in a true ligament. The authors conclude that this is a reflection of anterosuperior capsule. They believe it unlikely that the coracohumeral ligament plays a significant suspensory role in its physiologic state.

Gohlke F, Essigkrug B, Schmitz F: The pattern of the collagen fiber bundles of the capsule of the glenohumeral joint. *J Shoulder Elbow Surg* 1994;3:111-128.

The authors studied the capsule in 43 cadaver shoulders, describing the collagen fiber arrangement in differing sections of the capsule. The capsule was found to have a complicated structure with a complex pattern of collagen organization that differed from section to section.

Harryman DT II, Sidles JA, Harris SL, et al: The role of the rotator interval capsule in passive motion and stability of the shoulder. *J Bone Joint Surg* 1992;74A:53-66.

The authors used eight fresh frozen cadaver shoulders that were placed in a testing apparatus that had a 6° of freedom position sensor and a 6° of freedom force and torque transducer so that glenohumeral rotations and translations could be measured from applied loads. Measurements were taken with an intact, then vented capsule, and then with a sectioned rotator cuff interval, and with an imbricated rotator cuff interval. The authors conclude that the function of the rotator interval capsule is to check the range of flexion, extension, adduction, and external rotation; and to check inferior translation of the glenohumeral joint in the adducted shoulder.

Hata Y, Nakatsuchi Y, Saitoh S, et al: Anatomic study of the glenoid labrum. *J Shoulder Elbow Surg* 1992;1:207-214.

The labrum was studied in 33 cadaver shoulders. The size of the glenoid and labrum of each specimen was measured. The authors found no significant correlation between the size of the labrum and that of the glenoid.

O'Brien SJ, Schwartz RS, Warren RF, et al: Capsular restraints to anterior-posterior motion of the abducted shoulder: A biomechanical study. *J Shoulder Elbow Surg* 1995;4:298-308.

The authors tested cadaver shoulders in a biomechanical testing apparatus to quantitate the contribution of the capsule in anterior-posterior translation of the abducted shoulder. The primary anterior-posterior stabilizer was found to be the inferior glenohumeral ligament complex. The study also quantified the normal amount of anterior-posterior translation in a cadaver model.

Ticker JB, Bigliani LU, Soslowsky LJ, et al: Inferior glenohumeral ligament: Geometric and strain-rate dependent properties. *J Shoulder Elbow Surg* 1996;5:269-279.

Using near-physiologic strain rates, the authors examined the tensile properties of the IGHL complex. The superior band and anterior axillary pouch provide viscoelastic stiffening to provide restraint to the humeral head. The inferior glenohumeral ligament complex was noted to be thickest from anterior to posterior and from proximal (glenoid) to distal (humeral) insertions.

Rotator Cuff

Clark JM, Harryman DT II: Tendons, ligaments, and capsule of the rotator cuff: Gross and microscopic anatomy. *J Bone Joint Surg* 1992;74A:713-725.

The authors studied the gross anatomy and histology of the capsule, ligaments, and rotator cuff from 32 cadaver shoulders. The rotator cuff structure was found to be a five layered structure, a composite of the capsule, the ligaments, and the tendons. This complex interweaving of layers is described both by gross anatomy and histology.

Lippitt SB, Vanderhooft JE, Harris SL, et al: Glenohumeral stability from concavity-compression: A quantitative analysis. *J Shoulder Elbow Surg* 1993;2:27-35.

Using an experimental setup that allowed measurement of joint position and compressive forces at the joint, the authors were able to study the stability provided by the compressive forces on the glenohumeral joint. The concavity-compression mechanism was found to be efficient in stabilizing the glenohumeral joint. With the labrum intact, the humeral head was able to resist tangential forces of up to 60% of the applied compressive load. The greater glenoid depth superiorly and inferiorly had a greater resistance to translation than did forces in the anterior posterior plane. Resection of the glenoid labrum reduced the effectiveness of this stabilizing mechanism by approximately 20%. Concavity-compression is an important mechanism for providing stability in the midrange of glenohumeral joint motion.

Wuelker N, Roetman B, Roessig S: Coracoacromial pressure recordings in a cadaveric model. *J Shoulder Elbow Surg* 1995;4:462-467.

The authors used computer regulation of servo-actuator forces to control cycles of glenohumeral joint motion in an experimental setup. Capacitive sensors were used to continuously record pressures underneath the coracoacromial vault during experimental motion. With the loss of force on the subscapularis and infraspinatus-teres minor muscles there was a significant 61% increase of recorded pressures in the coracoacromial vault. Lack of force of the supraspinatus only resulted in an insignificant change in the average coracoacromial pressures. With an anterior acromioplasty and coracoacromial ligament division the mean acromial pressures decreased by 5%.

Long Head of the Biceps Tendon

Itoi E, Motzkin NE, Moorey BF, et al: Stabilizing function of the long head of the biceps in the hanging arm position. *J Shoulder Elbow Surg* 1994;3:135-142.

Using an experimental setup that allowed measurement of three-dimensional position and force transducers, the authors used nine fresh frozen cadaver shoulders to investigate the function of the long head of the biceps tendon in a hanging arm position. Anterior-posterior displacement was significantly decreased by long head of biceps tendon loading. The stabilizing function of the long head of biceps tendon is influenced by arm position.

Refior HJ, Sowa D: Long tendon of the biceps brachii: Sites of predilection for degenerative lesions. *J Shoulder Elbow Surg* 1995;4:436-440.

The authors studied 104 cadavers to investigate the morphologic and cross-sectional anatomy of the long head of the biceps tendon, and to determine the site of potential degenerative lesions. The tendinous length and cross-sectional size are described. The narrowest anatomic enclosure, the distal biceps groove, appears to be the most prevalent site for degenerative changes in the long head of biceps tendon.

Subacromial Space

Holt EM, Allibone RO: Anatomic variants of the coracoacromial ligament. *J Shoulder Elbow Surg* 1995;4:370-375.

The authors measured and used histologic analysis in 50 cadaveric shoulders to analyze the coracoacromial ligament. They identified three main types of coracoacromial ligament based on their shape: quadrangular, Y-shaped, and a broad band type. The differing types of coracoacromial ligament were measured grossly and their thickness analyzed.

Ide K, Shirai Y, Ito H, et al: Sensory nerve supply in the human subacromial bursa. *J Shoulder Elbow Surg* 1996;5:371-382.

The authors used silver impregnation and immunohistochemical methods to map the neural elements of the subacromial bursa. Free nerve endings, pacinian corpuscles, and Ruffini endings were found predominantly on the roof side of the bursa along the coracoacromial arch.

Nicholson GP, Goodman DA, Flatow EL, et al: The acromion: Morphologic condition and age-related changes. A study of 420 scapulas. *J Shoulder Elbow Surg* 1996;5: 1-11.

Two hundred ten skeletal specimens (420 scapulas) from ages 21-70 were evaluated to determine the influence of age on the acromial morphologic condition. The mean acromial dimensions in men and women for length, width, and anterior thickness were noted. The acromial facet for the acromioclavicular joint was analyzed by size and inclination. Anterior acromial spur formation by visual inspection was noted to increase from 7% of specimens younger than 50 years to 30% of specimens older than 50 years. This was a significant age-dependent finding. The morphologic condition evaluated by outlet radiographs showed no statistically significant impact of age on morphologic condition. The authors conclude that the variations seen in acromial morphology are not acquired from age-related changes and that morphology contributes to impingement disease independent of, and in addition to, age-related processes.

Ogata S, Uhthoff HK: Acromial enthesopathy and rotator cuff tear: A radiologic and histologic postmortem investigation of the coracoacromial arch. *Clin Orthop* 1990;254:39-48.

The authors studied 76 autopsy specimens for changes at the coracoacromial ligament insertion on the undersurface of the acromion. They noted that spur formation began in the insertion of the coracoacromial ligament as a result of endochondral ossification.

Soslowsky LJ, An CH, Johnston SP, et al: Geometric and mechanical properties of the coracoacromial ligament and their relationship to rotator cuff disease. *Clin Orthop* 1994;304:10-17.

The geometric and biomechanical properties of the coracoacromial ligament were studied in 20 fresh frozen specimens. Ten had rotator cuff tears, and ten had intact cuffs. Changes in the dimensions and material properties of the ligaments were seen between torn and intact specimens.

Soslowsky LJ, Flatow EL, Bigliani LU, et al: Stabilization of the glenohumeral joint by articular contact and by contact in the subacromial space, in Matsen FA, Fu FH, Hawkins RJ (eds): *The Shoulder: A Balance of Mobility and Stability.* Rosemont, IL, American Academy of Orthopaedic Surgeons, 1993, pp 107-124.

The authors in this chapter report their results of stereophotogrammetry measurements on the rotator cuff contact in the subacromial space on the undersurface of the acromion. They noted that the acromiohumeral interval decreased continuously with arm elevation. The pattern of contact on the undersurface of the acromion moved from the anterolateral border to medial and posterior with increasing arm elevation.

Vangsness CT Jr, Enniss M, Taylor JG, et al: Neural anatomy of the glenohumeral ligaments, labrum, and subacromial bursa. *Arthroscopy* 1995;11:180-184.

The authors obtained autopsy specimens of shoulders from 8 cadavers. The shoulder ligaments, glenoid labrum, and subacromial bursa were stained with a gold chloride stain for showing nerve endings. The subacromial bursa showed diffuse copious free nerve endings. More complex mechanoreceptors were not seen in the bursal tissue. However, these complex mechanoreceptors were identified in the superior, middle, inferior, and posterior glenohumeral ligaments. Specialized proprioceptive nerve endings were also found in the coracoclavicular and coracoacromial ligaments. The glenoid labrum showed no evidence of any mechanoreceptors. Occasional free nerve endings, were noted in the peripheral half of the fibrocartilaginous labrum.

Scapulothoracic Articulation

Ruland LJ III, Ruland CM, Matthews LS: Scapulothoracic anatomy for the arthroscopist. *Arthroscopy* 1995;11:52-56.

The authors studied eight unembalmed cadaveric shoulders by anatomic dissection, followed by anatomic dissection after arthroscopy. They describe the anatomy in the scapulothoracic space as being divided into two spaces with a well-defined bursa in the serratus anterior space. Critical neurovascular structures in relationship to possible arthroscopic approaches are also described.

2
Biomechanics of Glenohumeral Stability

John E. Kuhn, MD

Introduction

The glenohumeral joint has evolved to allow for more motion than any other joint in the human body. The advantages of an increased range of motion are accompanied by a loss of constraint and inherent stability. As such, the human shoulder is also the most frequently dislocated joint. The wide variation in shoulder motion between individuals makes the concepts of laxity and instability confusing. Many definitions of instability have been offered, ranging from the failure to keep the humeral head centered in the glenoid to exceeding the limits of motion of the glenohumeral joint. The major distinguishing feature of instability is that, unlike laxity, it is associated with symptoms.

Many mechanisms have been described in the maintenance of shoulder stability, although their degree of involvement remains unclear. Although these components clearly work in concert to maintain stability, they can be divided into static and dynamic categories.

Static Contributors to Glenohumeral Stability

Humeral Version

In the general population, the articular surface of the proximal humerus is inclined superiorly, with neck shaft angles averaging between 130° and 140°. In addition, the humeral head is retroverted 30° relative to the transepicondylar axis of the elbow (Fig. 1). The role that variation of these anatomic features plays in the development of instability is unclear. Although some studies have shown no differences in the degree of retroversion in normal patients compared to those with anterior instability, other studies have shown significantly less retroversion in patients with anterior glenohumeral instability. Although a few surgeons have performed rotational osteotomies of the humerus to treat recurrent instability, the role of humeral head version in shoulder stability is not fully understood. In Weber's rotational osteotomy for recurrent anterior instability, a Putti-Platt capsulorrhaphy was performed concomitantly.

Glenoid Version

In the resting position, the scapula is oriented 30° to 45° anterior to the coronal plane. The glenoid fossa is oriented in 7° of retroversion relative to the scapula in 75% of individuals, with a great degree of variation in the remaining 25%. Most authors agree that in the resting position, the glenoid fossa has a 5° superior tilt (Fig. 2). The superior tilt of the scapula has been shown repeatedly to play a role in controlling inferior humeral head translation; however, the role of glenoid version in anteroposterior instability remains unclear. Some studies have shown that patients with anterior instability have relatively more anteversion of the glenoid than normal, and

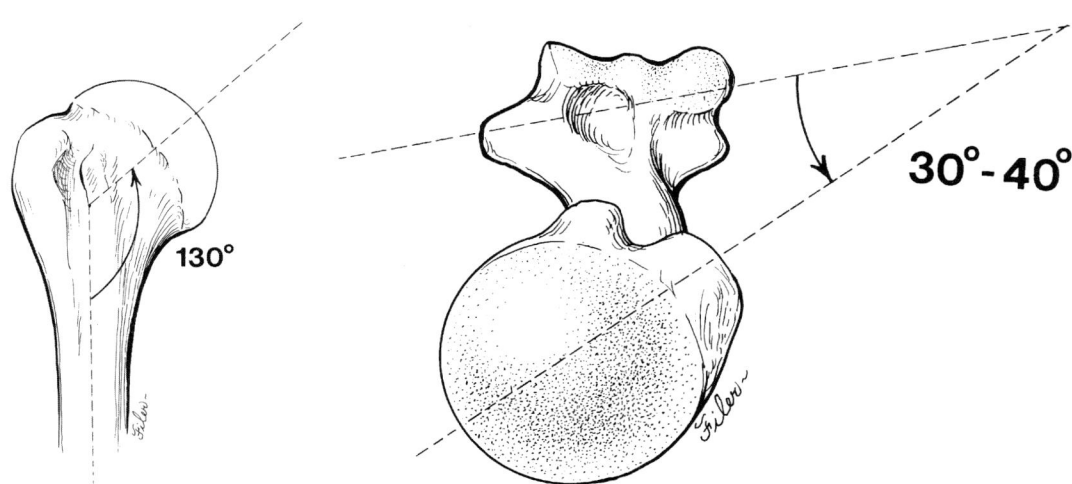

Fig. 1 Humeral version. The neck shaft angle of the humerus is dorsally inclined between 130° and 140°, whereas the humeral head is retroverted between 30° and 40°. Less retroversion in some studies has been associated with anterior glenohumeral instability. (Reproduced with permission from Warner JJP: The gross anatomy of the joint surfaces, ligaments, labrum, and capsule, in Matsen FA III, Fu FH, Hawkins RJ (eds): *The Shoulder: A Balance of Mobility and Stability.* Rosemont, IL, American Academy of Orthopaedic Surgeons, 1993, pp 7-28.)

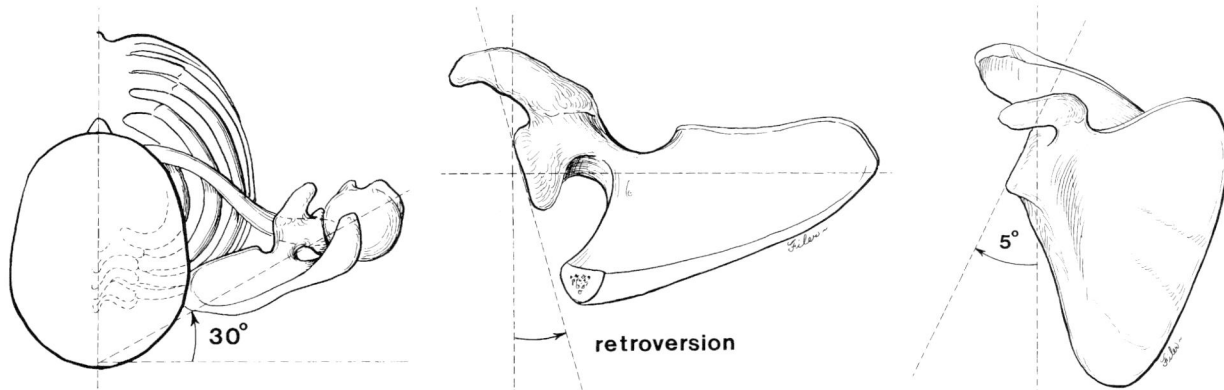

Fig. 2 Scapular and glenoid version. The scapula is oriented 30° to 45° anterior to the coronal plane (**left**), the glenoid fossa is oriented in approximately 7° of retroversion (**center**), with approximately 5° of superior tilt in most individuals (**right**). Some studies have shown more anteversion of the glenoid in patients with instability. (Reproduced with permission from Warner JJP: The gross anatomy of the joint surfaces, ligaments, labrum, and capsule, in Matsen FA III, Fu FH, Hawkins RJ (eds): *The Shoulder: A Balance of Mobility and Stability.* Rosemont, IL, American Academy of Orthopaedic Surgeons, 1993, pp 7-28.)

similarly, patients with posterior instability have relatively more retroversion of the glenoid than normal. Other studies have failed to show these relationships. Although glenoid osteotomy for posterior instability has been advocated by many, the lack of reproducible reference points and uniform conclusions makes it difficult to appreciate the role of glenoid version in clinical shoulder instability.

Surface Area and Articular Conformity

Although most agree that the articulating surface of the humeral head is large relative to the much smaller glenoid, there is controversy regarding the nature of that contact area. Saha described three types of humeral-glenoid articulations, based on the radius of curvature. In type A, the glenoid radius of curvature is larger than that of the humerus; in type B, the radii of curvatures match, leading to joint conformity; and in type C, the radius of curvature of the humerus is larger than that of the glenoid. Other anatomic studies, as well as magnetic resonance imaging and computed tomography, tend to show matching radii of curvature with joint conformity. Recent work by Soslowsky and associates, using stereophotogrammetry techniques, accurately defined the three-dimensional articular surfaces of the glenoid and humerus. This method has shown the articular surfaces to be nearly perfectly congruent, with deviations in the radii of curvature of less than 1% and the surfaces to be congruent within 3 mm. This situation results from relatively thicker articular cartilage at the periphery of the glenoid and thin cartilage in the center. The humeral articular cartilage, on the other hand, is thicker centrally and thinner at the periphery. These findings suggest that the humeral head maintains relatively uniform contact with the glenoid surface throughout shoulder motion. If the glenohumeral joint is highly congruent, then physiologic motion might be expected to fit a ball and socket model, with limited translation occurring during shoulder motion. Some studies using simulated muscle forces in cadavers have demonstrated this to be accurate.

Other studies, however, have demonstrated that passive glenohumeral motion results in translation of the humeral head on the glenoid, with anterior translation accompanying glenohumeral flexion, and posterior translation accompanying extension. These studies suggest that coupled translation accompanies all glenohumeral motions, particularly in the middle to extreme ranges of motion.

Taken together, these studies suggest that the glenohumeral joint is a congruent joint, yet because the glenoid is significantly smaller than the humeral head and thus shallow, translations can occur and instability can develop.

The Glenoid Labrum

The glenoid labrum acts as a static stabilizer of the glenohumeral articulation by deepening the glenoid socket by 9 mm in the superior-inferior direction, and by 5 mm in the anterior-posterior plane. This deepening accounts for up to 50% of the depth of the glenoid cavity. By deepening the glenoid socket, the labrum serves three purposes: it increases the surface area for contact with the humeral head; it creates a buttress, limiting translation of the humeral head by requiring it to lift away from the glenoid in order for subluxations to occur; and it serves as an attachment site for the glenohumeral ligaments. Hara and colleagues have shown that the labrum is weakest in the 4 o'clock position and that when loaded to failure under tension, the labrum becomes detached in the fibrous connective tissue close to the hyaline articular cartilage. Clinically, labral lesions are often associated with traumatic glenohumeral instability, yet biomechanical studies in which an isolated Bankart lesion was created have not produced significant increases in humeral translation on the glenoid, suggesting that other factors (such as plastic deformation of the glenohumeral ligaments) may be required for recurrent instability.

Intra-Articular Pressure

A number of studies have demonstrated that venting a cadaver glenohumeral joint will allow for passive translations in any direction with less force than that required for the nonvented shoulder. The normal glenohumeral joint is a closed system of finite volume. A slightly negative intra-articular pressure exists in the normal shoulder. Translations or distractions of the glenohumeral joint could increase joint volume and further decrease intra-articular pressure, and should help to improve glenohumeral stability. The magnitude of this effect is dependent on the position of the arm. In the abducted and externally rotated shoulder, the effect of intra-articular pressure is small compared to the static restraints of the glenohumeral ligaments, which in this case prevent humeral head translation. Negative intra-articular pressure may have a role in centering the humeral head, particularly in the neutral or early ranges of motion. However, the amount of stability provided by this mechanism, relative to other stabilizing mechanisms, is not clear.

The Glenohumeral Ligaments and Capsule

Thickenings in the shoulder capsule have been identified and described for many years, yet only recently have the functional, anatomic, and material properties of these ligaments been investigated. Histologic analysis has determined that these ligaments are comprised of collagen fiber bundles arranged in several layers of differing thickness and orientation. Although the posterior capsule has a simple pattern of radial and circular fibers, most areas of the glenohumeral capsule and ligaments demonstrate a more complex pattern of cross linking. The complex nature of the capsule suggests that it could be considered a cylinder. Nevertheless, most studies have investigated the individual components of the capsule through ligament cutting studies and strain gauge analysis in an effort to understand these static restraints. The ligaments that have been studied most thoroughly include the superior glenohumeral, coracohumeral, middle glenohumeral, and inferior glenohumeral ligament complex (Fig. 3).

Superior Glenohumeral Ligament and Coracohumeral Ligament The superior glenohumeral ligament is found in the rotator interval (that area bounded by the anterior border of the supraspinatus and the superior border of the subscapularis), parallel to the much larger, extra-articular coracohumeral ligament. The superior glenohumeral ligament originates from the superior rim of the glenoid at the supraglenoid tubercle just anteroinferior to the biceps tendon and inserts onto the lesser tuberosity of the humerus medial to the bicipital groove. It is variable in size and is found in over 90% of specimens. Unlike the coracohumeral ligament, histologic analysis of the superior glenohumeral ligament has shown it to be comprised of longitudinally arranged collagen bundles in a true ligament fashion.

Biomechanical studies have included strain gauge analysis and ligament cutting experiments and have determined that the superior glenohumeral ligament is a primary restraint to external rotation in the adducted or slightly abducted arm, is a primary restraint to inferior translation in the adducted arm, and is a secondary restraint to posterior translation in the adducted, flexed, and internally rotated shoulder.

The coracohumeral ligament had traditionally been considered a more significant structure. It is an extra-articular, dense, fibrous structure that histologically is a thickened fold-

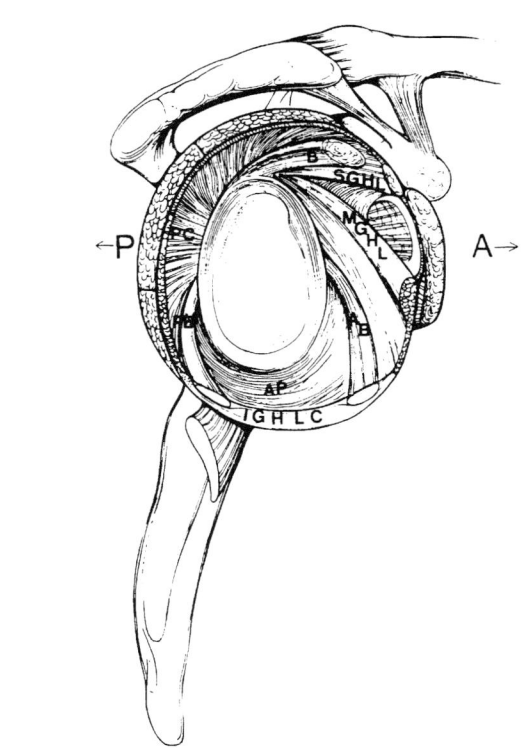

Fig. 3 The glenohumeral ligaments. The anterior aspect of the shoulder is to the right. The ligaments include the superior glenohumeral ligament (SGHL), the middle glenohumeral ligament (MGHL), and the inferior glenohumeral ligament (IGHL), which includes the superior band, anterior axillary pouch, and posterior axillary pouch. (Reproduced with permission from Ticker JB, Bigliani LU, Soslowsky LJ, et al: Inferior glenohumeral ligament: Geometric and strain-rate dependent properties. *J Shoulder Elbow Surg* 1996;5:269-279.)

ing of the shoulder capsule without the ligamentous organization of parallel bundles of collagen fibers. The coracohumeral ligament originates from the lateral border of the base of the coracoid process and divides into two bands. One band inserts into the greater tuberosity and tendinous anterior edge of the supraspinatus. The other band inserts on the lesser tuberosity and superior border of the subscapularis. The cross-sectional area of the coracohumeral ligament (53.7 ± 3.2 mm^2) is much greater than that of the superior glenohumeral ligament (11.3 ± 1.6 mm^2).

The coracohumeral ligament is thought to be a primary restraint to inferior translation of the adducted arm and to external rotation. These effects are somewhat additive, as cadaver-based biomechanical evaluations of inferior glenohumeral translation have demonstrated that the restraint provided by the coracohumeral ligament is more pronounced with external rotation, and that with the neutral or internally rotated shoulder, the coracohumeral ligament restraint is not great. The coracohumeral ligament is also thought to be a restraint to posterior instability with the arm in the adducted, forward flexed, and neutral to internally rotated position. With increased internal rotation of the flexed humerus, the inferior glenohumeral ligament becomes the significant restraint to posterior humeral translation.

In comparing material properties of isolated specimens of the coracohumeral and superior glenohumeral ligaments, the coracohumeral ligament has greater stiffness (36.7 ± 5.9 N/mm) and ultimate load (359.8 ± 40.3 N) than the superior glenohumeral ligament (17.4 ± 1.5 N/mm and 101.9 ± 11.5 N, respectively). The coracohumeral ligament, which fans out distally to converge with the rotator cuff tendons, fails proximally (near the coracoid) in bone-ligament-bone testing, whereas the superior glenohumeral ligament tends to fail distally as it thins near the humeral insertion. Interestingly, coracohumeral ligament stiffness and ultimate load values are higher than those reported for the inferior glenohumeral ligament complex, and significant elongation of the coracohumeral ligament (36%) occurs prior to failure.

Middle Glenohumeral Ligament The anatomy of the middle glenohumeral ligament is highly variable, poorly defined in 10% of shoulders and absent in up to 30%. Its origin may be the anterior-superior labrum, the scapular neck, or the supraglenoid tubercle, usually below the superior glenohumeral ligament and above the anterior band of the inferior glenohumeral ligament. The middle glenohumeral ligament inserts just anterior to the lesser tuberosity with the subscapularis. Two morphologic variations—a cord-like structure, clearly delineated from the anterior band of the inferior glenohumeral ligament, and a sheet-like structure, blending with the anterior band of the inferior glenohumeral ligament—have been described. The middle glenohumeral ligament may be extremely well developed and insert onto the biceps tendon, with a portion of the underlying anterior-superior labrum absent.

The middle glenohumeral ligament is a primary stabilizer to anterior translation with the arm abducted to 45°. It is also thought to be important in limiting external rotation at 60° and 90° of abduction. It may be a secondary stabilizer for inferior translation in the adducted arm.

Inferior Glenohumeral Ligament Complex The inferior glenohumeral complex, a triangular structure of varying thickness, comprises the inferior shoulder capsule. It has been evaluated histologically and has a substantially thicker area anteriorly called the anterior or superior band. A similar thickening posteriorly has been described by some. The entire structure seems to be thicker near the glenoid than the humerus.

The superior band originates from the glenoid labrum in the 2 to 4 o'clock positions and the posterior band, if present, from the 7 to 9 o'clock positions. The inferior glenohumeral ligament complex runs laterally to the humeral head between the subscapularis and the triceps. O'Brien and associates liken the inferior glenohumeral ligament complex to a hammock. In the abducted shoulder, external rotation will place the inferior glenohumeral ligament anteriorly, which will then restrain anterior translation of the humeral head. Correspondingly, internal rotation will direct the inferior glenohumeral ligament posteriorly, which will then restrain posterior translation of the humerus (Fig. 4). This finding has been confirmed by Blasier and associates, who also found that the

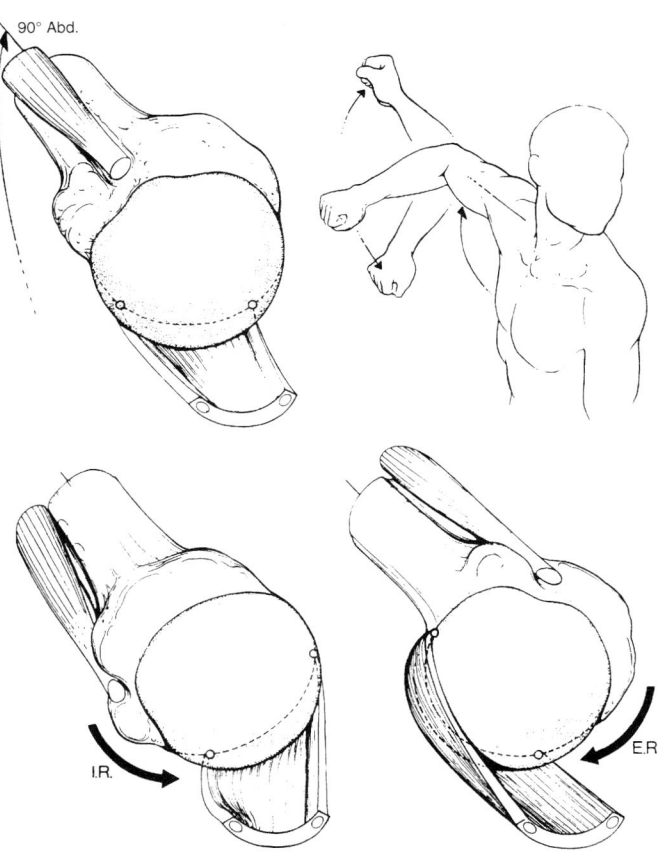

Fig. 4 The inferior glenohumeral ligament complex. In the abducted but neutral position, the inferior glenohumeral complex tightens inferior to the joint **(top left)**. When externally rotated, the inferior glenohumeral ligament complex moves anteriorly, preventing anterior humeral head translation **(bottom right)**. When internally rotated, the inferior glenohumeral ligament complex moves posteriorly, preventing posterior translations of the humeral head **(bottom left)**. IR = internal rotation; ER = external rotation. (Reproduced with permission from O'Brien SJ, Neves MC, Arnoczky SP et al: The anatomy and histology of the inferior glenohumeral ligament complex of the shoulder. *Am J Sports Med* 1990;18:449-456.)

restraining effect of the inferior glenohumeral ligament in preventing posterior humeral translation of the adducted, forward elevated, internally rotated arm was greater than that of the coracohumeral ligament.

The material properties of the inferior glenohumeral ligament complex have been evaluated by Bigliani and associates. With slow strain rates, the anterior axillary pouch portion fails at a higher strain than the superior band portion or the posterior axillary pouch portion. In addition, the midsubstance of the ligament demonstrates a lower strain to failure than the entire bone-ligament-bone preparation, suggesting that significant strain occurs at the insertion of the ligament. Failure at the glenoid insertion occurs most frequently, followed by failure at the ligament midsubstance, then the humeral insertion. The stress at failure for this slow strain rate is similar for all three portions of the inferior glenohumeral ligament complex, averaging 5.5 MPa. This value is lower than those reported for other soft tissues such as the anterior cruciate ligament and the patellar tendon.

Ticker and colleagues performed similar testing of the inferior glenohumeral ligament components under more rapid strain rates of 10% per second. They found that the superior band has greater tensile strength at failure (62.63 ± 9.78 MPa) than either the anterior axillary pouch (47.75 ± 17.89 MPa) or the posterior axillary pouch (39.97 ± 13.29 MPa). As with slow strain rates, greater strain was observed near the bony insertion sites of the specimen than in the midsubstance of the tissue. When compared to earlier work, in which slower strain rates were used, the inferior glenohumeral ligament complex responded to increased strain rates with increased strength and stiffness. Therefore, it can be concluded that the superior band of the inferior glenohumeral ligament complex is a significant static restraint to anterior-inferior translation of the humeral head in the abducted externally rotated humerus.

Dynamic Contributors to Glenohumeral Stability

The muscles of the rotator cuff and the long head of the biceps muscle provide dynamic stability to the glenohumeral joint in a variety of ways.

Joint Compression

Numerous studies have shown that contraction of the rotator cuff muscles will compress the humeral head into the glenoid, resulting in an increase in the force required to translate the humeral head. Biomechanical studies have shown that when the rotator cuff is activated, the joint compression effect seems to be more important than the static capsular constraints in stabilizing the glenohumeral joint.

In a series of studies by Blasier and associates, physiologic loads of the rotator cuff were simulated and were shown to have a major stabilizing effect on the glenohumeral joint. If tension on any one component of the cuff was removed, however, increased anterior humeral translation occurred with less force regardless of which component was omitted. This suggests the entire cuff acts in concert to provide joint compression and stability. In related experiments, the entire rotator cuff has been shown to have stabilizing effects in limiting posterior and inferior translations of the humeral head.

Individual Components of the Rotator Cuff

Individual components of the rotator cuff may play an important role in maintaining glenohumeral stability, particularly in the unstable shoulder. Using electromyography, it has been shown that throwing athletes with anterior instability have demonstrable weakness during internal rotation. Because ruptures of the subscapularis have been noted in older patients with recurrent dislocations, some authors suggest that the subscapularis may play a role in preventing anterior instability, particularly in the lower ranges of abduction. Similarly, the infraspinatus and teres minor may have similar effects on posterior instability.

Finally, a posterior injury from anterior dislocation has been described by Codman and, later, by McLaughlin in which anterior dislocation is accompanied by supraspinatus and infraspinatus tendon tears. This condition is common in older people with anterior glenohumeral dislocations, and in patients with greater tuberosity fractures accompanying anterior glenohumeral dislocations.

Blasier and associates evaluated the role of individual components of the rotator cuff and their effect on posterior instability in a cadaver model, and found that the subscapularis provided the most resistance to posterior subluxation of the humerus in the adducted, forward elevated, and internally rotated arm. Using the same apparatus to evaluate inferior humeral translation, they found that the supraspinatus was an important restraint to inferior translation, and that the subscapularis and external rotators initially tended to reduce the force necessary to create inferior translation of the humeral head, demonstrating initial inferior destabilization. With further inferior subluxation, the internal and external rotators improve in their stabilizing effect, presumably through concavity compression.

Preloading Glenohumeral Ligaments

The muscles of the rotator cuff may serve in a dynamic way to pre-tension the glenohumeral ligament complex. Histologic analysis of the shoulder capsule has demonstrated that the rotator cuff tendons insert onto and intermingle with the shoulder joint capsule at the humerus. Stretch receptors, Ruffini end organs, and pacinian corpuscles have been identified in the capsuloligamentous structures. Although the glenohumeral joint capsule and its ligaments are relatively lax in the early and midranges of shoulder motion, it has been suggested that contraction of the rotator cuff components may activate these sensors and dynamize, or preload, the ligaments through complex reflex arcs. Similarly, these receptors may act to trigger the activation of specific cuff components through reflex arcs to protect the ligaments in which the stretch receptors are found. These reflex arcs have recently been demonstrated in a feline model.

Proprioception

The specialized nerve endings discussed above may also provide the glenohumeral joint with proprioception, another component of dynamic stabilization of the glenohumeral joint. Studies evaluating proprioceptive ability in humans have determined that subjects with clinical laxity have significantly less proprioceptive skills than normal subjects. In addition, subjects are more sensitive to proprioception when the shoulder is near the limits of motion, and during external rotation. In one study, the injection of lidocaine into the glenohumeral joint resulted in increased passive translation in normal subjects. Patients with known anterior instability have less proprioceptive ability than normal subjects; however, proprioception can be restored after surgical repair. These studies suggest that proprioception, through reflex mechanisms or even cortical mechanisms, may have an important role in glenohumeral stability, particularly in the abducted and externally rotated shoulder.

The Biceps Tendon

Many studies have investigated the role of the long head of the biceps in shoulder stability. Like the rotator cuff, the long

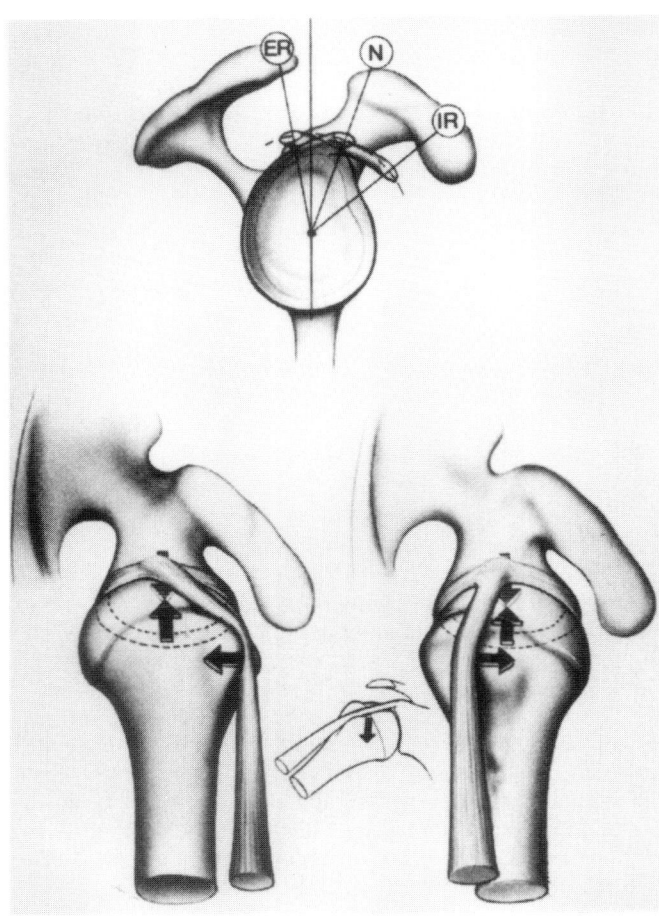

Fig. 5 The biceps tendon. Contraction of the biceps tendon is thought to influence glenohumeral stability by joint compression, and as a static restraint **(top)**. In internal rotation, the biceps moves anteriorly, and limits anterior translation **(bottom left)**. In external rotation, the biceps moves posteriorly, and limits posterior translation **(bottom right)**. ER = external rotation; N = neutral; IR = internal rotation. (Reproduced with permission from Pagnani MJ, Deng XH, Warren RF, et al: Role of the long head of the biceps brachii in glenohumeral stability: A biomechanical study in cadavera. *J Shoulder Elbow Surg* 1996;5:255-262.)

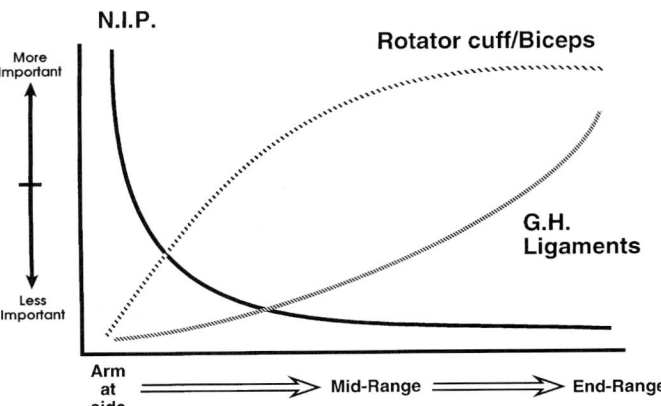

Fig. 6 The relative roles of the components of glenohumeral stability. The components of glenohumeral stability work in concert, yet with the arm in neutral position, negative intra-articular pressure (NIP) seems to be important, with the rotator cuff becoming more important in the midrange of motion, and the glenohumeral (GH) ligaments becoming more important nearer the limits of motion. (Reproduced with permission from Warner JJP, Flatow EL: Anatomy and biomechanics, in Bigliani LU (ed): *The Unstable Shoulder.* Rosemont, IL, American Academy of Orthopaedic Surgeons, 1996, pp 1-26.)

head of the biceps can increase joint compression and may increase the force required to translate the humeral head. In a study by Rodosky and associates, sectioning of the long head of the biceps tendon in the abducted externally rotated arm resulted in an increase in strain in the inferior glenohumeral ligament. Pagnani and associates have demonstrated that the stabilizing role of the biceps tendon seems to be dependent on position. When the arm is internally rotated, tension on the biceps diminishes anterior humeral head translation. Conversely, when the arm is externally rotated, the biceps limits posterior translation (Fig. 5). The biceps' effect on stability is more pronounced with the arm in the lower and middle elevation angles.

In testing restraints to posterior translation of the adducted, forward-flexed, and internally rotated humerus, it has been shown that the long head of the biceps may have the potential for a destabilizing effect. In testing inferior translation, the biceps, like the supraspinatus, functions to restrain inferior translation.

The Scapular Rotators

Although the glenoid is small, it can be thought of as a platform that supports the humeral head. Its position relative to the humeral head and the forces that may create instability is critical. The position of the scapula is controlled by the scapular rotators, which are the muscles connecting the scapula to the torso, and include the trapezius, rhomboids, latissimus dorsi, serratus anterior, and levator scapulae. Abnormal function of these muscles, which results in altered scapulothoracic motion, may be related to glenohumeral instability. Scapular winging has been described as a feature of patients with anterior instability. Warner and associates, using Moiré topography, found that scapulothoracic dysfunction was common in a population of patients with shoulder instability. In addition, in a number of large series of patients with scapular winging, shoulder instability has been described as a secondary symptom. If the scapular rotators are unable to position the glenoid effectively, particularly by rotating the scapula upward during arm elevation, the glenoid may not be in position to act as a stable platform for the humeral head, and instability may result.

Relative Importance of the Various Components to Glenohumeral Stability

The various components of glenohumeral stability identified to date clearly have a role in maintaining shoulder stability (Fig. 6); however, more work is necessary in order to evaluate the relative roles of each of the different components. Nevertheless, it seems that the position of the arm is critical in determining which factors become important in stability; with the arm in a neutral position, intra-articular pressure and muscles play a major role. In the midrange of motion, the rotator cuff seems to have an increased role in shoulder stability, and in extremes of motion, the glenohumeral ligaments become important. Clearly, further study is required.

Selected Bibliography

Bigliani LU, Pollock RG, Soslowsky LJ, et al: Tensile properties of the inferior glenohumeral ligament. *J Orthop Res* 1992;10:187-197.

In 16 cadaver specimens, the inferior glenohumeral ligament was divided into bone ligament-bone preparations for the superior band, the anterior axillary pouch, and the posterior axillary pouch. Specimen dimensions were measured, and the specimens were uniaxially loaded to failure under relatively slow rates (0.04 mm/s and 0.004 mm/s). The inferior glenohumeral ligament was found to be thicker in the anterosuperior region than in the posteroinferior region. The anterior axillary pouch specimens failed at a higher strain (34%) than the superior band specimens (24%) and the posterior axillary pouch specimens (27%). Failure occurred at the glenoid insertion (40%), the ligament substance (35%), and the humeral insertion (25%), with significant capsular stretching occurring before failure. The midsubstance of the ligaments failed at significantly less strain (11%) than the entire specimen (27%), suggesting larger strain occurs near the insertion sites. The stress at failure was similar for all three regions of the inferior glenohumeral ligament (5.5 MPa), which is much less than that reported for the anterior cruciate ligament and the patellar tendon.

Blasier RB, Soslowsky LJ, Malicky DM, et al: Posterior glenohumeral subluxation: Active and passive stabilization in a biomechanical model. *J Bone Joint Surg* 1997;79A:433-440.

Specimens with rotator cuff forces applied were tested in the forward-flexed, adducted position with varying rotation and a posterior force used to create posterior humeral head subluxation. The authors demonstrated that all cuff muscles contribute to glenohumeral stability; however, the subscapularis provided the most resistance to posterior humeral translation. The effect of the long head of the biceps tendon was position-dependent, and actually had a destabilizing effect with increased internal rotation. With greater displacement, the coracohumeral ligament was an important restraint in neutral rotation, and increased internal rotation enlisted the inferior glenohumeral ligament as a major restraint to posterior humeral translation.

Boardman ND III, Debski RE, Warner JJP, et al: Tensile properties of the superior glenohumeral and coracohumeral ligaments. *J Shoulder Elbow Surg* 1996;5:249-254.

This article is a biomechanical evaluation demonstrating that the coracohumeral ligament has a greater cross-sectional area, greater stiffness, and greater ultimate load than the superior glenohumeral ligament, suggesting the coracohumeral ligament is an important stabilizer in the shoulder.

Cooper DE, O'Brien SJ, Arnoczky SP, et al: The structure and function of the coracohumeral ligament: An anatomic and microscopic study. *J Shoulder Elbow Surg* 1993;2:70-77.

Although the coracohumeral ligament is considered important in glenohumeral stability, the authors have demonstrated that it is not a true ligament, and histologically appears to be a folding of the capsule.

Gibb TD, Sidles JA, Harryman DT II, et al: The effect of capsular venting on glenohumeral laxity. *Clin Orthop* 1991;268:120-127.

This article is one of many studies demonstrating that the vented shoulder has significantly more glenohumeral translation than the shoulder with an intact capsule.

Gohlke F, Essigkrug B, Schmitz F: The pattern of the collagen fiber bundles of the capsule of the glenohumeral joint. *J Shoulder Elbow Surg* 1994;3:111-128.

This evaluation of the macroscopic anatomy and architecture of the collagen fiber bundles demonstrates a complex arrangement of interlinking between different components of the glenohumeral capsule and suggests that the capsule functions as a cylinder.

Hara H, Ito N, Iwasaki K: Strength of the glenoid labrum and adjacent shoulder capsule. *J Shoulder Elbow Surg* 1996;5:263-268.

By sectioning the capsule and labrum in a cadaver model, the authors have demonstrated that the anterior-inferior portion of the labrum is relatively weak.

Harryman DT II, Sidles JA, Clark JM, et al: Translation of the humeral head on the glenoid with passive glenohumeral motion. *J Bone Joint Surg* 1990;72A:1334-1343.

Passive motion of the humeral head on the glenoid resulted in obligate translations at the mid and end ranges of motion. Glenohumeral flexion caused obligate anterior translation, and extension caused posterior translation.

Harryman DT II, Sidles JA, Harris SL, et al: The role of the rotator interval capsule in passive motion and stability of the shoulder. *J Bone Joint Surg* 1992;74A:53-66.

A ligament sectioning and imbrication study showing that the rotator interval limits inferior and posterior translation is presented.

Lippit SB, Vanderhooft JE, Harris SL, et al: Glenohumeral stability from concavity-compression: A quantitative analysis. *J Shoulder Elbow Surg* 1993;2:27-35.

The authors present a biomechanical study demonstrating the significant effect of the labrum on glenohumeral stability.

Malicky DM, Soslowsky LJ, Blasier RB, et al: Anterior glenohumeral stabilization factors: Progressive effects in a biomechanical model. *J Orthop Res* 1996;14;282-288.

This model studied the stabilizing effects of muscles and ligaments simultaneously. The supraspinatus and subscapularis were important muscles for resisting anterior subluxations. The glenohumeral ligaments were important in the adducted and externally rotated arm.

O'Brien SJ, Neves MC, Arnoczky SP, et al: The anatomy and histology of the inferior glenohumeral ligament complex of the shoulder. *Am J Sports Med* 1990;18:449-456.

An evaluation of the gross and histologic anatomy of the inferior glenohumeral ligament complex in the shoulder is presented.

Pagnani MJ, Deng XH, Warren RF, et al: Role of the long head of the biceps brachii in glenohumeral stability: A biomechanical study in cadavera. *J Shoulder Elbow Surg* 1996;5:255-262.

In a cadaver model, application of force to the biceps creates a joint compressive load and helps to stabilize the glenohumeral joint. This effect is more pronounced in lower and middle ranges of elevation, and humeral rotation affects this phenomenon.

Rodosky MW, Harner CD, Fu FH: The role of the long head of the biceps muscle and superior glenoid labrum in anterior stability of the shoulder. *Am J Sports Med* 1994;22:121-130.

In a cadaver model of the arm in abduction and external rotation, with simulated rotator cuff forces, activation of the biceps increases the resistance to torsion forces and decreases the stress on the inferior glenohumeral ligament.

Soslowsky LJ, Flatow EL, Bigliani LU, et al: Articular geometry of the glenohumeral joint. *Clin Orthop* 1992;285:181-190.

The authors present an elegant model to assess the glenohumeral articular geometry in three dimensions. The glenohumeral joint is congruent with similar radii of curvature for the humeral head and the glenoid.

Soslowsky LJ, Flatow EL, Bigliani LU, et al: Quantitation of in situ contact areas at the glenohumeral joint: A biomechanical study. *J Orthop Res* 1992;10:524-534.

The authors present a stereophotogrammetric method for determining articular contact at the glenohumeral joint through a range of motion. The authors demonstrate contact migration on the humeral head cartilage surface and more uniform contact on the glenoid cartilage surface.

Soslowsky LJ, Malicky DM, Blasier RB: Active and passive factors in inferior glenohumeral stabilization: A biomechanical model. *J Shoulder Elbow Surg*, 1997;6:371-379.

The authors applied rotator cuff forces to the individual tendons and performed ligament cutting to determine the effect of individual components of the cuff and glenohumeral ligament/capsule in preventing inferior translation. Their results demonstrate that the coracohumeral ligament and the inferior glenohumeral ligament are effective static restraints, particularly in external rotation. Interestingly, the supraspinatus and biceps were the most significant rotator cuff restraints to inferior translation, suggesting that the biceps may not have a role in acting as a humeral head depressor.

Speer KP, Deng X, Borrero S, et al: Biomechanical evaluation of a simulated Bankart lesion. *J Bone Joint Surg* 1994;76A:1819-1826.

Using a cadaver model, the authors created a Bankart lesion and evaluated anterior glenohumeral translation. Their data suggest that the Bankart lesion alone cannot be responsible for instability, and other factors, such as permanent deformation of the glenohumeral capsule, must also be involved.

Ticker JB, Bigliani LU, Soslowsky LJ, et al: Inferior glenohumeral ligament: Geometric and strain-rate dependent properties. *J Shoulder Elbow Surg* 1996;5:269-279.

When testing isolated specimens from the inferior glenohumeral ligament complex at relatively high strain rates (10% per second), the anterior or superior portion of the complex had relatively greater stiffness than the axillary or posterior portions. The posterior portion had a relatively lower tensile stress at failure than the other two portions. Strain at the midsubstance was always less than the bone-to-bone strain, suggesting that tissue near the insertion of the ligaments will experience greater strain than in the midsubstance.

Turkel SJ, Panio MW, Marshall JL, et al: Stabilizing mechanisms preventing anterior dislocation of the glenohumeral joint. *J Bone Joint Surg* 1981;63A:1208-1217.

This article is a classic study that demonstrates that the middle glenohumeral ligament functions as a primary stabilizer for anterior instability at 45° of abduction and limits external rotation in mid abduction. The importance of the inferior glenohumeral ligament in the abducted externally rotated humerus is demonstrated.

Warner JJ, Deng XH, Warren RF, et al: Static capsuloligamentous restraints to superior-inferior translation of the glenohumeral joint. *Am J Sports Med* 1992;20:675-685.

A ligament-cutting experiment demonstrates that the superior glenohumeral ligament is the primary restraint to inferior translation of the adducted shoulder, and the coracohumeral ligament does not play a significant suspensory role. The inferior glenohumeral ligament complex becomes important in limiting inferior translation with increased abduction of the glenohumeral joint.

Warner JJ, Micheli LJ, Arslanian LE, et al: Scapulothoracic motion in normal shoulders and shoulders with glenohumeral instability and impingement syndrome: A study using Moiré topographic analysis. *Clin Orthop* 1992;285:191-199.

Moiré topographic analysis employed to evaluate scapulothoracic asymmetry demonstrated that patients with instability had significantly more asymmetry. Although it is not clear if this is a primary or secondary phenomenon, this study emphasizes the importance of the scapulothoracic articulation in shoulder stability.

3

Basic Science of the Rotator Cuff

James E. Carpenter, MD

The rotator cuff has a central role in mechanics and function of the shoulder, and its biomechanics, along with the biology of aging, degenerative processes, and injury repair, play a predominant role in our knowledge of basic science of the shoulder. It is clear that the rotator cuff does not function alone; it is part of a complex system of muscles, ligaments, and joints that affect shoulder movement. Electromyographic studies of muscle contractions during various activities have demonstrated this complex arrangement. The rotator cuff is the part of this system that is most frequently injured and dysfunctional in individuals presenting with shoulder pain. In addition to assessment of structure and biomechanics, knowledge of the biochemistry of normal cuff tendons helps in understanding how these structures are suited for their unique function and affected by injury and disease.

Supraspinatus

The supraspinatus muscle is a fusiform muscle originating from the scapula in a fossa superior to the scapular spine. It is innervated by the suprascapular nerve, which travels through the suprascapular notch on its course from the brachial plexus. The nerve can be subjected to compression in the notch as it passes beneath the suprascapular ligament. As the supraspinatus muscle passes laterally, it courses beneath the coracoacromial arch and inserts onto the greater tuberosity of the humerus. The space defined by the acromion superiorly, the humeral head inferiorly, the scapular spine posteriorly, and the coracoacromial ligament anteriorly is known as the supraspinatus outlet. The supraspinatus tendon must pass through this outlet to its insertion. As such, it can be compressed between the unyielding humeral head and the overlying coracoacromial arch. Compression of the tendon has been implicated in the pathogenesis of cuff disease.

As the supraspinatus tendon nears its insertion, it fuses with the infraspinatus tendon posteriorly, making any distinction between the two impossible. Although the majority of the supraspinatus tendon's fibers insert onto the greater tuberosity, some fibers course posteriorly to merge with those of the infraspinatus, while others extend anteriorly toward the rotator interval. The rotator interval is the space between the anterior portion of the supraspinatus and the superior portion of the subscapularis (Fig. 1). Medially, the coracoid projects through the rotator interval. The tendon from the long head of the biceps passes through the interval to its attachment on the glenoid. The fibers from the supraspinatus join with fibers from the subscapularis to form a sheath around the biceps tendon. Fibers of the coracohumeral ligament extend from the coracoid to the rotator interval and the supraspinatus, contributing to the cuff-capsule complex (Fig. 2). Through this complex, the supraspinatus muscle is attached not only to the

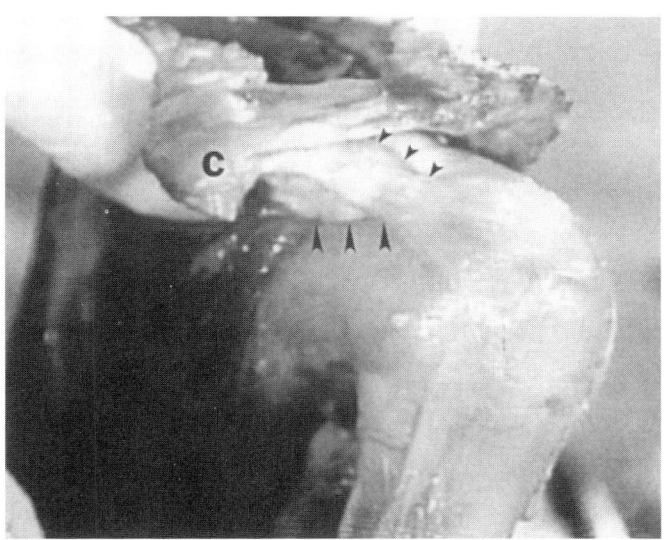

Fig. 1 Anterosuperior view of the rotator cuff in a left shoulder. The arrowheads indicate the edges of the supraspinatus and subscapularis tendons with the rotator interval being the space between these edges. The coracohumeral ligament can be seen overlying this interval. The "c" in the figure denotes the coracoid process. (Reproduced with permission from Harryman DT II, Clark JM Jr: Anatomy of the rotator cuff, in *Rotator Cuff Disorders*. Baltimore, MD, Williams & Wilkins, 1996, pp 23-35.)

greater tuberosity, but to the other cuff structures as well. Muscular contractions can thus tension the adjacent cuff and capsule in addition to applying force to the greater tuberosity.

The supraspinatus has several kinematic functions. Because of its position close to the humeral head, it has a small moment arm. Most importantly, it acts to depress and centralize the humeral head. The supraspinatus contributes to humeral elevation in concert with the deltoid and other muscles. Because of its relatively small size and short moment arm, its contribution is small comparatively; however, it is thought to play a key role in stabilizing the head during early elevation and abduction. Additionally, as the supraspinatus can tension the superior capsular-cuff complex, it resists inferior subluxation of the humerus and can assist in compression of the humeral head into the glenoid cavity, providing joint stability.

Infraspinatus

The infraspinatus muscle arises from the scapular fossa inferior to the scapular spine and is innervated by the

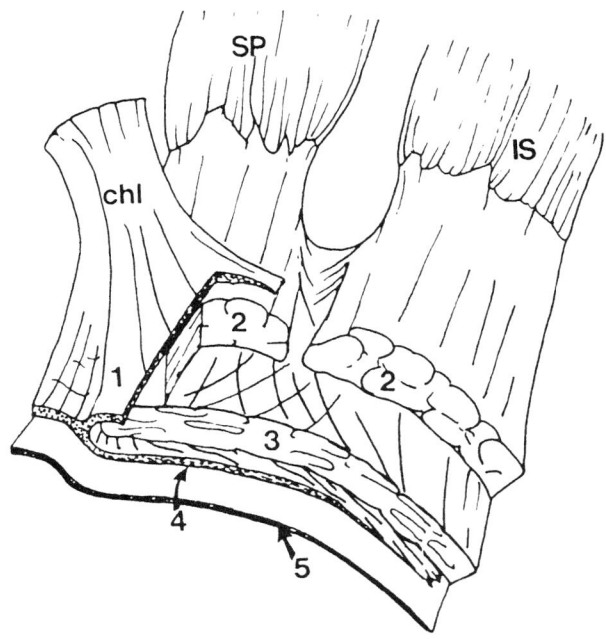

Fig. 2 A schematic of the relationship between the coracohumeral ligament and the superior portion of the rotator cuff. Note that the coracohumeral ligament fibers extend over the most superficial portion of the cuff and send fibers through the rotator interval and down along the deep cuff just above the joint capsule. chl = coracohumeral ligament; SP = supraspinatus; IS = infraspinatus; 1 = most superficial layer of the cuff capsule complex; 2 = second layer composed of true rotator cuff tendons; 3 = intermediate cuff layer; 4 = deep extension of coracohumeral ligament, circumferential fibers; 5 = glenohumeral joint capsule. (Reproduced with permission from Clark JM, Harryman DT II: Tendons, ligaments, and capsule of the rotator cuff: Gross and microscopic anatomy. *J Bone Joint Surg* 1992;74A:713-725.)

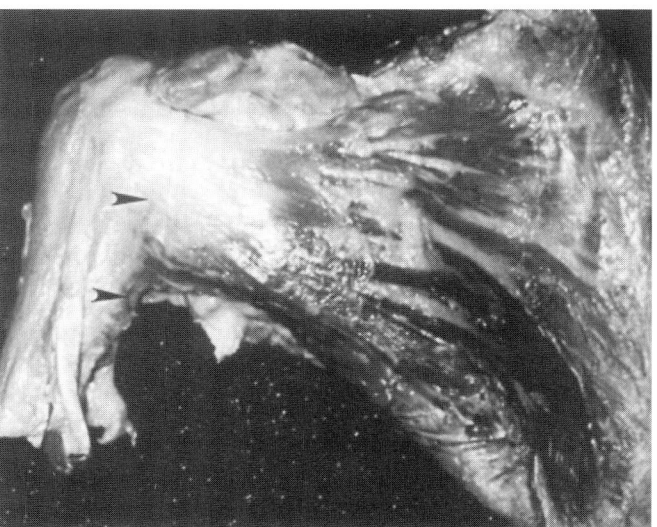

Fig. 3 Anterior view of the subscapularis tendon in a right shoulder. The superior portion of the subscapularis inserts as a well-defined tendon into the lesser tuberosity. The inferior portion of the muscle inserts as muscular fibers directly onto the humerus, as shown by the arrowheads. Reproduced with permission from Harryman DT II, Clark JM Jr: Anatomy of the rotator cuff, in *Rotator Cuff Disorders*. Baltimore, MD, Williams & Wilkins, 1996, pp 23-35.)

suprascapular nerve. To reach the infraspinatus, the nerve must pass around the base of the scapular spine at the spinoglenoid notch. At this point the nerve is vulnerable to injury during surgical mobilization of the cuff during rotator cuff repair, as well as from nonsurgical events. Denervation at this level has been found to occur not infrequently in certain athletes, especially volleyball players, and is likely to occur as a result of a repeated injury.

The infraspinatus has an intramuscular raphe dividing it into an upper and lower portion. This raphe, seen as a light-colored stripe at surgery, can be used as the point at which to split the muscle for access to the posterior glenohumeral joint and capsule without significant risk of nerve injury. It may be an easier plane to find than the true internervous plane between the infraspinatus and teres minor. Laterally, the fibers of the infraspinatus insert onto the greater tuberosity, posterior to the supraspinatus. Near the insertion, some of the fibers diverge to blend with the supraspinatus anteriorly and the teres minor inferiorly. Through these interconnections with the adjacent cuff tendons, the muscle of the infraspinatus can tension the entire posterosuperior cuff-capsule complex.

The primary action of the infraspinatus is to externally rotate the humerus. Because it is the most powerful of the humeral external rotators, individuals with cuff tears that extend into the infraspinatus frequently present with profound loss of external rotation strength. The infraspinatus also contributes to joint stability by forming a barrier to posterior translation as well as by compressing the humeral head into the glenoid concavity.

Teres Minor

The teres minor is the smallest and least clinically important of the cuff muscles. It originates from the lower border of the scapula and inserts on the most inferior portion of the greater tuberosity. It receives its innervation from a branch of the axillary nerve as it courses through the quadrangular space. Thus, a true internervous plane exists between the infraspinatus and the teres minor for surgical approaches. The teres minor acts as an external rotator of the humerus.

Subscapularis

The subscapularis is the largest and most powerful of the cuff muscles. It originates from the subscapularis fossa, which comprises nearly the entire anterior scapula. The subscapularis is a multipennate muscle that inserts onto the lesser tuberosity of the humerus. The majority of the muscle inserts through a tendinous attachment that fuses with the joint capsule near the humerus. An inferior third inserts as muscular fibers directly onto the humerus and joint capsule (Fig. 3).

The muscle is innervated by the upper and lower subscapular nerves, though the upper nerve is of primary importance. Similar to other cuff tendons, the fibers of the subscapularis tendon merge with those of the joint capsule and glenohumeral ligaments as they extend laterally. In addition, at the superior edge, fibers interconnect with those of the supraspinatus in the rotator interval. In this region, they contribute to the sheath around the biceps tendon.

The subscapularis is a strong internal rotator of the humerus. It acts with other muscles (eg, pectoralis major, latissimus dorsi, teres major, anterior deltoid) to create a powerful internal rotation motion. Because of the contributions of the other muscles, it is difficult to isolate subscapularis function on physical examination. Lift-off of the hand from the back with the arm starting in internal rotation is the best technique to isolate subscapularis function. In addition to producing internal rotation, the subscapularis acts to depress the humeral head and stabilize the head into the glenoid cavity. The subscapularis has exhibited passive resistance to anterior subluxation in the abducted externally rotated position.

Microstructure

As the individual tendons extend toward the humerus, instead of inserting as individual tendons, they intersect and blend with fibers from adjacent tendons. Through these connections, loads are transmitted transversely across the cuff and significant shear forces occur. This arrangement may have importance in the initiation of cuff tears. Where these tendon fibers insert, a five-layer structure to the superior cuff-capsule complex has been described. In this scheme, starting from the bursal surface (Fig. 4), layer one is composed of the superficial portion of the coracohumeral ligament. Layer two is seen as closely packed parallel tendon fibers grouped in large bundles extending directly from the muscle bellies to the humeral insertions and likely is the primary load-carrying portion of the cuff tendons. The third layer is also thick and tendinous, but has smaller fascicles and a less uniform orientation. Layer four is comprised of loose connective tissue in which thick bands of collagen run perpendicular to the primary fiber orientation of the cuff tendons. This layer is also the deep extent of the coracohumeral ligament and has been variously described as a transverse band, a pericapsular band, or a rotator cable by different authors (Fig. 5). As such, it may play a role in distributing forces between portions of the cuff. Layer five is the true capsular layer and forms a continuous layer from the glenoid to the humerus.

Vascularity

The supraspinatus tendon receives its blood supply primarily from the suprascapular artery. Some authors report contributions from the posterior humeral circumflex near its insertion, whereas others identify a blood supply from the anterior humeral circumflex and subscapular arteries. Classic studies by Codman identified a "critical zone" at the supraspinatus tendon insertion as a region that has an inadequate blood supply. More recently, a sparse vascular distribution at the articular side of the supraspinatus tendon and a well-vascularized bursal side has been demonstrated. In uninjured cuff tendons it appears that this "critical zone" is actually well vascularized with many anastomoses. It has been suggested that an interruption of perfusion might be caused by pressure on the tendon from the humeral head below and coracoacromial arch above. This pressure might "wring out the blood supply to these tendons" when the arm is at the side, thus providing an extrinsic explanation for a diminished blood supply.

It appears that the normal supraspinatus tendon is well vascularized. However, injury, degeneration, tension in the cuff from muscular contraction, or compression of the cuff against the coracoacromial arch may lead to an area of inadequate blood supply.

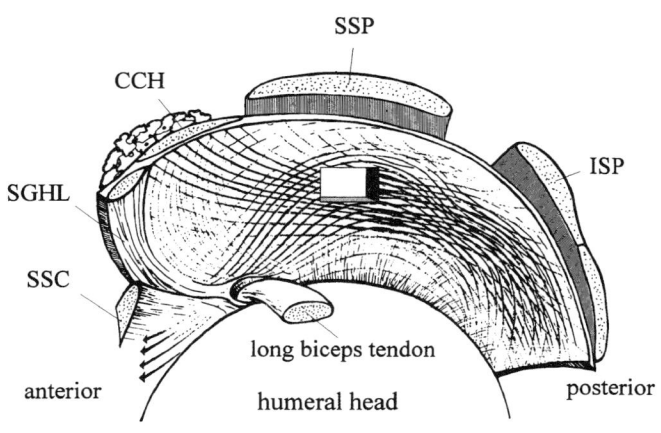
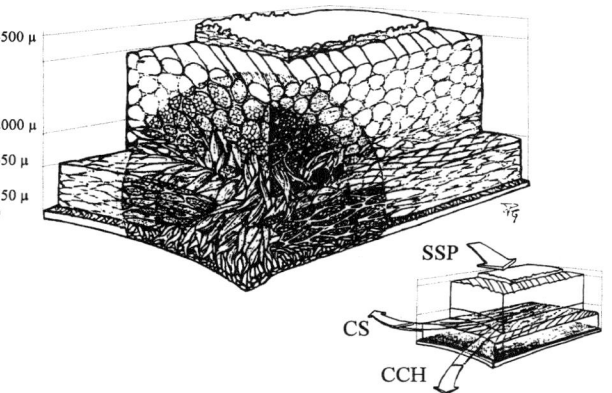

Fig. 4 A cross-sectional view of the superior shoulder cuff-capsule joint complex. This structure has generally been considered to be comprised of five layers. Variation in tissue properties and loads between layers may contribute to shear forces along these planes, which may be a factor in initiation of rotator cuff tears. SGHL = superior glenohumeral ligament; CCH = coracohumeral ligament; SSP = supraspinatus; SSC = subscapularis; ISP = infraspinatus; CS = circular system of fiber bundles. (Reproduced with permission from Gohlke F, Essigkrug B, Schmitz F: The pattern of collagen fiber bundles of the capsule of the glenohumeral joint. *J Shoulder Elbow Surg* 1994;3:111-128.)

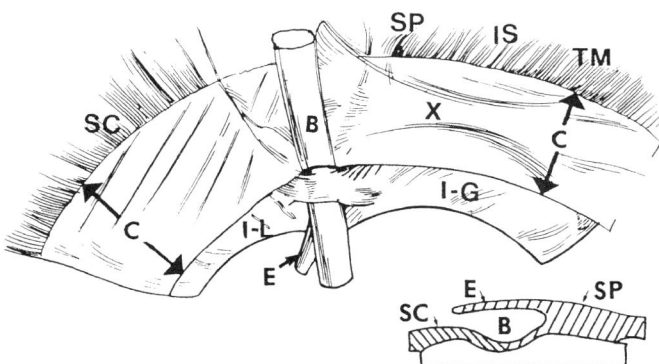

Fig. 5 Schematic of the joint capsule and cuff from the articular side. Note the thickened portion of superior capsule (X). This transverse band may contribute to dispersion of forces across adjacent portions of the rotator cuff. It may play a role in adequate force transmission, even in the face of a full-thickness cuff tear. Both the supraspinatus and subscapularis contribute to the floor of the biceps sheath, whereas the supraspinatus contributes the superior or roof portion. C = capsule; SC = subscapularis; B = biceps; E = extension from supraspinatus tendon; SP = supraspinatus; IS = infraspinatus; I-L = insertions on lesser tuberosity; I-G = insertions on greater tuberosity; TM = teres minor; X = transverse band. (Reproduced with permission from Clark JM, Harryman DT II: Tendons, ligaments, and capsule of the rotator cuff: Gross and microscopic anatomy. *J Bone Joint Surg* 1992;74A:713-725.)

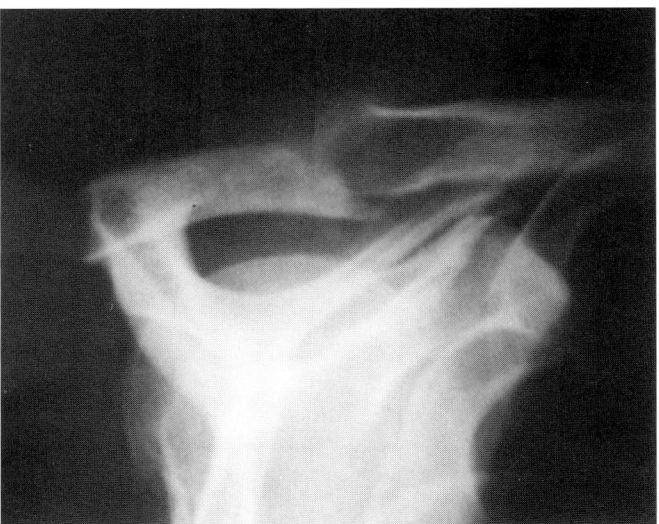

Fig. 6 A lateral or outlet view radiograph demonstrating the presence of a spur, which compromises the space available for the supraspinatus tendon. This significant acromial spur was present in the absence of a full-thickness rotator cuff tear.

Coracoacromial Arch

A review of rotator cuff anatomy is incomplete without a description of the coracoacromial arch. This structure comprises the roof above the supraspinatus tendon and defines the outlet or space through which this tendon must pass. There are a number of reports that discuss the variation in the shape of the acromion. When viewed from the lateral side, the acromion may be relatively flat, gently curved, or may have a hooked or pointed anterior edge (Fig. 6). These variations have important implications in the pathogenesis of cuff tears and in the treatment of individuals with cuff pathology. Attached to its anterior-inferior edge is the well-defined coracoacromial ligament. This ligament extends in two bands, a medial band and a more clinically significant lateral band, to the coracoid process. The lateral band attaches primarily to the coracoid, but the lateralmost fibers merge with fibers of the conjoined tendon and extend distally with them.

Variations in the histology, geometry, and biomechanics of the coracoacromial ligament have been found in relation to cuff tears, suggesting that it, too, may play a role in cuff disease. Thus, this series of structures (acromion, coracoacromial ligament, coracoid) form a rigid arch above the supraspinatus tendon and may compress the underlying tendon, contributing to tendon injury (Fig. 7).

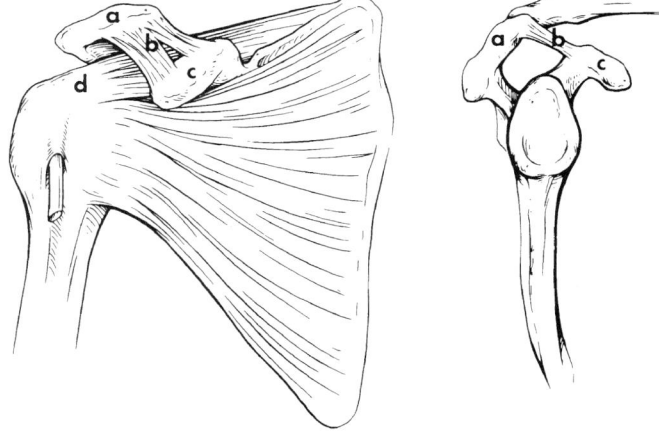

Fig. 7 **Left,** Anterior view of the right shoulder demonstrating the coracoacromial arch positioned over the supraspinatus tendon. **Right,** Lateral view of the scapula and coracoacromial ligament demonstrating the enclosed arch of the supraspinatus outlet through which the supraspinatus tendon must pass. a = acromion, b = coracoacromial ligament, c = coracoid, d = supraspinatus tendon. (Reproduced with permission from Soslowsky LJ, An CH, Johnston SP, et al: Geometric and mechanical properties of the coracoacromial ligament and their relationship to rotator cuff disease. *Clin Orthop* 1994;304:10-17.)

Biomechanics

Inman and associates were one of the early groups to measure the role of the rotator cuff in shoulder function. In finding that the cuff muscles were all active during most shoulder motions, they supported the concept of force couples around the glenohumeral joint. Employing this concept, groups of muscles work together to balance each others' unwanted actions to produce the desired effect (Fig. 8). For example, the cuff muscles depress and stabilize the humeral head at the

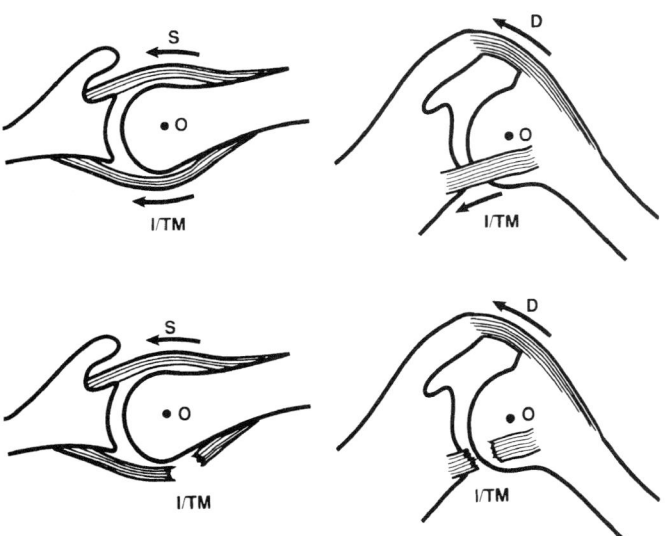

Fig. 8 **Top,** Intact force couples in the horizontal and vertical planes allow for normal rotation of the humeral head within the glenoid. **Bottom,** When one component of the force couple is lost, there is imbalance in the muscle forces and abnormal kinematics. S = subscapularis; I/TM = infraspinatus/teres minor; D = deltoid; O = center of rotation. (Reproduced with permission from Friedman RS, Knetsche RP: Biomechanics of the rotator cuff, in *Rotator Cuff Disorders.* Baltimore, MD, Williams & Wilkins, 1996, pp 45-56.)

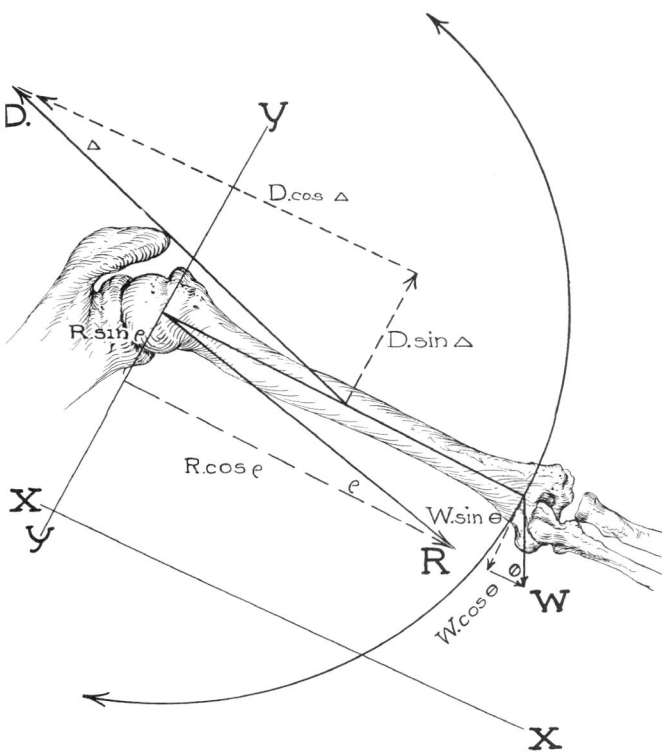

Fig. 9 A simplistic free body diagram of the shoulder. D = deltoid force; W = weight of the arm; R = reaction force. (Reproduced with permission from Inman VT, Saunders JB, Abbott LC: Observations on the function of the shoulder joint. *J Bone Joint Surg* 1944;26A:1.)

same time the deltoid acts to elevate the arm. When one of these forces is eliminated through injury or paralysis, this coupling is lost and abnormal mechanics result.

In order to investigate these concepts experimentally, a number of mathematic, analytic, and cadaveric shoulder models have been employed. Simple two-dimensional free-body models such as that presented by Inman (Fig. 9) including only one or two muscle forces have been used to approximate deltoid, cuff, and joint reactive forces. These studies suggest that very significant forces, on the order of body weight, can be generated at the shoulder because of the long lever arm of the upper extremity (Fig. 10). The cadaveric models are most helpful because they use the entire glenohumeral joint while simulating muscle forces of portions of the cuff and deltoid, and the long head of the biceps. By individually adjusting the tension on the tendon stumps, different arm positions can be achieved and studied (Fig. 11).

Modifications of these structures and forces can then be used to study abnormal conditions, most specifically cuff tears, cuff paralysis, and alterations in the coracoacromial arch. Although the techniques of simulating forces as well as measuring translations vary, the results found among these models are similar. The importance of the supraspinatus at the initiation of abduction is confirmed. As shown in Figure 12, when paralysis of the supraspinatus is simulated (but the cuff is still intact) the force required by the middle deltoid to abduct the arm in the scapular plane increases by 100% at the initiation of abduction, but is not increased at all beyond 90° of abduction. Interestingly, there is little superior translation of the humeral head with this simulated supraspinatus paralysis when compared to experimental cuff tears. This "spacer" effect of the superior cuff may occur because of the presence of the tendon in the subacromial space, blocking translation, or because forces from adjacent cuff muscles are transmitted to the intact superior capsule and cuff.

Actual cuff tears have been simulated by creating defects in the supraspinatus tendon and measuring the changes in kinematics. Several studies have demonstrated that small cuff tears that do not involve the infraspinatus or subscapularis have little effect on superior translation of the humeral head or on the degree of abduction achievable. This is particularly true if the biceps force is intact. This finding helps to explain why shoulder function may be normal in many individuals with small or moderate tears. Under these conditions, the force couple provided by the anterior and posterior portions of the intact cuff is adequate despite a defect in the superior cuff. The transverse band that is found in the superior capsule-cuff complex (called the rotator cable by some authors) may provide the link necessary between the intact portions of the cuff. However, if the tear is massive (involving two or three tendons), then a significant alteration in kinematics is seen. There is also loss of the normal force couple, resulting in significant superior translation of the humeral head and limitation of abduction. Anatomic repair of these tears can result in

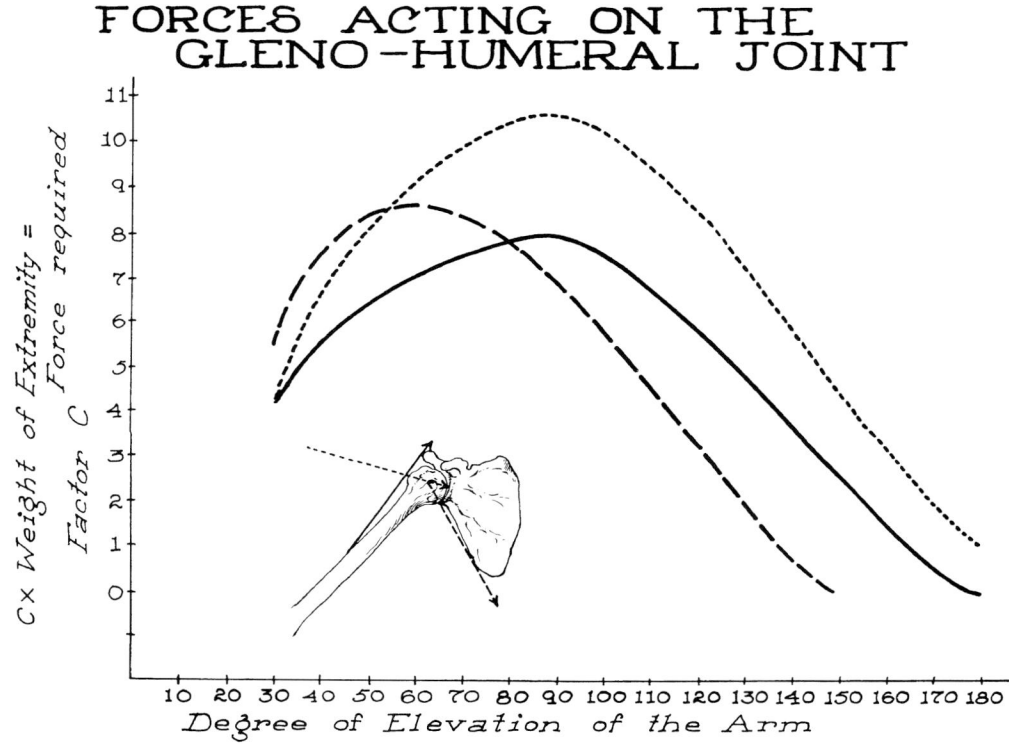

Fig. 10 Results from a simple two-dimensional free body analysis of the glenohumeral joint. This model demonstrates the large forces generated by the deltoid and at the glenohumeral joint. In turn, these forces must be counteracted by inferiorly directed muscle forces for joint stabilization to occur. (Reproduced with permission from Inman VT, Saunders JB, Abbott LC: Observations on the function of the shoulder joint. *J Bone Joint Surg* 1944;26A:1.)

a return to normal kinematics. It has been proposed that partial repair may restore function when complete repair cannot be achieved.

Cadaveric models have also helped to define the role of the long head of the biceps tendon. The biceps may function as a shoulder joint stabilizer, but its action depends on joint position. In the presence of large or massive cuff tears, activation of biceps force reduces pathologic motion and can restore function. These findings suggest that preservation of the biceps during surgical repair of cuff tears may be important.

Recently, the effects of acromioplasty and coracoacromial ligament excision have been modeled. As might be expected, when the humeral head is pushed superiorly it will translate further if the anterior acromion and coracoacromial ligament are removed. In more detailed analysis with simulated cuff function, significant changes in kinematics occurred following coracoacromial ligament removal only with a concomitant large or massive cuff tear. This effect may occur because of loss of contact with the undersurface of the acromion or from loss of tethering of the anterior tip of the acromion to the coracoid. These studies help confirm clinical observations that in some cases of massive or irreparable cuff tears, coracoacromial ligament resection results in significantly greater superior translation of the humeral head. In order to avoid this difficult clinical problem, preservation or reattachment of the coracoacromial ligament during surgical repair of large or massive tears has been recommended.

Although these models go a long way toward improving understanding of rotator cuff function in normal and pathologic conditions, a number of limitations exist. Most important is the relationship of these findings to clinical symptoms. It is not known whether or not superior translation is related to shoulder pain. Similarly, the complex effects of pain on muscle inhibition cannot be accurately modeled.

Although much is known about the kinematics of the rotator cuff at the whole joint level, less information is available about the mechanical properties of the individual tendons. This is true in part because it is difficult to isolate and test identifiable portions of the rotator cuff with the large number of varying fiber orientations and interactions. Because of its predominant importance in cuff pathology and mechanics, the supraspinatus tendon has been evaluated by several techniques. It has been divided into anterior, middle, and posterior bands and studied biomechanically. Using this technique, the posterior third of the supraspinatus tendon was found to be significantly thinner than either the anterior or middle thirds, whereas the ultimate load and stress are significantly greater for the anterior portion than the middle or posterior portion. The modulus of elasticity is greater in the anterior third than in the middle or posterior portions (Fig. 13). It appears that

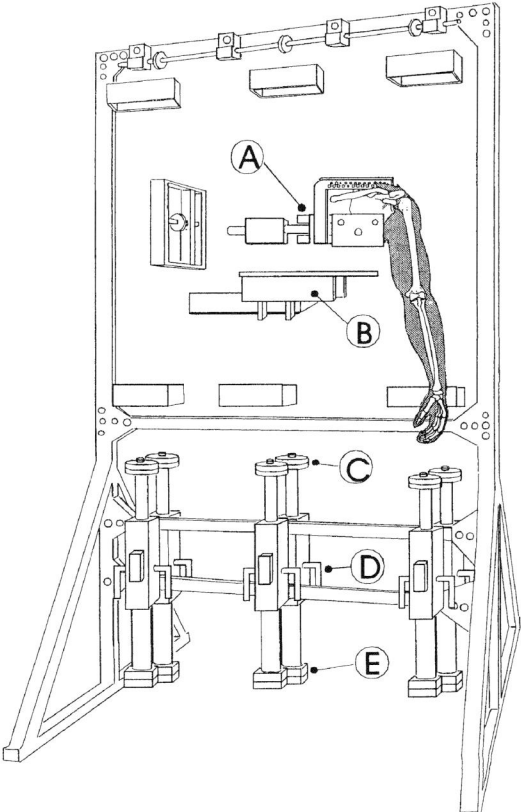

Fig. 11 The University of Pittsburgh dynamic shoulder testing apparatus. The entire upper extremity hangs free while the scapula is stabilized. Computer-controlled load actuators simulate load of the four rotator cuff muscles as well as the three portions of the deltoid. The arm is free to move in any direction while displacements and forces can be measured dynamically. (Reproduced with permission from Thompson WO, Debski RE, Boardman ND III, et al: A biomechanical analysis of rotator cuff deficiency in a cadaveric model. *Am J Sports Med* 1996;24:286-292.)

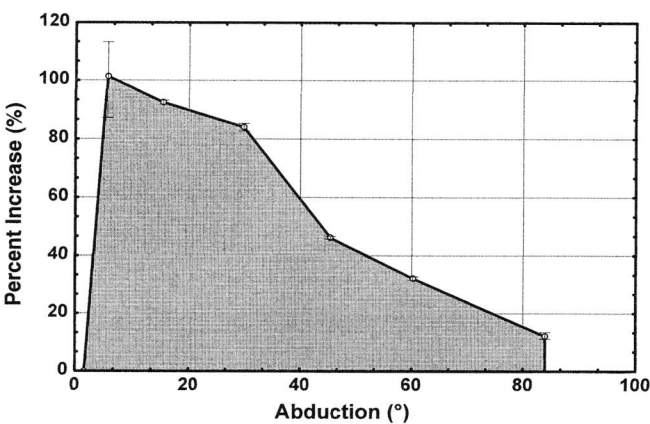

Fig. 12 Deltoid force required to achieve various positions of shoulder abduction with simulated paralysis of the supraspinatus muscle. This indicates that loss of the supraspinatus is most significant at the initiation of abduction and that at greater than 90° of abduction there is no effect on the deltoid from loss of supraspinatus force. (Reproduced with permission from Thompson WO, Debski RE, Boardman ND III, et al: A biomechanical analysis of rotator cuff deficiency in a cadaveric model. *Am J Sports Med* 1996;24:286-292.)

the anterior portion of the supraspinatus tendon is mechanically the strongest and seems to perform the primary load transmission from the supraspinatus muscle.

Mechanical properties within the supraspinatus tendon have also been evaluated between the articular and bursal sides of the tendon. It has been demonstrated that the bursal side of the supraspinatus tendon has a lower modulus of elasticity, yet a higher ultimate strain and stress, compared to the articular side of the supraspinatus. On this basis it can be suggested that the articular side of the supraspinatus tendon is more susceptible to mechanical failure in tension than is the bursal side if subjected to the same load. It is likely that differences in fiber bundle orientation and matrix composition within these two portions of the capsule are responsible for these differences in mechanical properties. The regional variations in mechanical strength may help explain the

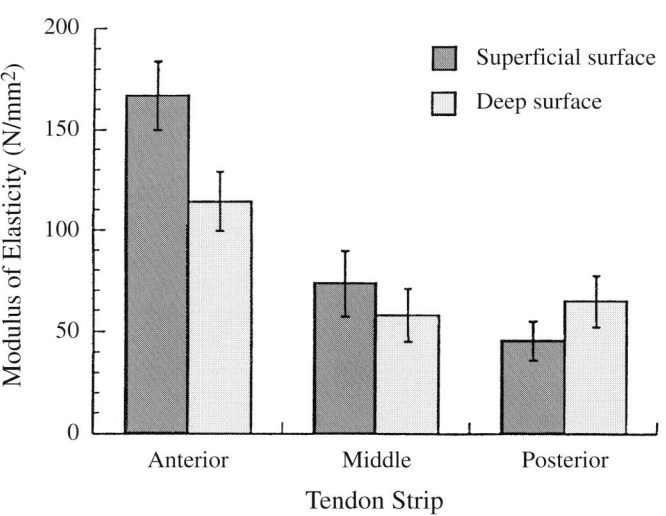

Fig. 13 Biomechanical assessment of the anterior, middle, and posterior thirds of the supraspinatus tendon demonstrate that the anterior portion is the thickest and has the highest modulus of elasticity. These data indicate that the majority of load transmission probably occurs through this anterior third. (Reproduced with permission from Itoi E, Berglund LJ, Grabowski JJ, et al: Tensile properties of the supraspinatus tendon. *J Orthop Res* 1995;13: 578-584.)

development of partial thickness rotator cuff tears, especially because they seem to occur more commonly on the articular surface.

Biochemistry

Tendons contain collagen with several types of cross-linking and small amounts of elastin, glycosaminoglycans (GAG), and proteoglycans, along with water. The collagen present in normal tendon is predominantly type I (> 95%), with small amounts of types III and V. Conditions of tendon injury and repair prompt an increase in the amount of type III collagen, which is thought to be responsible for early stabilization of the extracellular matrix. Type III collagen has been found to be increased at the margins of rotator cuff tears as well as in biopsy specimens from patients with chronic tendinitis without full-thickness tears. Cells producing type I collagen have been found at the proximal margin of torn supraspinatus tendons. These findings indicate active new matrix synthesis, consistent with tissue remodeling and wound healing in the injured supraspinatus tendon. The amount of type III collagen present in the supraspinatus tendon may be an indicator of the degree of tendon injury and repair activity.

Other constituents of the cuff tendons have been shown to be altered in rotator cuff disease. Fibrocartilaginous regions have been demonstrated in various tendons throughout the body that are subjected to compressive loading, such as where tendons wrap around bone in these regions. There is an increased amount of GAG associated with several proteoglycans, including aggrecan, which is typically found in cartilage. In normal human rotator cuff tendons there has been reported an increased GAG content compared to that of the tensile portion of the biceps tendon. This finding suggests that the cuff tendons have adapted to loads other than pure tension, possibly from compression against the coracoacromial arch. Histologically, no fibrocartilage regions are evident in normal tendon. In contrast, histologic specimens from aged cadaveric cuff tendons have been found to have GAG infiltration and fibrocartilaginous transformation. Biopsy specimens from patients with symptomatic cuff tendinopathy have had increased amounts of GAG compared to specimens from normal cadaveric cuff tendons. These findings suggest that the supraspinatus, which has a greater amount of GAG than other tendons (which are subject to only tensile loads), undergoes further fibrocartilaginous change when affected by chronic tendinitis.

Rotator Cuff Injury

Injuries to the rotator cuff are common. The most dramatic and most studied of these injuries is a complete, full-thickness tear. Such tears almost inevitably involve the supraspinatus tendon and may also involve the infraspinatus, teres minor, subscapularis, and/or the long head of the biceps tendon. However, partial tears and tendinopathy without definable tears are also common findings. It is generally thought that these entities represent different presentations of the same disease process; however, this theory has not been established.

Pathology

Studies on the histopathology of rotator cuff disease have primarily relied on tissue from the subacromial bursa and the supraspinatus tendon in patients undergoing rotator cuff surgery for full-thickness cuff tears. There is a significant proliferation of reparative tissue around the edges of the tendon and in the surrounding bursal tissue, with degenerative changes occurring within nearby tendon. True inflammatory infiltrates have not been predominant in these tissues, making the term "tendinitis" not the most appropriate. Rotator cuff tendinosis is the most appropriate term based on the pathology seen. These samples have generally been obtained from tissue adjacent to cuff tears, and may not be characteristic of supraspinatus tendinopathy in the absence of tendon rupture.

Unfortunately, biopsy specimens from a large number of patients with cuff disease in the absence of significant cuff tearing have not been available. Less than 20% of cadaveric tendons studied by one group show histologic abnormalities before the age of 40; this number increases to approximately 50% later in life. The tendon alterations found have included GAG infiltration, fibrocartilaginous transformation, loss of the waviness and organization in the collagen fibers, and degenerative changes. When the histologic changes are evaluated in biopsy specimens from patients with "rotator cuff

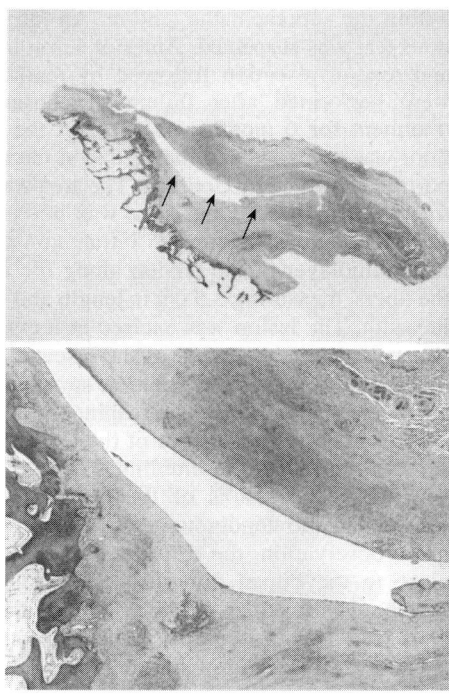

Fig. 14 Top, En bloc section of the supraspinatus insertion with a partial cuff tear. This intratendinous tear (arrows) extends nearly through to the bursal surface. **Bottom,** In this close-up view, the tear extends between layers of the tendon and is lined by a single layer of cells with no evidence of defect closure. (Reproduced with permission from Fukuda H, Hamada K, Nakajima T, et al: Pathology and pathogenesis of the intratendinous tearing of the rotator cuff viewed from en bloc histologic sections. *Clin Orthop* 1994;304:60-67.)

tendinitis," there are changes that are consistent with new matrix synthesis, tissue remodeling, and wound healing. These findings are similar to those seen in biopsy specimens from patients with lateral epicondylitis of the elbow. Compared to those from normal tendons, biopsy specimens from supraspinatus tendons in patients with rotator cuff disease have an increased concentration of GAG.

Microscopic study of specimens from patients with partial-thickness rotator cuff tears may represent the earlier stages of cuff disease before a full-thickness tear develops. As such, study of these specimens may give insight to the pathogenesis of cuff disease. Partial tears have been found to be most commonly bursal-sided, but can also be articular-sided, or intratendinous. They generally demonstrate a loss of the wavy fiber pattern, collagen fiber disruption, the presence of a granulation tissue response, and vascular proliferation intermixed with areas of degeneration. The proximal stumps appear rounded and avascular with little repair response, whereas hypervascularity and granulation tissue are present at the insertion and distal stumps. The tears extend horizontally between layers of the cuff-capsule complex, generally in the midlayer of the tendon (Fig. 14). It is postulated that shear forces within the tendon are responsible for this type of tearing. Despite the proliferative tissue around these partial tears, healing or closure of the defects is not apparent.

Etiology of Cuff Disease

Those studies that have attempted to address mechanisms of chronic rotator cuff injury can be grouped by whether they support an intrinsic or extrinsic mechanism. Intrinsic tendon injury originates within the tendon from direct tendon overload or tendon degeneration. Extrinsic tendon injury is caused by compression against surrounding structures, most specifically the coracoacromial arch. Depending on which mechanism is dominant in a particular injury, different approaches toward prevention and treatment of rotator cuff disease might be appropriate.

Studies supporting intrinsic mechanisms have included vascular and anatomic investigations, as well as evaluations of overuse syndromes. The critical zone described earlier was thought to represent a region of poor vascularity that was at risk for injury and that had little capacity for repair. Subsequent studies on the vascular supply to the supraspinatus tendon show an adequate blood supply in normal tendons. However, aging, injury, or external compression may diminish perfusion, setting up conditions for rotator cuff disease. Histologically, regions adjacent to cuff tears have demonstrated degenerative changes within the tendon. These changes may precede the tear, making the tendon intrinsically more susceptible to further injury and eventual tearing.

Studies supporting the extrinsic mechanisms of cuff tear pathogenesis have implicated impingement against the undersurface of the acromion and the coracoacromial ligament as the primary factors for causing these tears. It is likely that if external compression of the rotator cuff tendons is a mechanism for rotator cuff disease, then variations in the anatomy of the coracoacromial arch would be important in the disease pathogenesis. In comparing cadavers with rotator cuff tears to those without tears, it has been found that specimens with type III or hooked acromia (projecting further into the subacromial space) had an increased likelihood of association with a full-thickness cuff tear, compared to a type I or flat acromion. Similarly, a study of patients with symptomatic rotator cuff disease found an increased prevalence of a hooked or type III acromion. Quantitative assessment of the geometric area of the supraspinatus outlet has demonstrated a correlation between rotator cuff tears and a reduced space for the supraspinatus.

Changes in the coracoacromial ligament can also reduce the supraspinatus outlet area, creating an extrinsic compression on the cuff. Histologically, the ligament is more disorganized,

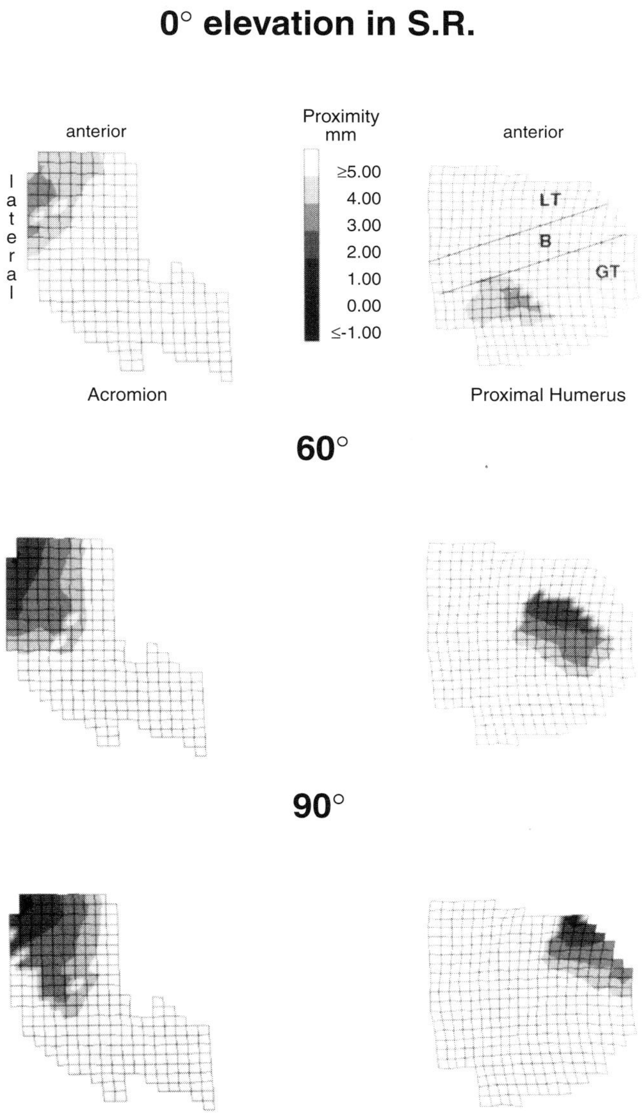

Fig. 15 Surface contact maps demonstrating the areas of contact between the undersurface in the acromion at zero, 60°, and 90° of elevation. Contact occurs between the greater tuberosity and the anterior lateral portion of the acromion. This contact area increases as the arm is abducted. SR = starting rotation; LT = lesser tuberosity; B = biceps; GT = greater tuberosity. (Reproduced with permission from Soslowsky LJ: Studies on diarthrodial joint biomechanics with special reference to the shoulder. New York, NY, Columbia University, 1991. Thesis.)

with a loss of normal collagen fiber orientation in shoulders with rotator cuff tears. There is a shortening and thickening of the coracoacromial ligament in shoulders with rotator cuff tears compared to shoulders without cuff tears. Biomechanically, there is a decrease in the elastic modulus of the ligament, but because of a greater cross-section there is no change in the overall structural properties. Such studies clearly demonstrate alterations in the anatomy and biomechanics of the coracoacromial arch in association with rotator cuff tears, yet it cannot be determined if these changes lead to tears through compression on the supraspinatus tendon or occur as a result of altered loading after a cuff tear.

In analysis of subacromial contact, it has been demonstrated that the undersurface of the acromion and the rotator cuff tendon are closest between 60° and 120° of humeral elevation (Fig. 15). Because this range represents the typically painful arc of motion in patients with cuff disease, it has been hypothesized that extrinsic compression of the cuff tendons against the acromion and coracoacromial ligament may be responsible for this pain. The contact occurs at the anterior-inferior portion of the acromion at the attachment of the coracoacromial ligament. These areas of contact have been shown to be increased in shoulders with hooked or type III acromions. Furthermore, simulated acromioplasty can reduce the contact area. Direct pressure measurements have been made on the undersurface of the acromion in cadavers, demonstrating greatest contact pressures at the anterior-inferior portion of the acromion at the attachment of the coracoacromial ligament (Fig. 16).

Thus, there exists evidence for both intrinsic and extrinsic mechanisms for rotator cuff disease. It can be stated with certainty that changes occur in both the cuff tendons and the coracoacromial arch in rotator cuff disease. Whether the tendon changes are initiated within the tendon and then through altered mechanics effect change in the arch structures or are a result of compression from primary arch abnormalities cannot be determined from these studies. Surgeons have tended to focus on the extrinsic causes because it is there that surgical corrections can be most easily entertained.

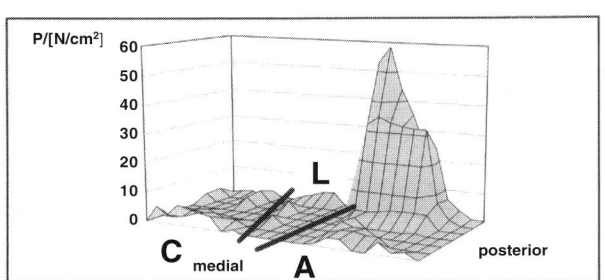

Fig. 16 Direct pressure measurements from the undersurface of the acromion in the cadaver model demonstrate greatest pressure between the greater tuberosity and the anterolateral portion of the acromion at the insertion of the coracoacromial ligament. A = acromion; C = coracoid; L = coracoacromial ligament. (Reproduced with permission from Wuelker N, Roetman B, Roessig S: Coracoacromial pressure recordings in a cadaveric model. *J Shoulder Elbow Surg* 1995;4:462-467.)

In an effort to more rigorously test these various hypotheses of cuff disease etiology, an animal model has been proposed. The advantage of using an animal model is that a known condition or injury can be applied to the shoulder and the response followed and measured. The rat model is ideal because of the anatomic similarity of the supraspinatus tendon and acromion to that of the human. With this model, histologic changes consistent with tendinosis have been observed after either an intrinsic injury (collagenase injection), an extrinsic compression (tendon graft wrapped around the acromion), or a combination of alterations. These changes would suggest that injuries may occur from either mechanism or from a combination of intrinsic and extrinsic factors.

Selected Bibliography

Bigliani LU, Ticker JB, Flatow EL, et al: The relationship of acromial architecture to rotator cuff disease. *Clin Sports Med* 1991;10:823-838.

Burkhart SS: Reconciling the paradox of rotator cuff repair versus debridement: A unified biomechanical rationale for the treatment of rotator cuff tears. *Arthroscopy* 1994;10: 4-19.

Clark JM, Harryman DT II: Tendons, ligaments, and capsule of the rotator cuff. *J Bone Joint Surg* 1992;74A:713-725.

In this classic study of the microstructure of the rotator cuff and especially the superior cuff-capsular complex, the interconnections between the cuff tendons, the coracohumeral ligament, and glenohumeral ligaments are detailed. A five-layered scheme to the structure of the superior cuff is also presented.

Flatow EL, Soslowsky LJ, Ticker JB, et al: Excursion of the rotator cuff under the acromion: Patterns of subacromial contact. *Am J Sports Med* 1994;22:779-788.

Using stereophotogrammetry, the region of contact between the undersurface of the acromion and the rotator cuff was determined in various arm positions in an anatomic model. The anterior-inferior portion of the acromion was the primary area of contact. The area increased with humeral elevation and with hooked or curved acromia.

Fukuda H, Hamada K, Nakajima T, et al: Pathology and pathogenesis of the intratendinous tearing of the rotator cuff viewed from en bloc histologic sections. *Clin Orthop* 1994;304:60-67.

This study provides an unsurpassed histologic analysis of partial tears in the supraspinatus tendon from actual patients treated surgically for symptomatic cuff disease. Because these partial tears may represent early phases of cuff disease, they may provide helpful data on the initiation of cuff tears.

Golhke F, Essigkrug B, Schmitz F: The pattern of the collagen fiber bundles of the capsule of the glenohumeral joint. *J Shoulder Elbow Surg* 1994;3:111-128.

A detailed study of the structure of the glenohumeral joint capsule-rotator cuff complex is presented. The authors provide an analysis of the glenohumeral ligaments and the interactions between the cuff and capsule. Their findings suggest that significant shear forces occur within the cuff-capsule complex that may represent an etiology for initiation of cuff tears.

Howell SM, Imobersteg AM, Seger DH, et al: Clarification of the role of the supraspinatus muscle in shoulder function. *J Bone Joint Surg* 1986;68A:398-404.

Inman VT, Saunders JB, Abbott LC: Observations on the function of the shoulder joint. *J Bone Joint Surg* 1944;26A:1-30.

Itoi E, Berglund LJ, Grabowski JJ, et al: Tensile properties of the supraspinatus tendon. *J Orthop Res* 1995;13:578-584.

In this study, the supraspinatus tendon is subdivided into an anterior, middle, and posterior portion. The anterior third of the tendon is the largest and strongest portion of the cuff and is likely performing the primary mechanical function.

McLaughlin HL, Asherman EG: Lesions of the musculotendinous cuff of the shoulder. *J Bone Joint Surg* 1951;33A:76-86.

Neer II CS: Anterior acromioplasty for the chronic impingement syndrome in the shoulder: A preliminary report. *J Bone Joint Surg* 1972;54A:41-50.

Nicholson GP, Goodman DA, Flatow EL, et al: The acromion: Morphologic condition and age-related changes. A study of 420 scapulas. *J Shoulder Elbow Surg* 1996;5:1-11.

In studying over 200 specimens from the Cleveland Museum of Natural History, this group found that variations in the shape of the acromion were independent of age and appeared to be a primary anatomic characteristic, whereas spur formation at the anterior acromion was related to age.

Riley GP, Harrall RL, Constant CR, et al: Glycosaminoglycans of human rotator cuff tendons: Changes with age and in chronic rotator cuff tendinitis. *Ann Rheum Dis* 1994;53:367-376.

Glycosaminoglycan content was significantly greater in the supraspinatus tendon of normal shoulders than in the distal portion of the long head of the biceps tendon. In specimens from patients with tendinitis, there was evidence of acute inflammation and new matrix synthesis. This new approach toward understanding rotator cuff disease through changes in the biochemistry of the cuff tendons may help in understanding the effects of aging as well as delineate intrinsic changes in the cuff associated with cuff disease.

Soslowsky LJ, An CH, Johnston SP, et al: Geometric and mechanical properties of the coracoacromial ligament and their relationship to rotator cuff disease. *Clin Orthop* 1994;304:10-17.

In a comparison of shoulders with and without cuff tears, there were significant differences in the properties of the coracoacromial ligament. In shoulders with cuff tears the ligaments were shorter, had greater cross-sectional area, and had a lower modulus of elasticity.

Soslowsky LJ, Carpenter JE, Debano CM, et al: Development and utilization of an animal model for investigations on rotator cuff disease. *J Shoulder Elbow Surg* 1996;5:383-392.

Using a set of anatomic and functional criteria, various animal models were evaluated for their appropriateness for studying rotator cuff disease. The rat was selected as the most acceptable animal model. Using intrinsic and extrinsic alterations to the supraspinatus tendon, histologic alterations were evaluated in the rotator cuff. Changes consistent with tendon injury and a reparative response were found from intrinsic injury and extrinsic compression, as well as from a combination of alterations.

Thompson WO, Debski RE, Boardman ND III, et al: A biomechanical analysis of rotator cuff deficiency in a cadaveric model. *Am J Sports Med* 1996;24:286-292.

A detailed study on the kinematics of the rotator cuff in normal conditions and with simulated cuff tears is presented. The sophisticated cadaveric model used is an excellent example of a whole joint approach toward understanding cuff mechanics in normal and disease states. The findings presented here are directly applicable to the clinical situation.

Wuelker N, Roetman B, Roessig S: Coracoacromial pressure recordings in a cadaveric model. *J Shoulder Elbow Surg* 1995;4:462-467.

The kinematics of the rotator cuff are studied using a computer-controlled cadaveric shoulder model. The contact pressures developed between the undersurface of the coracoacromial arch and the rotator cuff are analyzed. The greatest pressures were found under the anterior portion of the acromion, an area long referred to as the impingement region.

Zuckerman JD, Kummer FJ, Cuomo F, et al: The influence of coracoacromial arch anatomy on rotator cuff tears. *J Shoulder Elbow Surg* 1992;1:4-14.

A detailed study of 140 cadaver shoulders correlating cuff tears to geometric measures of arch anatomy is presented. The supraspinatus outlet area was found to be 22.5% smaller in shoulders with cuff tears.

4

Shoulder Kinematics and Kinesiology

Bruce D. Beynnon, PhD, Claude E. Nichols, MD, and John E. Novotny, MS

Introduction

The primary role of the shoulder is to convey the forces and moments at the hand and forearm to the torso. In contrast to other joints, the shoulder must be able to handle a great variation of loads, from holding a pencil to lifting a barbell. It must be able to carry loads through large ranges of possible motions and at rates of motion that vary from delicate to explosive.

Loads and moments are carried through the shoulder complex in three ways. The first is through contact between articular surfaces of the joints. This is the case for the sternoclavicular, acromioclavicular, and glenohumeral joints. The fourth articulation of the shoulder complex, the scapulothoracic, does not involve contact of articular surfaces but only muscular connections. The second method of load transmission is through the soft tissues such as the ligaments, joint capsules, and the labrum that span and surround the articulations. The third means is through the active control of the 18 muscles that cross the four articulations of the shoulder complex. The muscles provide the primary stability under shoulder loading and drive all the motions that occur. Alteration of any one of these three methods may result in instability, pain, and loss of function.

Because the ability to measure loads in biologic tissues is limited, the resulting motions caused by the applied loads usually are measured in biomechanical research. The measurement of motion without regard to the forces causing it is termed kinematics. Shoulder complex kinematics have been investigated in both in vivo and in vitro conditions.

Descriptions of Shoulder Motion

In assessing joint kinematics, the motion of the body segment of interest is measured relative to a fixed or bony landmark in another body segment. The methods for defining these bony landmarks and coordinate systems in the torso, scapula, clavicle, and humerus are not universal, making comparisons between different studies difficult. In general, the motion to be described for the shoulder is that of the rotation of the humerus, and it is often referenced to the torso for whole body motions such as throwing. For in vitro studies in which the scapula is accessible, the glenohumeral motion is often measured and referenced to the scapula. The motions of the clavicle and the scapula relative to the torso have not been well defined because bony reference points are difficult to define in vivo.

Methods for describing humeral rotation relative to the torso are varied. Different terms have been used in clinical examinations such as abduction and adduction for motion in the coronal plane of the torso, forward flexion and extension for motion in the sagittal plane, horizontal flexion and extension in the horizontal plane, and internal and external rotation of the humerus relative to its long axis. Difficulties in describing humeral motion, such as Codman's paradox, have driven the need for more precisely defined motion descriptions.

A global analogy has been used to describe the rotational orientation of the humerus relative to the torso (Fig. 1). The position of the elbow on the humerus is defined by two values, the plane of elevation and the angle of elevation, which can be visualized as the longitude and latitude of a globe centered at the humeral head. With the elbow flexed to 90°, the amount of internal and external rotation is defined as the angle of the forearm relative to the lines of latitude. With this method, though, the classic anatomic position remains undefined. Mathematically, translation between any two coordinate systems can also be presented numerically as a three element by three element matrix known as the rotation matrix, or matrix of direction cosines.

Two more methods used to quantify not only humeral rotation but also humeral translation are the Eulerian coordinate system and the screw-displacement axis system. The Eulerian system (Fig. 2) is a three-dimensional description of the

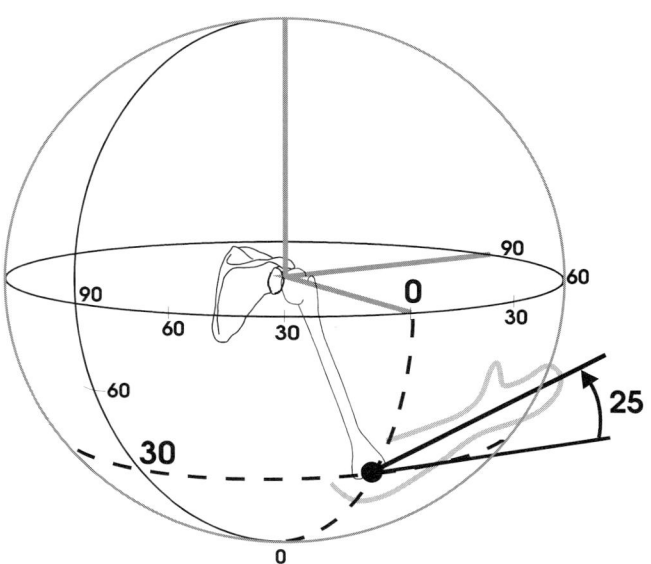

Fig. 1 Global analogy for defining humeral orientation, in this case for glenohumeral motion. The plane of elevation is 0° as measured from the plane of the scapula, and the angle of elevation is 30° from vertical. The amount of external rotation is 25°, as measured by the angle that the flexed forearm makes to the lines of latitude of the globe as shown.

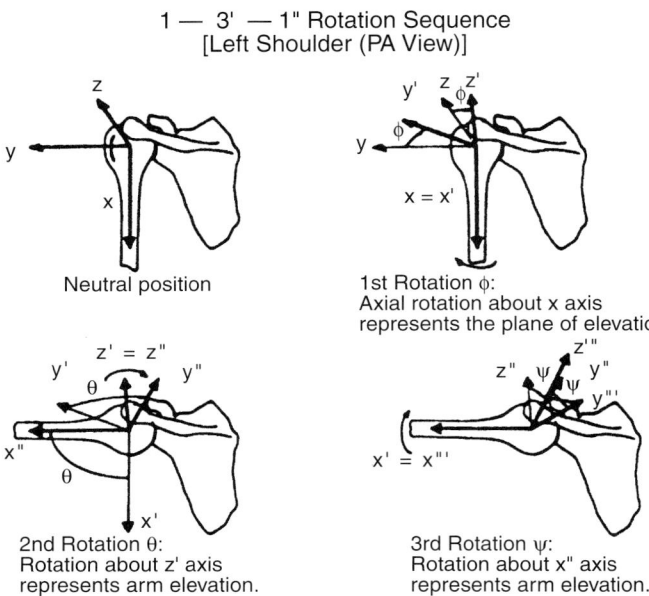

Fig. 2 The Eulerian coordinate system applied to the glenohumeral joint. The orientation of the humerus relative to the glenoid is defined by the sequence-dependent Eulerian angles. (Reproduced with permission from Morrey BF, An KN: Biomechanics of the shoulder, in Rockwood CA, Matsen FA III (eds): *The Shoulder*. Philadelphia, PA, WB Saunders, 1990, pp 208-245.)

relative position of the humerus in space and requires three angular rotations and three linear translations. These motions can be referenced to anatomic planes and are clearly understood. The position of the humerus relative to the glenoid is described by the displacement of the humeral coordinate system relative to the glenoid system. The description of joint orientation, though, is dependent on the sequence of rotation of the humeral coordinate system relative to a thoracic or glenoid coordinate system.

In the screw-displacement axis system, the difference from one position of the humerus relative to the scapula to another such position is defined by a rotation of the humerus about a given axis and a translation along that axis. The position of the axis and the translation can be calculated provided that three reference points on the moving humerus can be followed. In contrast to the Eulerian coordinate system, the screw-displacement axis system has the advantage of being independent of the coordinate systems chosen. However, this description of motion may be difficult to interpret relative to clinical descriptions of joint motion.

Four basic groups of study techniques are used to describe shoulder function. The first group consists of techniques that use planar or biplanar radiographs to observe bony motion. The second group includes in vitro or in vivo studies applying known forces, simulated muscle forces, or given motion patterns. The third group includes various mathematical models of shoulder function. The fourth group measures muscle electromyography (EMG) around the shoulder in activities from rehabilitation exercises to swimming.

Radiographic Techniques

Two-dimensional techniques using radiographs have been used to define humeral and scapular motion relative to the torso in the plane of the radiographic film. These techniques have the advantage of directly measuring shoulder kinematics in vivo. Unfortunately, the motion information measured is purely static because the arm must be still during radiographic exposure. Also, the definition of bony coordinate systems can be difficult and add to errors in measurement.

Classically, the angle between the spine of the scapula and the humeral shaft measured during abduction or forward flexion was used to describe the scapulohumeral rhythm during glenohumeral elevation. The scapula was found to move inconsistently during the first 30° of upward motion and then in a constant 2:1 ratio of humeral to scapular motion until maximal elevation. These observations demonstrated the importance of the scapulothoracic articulation with regard to total shoulder motion; however, subsequent studies have defined this relationship in the scapular plane, which is a fundamental plane of motion. The plane of the scapula is oriented 30° to 45° anterior to the coronal plane. In this coordinate system, a 5:1 ratio of humeral-scapular motion has been observed, although this value remains a source of controversy.

During elevation in the scapular plane, the center of rotation of the humerus is located within 6 mm of the center of the humeral head at all times except in subjects with previous shoulder injuries. In the horizontal plane the humeral head is found to remain centered in the glenoid, suggesting that the ball and socket mechanism of the glenohumeral joint is maintained.

To overcome the problems of representing three-dimensional motion with a two-dimensional radiograph, biplanar radiographs and stereophotogrammetry have been used to describe the shoulder rhythm in vivo, finding a highly reproducible pattern within individual subjects. Tantalum markers placed into the humerus, clavicle, and scapula facilitate definition of the bony coordinate systems and increase the accuracy of the measurements made.

In Vitro and In Vivo Studies

Various experimental techniques using direct measurement of bony motion have provided detailed information on shoulder kinematics. Mechanical studies on cadaveric tissues provide a controlled environment to test difficult-to-measure joint kinematics and to investigate the effects of joint surface and soft-tissue restraints. Most of this research has been focused on the glenohumeral joint. Some in vitro experiments also include simulated muscle forces at the rotator cuff, deltoid, or biceps. Although the scapulothoracic articulation is purely muscular, some attempts have been made to simulate the motion of the scapula on the torso during in vitro glenohumeral testing. Clearly, in vivo studies would provide true physiologic conditions of joint loading and muscular control, but the methods needed to perform these studies are invasive. Kinematic studies with camera systems are useful for analysis of in vivo whole body motions, but often at the expense of measurement accuracy.

Techniques to measure the position and orientation of the glenohumeral joint using an electromagnetic tracking system have been applied to study glenohumeral elevation in vitro. These three-dimensional measurements have identified the maximum elevation of the humerus to be 120°, occurring 23° anterior to the scapular plane regardless of whether the arm is in neutral, internal, or external rotation. This technique has been used to examine humeral head translation while applying anterior-posterior drawer and superior-inferior translational forces to the humerus in vitro. The humeral head translates the most anteriorly in the neutral position. In internal rotation, a significantly reduced anterior-posterior range of motion is observed.

Analyzing the role of the capsular restraints has led to the identification of secondary rotations occurring during primary rotations. These "confounding" or coupled rotations include external rotation and abduction during flexion, external rotation and adduction with extension, and flexion and external rotation with abduction.

The translation of the humeral head has been studied in vitro using an electromagnetic tracking system, noting that during flexion under manual loading the humeral head translates anteriorly, and during extension, it moves posteriorly. These translations are described as obligate because they are forced to occur during rotational motion and are presumably caused by the asymmetrical tightening of the glenohumeral capsule. Shortening the capsule restricts motion, while cutting or lengthening the capsule increases translations.

Similar techniques have been performed in vivo to identify differences in translations during clinical stability tests, including the fulcrum, anterior-posterior drawer, sulcus, and push-pull tests in both normal subjects and patients with documented instability. The wide variation in translations found, both in normal and clinically unstable shoulders, indicates that measurements of translations during clinical testing may not be a sufficient indication of instability or pathologic translations.

Other techniques to quantify in vitro kinematics include the use of modified materials testing systems and biplanar sliding tables. With these techniques, the orientation of the scapula and humerus are fixed at given angles of abduction, flexion-extension, and internal-external rotation, constraining the joint. The humerus is then translated with 3° of freedom. Using sequential cutting techniques, superior-inferior translation was observed to be greatest with the arm at 0° of abduction compared to 90°. Anterior-posterior translations have also been measured in intact specimens and in those with a simulated Bankart lesion. Under normal conditions, the anterior-posterior translation is maximal at 45° of elevation and neutral rotation.

Various devices have been developed to investigate the role of muscular forces across the glenohumeral joint in vitro. In vitro glenohumeral kinematics with the application of simulated muscle forces through the tendons of the rotator cuff muscles has permitted investigators to examine the role of dynamic structures in controlling shoulder kinematics. Dynamic simulation of the cocked position of throwing shows that the infraspinatus/teres minor complex offers resistance to anterior translation at both lower and higher magnitudes of external rotation force. The subscapularis offers resistance only at lower force levels. Similarly, during abduction and external rotation with forces applied to the tendon of the long head of the biceps and the tendons of the rotator cuff muscles, the biceps force resists external rotation by increasing joint stiffness by 32%. Applied muscle forces, tendon excursions, and glenohumeral kinematics have been monitored during abduction in the scapular plane using dynamic muscle forces. When the ratio of force applied to the middle deltoid and supraspinatus tendons while achieving maximum abduction favors the deltoid, smaller forces are required in the other tendons during that motion. Elevation of the glenohumeral joint decreases 16% when the forces applied to the subscapularis and infraspinatus/teres minor muscles are eliminated.

Contact between the articular surfaces of the glenohumeral joint has been examined, varying the rotator cuff and deltoid tendon forces and the line of action of the weight of the arm to simulate the movement of the scapula during elevation. Stereophotogrammetry techniques were used to describe the articular surfaces and, combined with the kinematic data during elevation, define the areas of surface contact. With increasing elevation in external rotation, the humeral head contact on the glenoid surface shifts posteriorly. In rotating from neutral to internal rotation, humeral head contact on the glenoid moves from an inferior, anterior position to a superior, posterior position.

Mathematical Models

A number of mathematical models of the complete shoulder mechanism have been developed. A model of this type seeks to describe a complex system, such as the shoulder, using clearly defined mathematical expressions. These expressions are representations of how the joints, ligaments, and muscles function, and are based on information obtained from in vivo or in vitro experiments. Modeling allows for the investigation of physical variables or situations that are difficult or impossible to study experimentally. The validity of a given model and the assumptions used to formulate it for a particular situation should be considered when applying their results to clinical conditions.

The recent models generally deal with all of the articulations of the shoulder and how the musculature behaves under certain motion and loading patterns. Each model begins with a generalized geometry to describe the bony architecture and locations of the muscle origins and insertions. Each muscle of interest is given certain force-producing properties based on its physiologic cross-sectional area or other relevant factors. Finally, a cost function is applied to the muscular system that describes the control strategy that will be used to achieve the task of interest.

A model of the shoulder complex has been proposed for use in the design of multisegmental human body models and anthropometric dummies. Optimization of the model was used to describe the limits of humeral motion with elliptical cones. A complex dynamic model has also been developed to investigate muscle forces during abduction of the humerus. This model includes extensive development of inertial, geometric, and muscle contraction parameters. In vivo kinematic and electromyographic data were also incorporated to drive the model and for validation purposes.

In studies of whole body shoulder motion, a high-speed motion analysis system has been used to record the fast ball throws of baseball pitchers. Information was reported for range of motion and velocity of the humerus relative to the torso. The humerus remained abducted at around 100° throughout motion. There is 30° to 0° of horizontal abduction before release. Explosive motion occurs as the arm externally rotates relative to the body from full horizontal external rotation to release with a mean maximum velocity of 6,940°/sec at release. This information was used in an inverse dynamics model to predict joint forces and torques at the shoulder. In a similar study, motion analysis was also used to determine angular velocities and accelerations at the shoulder and elbow for input into a kinetic chain model of throwing.

Electromyography

EMG measurements in the muscles of the shoulder have been performed for a number of activities and athletic skills. Generally, a correlation between the magnitude of the EMG signal and the force output of the muscle is measured for a given activity that isolates the muscle and produces a maximal voluntary contraction, usually isometrically. Many investigators believe that this approach indirectly measures the contribution of the muscle to the overall joint function. Relating EMG data with kinematic information can provide information on the muscular coordination and, it is thought by some, the forces required to throw, row, or stroke.

There are, however, concerns about making these associations between muscle force and EMG data because nonlinearities have been found between the two as a result of the length of the muscle and the velocity of contraction. As a result, calibrations of muscle force to EMG using static, isometric loading patterns may not provide an accurate representation of dynamic conditions. Technical difficulties in the initial placement of fine-wire electrodes and their movement within muscles during contraction may also result in signal variation and misrepresentation of overall muscle function. Surface electrodes attempt to avoid these problems by averaging EMG activity over the muscle body, but are sometimes affected by signal cross-talk from other muscles. Also, in order to understand the forces and moments applied across the joints of the shoulder complex by its muscles, geometric considerations such as the locations of origins and insertions, the orientations of the muscle fibers, and the muscle moment arms must be known. Information on these parameters has been presented for use in a mathematical model of the shoulder complex, but has not been applied to EMG-based studies.

Baseball pitching has been extensively examined using EMG analysis and a fast-speed camera system. In a series of studies, indwelling, fine-wire electrodes were used to record electrical activity of many muscles around the shoulder. A compilation of EMG results from a series of studies has been presented for the scapular, glenohumeral, elbow, forearm, wrist, and finger muscles during throwing.

In comparisons between professional and amateur pitchers, two different groups of muscles were identified as acting during the cocking and acceleration phases of throwing (Fig. 3). The first group was more active during the early and late cocking stages and includes the deltoid, trapezius, supraspinatus, infraspinatus, teres minor, and biceps brachii. The second group consisted of the subscapularis, serratus anterior, pectoralis major, latissimus dorsi, and triceps and was active to propulse the arm forward during acceleration. Greater activity was found in the supraspinatus, infraspinatus, and biceps

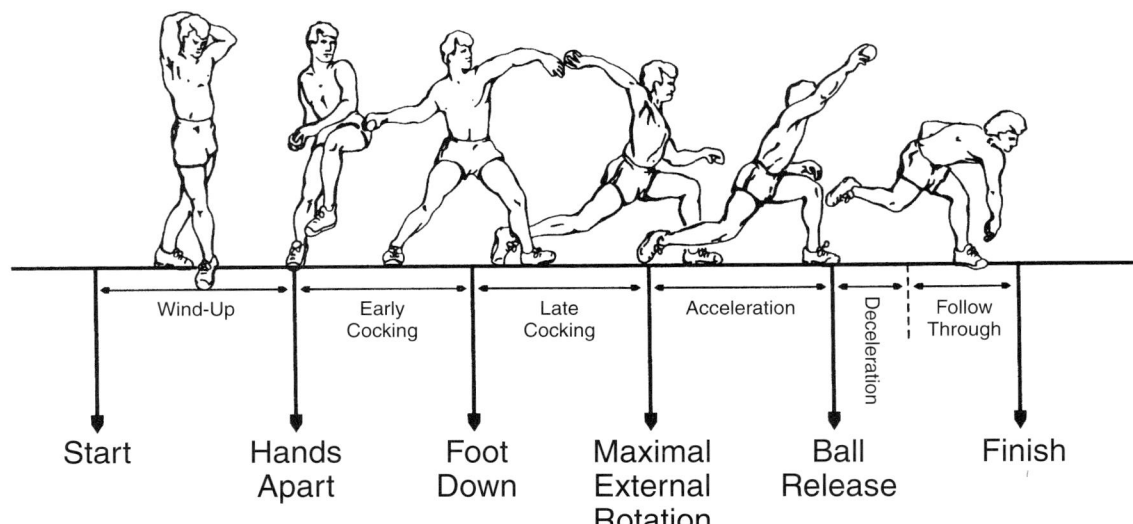

Fig. 3 The six phases of throwing are defined for the baseball pitch, from left to right: wind up, early cocking, late cocking, acceleration, deceleration, and follow-through. (Reproduced with permission from DiGiovine NM, Jobe FW, Pink M, et al: An electromyographic analysis of the upper extremity in pitching. *J Shoulder Elbow Surg* 1992;1:15-25.)

brachii during cocking in amateurs compared to professionals, while professionals fired the subscapularis and latissimus dorsi more in acceleration.

In patients with anterior instability, the EMG showed significantly more activity for the supraspinatus in late cocking and in the biceps during acceleration, possibly indicating that these muscles act to control anterior translations. Less activity was seen in the pectoralis major, subscapularis, and serratus anterior in late cocking, and also in the subscapularis, latissimus dorsi, and serratus anterior in acceleration. These muscles are thought to be responsible for internal rotation of the humerus and protraction of the scapula during these phases of throwing. Loss of this muscular activity could require other soft-tissue restraints to carry these loads, and this increased loading might lead to their injury.

In the same manner, the EMG patterns of swimmers were observed in normal subjects and compared to those with painful shoulders. During the butterfly stroke, in the painful shoulder subjects, hand entry was wider, causing more activity of the posterior deltoid. There was also a significant decrease in activity in the teres minor and serratus anterior throughout pull-through, indicating loss of scapular stability, perhaps because of fatigue, and an inability to balance the powerful pull of the pectoralis major. During the breaststroke, significantly increased activity was seen in the subscapularis during pull-through in patients with painful shoulders. Decreased activity in the upper trapezius, supraspinatus, and middle deltoid and increased activity in the latissimus dorsi was evident during recovery. Similar analyses have been performed during tennis swings to evaluate serving, forehand stroke, and backhand stroke in normal subjects, during the golf swing in men and women professionals, and during a general rehabilitation program on normal subjects and one tailored for baseball throwers.

Summary

More than any other joint complex in the body, the role of muscular stabilization is paramount in the shoulder. As a result, the wide range of in vitro muscular force experiments, mathematical models of muscle actions, and EMG studies of muscular activity are all adding important information, yet the limitations and assumptions of these experimental techniques is problematic. Advances in this area could be invaluable in planning rehabilitation exercises and in gathering further information in studying the activities of daily living that are more often a problem in the general population. The information available to describe shoulder kinesiology comes from various different techniques and is focused on a wide range of specialized topics. The challenges to the clinician, surgeon, and researcher are to synthesize this into a comprehensive view of shoulder function that can be applied to the individual patient under care. It is clear that further work is necessary to understand even normal shoulder function.

Selected Bibliography

Descriptions of Shoulder Motion

An KN, Browne AO, Korinek S, et al: Three-dimensional kinematics of glenohumeral elevation. *J Orthop Res* 1991;9:143-149.

Pearl ML, Harris SL, Lippitt SB, et al: A system for describing positions of the humerus relative to the thorax and its use in the presentation of several functionally important arm positions. *J Shoulder Elbow Surg* 1992;1: 113-118.

A system using a global analogy is used to present humeral to thoracic positions based on the plane of humeral elevation and the angle of elevation within this plane. Internal-external rotation is the angle of the flexed forearm to the lines of latitude.

Spoor CW, Veldpaus FE: Rigid body motion calculated from spatial co-ordinates of markers. *J Biomech* 1980;13:391-393.

Radiographic Techniques

Hogfors C, Peterson B, Sigholm G, et al: Biomechanical model of the human shoulder joint: II. The shoulder rhythm. *J Biomech* 1991;24:699-709.

Poppen NK, Walker PS: Normal and abnormal motion of the shoulder. *J Bone Joint Surg* 1976;58A:195-201.

In Vitro and In Vivo Studies

Cain PR, Mutschler TA, Fu FH, et al: Anterior stability of the glenohumeral joint: A dynamic model. *Am J Sports Med* 1987;15:144-148.

Harryman DT II, Sidles JA, Harris SL, et al: Laxity of the normal glenohumeral joint: A quantitative in vivo assessment. *J Shoulder Elbow Surg* 1992;1:66-75.

Harryman DT II, Sidles JA, Harris SL, et al: The role of the rotator interval capsule in passive motion and stability of the shoulder. *J Bone Joint Surg* 1992;74A:53-66.

Kinematics of the glenohumeral joint were studied in vitro for planar rotations of the humerus and clinical examinations with the rotator interval normal, sectioned, and imbricated. Anterior obligate translations, those translations of the humeral head across the glenoid that occur with flexion, were increased by sectioning of the interval and were reduced by imbrication.

Itoi E, Motzkin NE, Morrey BF, et al: Contribution of axial arm rotation to humeral head translation. *Am J Sports Med* 1994;22:499-503.

Lippitt SB, Harris SL, Harryman DT II, et al: In vivo quantification of the laxity of normal and unstable glenohumeral joints. *J Shoulder Elbow Surg* 1994;3:215-223.

Motion at the glenohumeral joint is measured in vivo during clinical exams in normal subjects and patients with clinical instabilities. Due to wide variations in the results, it is felt that motion analysis during clinical exams cannot differentiate between the subject conditions.

McMahon PJ, Debski RE, Thompson WO, et al: Shoulder muscle forces and tendon excursions during glenohumeral abduction in the scapular plane. *J Shoulder Elbow Surg* 1995;4:199-208.

Rodosky MW, Harner CD, Fu FH: The role of the long head of the biceps muscle and superior glenoid labrum in anterior stability of the shoulder. *Am J Sports Med* 1994;22:121-130.

A device applying forces to the tendons of the rotator cuff and long head of the biceps was used to move the glenohumeral joint in abduction, where it was then loaded with an external rotation torque. Increasing forces applied to the long head of the biceps increased torsional rigidity, which was lost after a simulated superior labral lesion.

Soslowsky LJ, Flatow EL, Bigliani LU, et al: Quantitation of in situ contact areas at the glenohumeral joint: A biomechanical study. *J Orthop Res* 1992;10:524-534.

Information from stereophotogrammetry was used to define articular surfaces of the humeral head and glenoid and was combined with data from in vitro joint testing with abduction including simulated scapular inclination and either internal or external rotation. Different areas of contact between the surfaces were found for each condition with only a small portion of the humeral head in contact at any one position.

Speer KP, Deng X, Borrero S, et al: Biomechanical evaluation of a simulated Bankart lesion. *J Bone Joint Surg* 1994;76A:1819-1826.

Translation of the humerus on the glenoid is studied in vitro at fixed angles of elevation and internal-external rotation in specimens with a simulated Bankart lesion. Detachment of the anterior capsule did not result in significantly increased anterior translation, indicating that perhaps other mechanisms such as capsular elongation may also need to be present to produce dislocation.

Mathematical Models

Engin AE, Tumer ST: Three-dimensional kinematic modelling of the human shoulder complex: Part I. Physical model and determination of joint sinus cones. *J Biomech Eng* 1989;111:107-112.

Feltner ME: Three-dimensional interactions in a two-segment kinetic chain: Part II. Application to the throwing arm in baseball pitching. *Int J Sports Biomech* 1989;5:420-450.

Fleisig GS, Andrews JR, Dillman CJ, et al: Kinetics of baseball pitching with implications about injury mechanisms. *Am J Sports Med* 1995;23:233-239.

Using information from kinematic studies and an inverse dynamic model of the body, forces and moments in the upper extremity were calculated for baseball pitching. Two critical points of the throwing motion were determined, one just before maximum external rotation and one shortly after release, when loads on the shoulder and elbow were very high and may be related to injury mechanisms.

Tumer ST, Engin AE: Three-dimensional kinematic modelling of the human shoulder complex: Part II. Mathematical modelling and solution via optimization. *J Biomech Eng* 1989;111:113-121.

Van der Helm FC: A finite element musculoskeletal model of the shoulder mechanism. *J Biomech* 1994;27:551-569.

A finite element model of the shoulder joint containing four bones, three joints, three extracapsular ligaments, the scapulothoracic gliding plane and 20 muscles or muscle parts was formulated. Surface EMG could only verify the model in a qualitative sense, because the force-to-length relationships of the muscles are unknown.

Electromyography

DiGiovine NM, Jobe FW, Pink M, et al: An electromyographic analysis of the upper extremity in pitching. *J Shoulder Elbow Surg* 1992;1:15-25.

The muscle firing patterns of 29 muscle bellies of the shoulder, arm, elbow, wrist and fingers during five phases of baseball pitching are compiled.

Glousman R, Jobe F, Tibone J, et al: Dynamic electromyographic analysis of the throwing shoulder with glenohumeral instability. *J Bone Joint Surg* 1988;70A:220-226.

Kelly BT, Kadrmas WR, Kirkendall DT, et al: Optimal normalization tests for shoulder muscle activation: An electromyographic study. *J Orthop Res* 1996;14:647-653.

Four manual muscle testing positions were identified from a set of 27 that elicited maximal EMG activity in eight muscles of the shoulder. These positions are offered for use in standardizing as a means of EMG normalization among different studies of the shoulder.

Pink M, Jobe FW, Perry J, et al: The normal shoulder during the butterfly swim stroke: An electromyographic and cinematographic analysis of twelve muscles. *Clin Orthop* 1993;288:48-59.

Van der Helm FC, Veeger HE, Pronk GM, et al: Geometry parameters for musculoskeletal modelling of the shoulder system. *J Biomech* 1992;25:129-144.

5

Basic Science Considerations in Glenohumeral Arthroplasty and Proximal Humeral Fractures

A. Marc Tetro, MD, FRCSC and Ken Yamaguchi, MD

Relevant Anatomy and Biomechanics of the Shoulder Joint

Normal glenohumeral motion is more complex than it appears. In their classic article, Poppen and Walker described the mechanics of normal glenohumeral motion with the contribution (2:1 ratio) of the glenohumeral and scapulothoracic motion relationship altered at the extremes of elevation. During the first 30° of elevation, the motion is predominantly glenohumeral, with an associated 3 mm of superior translation. In the final 60° of motion, the contributions of the glenohumeral and scapulothoracic joints are approximately equal (1:1 ratio). Because the center of humeral motion remains relatively constant, the shoulder has been termed a ball-and-socket joint.

In order to achieve this motion, the glenohumeral joint has developed with minimal constraint and relatively limited contact area between the two articulating surfaces (glenoid covering only 25% to 30% of the humeral head). The conformity of the glenohumeral joint is therefore important in its relationship to joint biomechanics and the ball-and-socket mechanism. Traditionally, the glenoid was deemed to be "flatter" than the humerus with a larger radius of curvature (by radiographic analysis). However, with the use of stereophotogrammetry, the glenohumeral joint has been found to have a high degree of conformity and true ball-and-socket kinematics (Fig. 1, Table 1). The humerus and reciprocal glenoid articular surfaces are almost perfect spheres, with the glenoid having thick articular cartilage at its margins and very thin cartilage centrally to make the radius of curvature very similar on the two surfaces. The radius of curvature of the glenoid is only 2 mm larger than that of the humerus. Additional conformity and surface contact is imparted by the glenoid labrum. In contrast, Harryman and associates have noted obligate humeral translation occurring with normal glenohumeral motion, suggesting a slight deviation from true ball-and-socket kinematics. The importance of these differing views relates to the degree of joint conformity in prosthetic design. Although different arthroplasty designs offer choices in the degree of joint conformity, the relative contribution of each theory has not yet been resolved.

The lateral humeral offset is defined as the distance from the lateral coracoid margin to the lateral aspect of the greater tuberosity (Fig. 2). Iannotti studied the normal glenohumeral relationships and noted a very strong correlation between the size of the humeral head and the lateral humeral offset. The humeral offset is thought to accurately represent the moment arm of the deltoid and supraspinatus muscles and therefore has a direct correlation to shoulder function. Proper re-

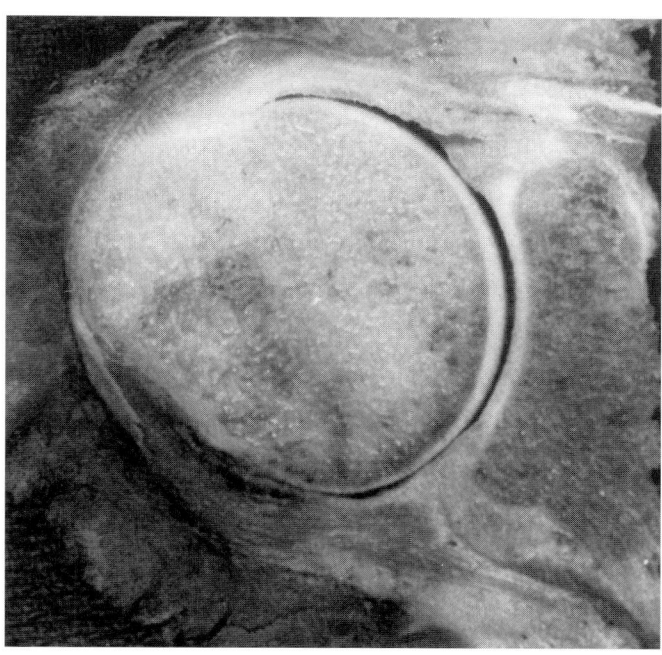

Fig. 1 A coronal section of a cadaver specimen representing a similar image achieved with stereophotogrammetry. Note the congruity of the articular surfaces with the glenoid having thicker cartilage peripherally. (Reproduced with permission from Soslowsky LJ, Flatow EL, Bigliani LU, et al: Articular geometry of the glenohumeral joint. *Clin Orthop* 1992;285:181-190.)

Table 1. The radius of curvature results for female cadavera as measured by stereophotogrammetry

Specimen	Cartilage Radius of Curvature	Bone Radius of Curvature
Humeral head	23.37 ± 1.69 (n = 16)	23.15 ± 2.09 (n = 13)
Glenoid	23.62 ± 1.56 (n = 13)	30.28 ± 3.16 (n = 5)

creation of the lateral humeral offset, along with soft-tissue balancing, may help to optimize the postoperative muscular function (moment arm).

The glenohumeral joint has often been referred to as a nonweightbearing joint, but joint reaction forces at 90° of abduction are equal to 89% of body weight. Further, with a 5-kg

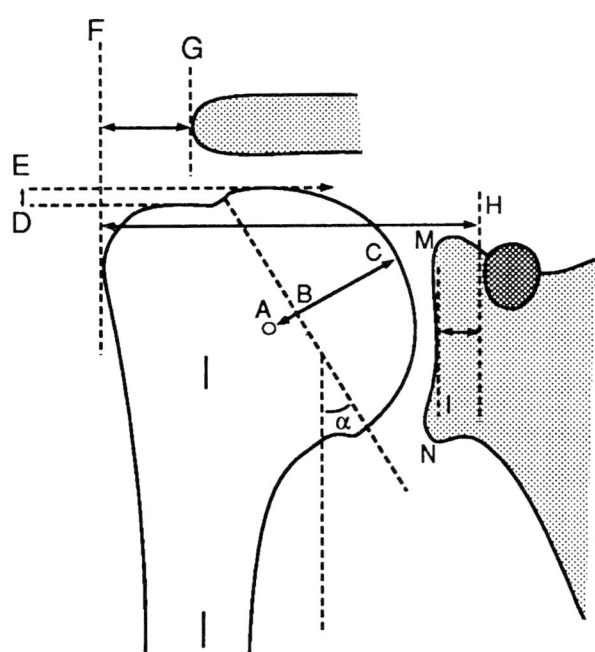

Fig. 2 The normal glenohumeral relationships, with the humeral offset depicted by the distance F to H, the thickness of the humeral head from B to C, and the center of the humeral head is C. Note the superior position of the humeral head proximal to the greater tuberosity (D to E). (Reproduced with permission from Iannotti JP, Gabriel JP, Schnek SL, et al: The normal glenohumeral relationships: An anatomical study of one hundred and forty shoulders. *J Bone Joint Surg* 1992;74A:491-500.)

weight in the outstretched hand (90° shoulder abduction), the joint reaction force is 2.5 times body weight. The transmission of a large amount of force through the glenoid has significant implications when considering shoulder arthroplasty. The joint reaction forces vary with shoulder abduction. At 0° of abduction, the force is directed inferiorly, but it changes to superior direction at 60° and returns to inferior again at 150° of elevation. These forces are often transmitted to the glenoid in a nonperpendicular plane, with the maximal shear force occurring at between 30° to 60° of abduction. Coincidentally, this arc of abduction is where the rotator cuff is most active, "containing" the humerus over the glenoid while the deltoid contracts. Without rotator cuff function, the humerus would translate superiorly and impinge on the undersurface of the acromion, and thereby limit shoulder motion. Therefore, rotator cuff function is very important to obtaining normal motion.

The rotator cuff is the primary restraint that maintains the humeral head over the glenoid cavity and resists the action of the deltoid shear force. However, in the shoulder with a deficient rotator cuff, the coracoacromial ligament is very important as a secondary static restraint to prevent superior migration of the head. This restraint may provide a new fulcrum for the shoulder in the absence of rotator cuff function.

Prosthetic Design Considerations of Glenohumeral Arthroplasty

The majority of the total shoulder replacements currently in use today employ an unconstrained design with good and excellent results reported at the mid-term follow-up. Constrained shoulder replacements have the same difficulties as other constrained joint replacements, with loosening and mechanical failure rates of 30% to 50%, caused primarily by increased stress transfer to the bone-prosthesis interface. Moreover, there have been many instances of materials failure and instability in constrained designs. As such, constrained total shoulder arthroplasties have largely been abandoned.

The Humeral Component

Humeral component failure, defined as a symptomatic loose component, is very uncommon. Approximately 1% of all glenohumeral arthroplasties are classified as failures using this criterion. However, the design and appropriate position of the humeral prosthesis do have an impact on outcome and restoration of normal function.

Fixation

Recent reviews show that radiolucent lines occur in approximately 14% (range, 1% to 44%) of humeral arthroplasties, but the rate of clinically symptomatic loose humeral components requiring revision is less than 1% (Table 2). Regardless of the choice between cemented and uncemented components, the rate of symptomatic loosening is very low. Press-fit fixation appears sufficient unless there are patient-specific concerns about rotational stability, subsidence, or bone quality. With cemented humeral components, cementing technique generally follows guidelines gained from experience with hip arthroplasty. Although not shown to be beneficial, third-generation cementing techniques are generally recommended (pulse lavage of humerus, drying of bone surfaces, cement restrictor, and vacuum mixing of cement with pressure insertion).

The literature would suggest that bone or tissue ingrowth prostheses are reliable as a mode of fixation in the humerus with results similar to those of cement fixation and with only rare reports of loose components. The highlights of optimizing bone ingrowth include: (1) porous prosthetic surface with pores in the range of 100 to 400 µm; (2) intimate bone-prosthesis interface; and (3) minimizing micromotion between bone and implant. In the hip and knee literature, much of the information about ingrowth is obtained at postmortem examination. To date, there is only one such report concerning the shoulder that suggests that this method is an effective means of fixation for the humeral component. Therefore, the decision on mode of fixation is surgeon- and case-dependent, with the outcomes being very similar to date.

The mode of fixation has impact not only on the fixation, but also on component alignment. Loose-fitting cemented humeral components, prior to cement polymerization, have six degrees of freedom of which the surgeon must be aware when positioning the stem. These include (1) medial/lateral displacement and (2) varus/valgus rotation (tilt) in the coronal plane; (3) anteroposterior displacement and (4) rotation in the

Table 2. Results of reported clinical series of various total shoulder prostheses with different modes of fixation

Component	Author	Follow-up* (years)	Humerus				Glenoid			
			Number	Fixation	Radiolucent Lines (%)	Component Failures (%)	Number†	Fixation	Radiolucent Lines (%)	Component Failures (%)
Neer II	Neer et al (1982)	3.1	194	Cement and pressfit	1	1	194 (15 MB)	Cement	30	3
	Cofield et al (1984)	3.8	73	Cement and pressfit	32	0	73	Cement	82	4
	Barrett et al (1987)	3.5	50	Cement and pressfit	8	0	50	Cement	74	8
	Figgie et al (1988)	5	50	Cement	0	0	50	Cement	36	6
	Barrett et al (1989)	5	133	Cement	0	0	133 (19 MB)	Cement	82	0
	Hawkins et al (1989)	3.3	70	Cement and pressfit	24	0	70	Cement	100	2.9
	Boyd et al (1991)	4.6	131	Cement and pressfit		0	131 (26 MB)	Cement	12	1.5
	Kelly (1994)	9.5	36	Cement and pressfit	55	5.6	36	Cement	66	5.6
Cofield	Cofield et al (1992)	4.3	31	Pressfit	29	6.5	32	Bone ingrowth	48	12.5
Dana	Amstutz et al (1988)	3.5	46	Cement		0	46	Cement	95	11
	Thomas et al (1991)	3.8	26	Cement		0	26	Cement	100	7.7
Custom	Figgie et al (1992)	5	27	Cement	0	0	27	Cement	26	0

* Most series report follow-up at 3 to 5 years postsurgery
† MB = metal-backed glenoid

sagittal plane; (5) proximal/distal positioning (height); and (6) axial rotation (version) in the transverse or axial plane. However, with press-fit humeral stems, the components fit snugly in the humeral canal and are obligated to follow the endosteal course. The surgeon can only control the version (axial rotation) and height of the component (with the anatomy of the canal orientation dictating the four degrees in the sagittal and coronal planes). Humeral version is only capable of providing less than 2 mm of difference on the effective combined neck plus head length (ie, humeral offset). Hence, the version of the humeral component has little effect on soft-tissue balancing and humeral offset. The height should be accurately controlled to ensure appropriate soft-tissue tensioning. Modular components may have an effect on the height of the humeral component. Recently, interest has been shown toward development of a posterior offset humeral head (4 mm posterior in relation to shaft) to allow more accurate restoration of normal anatomy. The effect of this design on glenohumeral arthroplasty function is unknown, with recent designs presently being tested in Europe.

Humeral Offset and Soft-Tissue Reconstruction

Restoration of the lateral humeral offset helps maintain the moment arms of the deltoid and rotator cuff muscles (Fig. 2). The joint line, and therefore fulcrum position, tends to be located 30% of the distance from the lateral base of the coracoid to the middle of the humeral canal (a location more convenient to assess prior to reconstruction). Accordingly, with plain radiographs, the normal "humeral offset ratio" is approximately 0.3. Using this information, preoperative planning may be improved in certain situations to better select the appropriate size components and help restore humeral offset.

Restoration of the offset by preoperatively templating the components (including use of the contralateral shoulder as a guide) may help in this regard. Intraoperatively, the superiormost aspect of the humeral prosthetic head should be above that of the greater tuberosity to avoid subacromial impingement. Proper offset can be approximated by restoring the lateral margin of the greater tuberosity to 1.5 to 2 cm lateral to the lateral margin of the acromion (arm at 0° of abduction, 0° of external rotation).

Although pain relief is usually satisfactory following shoulder arthroplasty, range of motion can be disappointing, mainly because of a loss of glenohumeral abduction. Optimization of the soft-tissue balancing (ie, humeral offset) may be a critical factor. This is particularly true when considering the reconstruction of the greater tuberosity in treatment of fractures.

Modular Components

The use of modular components has increased since the 1980s; this increase can be justified in the attempt to recreate normal alignment (offset) and soft-tissue balancing. In revision arthroplasty, conversion from hemiarthroplasty to a total arthroplasty may be less cumbersome because the modular head can be removed to allow glenoid preparation without removing the humeral stem. As with total hip arthroplasty, most humeral head components are fixed to the stem with a Morse taper interface. Some designs have incorporated a "reverse" Morse taper design to make glenoid revision easier (ie, the head is the "male" and the humeral stem "female").

Dissociation of the modular head and stem components has been a major concern; disengagement of the polyethylene liner from the metal-backed glenoid has been less frequently noted (Fig. 3). The events surrounding disassembly are different than those of the hip, with humeral head dissociation not reported to occur with reduction of a dislocation. Blevins and associates found that the major factor leading to dissociation was fluid left in the head-stem interface of a reverse Morse taper design at the time of surgery. Such fluid decreased the force required for dissociation by two thirds, allowing removal of the humeral head by hand. When considered in relation to the 12 reported disengagement cases, 11 of 12 occurred within 8 weeks postoperatively, and fluid in the interface was the most likely cause. A similar problem has not been reported with standard Morse taper designs. When the Morse taper elements are dry, the force required for dissociation is proportional to the impact force putting the head on the humeral stem. Both of these factors are within the surgeon's control.

Modularity in the lower extremity has been associated with corrosion between components and component fracture. In the shoulder, component fracture has not been seen but the concern of corrosion remains, because it may contribute to third body wear and long-term failure. However, there is no literature to date investigating this potential complication.

The Glenoid Component

One of the major concerns in glenohumeral arthroplasty is achieving and maintaining secure fixation of the glenoid component. The cause of failure, in general, relates to the limited volume and the relatively poor strength of bone available for prosthetic fixation. The present challenge is to design a prosthesis that minimizes the stress placed on the component and the component-bone interface, minimizes wear of the articulating surface, and optimizes the fixation into the glenoid vault. Despite the high prevalence of radiolucent lines about the glenoid component, actual clinical failure is much less common (Table 2). The frequency of unconstrained shoulder arthroplasty failure caused by glenoid loosening (requiring revision for symptomatic glenoid component failure) ranges from 0 to 12.5%. However, many of the follow-ups are short to mid-term at 3 to 5 years. Kelly recently reported a 5.6% revision rate at 9.5 years with the Neer unconstrained prosthesis. For this reason, to date there is very little information regarding the etiology of the loss of fixation of the glenoid component to the bone surface.

Radiolucent Lines and Component Failure

The clinical significance of radiolucent lines around the glenoid component is not clear because many patients with this radiographic finding are asymptomatic. The reported rate is extremely variable, ranging from 30% to 96% of the patients reviewed. Moreover, many of these lines have been noted in the immediate postoperative period, without subsequent progression. At this time, there is no standard way of describing a

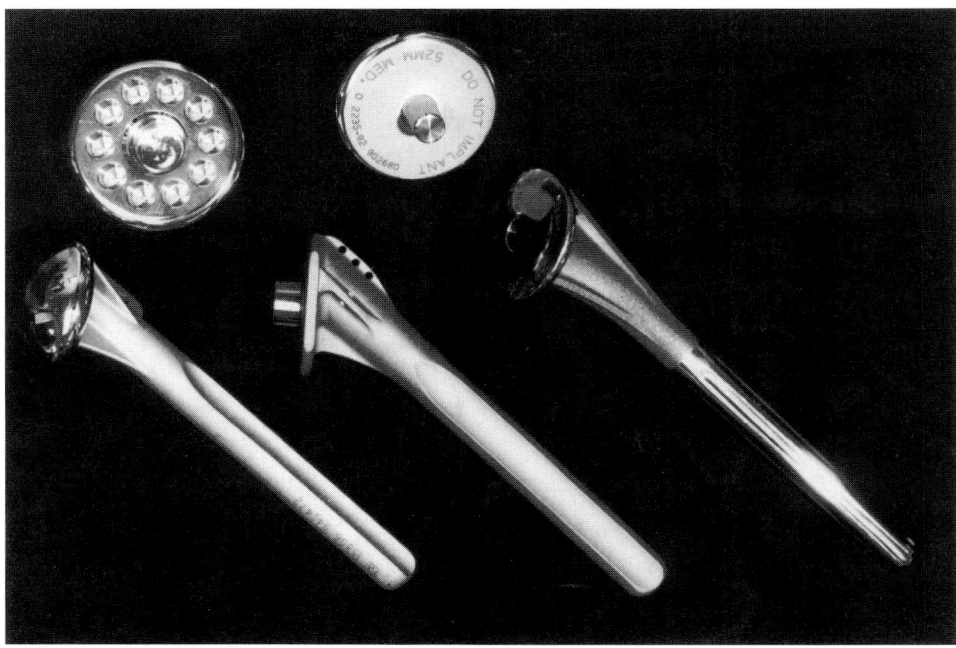

Fig. 3 A selection of commercially available humeral components highlighting the differences between a nonmodular humeral component **(left)**, a modular humeral component with regular Morse taper design **(center)**, and a modular humeral component with reverse Morse taper design **(right)**.

lucent line, and reproducible radiologic views are difficult to obtain. Findings of a progressive radiolucent line are suggestive of component loosening, an occurrence in 0 to 36% of cases.

Cement fracture, cement-prosthesis gapping, component shift, and component fracture are all indicative of component loosening or failure. The reported rates are from 0 to 23% with the two highest reported rates noted in bone ingrowth metal-backed components. Because the definitions of radiographic and clinical loosening are inconsistent, comparison of results is subjective and difficult.

In order to prevent or delay loosening, an understanding of the suspected modes of glenoid component failure (association with rotator cuff tears, posterior glenoid bond deficiency, and total shoulder instability) is important. To date there has been very little information presented concerning the importance of wear debris, osteolysis, and other contributors to aseptic loosening.

Failure of the glenoid component in the presence of a rotator cuff tear was first described by Franklin and associates in 1988. In a review of total shoulder arthroplasty with associated rotator cuff deficiency, they reported an increased rate of glenoid loosening as a result of the proximal humeral migration, with eccentric loading of the superior glenoid rim. This loading was believed to cause a "tilting" of the glenoid, and the term "rocking-horse glenoid" was coined for this mode of failure. With this concept in mind, Collins and associates recently investigated the effect of glenoid cavity bone preparation on glenoid component stability, while eccentrically loading the prosthetic cup. With removal of the articular cartilage plus glenoid preparation to obtain intimate contact between component and bone, the displacement of the component decreased by 50% with eccentric loads. Thus, it appears that careful preparation of the glenoid may improve initial stable fixation, even in the presence of rotator cuff tears.

Instability of the total shoulder arthroplasty has many similarities with rotator cuff deficiency, because the main reason for instability is a deficient cuff. The relationship of instability to loosening relates to edge loading of the glenoid (caused by unbalanced tensioning of soft tissues or malaligned components), which can cause rocking and tilting. If the humeral component dislocates, it is hypothesized that it may dislodge the glenoid component upon reduction.

In many presentations of arthritis (osteoarthritis, postinstability reconstruction arthritis, posttrauma, and some rheumatoid arthritis) the humeral head subluxates, causing glenoid erosion or bone loss. It was once believed that such defects could be reconstructed using polymethylmethacrylate cement. However, it is clear that the uncontained cement goes on to fracture, causing loosening and failure of the glenoid component. Similarly, if such defects are ignored, the glenoid component will not be adequately supported and may fail. The most common strategy for small to moderate posterior defects is to remove anterior bone. For large posterior bone loss, the best published success to date has been with the use of morcellized or structural bone grafts; however, former supporters of this technique are wavering in their support.

Thickness

Considering the glenoid anatomy, Iannotti noted that the distance from the base of the coracoid to the glenoid articular surface was relatively constant, being less than 5 mm in all cases studied. Therefore, the decision on the thickness of the glenoid component must consider the anatomy or risk lateralizing the joint line. A laterally translated articular surface may weaken the lever arms of the shoulder musculature and therefore may limit postoperative function. However, consideration must also be given to maximizing polyethylene thickness. Experience with lower extremity polyethylene wear properties has shown thicker polyethylene is associated with improved wear characteristics. The force transmitted across the glenohumeral joint is much less than the weightbearing joints of the lower extremity, though still often greater than body weight. Accordingly, polyethylene thickness has been less. Metal backing of the glenoid component adds to thickness and either minimizes polyethylene depth or increases lateral offset. As yet there is no reported literature evaluating the optimal polyethylene thickness (Fig. 4), but studies for

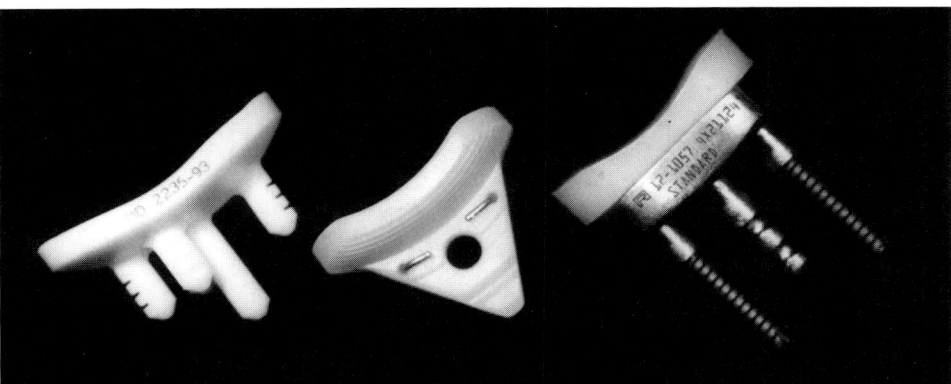

Fig. 4 A selection of commercially available glenoid components with the varying modes of glenoid fixation—all-polyethylene cemented peg style **(left)**, all-polyethylene cemented keel design **(center)**, bone ingrowth metal-backed design **(right)**. Note the relative thickness of the glenoid components.

metal-backed tibial components suggest that the polyethylene thickness should be at least 8 mm to avoid rapid wear.

Fixation

With cemented glenoid components being the most common, there is very little clinical information on which to base alternative fixation designs. However, there is some variation of cement fixation design, with the Neer prosthesis using a triangular keel construct, the Dana an inferiorly directed single stem, and the Global shoulder a multiple peg fixation system. Bone ingrowth, metal-backed glenoid prostheses have seen limited use, but reports of mid-term follow-up have been similar to that of the Neer cemented component.

Finite element studies of the glenoid have been employed to determine which variables are of importance with respect to component fixation. These studies have shown the best and most physiologic stress patterns of the glenoid component bone interface would be obtained with preservation of the subchondral bone, minimal reaming of the glenoid to obtain circumferential bone-component contact, and use of an all-polyethylene component (cemented) (Fig. 5). However, this is in contradiction of the previous results of Orr, who suggested that metal-backed components offered improved stress transfer to the bone.

There is very little information published to date on the merits of various glenoid component designs. One biomechanical study of the effect of peg fixation on sheer stress suggested that multiple small pegs conserve more bone stock, distribute stress more uniformly to the bone, and have stronger and stiffer shear fixation than prostheses with fewer, larger pegs. Finite element analysis suggests a stair-stepped or wedge design produces more natural stress transfer than the keel design (Fig. 5). Another report demonstrated that an inferiorly directed, rectangular stem design (eccentric) had increased bending stability when compared with the keel stem. However, the best long-term results have still been reported using the Neer (keel) design, which is considered the standard design.

Conformity of the Glenohumeral Articulation

Conformity considers the degree of any mismatch of the radius of curvature between the humeral and glenoid components. Although the biologic glenoid has often been said to have a larger radius of curvature than the humerus (2 to 4 mm), Neer elected to have the same radius of curvature for both components in his system. Severt and associates studied the effect of conformity and the constraint of the components in a biomechanical model. With glenohumeral translation believed to occur in the normal biomechanics, the imposition of matching radii of curvature increases the constraint of the system. As with constrained arthroplasties, this scenario may lead to early component loosening. Less conforming constructs (ie, mismatch of the radius of curvature) have less constraint and theoretically may be associated with lower stress on the component fixation. The situation of lower conformity, however, decreases the joint contact surface area and is associated with higher point contact stresses, which may lead to increased polyethylene wear. Harryman reported on a cadaveric study that analyzed the impact of increased conformity (same radii of curvature) versus lower conformity (glenoid radius 4 mm larger than humeral radius) on joint motion and translation (Fig. 6). It was found that if the soft tissue was appropriately tensioned, the degree of conformity had little impact on glenohumeral motion. Based on these results, the degree of conformity does not seem to affect motion. It may, however, affect wear and loosening rates.

Rotator Cuff Considerations

The condition of the rotator cuff is a critical factor in the outcome of a glenohumeral arthroplasty. Not only will its function affect the active motion of the shoulder, but the rotator cuff is also one of the prime stabilizers of the shoulder. Bigliani and associates recently reported on a homogenous group of patients with primary osteoarthritis. Ninety-seven percent of the patients had significant pain relief with an average active elevation of 160° at 3.3 years postoperatively. All patients in this group had normal rotator cuff and deltoid muscles. These results help to support the hypothesis that the main determinant of active shoulder motion is an intact rotator cuff and deltoid muscle group. However, the tasks and outcomes of reconstruction are very different in the shoulder with a deficient rotator cuff. Several reports describe active elevation of 100° to 110° or less in patients who are cuff-deficient.

Presently, there is much controversy regarding the method of treatment of the shoulder with a deficient rotator cuff. Humeral hemiarthroplasty is recommended by many; however, others still believe that pain relief is improved with the use of a glenoid component. The use of constrained total shoulder prostheses has been attempted, with predictably poor outcomes. "Biologic" resurfacing of the glenoid, in conjunction with hemiarthroplasty, has recently been suggested as an alternative. Using reflected capsule or fascia lata to resurface the glenoid, the short-term results of the hemiarthroplasty appear to be equivalent to those of total shoulder arthroplasty. However, there are concerns regarding progressive medialization with long-term follow-up. Use of a bipolar humeral component has been reported as a salvage procedure. At this time, basic science support is lacking for fibrocartilage incorporation of "biologic" resurfacing and biomechanical advantages for bipolar hemiarthroplasty.

Proximal Humeral Fractures

Proximal humeral fractures are very common, representing 5% to 7% of all fractures, and are particularly common in patients with osteoporosis. The most common mechanism of injury is a fall on an outstretched arm, resulting in an indirect fracture. Unlike many fractures of the lower extremity, 80% to 85% of all proximal humeral fractures are undisplaced or minimally displaced, and as such, require only a short course (2 to 3 weeks) of immobilization. In these cases, the prognosis is very good. As described by Neer, the four-segment classification has been the standard for evaluation and treatment of displaced proximal humerus fractures. Since that time, there has been a general paucity of basic science research on these fractures.

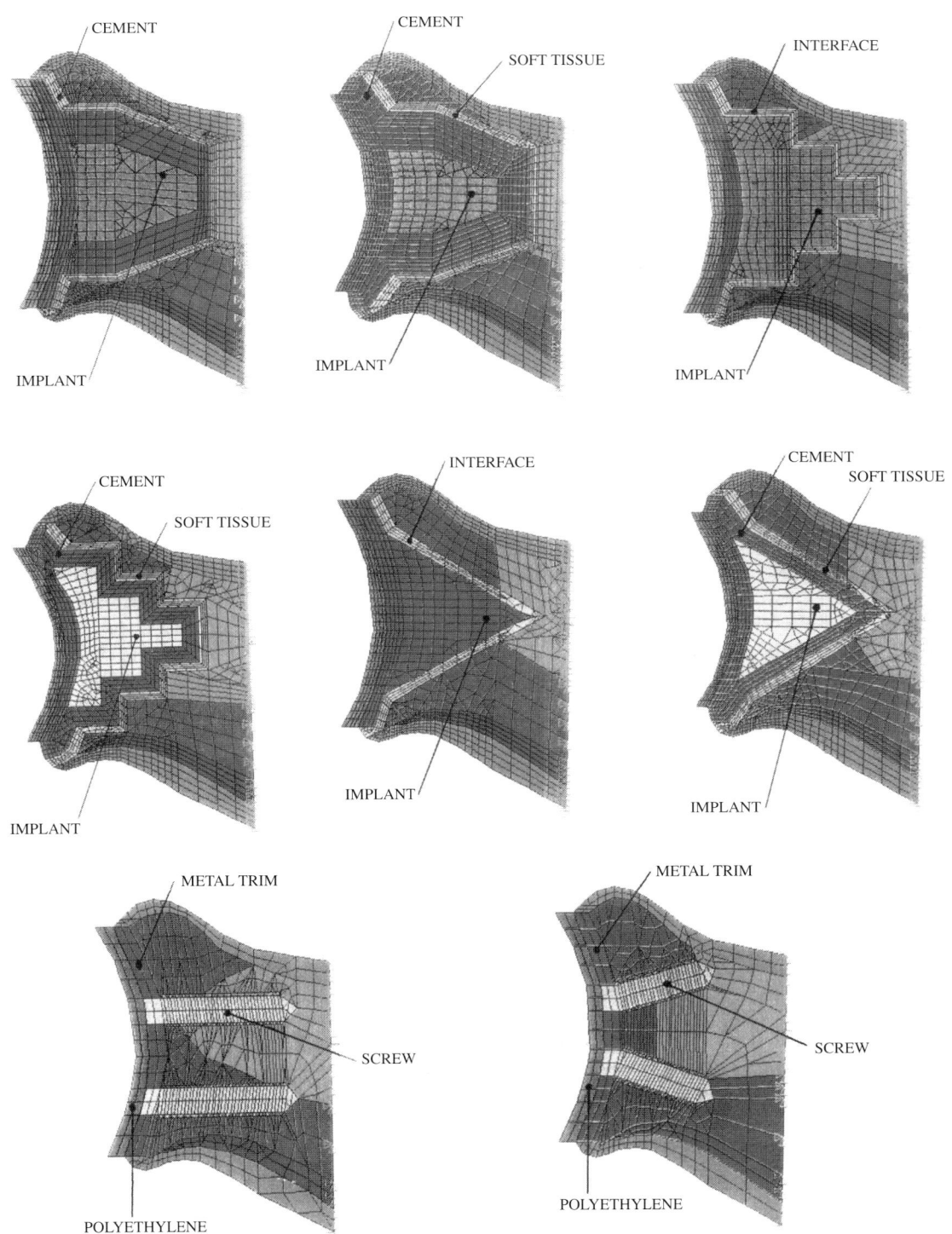

Fig. 5 Finite element study demonstrating the relative stress distribution of the various types of glenoid implants. The wedge and stair-stepped designs produce a more natural stress distribution. The presence of a soft-tissue layer causes increased stress. All-polyethylene implants provide a more physiologic stress transfer. (Reproduced with permission from Friedman RJ, Laberge M, Dooley RL, et al: Finite element modeling of the glenoid component: Effect of design parameters on stress distribution. *J Shoulder Elbow Surg* 1992;1:261-270.)

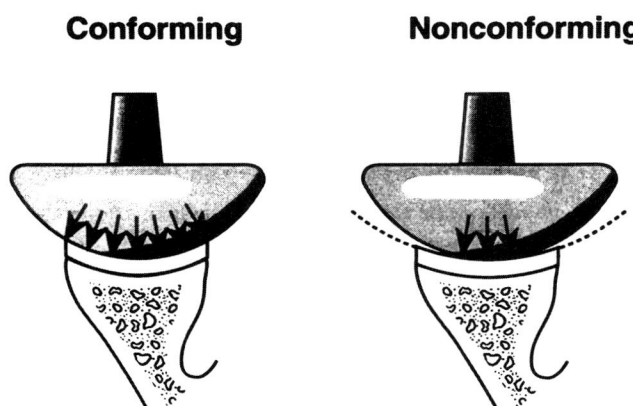

Fig. 6 The conformity of total shoulder arthroplasty components with **(left)** the humerus and glenoid component having the same radius of curvature and **(right)** the glenoid having a larger radius of curvature. (Reproduced with permission from Harryman DT, Sidles JA, Harris SL, et al: The effect of articular conformity and the size of humeral head component on laxity and motion after glenohumeral arthroplasty: A study in cadavera. *J Bone Joint Surg* 1995;77A: 555-563.)

Classification

An accurate diagnosis is the first step in formulating a treatment plan. Undisplaced fractures have good outcomes with conservative therapy, and classification systems are not necessary. The displaced fractures are more challenging and are generally classified to direct appropriate treatment. Presently, two classification systems have gained popularity. The Neer four-segment and the AO classification systems are the most popular. In the Neer classification, a fragment is counted as a "part" if it is displaced more than 1 cm or rotated more than 45°. The degree of displacement has prognostic implications relating to the damage of the blood supply, disruption of the rotator cuff, and potential for nonunion and malunion. Recent studies have questioned inter- and intraobserver variability and have raised questions on the usefulness of present classification systems. However, the research subjects varied widely in experience. Among experienced surgeons in these studies, concordance was quite good. Although such studies have demonstrated some limitations, the Neer classification is still considered the standard tool to classify upper humerus fractures. Observer agreement in these studies has been poor. This may demonstrate the need for better education and experience when evaluating these difficult fractures, rather than any deficiency with the classification system itself.

General Considerations for Open Reduction and Internal Fixation

The proximal humerus is somewhat unique in considerations for treatment with open reduction and internal fixation. In elderly patients and those with osteoporosis, the proximal humerus bone is often of poor quality. As such, classic methods of fixation with plate and screw techniques can result in failure of fixation because of the low pullout strength of the screws in bone. Hence, recommended techniques have bypassed proximal cancellous bone, employing wire or suture fixation of the relatively strong rotator cuff to distal cortical bone. Incorporation of intramedullary fixation with proximal suture or wire has been successful. However, mechanical testing of various internal fixation strategies is lacking.

Blood Supply of the Humeral Head and Osteonecrosis: Concerns in Three- and Four-Part Fractures

The blood supply to the humeral head is of interest, with reports of osteonecrosis frequently following three- and four-part proximal humeral fractures. The normal arterial anatomy of the humeral head has been described in cadaver perfusion studies. These studies have shown that the ascending branch of the anterior circumflex humeral artery and its intraosseous continuation, the arcuate artery, provide the main arterial supply to the humeral head and articular surface. The posterior circumflex artery supplies a small portion of the posteroinferior articular surface via the posteromedial branches (of the posterior circumflex humeral artery). Gerber noted a rich extraosseous anastomosis between the anterior circumflex humeral, posterior circumflex humeral, suprascapular, and thoracodorsal arteries, with the ascending branch of the anterior circumflex artery being the final common pathway supplying the arcuate artery. Therefore, in the event of injury to the anterior circumflex artery or distal portion of the ascending branch, collateral flow to the arcuate artery would be from these anastomoses.

Recently another rich intraosseous arterial anastomotic system was demonstrated that may help to perfuse the humeral head in the event of injury to the extraneous blood supply. Posteromedial vessels (branches of the posterior circumflex artery), in close association with the inferomedial capsule, were noted to have an intraosseous anastomosis to the arcuate artery and appeared to adequately perfuse the humeral head and articular surface. This situation may have implications in certain specific four-part fractures (primarily valgus-impacted) with the possibility of humeral head perfusion if the head fragment has 1 cm of the medial neck remaining intact with the head. This may help to explain the large variability in rates of osteonecrosis for four-part fractures (Table 3).

Table 3. Reports of the frequency of osteonecrosis occurring with four-part proximal humeral fractures

Author	No. of four-part fractures	% Osteonecrosis
Neer (1970)	8	75%
Lee and Hansen (1981)	19	21%
Sturzenegger et al (1982)	14	36%
Leyshon (1984)	8	75%
Jakob et al (1993)	19	26%
Darder et al (1993)	33	9%
Esser (1994)	8	0%

Osteonecrosis has long since been recognized as a significant problem with these complex fractures. Interestingly, the prevalence of osteonecrosis has not been constant, with rates varying from 20% up to 100%. With the knowledge of the tenuous blood supply to the proximal humerus, many have advocated limited open reduction and internal fixation (or even closed reduction) in order to minimize soft-tissue trauma, in hopes of maintaining the vascularity to the fragments. Recently, Gerber reported on the importance of accurate restoration of the humeral anatomy. Considering only patients with osteonecrosis following four-part proximal humeral fractures treated with open reduction and internal fixation (limited fixation), only those with a malreduction (and thus malunion) of fragments had a poor result (worse than with prosthetic replacement). However, even in the presence of osteonecrosis, those with accurate reduction and union had greater improvement in functional outcomes and pain scores when compared to those undergoing acute proximal humeral hemiarthroplasty.

Nonsurgical treatment can result in substantial residual displacement of the fracture fragments, resulting in functional impairment. Attempts by Neer to treat these fractures with open reduction and internal fixation resulted in a very high rate of osteonecrosis and poor functional outcomes. This scenario led to the recommendation for proximal humeral replacement in all four-part fractures. However, the functional result of proximal humeral hemiarthroplasty for fracture has not equaled results obtained for glenohumeral arthritis.

Selected Bibliography

Arntz CT, Jackins S, Matsen FA III: Prosthetic replacement of the shoulder for the treatment of defects in the rotator cuff and the surface of the glenohumeral joint. *J Bone Joint Surg* 1993;75A:485-491.

Ballmer FT, Lippitt SB, Romeo AA, et al: Total shoulder arthroplasty: Some considerations related to glenoid surface contact. *J Shoulder Elbow Surg* 1994;3:299-306.

Using two commercially available total shoulder arthroplasty systems, the authors performed a geometric study on the effect of glenoid surface contact on shoulder motion. In total shoulder arthroplasty, the range of shoulder motion allowing full surface contact (of the glenoid) is dependent on the component sizes and thus is a surgeon-controlled variable. When full contact does not occur, unwanted translation and irregular surface contact occurs and may contribute to abnormal stresses and wear of the glenoid component.

Ballmer FT, Sidles JA, Lippitt SB, et al: Humeral head prosthetic arthroplasty: Surgically relevant geometric considerations. *J Shoulder Elbow Surg* 1993;2:296-304.

Ten cadaveric humeri were studied to determine the geometric relationships of the native and prosthetic humeral articular surface in relation to the newly defined humeral reference axis. Changes in version of the press-fit stems were noted to have minimal effect on the soft-tissue tension. Soft-tissue release and head-neck size selection were the prime surgeon-determined factors to restore normal kinematics.

Brooks CH, Revell WJ, Heatley FW: Vascularity of the humeral head after proximal humeral fractures: An anatomical cadaver study. *J Bone Joint Surg* 1993;75B:132-136.

A cadaveric vascular injection study demonstrated the presence of significant intraosseous arterial anastomoses between the arcuate artery and the metaphyseal vessels of the proximal humerus and the posteromedial vessels of the posterior circumflex humeral artery. These collateral vessels may perfuse the humeral head in some four-part fractures.

Burkhead WZ, Hutton KS: Biologic resurfacing of the glenoid with hemiarthroplasty of the shoulder. *J Shoulder Elbow Surg* 1995;4:263-270.

Six patients underwent fascial resurfacing of the glenoid articular surface in conjunction with humeral hemiarthroplasty because of concerns of glenoid failure. The early results suggest equal function and pain relief compared with total shoulder arthroplasty and may be an alternative to glenoid resurfacing in the future.

Cofield RH: Total shoulder arthroplasty with the Neer prosthesis. *J Bone Joint Surg* 1984;66A:899-906.

Cofield RH, Daly PJ: Total shoulder arthroplasty with a tissue-ingrowth glenoid component. *J Shoulder Elbow Surg* 1992;1:77-85.

This article discusses a clinical trial reporting on 32 patients at a mean of 4 years 3 months following surgery in which a bone ingrowth glenoid component was used in conjunction with a Neer humeral head prosthesis. Five complications occurred, with four patients requiring reoperation for a failed glenoid component. Radiolucencies were present in 48% of the glenoid components.

Collins D, Tencer A, Sidles J, et al: Edge displacement and deformation of glenoid components in response to eccentric loading: The effect of preparation of the glenoid bone. *J Bone Joint Surg* 1992;74A:501-507.

In a cadaveric model, the effects of edge loading on an all-polyethylene glenoid total shoulder component were studied in relation to the preparation of the glenoid surface. Reaming to achieve intimate matching surfaces provided the least amount of component displacement and deformation.

Darder A, Darder A Jr, Sanchis V, et al: Four-part displaced proximal humeral fractures: Operative treatment using Kirschner wires and a tension band. *J Orthop Trauma* 1993;7:497-505.

Dines DM, Warren RF, Altchek, et al: Posttraumatic changes of the proximal humerus: Malunion, nonunion and osteonecrosis. Treatment with modular hemiarthroplasty or total shoulder arthroplasty. *J Shoulder Elbow Surg* 1993;2:11-21.

Friedman RJ, LaBerge M, Dooley RL, et al: Finite element modeling of the glenoid component: Effect of design parameters on stress distribution. *J Shoulder Elbow Surg* 1992;1:261-270.

A two-plane stress model of the natural glenoid was developed with finite element analysis to observe the loading conditions with different glenoid prosthetic stems. Based on the finite modeling, it was noted that (1) all-polyethylene implants optimize stress transfer; (2) the presence of soft tissue causes higher stress; and (3) stair-stepped and wedge designs produce more natural stress transfer compared with a keel design.

Gerber C, Schneeberger AG, Vinh T-S: The arterial vascularization of the humeral head: An anatomical study. *J Bone Joint Surg* 1990;72A:1486-1494.

Harryman DT, Sidles JA, Harris SL, et al: The effect of articular conformity and the size of humeral head component on laxity and motion after glenohumeral arthroplasty: A study in cadavera. *J Bone Joint Surg* 1995;77A:555-563.

A human cadaver model was used to analyze the effects of articular conformity and humeral head size in glenohumeral arthroplasty. Results indicate that the glenoid component radius of curvature of either 4 mm larger or the same radius as the humeral component had no significant impact on glenohumeral motion or stability, whereas oversized humeral heads markedly limit motion. The results suggest that prosthetic size selection and soft-tissue balancing are critical factors to motion and stability.

Hsu HC, Wu JJ, Chen TH, et al: The influence of abductor lever-arm changes after shoulder arthroplasty. *J Shoulder Elbow Surg* 1993;2:134-140.

Iannotti JP, Gabriel JP, Schnek SL, et al: The normal glenohumeral relationships: An anatomical study of one hundred and forty shoulders. *J Bone Joint Surg* 1992;74A:491-500.

Magnetic resonance imaging and cadaveric dissection of 140 shoulders was performed to delineate the normal anatomic relationships of the glenohumeral joint. Eighty-five percent of all measurements fell within eight fixed combinations of radius of curvature and thickness of humeral head. A strong correlation between lateral humeral offset and the size of the humeral head exists, suggesting reconstruction of the lateral humeral offset is important in optimization of the deltoid and rotator cuff moment arms.

Jacobson SR, Mallon WJ: The glenohumeral offset ratio: A radiographic study. *J Shoulder Elbow Surg* 1993;2:141-146.

Kelly IG: Unconstrained shoulder arthroplasty in rheumatoid arthritis. *Clin Orthop* 1994;307:94-102.

Mullaji AB, Beddow FH, Lamb GHR: CT measurement of glenoid erosion in arthritis. *J Bone Joint Surg* 1994;76B:384-388.

Forty-five arthritic shoulders (osteoarthritis and rheumatoid arthritis) and 19 normal shoulders were studied using computed tomography (CT) scans. In those shoulders with rheumatoid arthritis, nearly half of the glenoid was unsupported bone (mainly posteriorly). Similarly, in those with osteoarthritis, the glenoid surface anteroposterior dimension increased in size with osteophyte formation. The findings suggest that the CT scans can provide useful preoperative information for elective total shoulder arthroplasty.

Neer CS II: Displaced proximal humeral fractures: Part I. Classification and evaluation. *J Bone Joint Surg* 1970;52A:1077-1089.

Neer CS II: Displaced proximal humeral fractures: Part II. Treatment of three-part and four-part displacement. *J Bone Joint Surg* 1970;52A:1090-1103.

Neer CS II, Watson KC, Stanton FJ: Recent experience in total shoulder replacement. *J Bone Joint Surg* 1982;64A:319-337.

Norris TR, Green A, McGuigan FX: Late prosthetic shoulder arthroplasty for displaced proximal humerus fractures. *J Elbow Shoulder Surg* 1995;4:271-280.

Orr TE, Carter DR, Schurman DJ: Stress analyses of glenoid component designs. *Clin Orthop* 1988;232:217-224.

Sidor ML, Zuckerman JD, Lyon T, et al: The Neer classification system for proximal humeral fractures: An assessment of interobserver reliability and intraobserver reproducibility. *J Bone Joint Surg* 1993;75A:1745-1750.

Radiographs of 50 proximal humeral fractures (trauma series) were assessed by five different observers ranging in experience from second-year orthopaedic resident to shoulder specialist. Paired interobserver reliability was moderate (K = 0.48 to 0.52) with improved intraobserver reproducibility associated with increased experience (shoulder surgeon K = 0.83; radiologist K = 0.50)

Siebenrock KA, Gerber C: The reproducibility of classification of fractures of the proximal end of the humerus. *J Bone Joint Surg* 1993;75A:1751-1755.

Radiographs of 95 proximal humeral fractures were reviewed by five orthopaedic surgeons using the Neer and the AO/ASIF classification systems. Interobserver reliability was 0.40 for the Neer system (fair) and 0.53 for the AO/ASIF (moderate). Intraobserver reproducibility was 0.60 (moderate) and 0.58 (moderate), respectively.

Wirth MA, Rockwood CA Jr: Complications of shoulder arthroplasty. *Clin Orthop* 1994;307:47-69.

The authors identify and address the most common complications encountered in total shoulder arthroplasty. This includes, in decreasing order of frequency: instability, rotator cuff tear, ectopic ossification, glenoid loosening, intraoperative fracture, nerve injury, infection, and humeral component loosening.

Zyto K, Kronberg M, Broström L-Å: Shoulder function after displaced fractures of the proximal humerus. *J Shoulder Elbow Surg* 1995;4:331-336.

6

Evaluating Outcomes in the Treatment of Shoulder Disorders

John E. Kuhn, MD and Ralph B. Blasier, MD

Dr. Ernest Anthony Codman, a pioneer in shoulder surgery, also made advances in the study of outcomes of medical and surgical treatments. As early as 1914, Codman called for the standardized reporting of data so that outcomes at different hospitals could be compared. He discussed fiscal and clinical efficiency while identifying regional variations in medical service. Finally, he stressed the fundamental principle that the result to the patient is the central issue in determining the outcomes of medical and surgical treatments.

The recent emphasis on outcomes research has stemmed from the impression that too much money is being spent on health care in the United States. Results from research conducted in the 1970s and 1980s demonstrated that there is significant regional variation in the use of certain medical services. This implies that, in high-utilization areas, unnecessary or inefficient services are being provided, and in low-utilization areas, patients may not be receiving adequate medical care. In general, outcomes research requires standardization of data, allowing for comparison between institutions, and an emphasis on the patient's perception of the outcome of medical and surgical treatment.

A number of different assessments have been used to measure outcomes in patients with shoulder conditions. These tend to fall into a hierarchy of three different levels, including general health assessments, global shoulder assessments, and disease-specific evaluations (Outline 1). No single ideal assessment has yet been devised.

Although rarely done, all assessments should be tested for reliability and validity before clinical use. Test-retest reliability demonstrates that the assessment will produce the same results if given under the same conditions, and internal reliability demonstrates that an assessment evaluating similar conditions will produce similar results. Validity assures that the assessments measure outcomes accurately. The three approaches used to measure validity include content validity, which determines if all of the important aspects of a condition are covered by the assessment; criterion validity, which assures that the scores produced by the assessment correlate with accepted standards; and construct validity, which demonstrates that the assessment produces results consistent with the existing understanding of the field, or with other assessments.

This chapter has been adapted from Kuhn JE, Blasier RB: Measuring outcomes in shoulder arthroplasty. *Semin Arthroplasty* 1995;6:245-264.

Outline 1. Scoring systems used to evaluate the shoulder

Quality of Life Measures
  Quality of Life Index
  Quality Adjusted Life Years
General Health Measures
  SF-36
  Arthritis Impact Measurement Scale
  Nottingham Health Profile
  Sickness Impact Profile
Global Shoulder Assessments
  Without Scoring Systems
    American Shoulder and Elbow Surgeons Assessment
    Simple Shoulder Test
  With Scoring Systems
    Imatani Scoring System
    Severity Index for Chronically Painful Shoulders
    Swanson Score
    Hospital for Special Surgery Shoulder-Rating Score
    UCLA End-Result Score
    Constant Score
    American Shoulder and Elbow Surgeons Index
    Shoulder Pain and Disability Index
Assessments for Specific Shoulder Conditions/Populations
  Instability
    Rowe Bankart Repair Scoring System
    Walch-Duplay Rating Sheet
  Impingement
    Hospital for Special Surgery Impingement Shoulder Rating Score
  The Athlete
    The Athletic Shoulder Outcome Rating Scale

(Reproduced with permission from Kuhn JE, Blasier RB: Measuring outcomes in shoulder arthroplasty. *Semin Arthroplasty* 1995;6:245-264.)

Quality of Life and General Health Assessments

In general, the quality of a patient's life is very difficult to assess. However, two such measures have gained some acceptance recently. The Quality of Life Index rates activity, daily living, health, support, and outlook on a numerical scale and scores each variable on a two-point scale. The Quality of Life Index was designed to assess the overall quality of life of patients with cancer and other chronic illnesses and is not particularly sensitive for patients with less severe complaints who are generally healthy. The Quality of Life Index may not be sensitive enough to evaluate the effect that a treatment for a shoulder condition may have on the patient's quality of life.

The Quality Adjusted Life Years (QALY) analysis is a measure of the patient's disability and distress. This measure

Table 1. Cost/benefit analysis using QALYs for various medical and surgical treatments, in US dollars

Medical Treatment	QALYs Gained	Total Cost* Per Patient	Cost per QALY
Scoliosis surgery-neuromuscular	17.01	4,851	285
Shoulder arthroplasty	0.945	972	1,029
Hip arthroplasty	4.0	4,410	1,102
Coronary artery bypass graft for left main artery	3.0	4,410	1,470
Hemodialysis	6.405	13,225	2,065
Kidney transplant	7.77	16,132	2,076
Scoliosis surgery-idiopathic	1.26	4,851	3,850
Coronary artery bypass graft for two-vessel disease	1.0	4,410	4,410
Continuous ambulatory peritoneal dialysis	3.57	19,858	5,562

*Cost as incurred in Great Britain, displayed in 1986 US dollars
(Adapted with permission from Williams A: The importance of quality of life in policy decisions, in Walker SR, Rosser RM (eds): *Quality of Life: Assessment and Application.* Lancaster, England, MTP Press Ltd, 1988, pp 279-290.)

Table 2. Point allocation for various components of global shoulder scoring systems*

Scoring System	Pain	Range of Motion	Strength	Function	Other-Item	Total
Imatani	40 (40%)	30 (30%)	—	30 (30%)-incl. weakness	—	100
Severity index	30 (30%)	—	15 (15%)	40 (40%)	Handicap - 15 (15%)	100
Swanson	10 (33.3%)	10 (33.3%)	—	10 (33.3%)	—	30
HSS	30 (30%)	25 (25%)	15 (15%)	30 (30%)	—	100
UCLA	10 (28.6%)	5 (14.3%)	5 (14.3%)	10 (28.6%)	Satisfaction - 5 (14.3%)	35
Constant	15 (15%)	20 (20%)	25 (25%)	20 (20%)	—	100
ASES index	50 (50%)	—	—	50 (50%)	—	100
SPADI	38.4%	—	—	61.6%	—	100

*Percentages indicate the relative weight given to each component of the scoring systems.

attempts to derive a global benefit measurement for any treatment by combining the value of the patient's quality of life and any extra life expectancy gained by the treatment. The numerical value generated by this formula can be used to compare different types of treatments for any diagnostic condition and can be used as a means of determining the patient benefit derived from a medical treatment relative to its financial cost (Table 1). Unfortunately, this assessment is heavily dependent on increases in life expectancy derived from a treatment and, as such, may not be applicable to measuring the effect of orthopaedic shoulder treatment. Nevertheless, this measure has been used to assess the value of shoulder arthroplasty relative to cost, and has been used to compare the value of other types of treatment for various disorders. This measure has already been used to determine the allocation of funds for specialty health care in Great Britain.

A general outcome measure is an assessment of the patient's overall health. The SF-36 questionnaire measures eight different aspects of subjective health perception and scores each on a 100-point scale. The areas measured are: (1) limitation in physical activities; (2) limitation in social activities; (3) limitations caused by physical health problems; (4) limitations caused by mental health problems; (5) general mental health; (6) bodily pain; (7) vitality; and (8) general health perception. The SF-36 assessment has been well validated and has been successful in evaluating a number of medical conditions. With regard to the shoulder, however, the SF-36 form does not seem to correlate well with other measures of shoulder disability, and as such, should not be used as the only measure of outcome to assess the results of shoulder treatment.

Global or Universal Shoulder Assessments

The shoulder assessment tools proposed in Outline 1 are designed to be applied to all disorders of the shoulder. Some produce a final numerical grade that allows statistical comparison of the overall preoperative and postoperative condition of the shoulder and allows for comparison of different methods of treatment. Other assessments serve as guides, assuring that none of the important elements in the evaluation of the outcome are neglected, while others are designed to be as simple as possible.

Some global scoring assessments emphasize pain, and others place more emphasis on function or range of motion (Table 2). Because the modern emphasis in outcomes research concerns the patient's perception of his or her condition, these scoring systems may not be applicable to the usual outcomes research. No published overall shoulder scoring system has yet been universally accepted. The various global shoulder assessments are discussed below.

Imatani Scoring System

The Imatani scoring system, originally developed to assess outcomes of treatment of young patients with acromioclavicular joint injuries, has also been used in Europe for the general evaluation of the shoulder. This scoring system is heavily biased toward pain and the patient's assessment of strength.

The Swanson Scoring System

The scoring system proposed by Swanson and colleagues was originally used to evaluate results following arthroplasty of the shoulder with the Swanson Bipolar Implant. In this system, equal weighting of ten points is given to pain, range of motion, and activities of daily living, for a total of 30 points. The system does not include assessments of strength or stability. This system considers flexion and abduction as the most important motions, and less emphasis is placed on other motions. This scoring system has not been utilized in other shoulder assessment studies.

The Hospital for Special Surgery System for Assessing Shoulder Function

The Hospital for Special Surgery Assessment has been used primarily by the parent institution and has not gained wide acceptance elsewhere. This scoring system places the greatest emphasis on pain, but also places substantial emphasis on function. Joint stability is not a consideration. The pain evaluation is not completed by the patient, but rather is completed by the evaluating physician. This situation may introduce bias and make it difficult to compare reports prepared at different institutions or by different clinicians.

The UCLA Scores

The original UCLA Shoulder Assessment, presented in 1981, was employed to evaluate outcome after shoulder arthroplasty. The UCLA End-Result Score is a modification of and similar to the original UCLA Shoulder Assessment, but was originally used to evaluate patients with rotator cuff pathology. Both scoring systems are general enough to have been used as global shoulder evaluations. The UCLA End-Result Score has a more detailed and easier to follow assessment for range of motion and strength than the original UCLA Shoulder Assessment. The UCLA End-Result Score was one of the first scoring systems to include patient satisfaction in the evaluation criteria. The system adds five points of a total of 35 points if the patient is "satisfied and better." Most patients record that they are not satisfied before surgery and are "satisfied and better" after surgery, even if they do not perform well clinically, thus inflating the score. The UCLA score is simple, easy to interpret, easy to use, and is widely applied in the evaluation of shoulder conditions.

The Severity Index for Chronically Painful Shoulders

The Severity Index for Chronically Painful Shoulders, also known as the Shoulder Severity Index, was developed to assess patients with chronic, painful shoulder disabilities. This shoulder assessment allocates 30 points to pain, 40 points to function, 15 points to strength, and 15 points to a visual analog scale for daily handicap. Numerical adjustments are then made for chronic shoulder pain, and for elderly patients whose activity is limited or who have prosthetic replacements. This elaborate and fairly complicated rating system has been largely abandoned because simpler systems seem to be just as effective.

The Constant Score

The Constant Score is a general scoring system and has been validated by testing normal individuals as well as symptomatic patients. In validating this test, it was found that the normal scores decrease with age and vary with gender, and as such, scores should be age- and gender-adjusted before

Table 3. The Constant Score

Pain Score (15 points maximum)	
None	15
Mild	10
Moderate	5
Severe	0
Activities of Daily Living (20 points maximum)	
Activity level (10 points)	
Full work	4
Full recreation/sport	4
Unaffected sleep	2
Positioning (10 points)	
Up to waist	2
Up to xiphoid	4
Up to neck	6
Up to top of head	8
Above head	10
Range of Motion (40 points maximum)	
Forward elevation (10 points) and lateral elevation (10 points)	
0-30°	0
31°-60°	2
61°-90°	4
91°-120°	6
121°-150°	8
151°-180°	10
External Rotation (10 points)	
Hand behind head, elbow forward	2
Hand behind head, elbow back	2
Hand to top of head, elbow forward	2
Hand to top of head, elbow backward	2
Full elevation from top of head	2
Internal Rotation (10 points)	
Lateral thigh	0
Buttock	2
Lumbosacral junction	4
Waist (L3 vertebral body)	6
T12 vertebral body	8
Interscapular (T7 vertebral body)	10
Strength of Abduction (25 points maximum)	1 point/lb

(Reproduced with permission from Constant CR, Murley AHG: A clinical method of functional assessment of the shoulder. *Clin Orthop* 1987;214:160-164.)

reporting data. The Constant Scoring System has been reported to have low intraobserver error and is reproducible. The Constant Score gives 35 points for the subjective assessment and 65 points for the objective assessment. Previous statistical work would suggest that this is a reasonable distribution. Pain and function are given less emphasis, while range of motion is given more emphasis (Table 3). The Constant Scoring System has been adopted by the European Society for Surgery of the Shoulder and Elbow, and data presented to this society must use the Constant Score. However, the Constant Score has not been widely used in published reports, especially in American journals. Strength must be tested using a spring balance, and the exact technique to measure strength is not well defined.

The American Shoulder and Elbow Surgeons Standardized Shoulder Assessment and Shoulder Score Index

The Research Committee of the American Shoulder and Elbow Surgeons (ASES) has created a standardized method for evaluating the shoulder (Figs. 1-8). The goal of this effort

SHOULDER ASSESSMENT FORM			
AMERICAN SHOULDER AND ELBOW SURGEONS			
Name:		Date	
Age:	Hand dominance: R L Ambi	Sex: M F	
Diagnosis:		Initial Assess? Y N	
Procedure/Date:		Follow-up: M; Y	

Fig. 1 Demographic information. (Reproduced with permission from the American Shoulder and Elbow Surgeons Research Committee: A standardized method for the assessment of shoulder function. *J Shoulder Elbow Surg* 1994;3:347-352.)

PATIENT SELF-EVALUATION		
Are you having pain in your shoulder? (circle correct answer)	Yes	No
Mark where your pain is		
Do you have pain in your shoulder at night?	Yes	No
Do you take pain medication (aspirin, Advil, Tylenol etc.)?	Yes	No
Do you take narcotic pain medication (codeine or stronger)?	Yes	No
How many pills do you take each day (average)?	___ pills	
How bad is your pain today (mark line)? 0⌊_____⌋10 No pain at all Pain as bad as it can be		

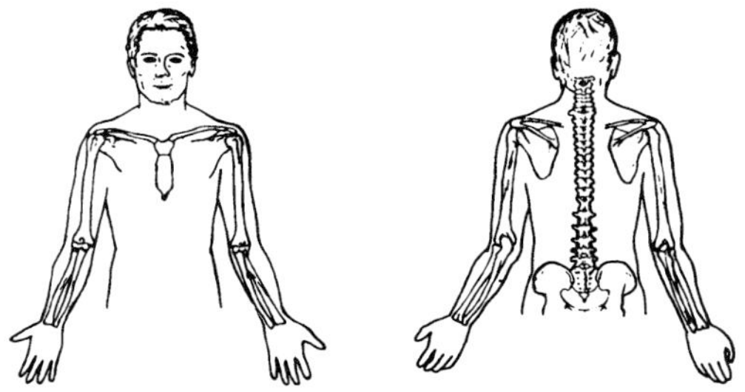

Fig. 2 Patient self-evaluation; pain questionnaire. (Reproduced with permission from the American Shoulder and Elbow Surgeons Research Committee: A standardized method for the assessment of shoulder function. *J Shoulder Elbow Surg* 1994;3:347-352.)

Does your shoulder feel unstable (as if it is going to dislocate)?	Yes	No
How unstable is your shoulder (mark line)? 0⌊_____⌋10 Very stable Very unstable		

Fig. 3 Patient self-evaluation; instability questionnaire. (Reproduced with permission from the American Shoulder and Elbow Surgeons Research Committee: A standardized method for the assessment of shoulder function. *J Shoulder Elbow Surg* 1994;3:347-352.)

Circle the number in the box that indicates your ability to do the following activities: 0 = **Unable** to do; 1 = **Very** difficult to do; 2 = **Somewhat** difficult; 3 = **Not** difficult		
ACTIVITY	RIGHT ARM	LEFT ARM
1. Put on a coat	0 1 2 3	0 1 2 3
2. Sleep on your painful or affected side	0 1 2 3	0 1 2 3
3. Wash back/do up bra in back	0 1 2 3	0 1 2 3
4. Manage toiletting	0 1 2 3	0 1 2 3
5. Comb hair	0 1 2 3	0 1 2 3
6. Reach a high shelf	0 1 2 3	0 1 2 3
7. Lift 10 lbs. above shoulder	0 1 2 3	0 1 2 3
8. Throw a ball overhand	0 1 2 3	0 1 2 3
9. Do usual work - List:	0 1 2 3	0 1 2 3
10. Do usual sport - List:	0 1 2 3	0 1 2 3

Fig. 4 Patient self-evaluation; activity of daily living questionnaire. (Reproduced with permission from the American Shoulder and Elbow Surgeons Research Committee: A standardized method for the assessment of shoulder function. *J Shoulder Elbow Surg* 1994;3:347-352.)

PHYSICIAN ASSESSMENT					
RANGE OF MOTION Total shoulder motion Goniometer preferred	RIGHT		LEFT	
	Active	Passive	Active	Passive
Forward elevation (Maximum arm-trunk angle)				
External rotation (Arm comfortably at side)				
External rotation (Arm at 90° abduction)				
Internal rotation (Highest posterior anatomy reached with thumb)				
Cross-body adduction (Antecubital fossa to opposite acromion)				

Fig. 5 Physician assessment; range of motion. (Reproduced with permission from the American Shoulder and Elbow Surgeons Research Committee: A standardized method for the assessment of shoulder function. *J Shoulder Elbow Surg* 1994;3:347-352.)

was to create a universal method to measure the condition of the shoulder, a method that would be easy to use, would assess activities of daily living, and would include a subjective component completed by the patient. This assessment is based primarily on the early work of Neer; however, many other scoring systems were reviewed during the development of this assessment.

The subjective or patient-completed assessment includes pain, symptoms of instability, and activities of daily living. Both pain and instability are graded on a ten-point visual analog scale. The functional assessment includes ten questions regarding activities of daily living. The patient grades his or her ability to perform each of these activities on a four-point scale. The objective or physician-completed part of the form reviews range of motion, specific physical findings, strength, and stability. Passive and active motion measurement includes forward elevation, cross-body adduction, external rotation with the arm at the side, and external rotation with the arm in 90° of abduction. Measurements of abduction were deliberately omitted. Strength is measured

SIGNS		
0 = none; 1 = mild; 2 = moderate; 3 = severe		
SIGN	Right	Left
Supraspinatus/greater tuberosity tenderness	0 1 2 3	0 1 2 3
AC joint tenderness	0 1 2 3	0 1 2 3
Biceps tendon tenderness (or rupture)	0 1 2 3	0 1 2 3
Other tenderness - List:	0 1 2 3	0 1 2 3
Impingement I (Passive forward elevation in slight internal rotation)	Y N	Y N
Impingement II (Passive internal rotation with 90° flexion)	Y N	Y N
Impingement III (90° active abduction - classic painful arc)	Y N	Y N
Subacromial crepitus	Y N	Y N
Scars - location:	Y N	Y N
Atrophy - location:	Y N	Y N
Deformity: describe	Y N	Y N

Fig. 6 Physician assessment; signs. (Reproduced with permission from the American Shoulder and Elbow Surgeons Research Committee: A standardized method for the assessment of shoulder function. *J Shoulder Elbow Surg* 1994;3:347-352.)

STRENGTH		
(record MRC grade)		
0 = no contraction; 1 = flicker; 2 = movement with gravity eliminated; 3 = movement against gravity; 4 = movement against some resistance; 5 = normal power.		
	Right	Left
Testing affected by pain?	Y N	Y N
Forward elevation	0 1 2 3 4 5	0 1 2 3 4 5
Abduction	0 1 2 3 4 5	0 1 2 3 4 5
External rotation (Arm comfortably at side)	0 1 2 3 4 5	0 1 2 3 4 5
Internal rotation (Arm comfortably at side)	0 1 2 3 4 5	0 1 2 3 4 5

Fig. 7 Physician assessment; strength. (Reproduced with permission from the American Shoulder and Elbow Surgeons Research Committee: A standardized method for the assessment of shoulder function. *J Shoulder Elbow Surg* 1994;3:347-352.)

using the five-level Medical Research Council Grades in forward elevation, abduction, internal rotation, and external rotation. Instability is graded on a four-point scale in three planes: anterior, posterior, and inferior. When presenting this form, the research committee recommended modifying or customizing it to fit the needs of individual clinicians. Although this may be a good suggestion for the clinician, standardized reporting of outcomes across institutions becomes difficult.

The Research Committee of the ASES has defined a subset of the Standardized Shoulder Assessment as the Shoulder Score Index. This index uses the subjective visual analog

INSTABILITY		
0 = none; 1 = mild (0-1 cm translation) 2 = moderate (1-2 cm translation or translates to glenoid rim) 3 = severe (>2 cm translation or over rim of glenoid)		
Anterior translation	0 1 2 3	0 1 2 3
Posterior translation	0 1 2 3	0 1 2 3
Inferior translation (sulcus sign)	0 1 2 3	0 1 2 3
Anterior apprehension	0 1 2 3	0 1 2 3
Reproduces symptoms?	Y N	Y N
Voluntary instability?	Y N	Y N
Relocation test positive?	Y N	Y N
Generalized ligamentous laxity?	Y N	
Other physical findings:		
Examiner's name: _____ _____ Date		

Fig. 8 Physician assessment; instability. (Reproduced with permission from the American Shoulder and Elbow Surgeons Research Committee: A standardized method for the assessment of shoulder function. *J Shoulder Elbow Surg* 1994;3:347-352.)

scale of pain for 50% of its total score and the activities of daily living questionnaire for the other 50%, producing a 100-point total.

The Simple Shoulder Test

Matsen and associates have developed an entirely subjective questionnaire that eliminates any physician-induced bias. The Simple Shoulder Test consists of 12 yes or no questions, completed by the patient in the office or at home. The questions involve the patient's belief that he or she can or cannot perform 12 tasks, graduated in the level of performance each task requires of the shoulder. Pain, instability, and weakness are evaluated indirectly through the questions, which assess the patient's perceived ability to perform different activities.

The Shoulder Pain and Disability Index

Like the Simple Shoulder Test, the Shoulder Pain and Disability Index is a patient-administered questionnaire that investigates the patient's perception of his or her shoulder. This evaluation uses visual analog scales to rate the patient's response to 13 questions; five evaluate pain, and eight evaluate disability. Scores for pain and disability are obtained; the pain score and the disability score are then averaged. This assessment is one of the few to have been validated and found to be reliable, with excellent criterion and construct validity.

The Athletic Shoulder Outcome Rating Scale

The Athletic Shoulder Outcome Rating Scale, developed by the Kerlan-Jobe clinic, is a global shoulder evaluation designed to improve the sensitivity of the assessment of the shoulder for the athletic population. A good result as determined by other assessments for the general population may not be an adequate result for an athlete.

Assessments for Specific Diseases

Many of the global shoulder assessments began as assessments for particular shoulder disorders, and through time have been applied in a more general fashion. The Swanson, Hospital for Special Surgery, and the original UCLA scores were all designed to evaluate the results of shoulder arthroplasty, and have since been applied to other conditions. Unfortunately, assessments that are centered on a surgical treatment may inappropriately combine patients with widely varying diagnoses (ie, degenerative arthritis, rheumatoid arthritis, and four-part fractures of the humeral head, all treated with arthroplasty) in the same group.

Other assessments originally described for a specific condition include the Imatani Score for acromioclavicular injury, and the modified UCLA score, which was originally used for the evaluation of surgical repair of rotator cuff tears. Similarly, a modification of the Hospital for Special Surgery score has been used to evaluate the results of anterior acromioplasty for impingement syndrome.

There are assessments for measuring the outcome of surgery for the treatment of traumatic glenohumeral instability. These include the Rowe score used in the United States, and the Walch-Duplay Score, which has been gaining acceptance in Europe. At this time there are no specific evaluations available concerning the diagnosis and treatment of multidirectional instability, posterior instability, rheumatoid arthritis, osteonecrosis, calcific tendinitis, adhesive capsulitis, or for the assessment of the treatment methods used in patients with fractures of the proximal humerus, clavicle, or scapula.

Evaluating Shoulder Outcomes: Recommendations

Recent work comparing different assessments has suggested that no one type of evaluation will prove to be adequate for all purposes. Instead, data may best be presented using two or all three levels of evaluation as described in Outline 1. The SF-36 general health assessment is gaining popularity in orthopaedics, and should probably be included in the assessment of patients undergoing shoulder treatment. With regard to global shoulder assessments, the ASES evaluation is currently preferred when presenting data in the United States, and the Constant assessment should be used when presenting results in Europe. When available, a diagnosis-specific or treatment-specific assessment may be added.

Selected Bibliography

Amstutz HC, Sew Hoy AL, Clarke IC: UCLA anatomic total shoulder arthroplasty. *Clin Orthop* 1981;155:7-20.

The UCLA Shoulder Assessment is presented.

Beaton DE, Richards RR: Measuring function of the shoulder: A cross-sectional comparison of five questionnaires. *J Bone Joint Surg* 1996;78A:882-890.

Five shoulder questionnaires including the Subjective Shoulder Rating Scale, Simple Shoulder Test, Modified American Shoulder and Elbow Surgeons Assessment, Shoulder Severity Index, and the Shoulder Pain and Disability Index were tested and found to have good reliability and validity except the Subjective Shoulder Rating Scale, which was not as reliable. The SF-36 was not believed to be sensitive to shoulder problems.

Codman EA: The product of a hospital. *Surg Gynecol Obstet* 1914;18:491-496.

Codman presents the classic and original discussion of outcomes research.

Constant CR, Murley AH: A clinical method of functional assessment of the shoulder. *Clin Orthop* 1987;214:160-164.

A description of and instructions for using this scoring system, which is popular in Europe, are presented.

Ellman H, Hanker G, Bayer M: Repair of the rotator cuff: End-result study of factors influencing reconstruction. *J Bone Joint Surg* 1986;68A:1136-1144.

The article presents a description of the UCLA End-Result Score.

Gerber C: Integrated scoring systems for the functional assessment of the shoulder, in Matsen FA III, Fu FH, Hawkins RJ (eds): *The Shoulder: A Balance of Mobility and Stability.* Rosemont, IL, American Academy of Orthopaedic Surgeons, 1993.

The Severity Index for Chronically Painful Shoulders is presented.

Imatani RJ, Hanlon JJ, Cady GW: Acute, complete acromioclavicular separation. *J Bone Joint Surg* 1975;57A:328-332.

A description of the Imatani Scoring System is presented.

Kuhn JE, Blasier RB: Measuring outcomes in shoulder arthroplasty. *Semin Arthroplasty* 1995;6:245-264.

This is a thorough review, with appendices of various scoring systems used in evaluating the shoulder.

Matsen FA III, Ziegler DW, BeBartolo SE: Patient self-assessment of health status and function in glenohumeral degenerative joint disease. *J Shoulder Elbow Surg* 1995;4:345-351.

The SF-36 components of bodily pain, physical functioning, and physical role fulfillment correlated best with the Simple Shoulder Test in patients with glenohumeral arthritis.

Richards RR, An KN, Bigliani LU, et al: A standardized method for the assessment of shoulder function. *J Shoulder Elbow Surg* 1994;3:347-352.

This article discusses the American Shoulder and Elbow Surgeons assessment form and provides instructions on its use.

Roach KE, Budiman-Mak E, Songsiridej N, et al: Development of a shoulder pain and disability index. *Arthritis Care Res* 1991;4:143-149.

The authors develop and validate a patient-administered assessment similar to the Simple Shoulder Test, with 13 questions for pain and disability, answered using a visual analog scale. This global assessment had excellent reliability and criterion validity.

Romeo AA, Bach BR Jr, O'Halloran KL: Scoring systems for shoulder conditions. *Am J Sports Med* 1996;24:472-476.

Evaluation of the Rowe, Modified Rowe, UCLA, and American Shoulder and Elbow Surgeons shoulder scores demonstrated significant variations in the scores generated for the same patients, and inter-rater reliability was poor, highlighting the fact that there is no accepted universal shoulder score.

Spitzer WO, Dobson AJ, Hall J, et al: Measuring the quality of life of cancer patients: A concise QL-Index for use by physicians. *J Chron Dis* 1981;34:585-597.

This article presents a description of the Quality of Life Index.

Swanson AB, DeGroot Swanson G, Sattel AB et al: Bipolar implant shoulder arthroplasty. *Clin Orthop* 1989;249: 227-247.

This article contains the description and instructions for use of the Swanson Shoulder Score.

Tibone JE, Bradley JP: Evalation of treatment outcomes for the athletic shoulder, in Matsen FA III, Fu FH, Hawkins RJ (eds): *The Shoulder: A Balance of Mobility and Stability.* Rosemont, IL, American Academy of Orthopaedic Surgeons, 1993, pp 519-530.

The Athletic Shoulder Outcome Rating Scale, as developed by the Kerlan-Jobe Clinic, is presented.

Ware JE Jr, Sherbourne CD: The MOS 36-item short-form health survey (SF-36): I. Conceptual framework and item selection. *Med Care* 1992;30:473-483.

This article discusses the SF-36 form and its design.

Warren RF, Ranawat CS, Inglis AE: Total shoulder replacement: Indications and results of the Neer non-constrained prosthesis, in Inglis AE (ed): American Academy of Orthopaedic Surgeons: *Symposium on Total Joint Replacement of the Upper Extremity.* St. Louis, MO, CV Mosby, 1982, pp 56-57.

A discussion of the Hospital for Special Surgery System for Assessing Shoulder Function is presented.

II
Instability and Athletic Injuries

Evan L. Flatow, MD
Section Editor

7

Clinical Assessment, Imaging, and Classification

Erin Boynton, MD, FRCSC and Anthony Miniaci, MD, FRCSC

Introduction

The shoulder is one of the most mobile joints in the body, responsible for positioning of the hand in space. This great requirement for mobility is reflected in glenohumeral joint structure and makes the joint prone to instability. Consequently, the glenohumeral joint is the most frequently dislocated large joint.

Understanding the key elements involved in instability through clinical examination and correlation of these findings with radiographic imaging should lead to improved classification systems and treatment protocols.

Pathophysiology of Instability

Both dynamic and static factors contribute to glenohumeral joint stability. During the midrange of motion when the capsular ligaments are lax, the rotator cuff and scapular muscles dynamically stabilize the glenohumeral joint by concavity-compression. Biomechanical analysis of the capsular ligaments has demonstrated that different parts of the capsule are important in preventing abnormal translations at the end range of motion. Depending on the position of abduction/adduction and rotation, different parts of the capsuloligamentous complex play a more dominant role. With the arm adducted, the superior capsule is more important to stability, whereas the inferior portion of the capsuloligamentous system is more important with the arm in abduction. The importance of the anterior and posterior portions of the capsule varies with the degree of glenohumeral rotation.

Traditional teaching has suggested that an "essential" pathologic lesion occurs with anterior shoulder instability. The Bankart lesion, or tear of the anterior band of the inferior glenohumeral ligament, was thought to be this lesion, and could be associated with humeral head impaction fractures (Hill-Sachs lesions) (Fig. 1), anterior glenoid deficiency or fracture (Fig. 2), and sometimes capsular laxity. Biomechanical analysis of glenohumeral joint stability after creating a Bankart lesion, however, has only demonstrated minimal increases in glenohumeral translation, and it was not possible to dislocate the glenohumeral joint until there had been significant injury to the posterior capsule. It appears that injury to both the anterior and posterior portions of the joint is required for dislocation to occur, which supports the circle concept of joint stability as described by Warren. There is, therefore, no single "essential" lesion of instability. Shoulder subluxation or dislocation may result in various injuries, ranging from frank tearing to plastic deformation of the ligaments, compression or avulsion fractures, or a combination of this pathology on opposite sides of the joint. An accurate understanding of the effect of injury to opposite sides of the capsu-

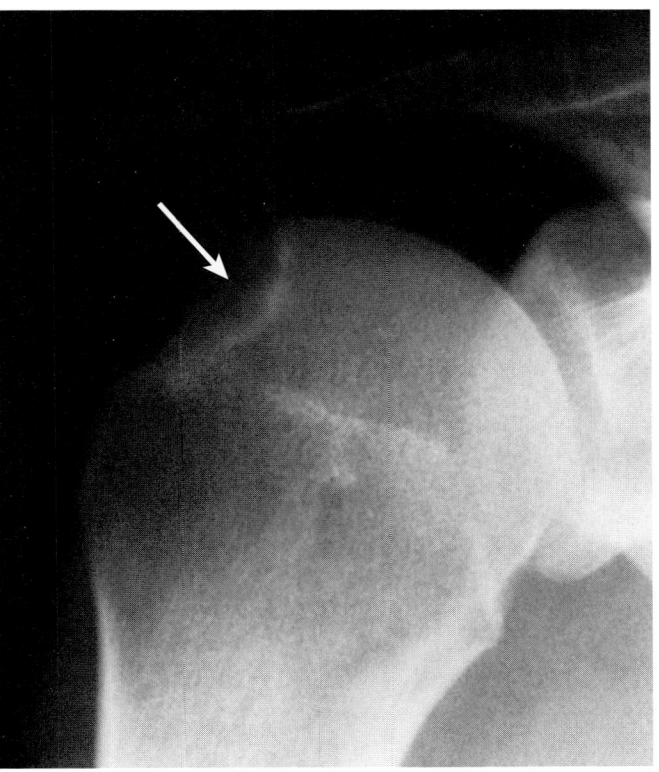

Fig. 1 Anteroposterior view of the shoulder demonstrating reduced glenohumeral joint with chronic Hill-Sachs lesion (*arrow*).

loligamentous complex on glenohumeral translation is critical in planning a therapeutic approach, and a precise understanding of pathology is important because it allows appropriate selection of both rehabilitation and surgical approaches to the treatment of the instability.

Clinical Evaluation

History and physical examination are critical in establishing the correct diagnosis in the patient with suspected instability. Information regarding direction, trauma, volition, and degree of instability is the mainstay of the history. The patient often feels a painful pop or slide as the shoulder either subluxates or completely dislocates. If the patient has had a frank dislocation, it is important to determine whether closed reduction was required or if spontaneous reduction occurred. The patient may be able to identify the direction of dislocation and

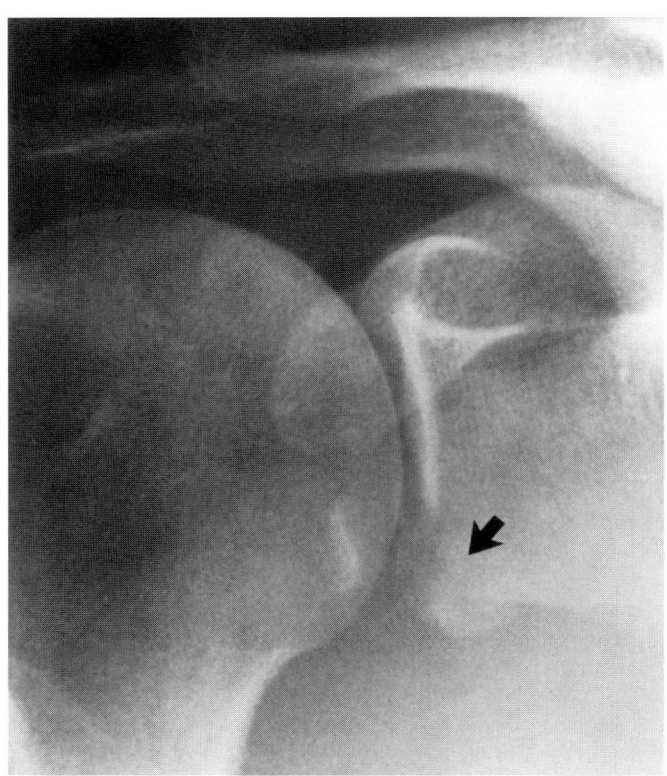

Fig. 2 Anteroposterior view of the glenohumeral joint demonstrating irregularity at the inferior portion, representing a bony Bankart lesion following anterior dislocation (*arrow*).

Although uncommon, some unusual forms of instability also need to be ruled out. Septic dislocation, neuromuscular disorders (eg, syringomyelia) or paralytic causes of instability (eg, Erb's palsy, traumatic brachial plexus lesions), congenital abnormalities (eg, hypoplastic glenoid), collagen abnormalities (Ehlers-Danlos syndrome) or postsurgical problems all need to be considered depending on the individual patient, specific conditions, and presenting complaint.

Examination of the patient with acute instability is important to confirm the diagnosis as well as the direction of dislocation. In the patient with an anterior dislocation, there is loss of the normal contour of the shoulder with squaring, and possibly an anterior fullness. The arm may be resting in slight abduction and external rotation and there will obviously be a significant restriction in range of motion, specifically a lack of internal rotation. Careful and thorough assessment is important because posterior dislocations are commonly missed during examination. Usually the patient presents with the arm at the side in adduction and internally rotated, with a visible and palpable fullness posteriorly. The key to the diagnosis is a lack of forward elevation and inability to externally rotate the arm, as well as loss of supination. Assessment of neurovascular function is essential, particularly axillary nerve function in the patient with anterior dislocation.

Following a complete history, a thorough physical examination is necessary to confirm the diagnosis of instability. Both shoulder girdles are inspected for previous scars, skin lesions, and muscular atrophy. General motion of the shoulder unit should be assessed for glenohumeral rhythm, scapulothoracic motion, and overall synchrony of motion. Palpation is performed to detect any tenderness of the joints of the shoulder girdle and should be done in an orderly fashion so that each joint, muscle, and bony prominence is examined. It is not common to find point tenderness around the shoulder in patients with recurrent instability unless there is associated rotator cuff pathology. Occasionally, overhead athletes with subtle instability may have posterior rotator cuff tenderness as well. Observation of active and passive range of motion is important to detect any contractures around the shoulder. Patients recovering from an acute dislocation, as well as overhead athletes with subluxation, may develop posterior capsular contractures that can accentuate impingement symptoms. Posterior capsular contracture can be detected with the arm in 90° of forward flexion and the forearm internally rotated or with the arm in 90° of abduction or by assessing loss of internal rotation as compared to the other side with the arm behind the back. When assessing for contractures and laxity, it is critical to examine both the affected and unaffected shoulder to determine baseline differences in degrees of laxity. It should be noted that in some overhead athletes a loss of internal rotation and increase in external rotation may be normal, and knowledge of this preexisting baseline is important to determine new pathology.

Instability Assessment

Special tests should be performed to accurately determine the direction(s) of instability. All patients are asked if they are capable of voluntarily demonstrating shoulder instability, and in those patients who can, multidirectional or posterior instability is usually the underlying problem (Fig. 3). Translation

which position causes apprehension. Determining the position that the arm was in at the time of dislocation will give a clue as to the direction of instability. Usually dislocation with the arm at or above 90° of forward flexion or abduction suggests anterior instability, whereas dislocation with the hand below the level of the shoulder suggests posterior instability. A similar relationship exists between internal rotation and posterior instability.

If a sensation of instability is the main complaint, it is somewhat easier to identify its pathology and cause than it is when pain is the presenting symptom, especially for some of the more subtle forms of instability, which can often have a more vague history and clinical picture. Jobe has recognized that some patients, particularly those younger than 30 years of age, may present with symptoms of "impingement" pain aggravated by overhead activity; however, it is unusual for patients younger than 30 years old to have primary rotator cuff pathology; therefore, signs of instability must be carefully sought. Rowe described the "dead arm syndrome" in young overhead athletes, in which the patients describe numbness, tingling, or weakness in the extremity during a specific activity. This complaint may be a clue to more subtle forms of anterior instability. The impingement pain that is secondary to the primary instability has been well described and documented and can be a result of labral pathology, capsular laxity, or rotator cuff overuse.

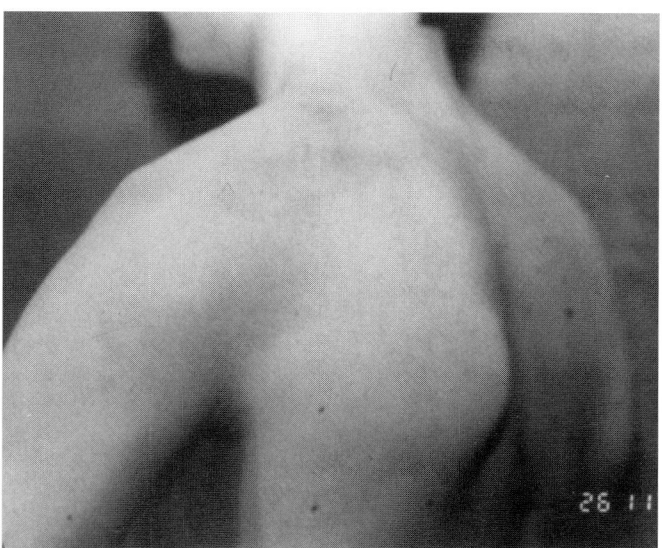

Fig. 3 Scapular winging in a patient who had multidirectional instability and laxity as the only diagnosis.

of the affected shoulder can be assessed by performing a drawer test. The patient is seated leaning slightly forward with the arm at the side, and is asked to relax the shoulder girdle. The examiner places a hand on the superior aspect of the acromion to stabilize the scapula and grasps the humeral head with the other hand. The humeral head is then translated anteriorly, posteriorly, and inferiorly and the degree of translation assessed. This can be done with the patient awake; however, Cofield and Irving have described a detailed examination of glenohumeral translation to be used under anesthesia. The technique provides useful information and can be adapted for use in the office. With the patient supine, the examiner grasps the patient's wrist and holds the arm in slight abduction and forward elevation such that the humeral head is centered on the glenoid. The examiner's other hand is used to grasp the humeral head and apply anterior, posterior, and inferior forces to detect humeral head translation. The arm is placed into different degrees of abduction and rotation to assess the integrity of the superior, inferior, anterior, and posterior portions of the capsuloligamentous complex.

Assessing generalized ligamentous laxity is often a necessary and important part of the examination and can be performed by measuring upper extremity joint laxity, elbow joint hyperextension > 5°, the ability to touch or place the thumb parallel to the forearm, and metacarpophalangeal joint hyperextension > 60°.

Anterior Stability Tests
Anterior instability can be evaluated by performing the anterior apprehension test. This maneuver can be performed with the patient supine or sitting and with the arm in 90° of abduction, with the elbow flexed 90°. The examiner's hand is placed on the superior aspect of the shoulder with the middle finger on the coracoid, the second finger on the anterior aspect of the humeral head, and the thumb on the posterior aspect of the humeral head. While an anteriorly directed force is applied to the humeral head, the arm is externally rotated. The patient with anterior instability will become apprehensive and will not allow the examiner to place the arm in the unstable position. In addition, the examiner can sometimes evaluate the degree of anterior translation. Several variations of the anterior apprehension test have been described, such as the Feagin maneuver, the crank test, and the fulcrum test. Jobe and Fowler have described the relocation test, which is a variation of the anterior apprehension test and is helpful in detecting more subtle forms of anterior instability when the patient presents with pain, instability, or both. With the patient supine, the examiner places the patient's arm in 90° of abduction and externally rotates the arm until the symptoms are reproduced. Alleviation of symptoms with posterior pressure may be suggestive of subtle anterior instability. Unfortunately, sometimes patients with primary rotator cuff pathology can also obtain pain relief with this maneuver, drawing into question the usefulness of the relocation test. Speer and associates have recently shown that with the arm in 90° of abduction the relocation test may not be helpful in distinguishing between instability and impingement when pain alone was considered, and the accuracy of the test was greater than 80% only when true apprehension was found. However, if the test is performed with maximal external rotation to the point of symptom production and taken in the context of subluxation and presenting history, this test can still be somewhat of a guide to the underlying cause of symptomatology.

Posterior Stability Tests
A posterior apprehension test can be performed with the patient supine and the arm in 90° of forward flexion while internally rotating the arm with a posteriorly directed force. The examiner may feel the humeral head subluxate or dislocate or the patient will complain of apprehension during this maneuver. With the patient in this position, a variation of this maneuver, termed the flexion pivot test, has also been useful. With the arm forward flexed to 90° and adducted, posterior pressure is applied. Posterior subluxation or dislocation may not necessarily be palpable at this point in patients with posterior instability. However, if the arm is slowly abducted at about 30° to 45°, the humeral head will reduce itself and produce a definitive clunk.

Inferior Stability Tests
Neer emphasized the importance of an inferior component of instability in patients with multidirectional and bidirectional instability. The sulcus test has been used in the diagnosis of inferior instability. The patient is relaxed with the arm at the side. The examiner pulls inferiorly on the arm and observes for any inferior translation of the humeral head by examining the space between the lateral acromion and the humeral head (the sulcus sign).

Impingement Tests
Impingement tests of the shoulder may be performed even in patients with instability to detect associated rotator cuff tendinopathy. These tests have been well described. The Neer

impingement test can be performed by placing one hand on the posterior aspect of the scapula to stabilize the shoulder girdle. The examiner takes the patient's arm by the wrist, and the arm is placed into full forward flexion. The patient will complain of pain at the extremes of forward flexion as the rotator cuff comes into contact with the rigid coracoacromial arch. The Hawkins test places the arm in 90° of forward flexion and forcefully internally rotates the arm, bringing the greater tuberosity in contact with the lateral acromion. Often an injection of the subacromial bursa combined with an impingement test (impingement injection test) can be both diagnostic and therapeutic in these patients. Range-of-motion testing of the cervical spine and a complete neurologic assessment should be performed on all patients who present with symptoms of instability.

The information obtained from clinical evaluation is needed to properly classify glenohumeral instability. A clear understanding of the type of instability is critical before surgical treatment can be recommended. If a patient is treated for unidirectional instability when in fact multidirectional instability is present, complications may arise and surgery fails. If classification of the instability is not possible, then adjuvant investigations including radiography, examination under anesthesia, fluoroscopy, and arthroscopy can add important information.

Radiographic Evaluation

Once a proper history and physical examination have been performed, additional information may be required to properly classify shoulder instability or detect associated pathology. When a patient presents with an acute dislocation of the glenohumeral joint, a trauma series consisting of three orthogonal views (true anteroposterior (AP), transcapular lateral, and axillary) is obtained (Fig. 4). These views are essential to establish the diagnosis and direction of dislocation. It is important to rule out associated fractures in the acute setting.

Special Views

Additional views may be added to further delineate pathology associated with recurrent instability; these include the West Point axillary view for glenoid rim fractures, an AP view with the shoulder in internal rotation, or a Stryker notch view (apical oblique view) for the assessment of Hill-Sachs lesions. It is important to rule out associated fractures or loose bodies and determine the presence and/or size of a bony Bankart lesion or Hill-Sachs lesion (Fig. 5) because these conditions may affect treatment and prognosis.

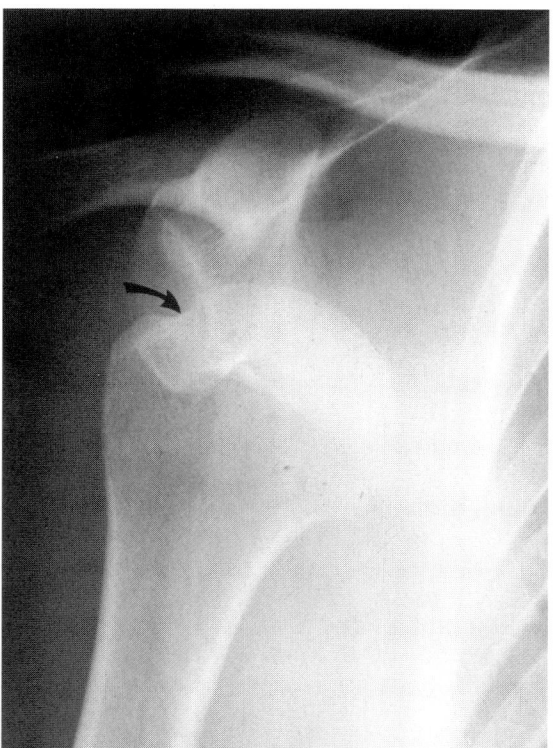
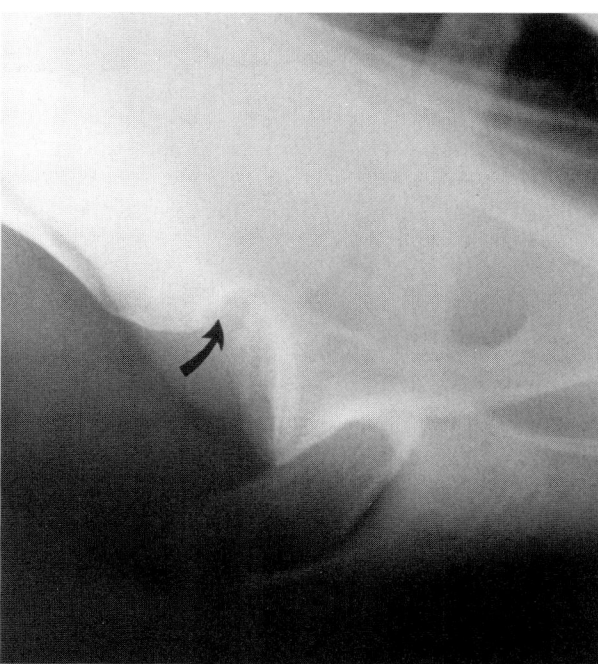

Fig. 4 Left, Anterior view of the anterior dislocation demonstrating an anteriorly dislocated shoulder with impaction of the posterolateral humeral head against the glenoid, creating a Hill-Sachs type of lesion (*arrow*). **Right,** Axillary view demonstrating an anterior dislocation of the shoulder. Arrow demonstrates a Hill-Sachs lesion created by the impact of the glenoid against the posterolateral aspect of the humeral head.

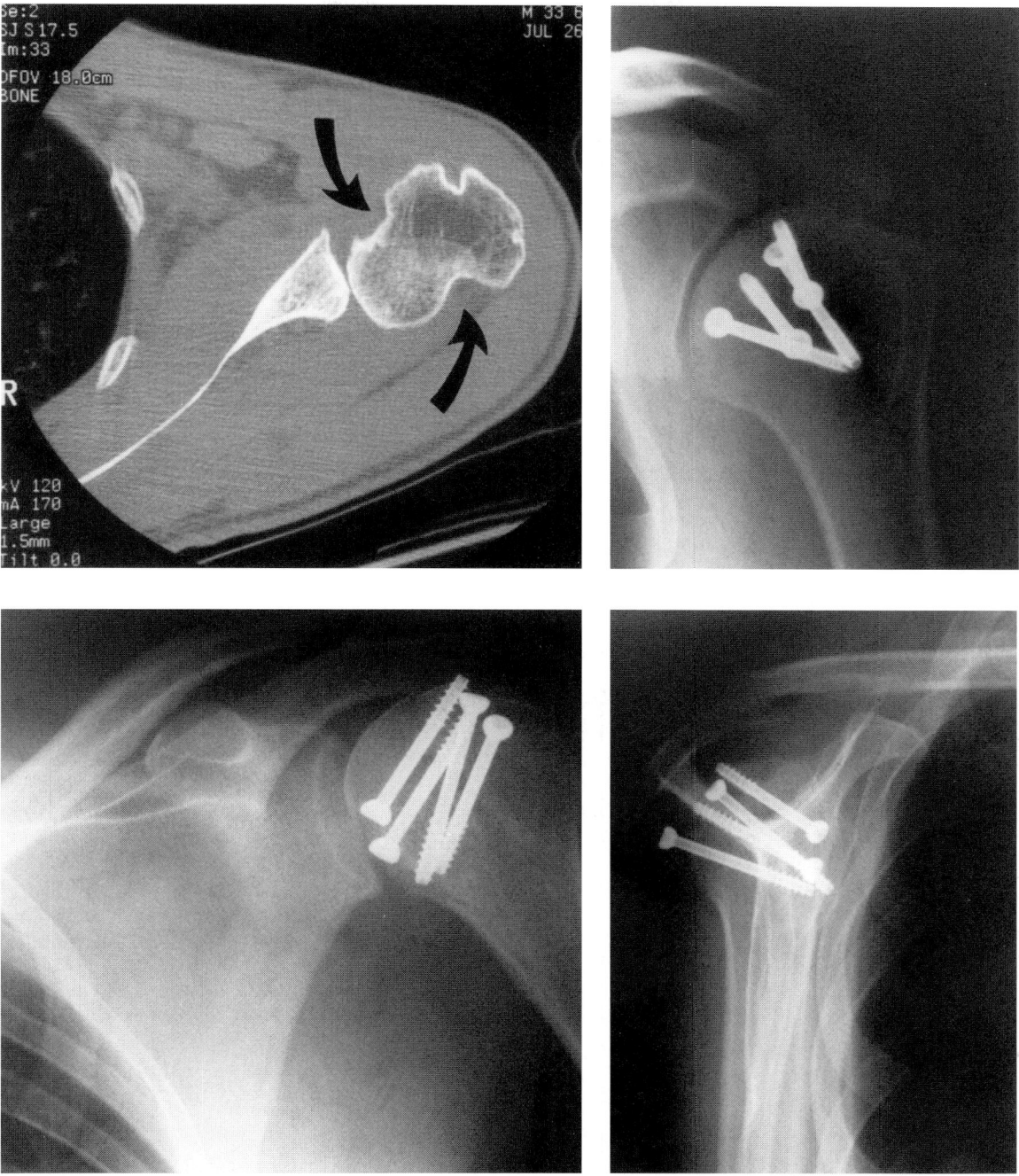

Fig. 5 **Top left,** Computed tomographic scan of a patient with recurrent anterior and posterior instability. The patient has both Hill-Sachs and reverse Hill-Sachs lesions (*arrows*), demonstrating instability. **Top right, bottom left** and **right,** Postoperative views of the same patient following allograft bone grafting of the Hill-Sachs and the reverse Hill-Sachs lesions to correct the instability.

Magnetic Resonance Imaging and Computed Tomographic Imaging

Computed tomographic (CT) arthrography, magnetic resonance imaging (MRI) (Fig. 6), or MRI arthrography are useful for determining any associated damage to the rotator cuff or Hill-Sachs lesions. Conflicting reports in the literature exist as to the sensitivity, specificity, and accuracy of these techniques, particularly in their ability to detect glenoid labral abnormalities. Early investigations of unstable shoulders with MRI were not very sensitive for the detection of labral pathology. Green and Christensen reported a prospective double-blind study of MRI findings that were correlated to surgical

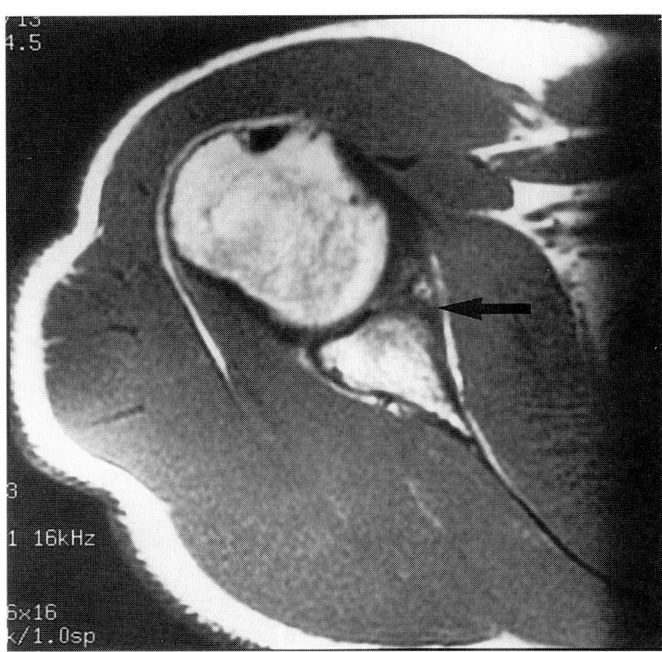

Fig. 6 Magnetic resonance imaging scan demonstrating a Bankart lesion in the anterior inferior portion of the glenoid.

reports. Diagnostic sensitivity and specificity were 75% and 100%, respectively, and the positive and negative predictive values were 100% and 41%, respectively, with an accuracy of 79%. Only 21% of labral abnormalities could be accurately classified with MRI, and it was concluded that the technique was not precise enough for surgical planning. The overall accuracy of MRI evaluation of labral lesions compared to surgical findings ranges from 76% to 90%. Techniques have improved with the development of MRI arthrography, with a reported diagnostic sensitivity of 90% and specificity of 93% for the detection of labral tears. Prospective comparison of MRI techniques has been shown to be superior to CT arthrography in the evaluation of labral pathology. A study performed by Morgan and associates prospectively evaluated MRI and CT-arthrotomography preoperatively. The findings of both investigations were confirmed at surgery. It was concluded that both techniques were equally successful in identifying biceps-labral lesions and intra-articular loose bodies. MRI demonstrated better diagnostic results in the evaluation of glenoid labral and humeral head lesions. Neither technique was consistent in the evaluation of capsular laxity. In the future, MRI may become more useful in the determination of specific injury to the capsuloligamentous complex following acute dislocation of the glenohumeral joint.

Glenohumeral Joint Stability and Classification Systems

A classification system is important in the diagnosis, prognosis, and treatment of instability. Traditional classification systems for shoulder instability are complex and based on multiple factors such as direction (anterior, posterior, multidirectional), timing (acute versus chronic), frequency (primary versus recurrent), traumatic versus atraumatic, degree (subluxation versus dislocation), voluntary versus involuntary, or habitual. All of these factors play an important role when considering management options. Unfortunately, too many classification systems exist and many do not address the exact nature of the pathology. For recurrent instability alone Cofield has estimated that between 24 and 54 subclassifications could be identified. A new anatomic classification system needs to be developed that reflects the specific pathology and more global nature of a glenohumeral dislocation.

Summary

An accurate diagnosis is required for the proper treatment of shoulder instability. Often the diagnosis can be established by history and physical examination. Additional information can be gained by radiographic imaging of the affected joint, which will help in the understanding of joint pathology. A thorough understanding of the zone of injury affecting opposite sides of the joint is critical to the development of more precise classification systems, which may guide future treatment.

Selected Bibliography

Clinical Evaluation

Bahr R, Craig EV, Engebretsen L: The clinical presentation of shoulder instability including on field management. *Clin Sports Med* 1995;14:761-776.

The classification and evaluation of the patient with shoulder instability is discussed.

Cofield RH: Physical examination of the shoulder: Effectiveness in assessing shoulder stability, in Matsen FA III, Fu FH, Hawkins RJ (eds): *The Shoulder: A Balance of Mobility and Stability.* Rosemont, IL, American Academy of Orthopaedic Surgeons, 1993, pp 331-343.

An excellent review of the main components required in the examination of the glenohumeral joint is presented, emphasizing the importance of examination of specific ligaments by detailed examination with the arm in various positions of abduction and rotation.

Gerber C, Ganz R: Clinical assessment of instability of the shoulder: With special reference to anterior and posterior drawer tests. *J Bone Joint Surg* 1984;66B:551-556.

Hawkins RJ, Bokor DJ: Clinical evaluation of shoulder problems, in Rockwood CA Jr, Matsen FA III (eds): *The Shoulder.* Philadelphia, PA, WB Saunders, 1990, pp 149-177.

The clinical evaluation of shoulder instability is discussed.

Jobe FW, Tibone JE, Jobe CM, et al: The shoulder in sports, in Rockwood CA Jr, Matsen FA III (eds): *The Shoulder.* Philadelphia, PA, WB Saunders, 1990, vol 2, pp 961-990.

Matsen FA III, Thomas SC, Rockwood CA Jr: Anterior glenohumeral instability, in Rockwood CA Jr, Matsen FA III (eds): *The Shoulder.* Philadelphia, PA, WB Saunders, 1990, pp 526-622.

Miniaci A, Dowdy PA, Fowler PJ: Clinical assessment of shoulder injuries, in Chan KM (ed): *Sports Injuries of the Hand and Upper Extremity.* New York, NY, Churchill Livingstone, 1995, pp 17-29.

The clinical assessment of shoulder injuries is reviewed.

Speer KP, Hannafin JA, Altchek DW, et al: An evaluation of the shoulder relocation test. *Am J Sports Med* 1994;22: 177-183.

Radiographic Evaluation

Garth WP Jr, Slappey CE, Ochs CW: Roentgenographic demonstration of instability of the shoulder: The apical oblique projection. A technical note. *J Bone Joint Surg* 1984;66A:1450-1453.

Green MR, Christensen KP: Magnetic resonance imaging of the glenoid labrum in anterior shoulder instability. *Am J Sports Med* 1994;22:493-498.

Gusmer PB, Potter HG: Imaging of shoulder instability. *Clin Sports Med* 1995;14:777-795.

The steps to take in evaluating the unstable shoulder to clarify the diagnosis and rule out associated pathology are presented.

Iannotti JP, Zlatkin MB, Esterhai JL, et al: Magnetic resonance imaging of the shoulder: Sensitivity, specificity, and predictive value. *J Bone Joint Surg* 1991;73A:17-29.

This study demonstrates that high-resolution MRI is an excellent noninvasive tool for the evaluation of the rotator cuff, with a sensitivity of 100% and 95% specificity. Imaging in the diagnosis of labral lesions was not well defined, with a sensitivity of 88% and specificity of 93%.

Jahnke AH Jr, Petersen SA, Neumann C, et al: A prospective comparison of computerized arthrotomography and magnetic resonance imaging of the glenohumeral joint. *Am J Sports Med* 1992;20:695-701.

Kieft GJ, Bloem JL, Rozing PM, et al: MR imaging of recurrent anterior dislocation of the shoulder: Comparison with CT arthrography. *Am J Roentgenol* 1988;150: 1083-1087.

Nelson MC, Leather GP, Nirschl RP, et al: Evaluation of the painful shoulder: A prospective comparison of magnetic resonance imaging, computerized tomographic arthrography, ultrasonography, and operative findings. *J Bone Joint Surg* 1991;73A:707-716.

This prospective study was conducted to determine which imaging modality was the most useful for preoperative assessment of patients with an unclear diagnosis and painful shoulders. The authors concluded that MRI and CT-arthrography were of equal value in the detection of glenoid labrum abnormalities and that MRI was superior to CT or ultrasonography in the evaluation of rotator cuff pathology.

Norris TR, Green A: Imaging modalities in the evaluation of shoulder disorders, in Matsen FA III, Fu FH, Hawkins RJ (eds): *The Shoulder: A Balance of Mobility and Stability.* Rosemont, IL, American Academy of Orthopaedic Surgeons, 1993, pp 353-367.

This chapter provides a good review of the imaging techniques available for the evaluation of shoulder disorders.

Palmer WE, Brown JH, Rosenthal DE: Labral-ligamentous complex of the shoulder: Evaluation with MR arthrography. *Radiology* 1994;190:645-651.

Palmer WE, Caslowitz PL: Anterior shoulder instability: Diagnostic criteria determined from prospective analysis of 121 MR arthrograms. *Radiology* 1995;197:819-825.

A prospective evaluation of glenohumeral instability with MRI-arthrography and correlation with surgical findings was performed on 121 patients. The authors concluded that MRI arthrographic abnormalities of the inferior labral-ligamentous complex correlated with anterior instability. However, capsular insertions were similar in both stable and unstable shoulders and, therefore, the role of capsuloligamentous incompetency without focal inferior labral-ligamentous abnormality was not useful in predicting instability.

Pavlov H, Warren RF, Weiss CB Jr, et al: The roentgenographic evaluation of anterior shoulder instability. *Clin Orthop* 1985;194:153-158.

Rokous JR, Feagin JA, Abbott HG: Modified axillary roentgenogram: A useful adjunct in the diagnosis of recurrent instability of the shoulder. *Clin Orthop* 1972;82:84-86.

Seeger LL: Magnetic resonance imaging of the shoulder. *Clin Orthop* 1989;244:48-59.

Classification Systems

Cofield RH, Irving JF: Evaluation and classification of shoulder instability: With special reference to examination under anesthesia. *Clin Orthop* 1987;223:32-43.

Ellman H, Gartsman GM: Pathogenesis and clinical evaluation of glenohumeral instability, in Ellman H, Gartsman GM (eds): *Arthroscopic Shoulder Surgery and Related Procedures.* Philadelphia, PA, Lea & Febiger, 1993, pp 255-271.

The definition of glenohumeral instability, along with review of pathology, clinical evaluation, and traditional classification systems, is presented. The glenohumeral classification system has been broadened to include an arthroscopic classification of shoulder instability.

Speer KP, Deng X, Borrero S, et al: Biomechanical evaluation of a simulated Bankart lesion. *J Bone Joint Surg* 1994;76A:1819-1826.

This article is an excellent review of the biomechanical consequences of ligament sectioning on glenohumeral translation, emphasizing the importance of the circle concept of joint stability. A Bankart lesion alone did not allow sufficient translation for dislocation to occur, suggesting that capsular stretch and laxity are also present in shoulders with recurrent dislocation.

Turkel SJ, Panio MW, Marshall JL, et al: Stabilizing mechanisms preventing anterior dislocation of the glenohumeral joint. *J Bone Joint Surg* 1981;63A:1208-1217.

8
Acute and Chronic Dislocations of the Shoulder

LTC Robert A. Arciero, MD and Maj Thomas M. Deberardino, MD

Acute Anterior Dislocation

The acute anterior shoulder dislocation is perhaps the most dramatic cause of instability of the shoulder. Frequently, considerable trauma is a prerequisite. The mechanism of injury usually is a force applied to a shoulder that is in an externally rotated and abducted position. This injury can occur in a fall or often can occur in contact/collision sports. For example, making a tackle with the arm abducted and externally rotated is a frequent cause of this injury in football.

Presentation and Examination

The patient presenting with an acute anterior dislocation has an easily appreciated loss of deltoid contour. The patient is in distress and usually complains of acute pain, with markedly decreased range of motion due to guarding. The affected arm is stabilized against the body with the opposite hand in a position of internal rotation and abduction. The patient will often state that the shoulder feels as though it has "slipped out of joint." It is important to obtain an accurate description of the mechanism of injury, which includes the arm position and magnitude of the forces involved, because this information will assist in determining direction.

The orthopaedist's examination of the patient must include a thorough neurovascular evaluation. Motor and sensory deficits involving the axillary nerve are noted in 5% to 35% of first-time anterior shoulder dislocations. Injuries to the brachial plexus, radial, musculocutaneous, or median nerves are much less common. Vascular injury (usually to the axillary artery) may occur either at the time of dislocation or reduction and is a reported complication in the elderly. The orthopaedist should be suspicious when examining an elderly patient with massive swelling or a rapidly expanding hematoma after an anterior shoulder dislocation. Consultation with a vascular surgeon, obtaining an angiogram, or both may be necessary. The presence and quality of both the radial and ulnar pulses are noted. A thorough neurovascular examination is imperative both before attempting reduction and after obtaining reduction. Areas of swelling, abrasion, laceration, obvious deformity or tenderness, and crepitus on palpation are noted. An evaluation of both passive and active range of motion of the shoulder, although difficult, is also performed. A detailed examination of the shoulder girdle should include inspection and palpation of the acromioclavicular and sternoclavicular joints. A suspected posterior dislocation of the sternoclavicular joint raises the possibility of significant vascular injury and should be treated as an emergency.

Radiographic Evaluation

Three views are routinely obtained to confirm the direction of the dislocation and to identify other concomitant bony in-

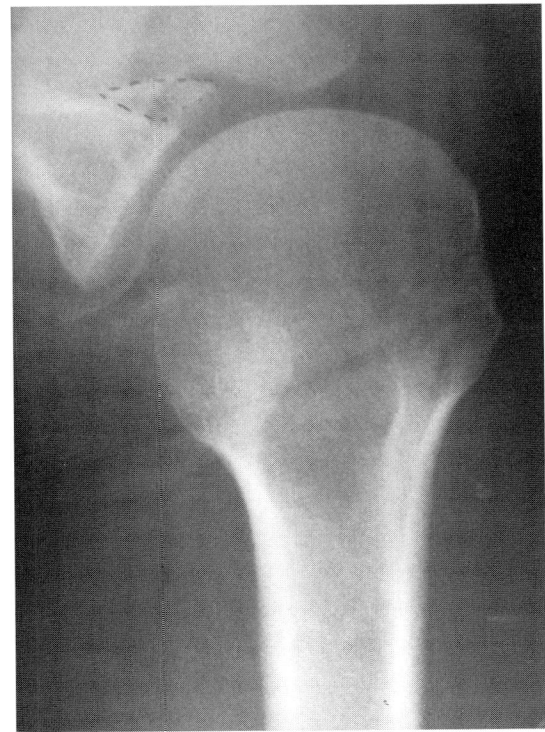

Fig. 1 West Point axillary radiograph demonstrating an acute, anterior glenoid rim fracture with displacement. (Reproduced with permission from Arciero RA: Acute traumatic anterior dislocation of the shoulder, in Bigliani LU (ed): *The Unstable Shoulder.* Rosemont, IL, American Academy of Orthopaedic Surgeons, 1996, pp 37-45.)

juries. The standard anteroposterior (AP) view, axillary or modified axillary view (West Point view), and a transcapular Y view will permit identification of associated glenoid rim fractures (Fig. 1), posterolateral humeral head defects (Hill-Sachs lesions), and fractures of the greater tuberosity (Fig. 2).

Initial Treatment

After completion of a thorough examination, initial treatment should be a closed reduction. Several techniques have been described in the literature that provide a safe means of obtaining a closed reduction. With the Stimson maneuver, the patient is placed prone on the examination table and 10 to 15 lb of weight are suspended from the wrist of the injured extremity. This gravity-assisted method may take up to 15 minutes to achieve reduction (Fig. 3, *left*). Rockwood has described a safe and efficient traction-countertraction method to obtain a shoulder reduction (Fig. 3, *right*).

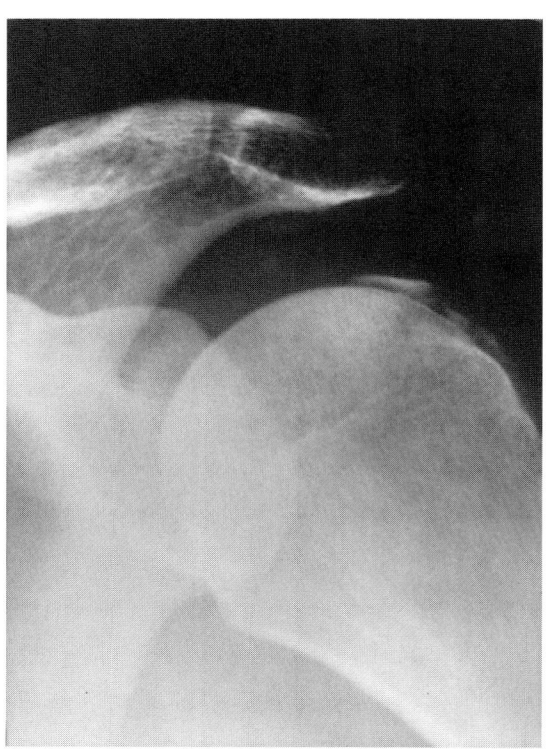

Fig. 2 Routine anteroposterior radiograph with the humerus in internal rotation demonstrating a greater tuberosity fracture after an initial dislocation. (Reproduced with permission from Arciero RA: Acute traumatic anterior dislocation of the shoulder, in Bigliani LU (ed): *The Unstable Shoulder.* Rosemont, IL, American Academy of Orthopaedic Surgeons, 1996, pp 37-45.)

Analgesia and/or intravenous (IV) sedation is used routinely in conjunction with the reduction maneuver unless the dislocation is evaluated immediately and reduced rapidly. Intravenous sedation is obtained with a narcotic or benzodiazepine. As an alternative to or in conjunction with intravenous sedation, intra-articular lidocaine injection has been described recently for analgesia. With this technique, 20 ml of 0.5% lidocaine is injected into the shoulder joint and subacromial space; 15 ml is placed into the intra-articular space, while 5 ml is placed more superficially in the subacromial space. This technique provides enough muscle relaxation and pain relief to achieve a gentle reduction.

After the reduction maneuver, the neurovascular examination is repeated and the results documented. In addition, postreduction radiographs are obtained and compared to the initial radiographs to evaluate the adequacy of the reduction and to determine whether further injury occurred during the reduction maneuver. A repeat physical examination within the first 10 days after injury is recommended. At this time, much of the acute pain and apprehension have resolved and a thorough examination may reveal concomitant soft-tissue injuries. This examination is especially important in patients older than 40 years of age. A dramatic increase in the rate of injury to other soft-tissue structures has been observed in this age group. Tears of the rotator cuff occur in 15% of patients older than 40 years who sustain an anterior shoulder dislocation. This rate increases to as high as 40% in patients older than 60 years. If at 4 weeks after injury there is no active abduction of the arm, a magnetic resonance imaging (MRI) scan and/or electromyogram may be necessary to confirm diagnosis of an associated rotator cuff tear or axillary nerve palsy.

When a suspected dislocation is witnessed on the athletic playing field, it is safe to consider an immediate gentle

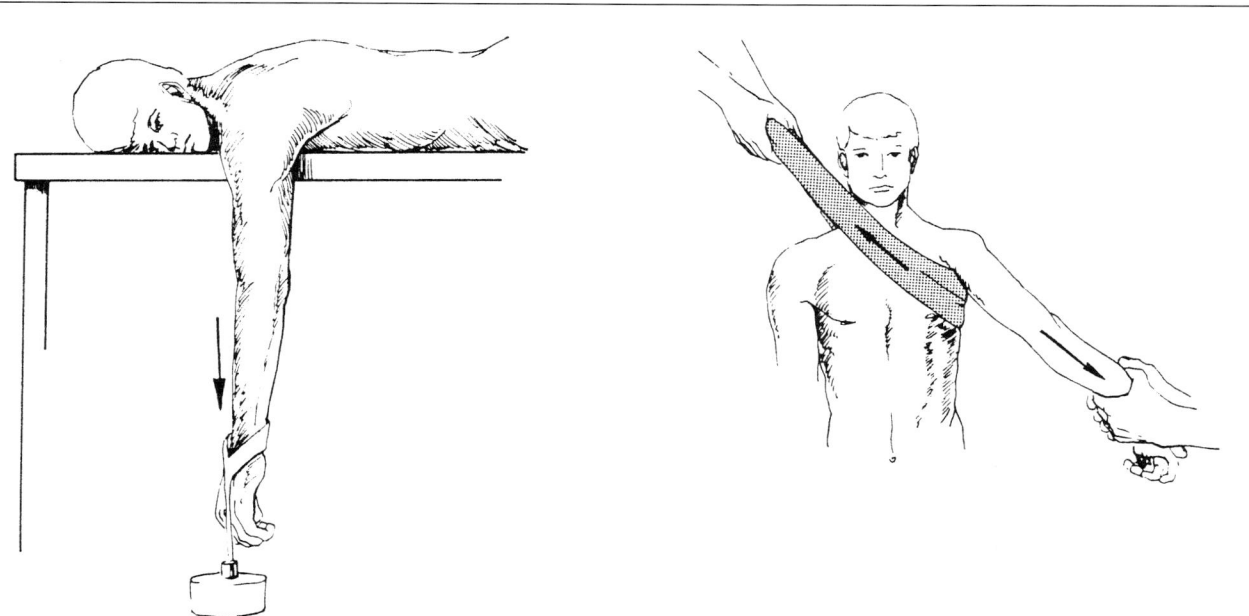

Fig. 3 Left, Gravity-assisted reduction of an anterior dislocation as described by Stimson. **Right,** Traction-countertraction method for reduction of an anterior dislocation of the shoulder. (Reproduced with permission from Warner JJP, Carborn DNM: Overview of shoulder instability. *Crit Rev Phys Rehab Med* 1992;4:145-198.)

reduction prior to obtaining radiographs. Experienced medical personnel can attempt reduction after noting the physical findings of loss of deltoid contour and the absence of crepitus. An on-the-field reduction attempt may easily be accomplished before the onset of pain and muscle spasm. Again, this procedure should not be carried out if fracture of the humeral neck or humeral head is suspected.

Natural History

Nonsurgical treatment is historically the treatment of choice for an acute, initial, traumatic anterior shoulder dislocation. This regimen usually consists of a period of immobilization, followed by a supervised rehabilitation program and restriction from return to athletics for a limited duration. The aim of this treatment is to allow soft-tissue healing, maximize strength of the dynamic stabilizers of the shoulder, and minimize recurrence.

Age and activity level are the most important prognostic factors regarding the risk of whether a patient with an acute dislocation will develop recurrent instability. In a review of over ten classic and more recent studies, the risk of recurrence is inversely proportional to the patient's age. Overall, the literature suggests a high recurrence rate in patients younger than 25 years of age who desire to continue athletic activity. In general, the risk of recurrent dislocation is as high as 95% in patients younger than 20 years of age, 50% to 75% in patients 20 to 25 years of age, less than 50% in patients older than 25 years, and less than 15% in patients older than 40 years.

In one study of over 100 patients, the overall recurrence rate was 66%. However, in athletes younger than 30 years of age the recurrence rate was 82%. Furthermore, recurrent subluxation was documented in 22% of patients. This study underscored the importance of age and activity as important factors for recurrent instability. In contrast, two studies have demonstrated much lower recurrence rates in young at-risk patients treated with 6 weeks of immobilization and a prolonged delay in return to athletic activity. Most recently, a 10-year follow-up study of 257 patients after the initial dislocation revealed a 48% recurrence rate, 20% with dislocation arthropathy, and a need for surgical stabilization in 23%. These authors found no increased success with longer periods of immobilization.

The literature regarding the natural history is confusing and is highlighted by retrospective reviews of the nonsurgical treatment. Many of these studies lack randomization, controls, and a functional performance evaluation, which is especially important in athletes and laborers. In addition, with the exception of two studies, there has been no documentation regarding recurrent subluxation after the initial dislocation. Recurrent subluxation affects functional return and frequently requires treatment after an anterior dislocation, especially in active patients.

In summary, patients younger than 25 years of age (particularly athletes) have high rates of recurrence with nonsurgical treatment. The recurrence rate will diminish in older patients to as low as 10% to 15% in patients older than 40 years.

Nonsurgical Treatment

The foundation of nonsurgical treatment includes immobilization, rehabilitation, and a delay in return to sport. Based on several studies, a period of 3 to 6 weeks of immobilization may be of some benefit to allow for soft-tissue healing. In the older patient, however, immobilization should be minimized to avoid stiffness. A supervised rehabilitation program with a delay in return to athletic activity until after full recovery of the internal rotators appears to be justified. In two earlier studies, immobilization of 6 weeks and a delay in return to full activity for another 6 weeks were thought to reduce recurrence.

Static and dynamic restraints provide for the normal stability of the glenohumeral joint. The capsule, ligaments, and bony architecture form the static system. The deltoid and muscles of the rotator cuff make up the dynamic restraint system. The goal of rehabilitation is to return the dynamic restraint system to its normal functional state while maintaining a safe environment for healing of the static restraints.

The primary goal of the initial phase of rehabilitation is to allow soft-tissue healing. Early controlled range of motion, still avoiding external rotation, may prevent glenohumeral contracture. Pendulum and Codman exercises are initiated as soon as possible. By stimulating mechanoreceptors in the capsule, early rehabilitation and motion may reduce pain. After time has been allotted for soft-tissue healing, it is imperative to maximize the efficiency of the dynamic stabilizers about the shoulder. A dysfunctional rotator cuff may result in abnormal glenohumeral motion, especially during forward elevation and abduction. This problem can lead to increased superior humeral head migration and result in secondary subacromial impingement. Therefore, isometric exercises directed toward the rotator cuff and deltoid muscle should be started as soon as pain permits. Several studies have stressed the concept of performing strengthening exercises in the plane of the scapula. This procedure is thought to minimize the tension applied to the injured anteroinferior capsular ligamentous structures and allow healing of the soft tissues.

The next phase of rehabilitation emphasizes the restoration of the dynamic stabilizers of the glenohumeral joint. The normal rotator cuff muscles work together to keep the humeral head centered within the glenoid fossa throughout the normal range of motion. Asynchronous firing of the rotator cuff muscles would also expose the static restraints of the shoulder to greater stress. A detailed rotator cuff strengthening program begins at 3 to 4 weeks. Rotator cuff strengthening initially focuses on isotonic exercises.

The external rotator muscles can be strengthened with a light dumbbell or elastic bands as the arm rotates externally about the axis of the adducted humerus. The patient lies on the uninvolved side. Low-speed isokinetic training is added after the patient begins to progress (Fig. 4, *left*).

Selective strengthening of the supraspinatus is best performed by light weight lifting in the plane of the scapula with the shoulder internally rotated (Fig. 4, *center*). The supraspinatus can also be isolated in the prone position with abduction lifts combined with slight external rotation.

The subscapularis is strengthened in a manner similar to that of the external rotators, with side-lying internal rotation lifts with dumbbells or against elastic band resistance. The patient, however, lies on the involved side (Fig. 4, *right*). As with the other cuff muscles, progressive isokinetic training is added as progress is made with isotonic strengthening.

In addition to the rehabilitation of the rotator cuff, the importance of restoring normal scapulothoracic motion,

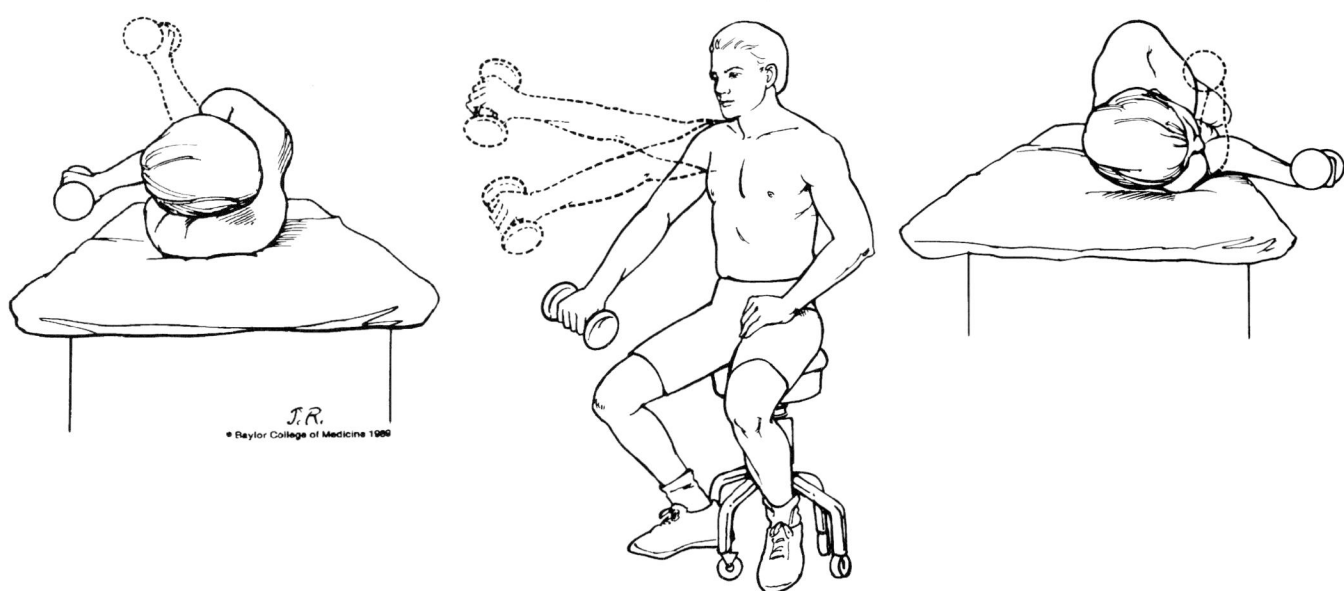

Fig. 4 **Left,** External rotation strengthening exercise. **Center,** Supraspinatus strengthening exercise. **Right,** Internal rotation strengthening exercise. (Reproduced with permission from Townsend H, Jobe FW, Pink M, et al: Electromyographic analysis of the glenohumeral muscles during a baseball rehabilitation program. *Am J Sports Med* 1991;19:264-272.)

especially in throwing athletes, has been the renewed focus of several recent studies. A stable scapula provides a solid base for rotation of the humerus and allows for maximal congruency between the humeral head and the normally positioned glenoid. The scapular strengthening regimen includes four specific exercises. Rowing emphasizes the rhomboids and the middle trapezius. The upper and lower trapezius and levator scapulae are addressed with scaption (elevation of the arm in scapular plane with external rotation of the humerus). The serratus is addressed with the push-ups with a plus (Fig. 5). The "plus" aspect of the push-up is achieved with maximal scapular protraction in the up position. The pectoralis minor and also the latissimus dorsi are strengthened with press-ups. Several investigators have shown that the biceps has an anterior stabilizing function. Therefore, it is important to incorporate strengthening of the biceps brachia into the rehabilitation program.

The goal of the final phase of rehabilitation is to prepare the athlete for return to sport-specific activities. Endurance training becomes important during this phase of rehabilitation. As the rotator cuff muscles and other muscles about the shoulder fatigue they lose their ability to perform as dynamic stabilizers. Thus, humeral head translation increases and the static restraints are exposed to greater stress.

In the past several years, plyometric exercise has been an effective addition to the shoulder rehabilitation program. Plyometric exercise is a quick powerful movement involving a prestretching of the muscle, thereby activating the stretch-shortening cycle. Many competitive sports demand athletes to perform upper extremity movements consisting of repeated stretch-shortening cycles. Therefore, plyometric exercise can be applied to the upper extremity to enhance the stretch-

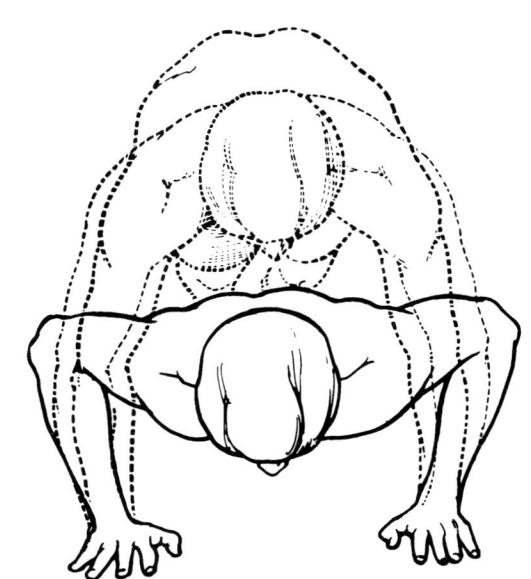

Fig. 5 Push-up plus. (Reproduced with permission from Pink M, Jobe FW: Shoulder injuries in athletes. *Clin Management* 1991;11:45.)

shortening cycle. The stretch-shortening cycle refers to the concept that muscle is stretched eccentrically before it contracts concentrically (eccentric-concentric coupling).

Plyometric exercise is theorized to improve muscle performance in several ways. Stress is applied to the elastic components by the eccentric loading. The tension of the resulting rebound force is thereby increased.

Another theory suggests the increased force production involves the inhibitory effect of the Golgi tendon organs. The Golgi tendon organs are located both at the proximal and distal myotendinous junctions and are sensitive to tension. They serve as a protective mechanism by limiting the force produced within a muscle. By desensitizing the Golgi tendon organs, the level of inhibition is raised, thereby allowing greater force production as greater loads are applied to the extremity.

Improved neuromuscular coordination may also explain the mechanism of increasing muscular performance with plyometric training. Investigators reason that the explosive movements incorporated into plyometric training may improve neural efficiency and therefore increase neuromuscular performance and maximize dynamic stabilization of the shoulder joint.

Sport-specific exercises form the nucleus of a well-designed plyometric program. Therefore, the retraining of the neuromuscular system is optimized. The upper extremity program contains four separate groups of exercises. The first group contains the warm-up exercises. The throwing movements, trunk exercises, and medicine ball wall exercises make up the remaining groups (Fig. 6).

Any rehabilitation program should stress the early and safe return of a normal range of motion, strengthening of the scapular stabilizing muscles about the shoulder, and strengthening of the rotator cuff. Despite these efforts, recurrent instability after the primary dislocation remains high in young patients, particularly athletes.

Surgical Treatment of the Initial Anterior Dislocation

Surgical treatment for recurrent shoulder instability is a well-accepted treatment option. A good or excellent outcome is achieved in most patients. Recently, the role of acute stabilization for the initial dislocation in the young athlete at risk for recurrence with nonsurgical treatment has been investigated. In several studies, arthroscopy has shown a low incidence of pure capsular tear and capsular hemorrhage in this clinical situation. Rather, several arthroscopic studies have documented the presence of a Bankart lesion and a hemarthrosis in greater than 90% of the cases after the initial traumatic dislocation. The capsulolabral complex representing the anterior portion of the inferior glenohumeral ligament has been found to be detached from the glenoid and exposing the scapular neck in the majority of cases (Fig. 7). This situation may be the optimum environment for success with an acute repair. Surgical treatment in this acute setting would take advantage of a hemarthrosis, the least degree of capsular injury, and provide an anatomic repair of the avulsed capsulolabral complex.

Arthroscopic stabilization of the acute, initial, traumatic anterior dislocation in a young athletic population has been evaluated in several studies. The presence of an acute Bankart lesion with excellent tissue quality and an unstable shoulder when examined under anesthesia have been hallmark features at surgery. Arthroscopic stabilization with early follow-up has significantly decreased the incidence of recurrent instability and the need for open stabilization procedures to treat any recurrence. In the second study of the initial anterior dislocation in cadets at the United States Military Academy (USMA), arthroscopic transglenoid suture repair was compared with nonsurgical treatment. In the arthroscopic repair group, the recurrence rate was 14% compared to 80% in the nonsurgical control group. The need for an open Bankart repair was 50% in the nonsurgical group compared to only one of 21 (4.8%) patients in the surgical group. These authors have reported on the use of arthroscopic stabilization using a bioabsorbable fixation device with similar results. Combining the results from several studies at the USMA, acute arthroscopic repair has

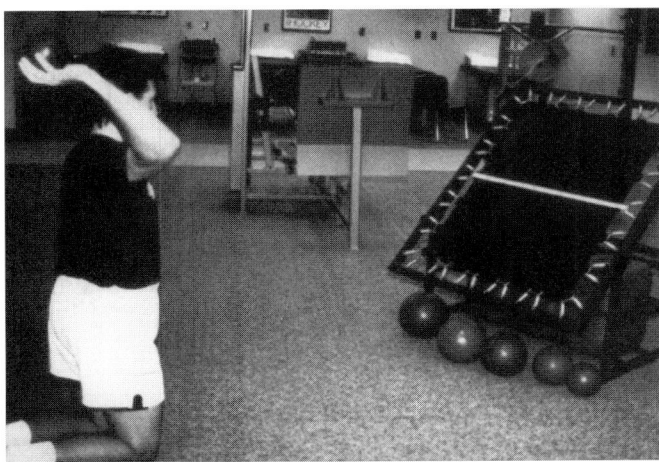

Fig. 6 Plyometric throwing drill in the kneeling position. (Reproduced with permission from Wilke IKE, Voight ML: Plyometrics for the shoulder complex, in Andrews JR (ed): *The Athlete's Shoulder.* New York, NY, Churchill Livingstone, 1994, p 563.)

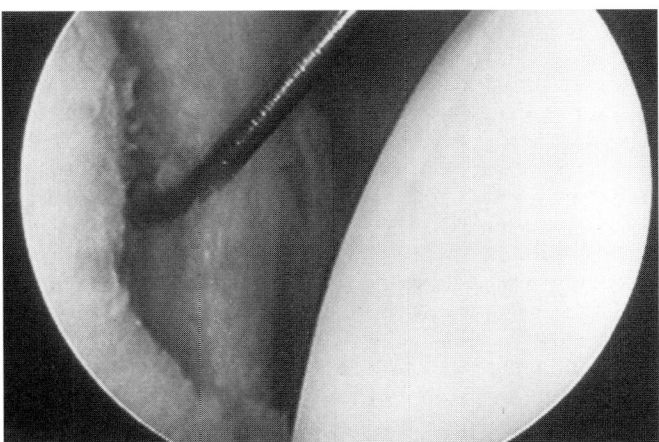

Fig. 7 Arthroscopic view of an acute, initial anterior dislocation in a right shoulder. Note the robust appearing labrum and tissue after the initial dislocation. (Reproduced with permission from Arciero RA: Acute traumatic anterior dislocation of the shoulder, in Bigliani LU (ed): *The Unstable Shoulder.* Rosemont, IL, American Academy of Orthopaedic Surgeons, 1996, pp 37-45.)

had an 88% success rate, whereas nonsurgical treatment has resulted in 85% of patients developing instability. Further long-term follow-up is necessary but it appears that the natural history has been reversed with early repair. The advantages of arthroscopic surgery appear to include significantly decreased incidence of recurrent instability, low surgical morbidity, and an increased return to preinjury athletic activity.

More recently the role of open primary surgical repair for acute, initial dislocations has been described. Preliminary results with early follow-up indicate the incidence of recurrent instability has been reduced to below 5%.

The acute management of the initial, traumatic, anterior shoulder dislocation should be tailored to the individual patient's age, activity demands and desire, and preinjury status of the shoulder. A majority of patients can be effectively managed with nonsurgical treatment as described above. Active patients between 18 and 24 years of age have a high incidence of recurrent shoulder instability. The consistent findings of a hemarthrosis and excellent tissue quality of the avulsed inferior glenohumeral ligament may constitute the ideal circumstance for acute repair. Early surgical intervention (open or arthroscopic) ensures an anatomic repair of the capsulolabral complex to the glenoid rim. Early results are encouraging and appear to significantly reduce the incidence of recurrent instability. Investigators have stressed, however, the importance of careful patient selection when considering acute surgical stabilization for initial anterior dislocations. Surgical management for the initial, traumatic dislocations can be considered for: (1) initial dislocations that require a reduction; (2) a young, athletic, high-demand patient (younger than 25 years of age) who is unwilling or unable to modify his or her lifestyle; (3) no prior shoulder subluxation or impingement history; (4) no neurologic injuries; and (5) no greater tuberosity fractures.

In addition, surgery may be indicated in the acute setting for the following specific situations: (1) a dislocation unable to be reduced by closed means; (2) a displaced greater tuberosity fracture > 1 cm; and (3) a large glenoid rim fracture > 20%.

Acute Posterior Shoulder Dislocation

Acute posterior shoulder dislocations are quite rare, accounting for only 5% of all shoulder dislocations. Unfortunately, however, the diagnosis is missed in nearly half of these injuries. Indirect forces from seizures or electric shocks are known to cause posterior shoulder dislocations. The stronger adductors and internal rotators (latissimus dorsi, pectoralis major, subscapularis, and teres major) induce adduction, flexion, and internal rotation during the generalized muscle contraction that occurs during electrical shock or seizure. These overpowering contractions lead to dorsal and posterior displacement of the humeral head with resultant posterior dislocation. A direct anterior blow to the shoulder joint or a fall on the adducted and outstretched arm can also lead to acute posterior shoulder dislocation.

Several cadaveric cutting studies have established the presence and significance of the various glenohumeral ligaments. They serve as static restraints at the limits of various shoulder motions and act synergistically to maintain normal humeral head translation and joint laxity. The posterior band of the inferior glenohumeral ligament is the major restraint to posterior translation with the arm in abduction. The anteriorly based superior and middle glenohumeral ligaments serve as secondary restraints to posterior translation with the arm abducted. In one study, however, complete dislocation did not occur until the superior and middle glenohumeral ligaments were sectioned along with the posterior band of the inferior glenohumeral ligament.

The underlying pathology of acute posterior instability is not as clearly defined in the literature as it is for acute anterior instability. A capsulolabral lesion (reverse Bankart lesion), capsular injury, a defect in the anterior medial humeral head (reverse Bankart lesion), excessive humeral head retroversion, posterior glenoid deficiency, and excessive glenoid retroversion have all been studied as risk factors for recurrent instability.

Presentation and Examination of Acute Posterior Dislocations

Patients with acute posterior traumatic dislocations of the shoulder usually complain of more pain than those with acute anterior dislocations. The arm is usually held against the body in adduction and internal rotation. This position combined with a lack of significant visual deformity can make initial recognition of a posterior dislocation difficult. A thorough directed physical examination, however, will reveal the correct diagnosis. Several key physical examination features of posterior dislocations have been described: (1) limited external rotation of the shoulder; (2) limited elevation of the arm; (3) posterior prominence of the shoulder; (4) flattening of the anterior aspect of the shoulder; and (5) prominence of the coracoid process.

In addition, a marked asymmetry of the shoulder contours can be appreciated, especially when viewing the shoulders from above and behind with the patient seated. This may be difficult in the obese or heavily muscled patient.

The hallmark feature of a posterior shoulder dislocation is limited external rotation, which occurs because the humeral head is fixed on the posterior glenoid rim/scapula. With time, the anteromedial based humeral head defect can enlarge from compression of the humeral head on the posterior rim of the glenoid.

As with acute anterior dislocations, it is essential to complete a thorough neurovascular examination on presentation. Neurovascular injuries and cuff tears, however, are much less common after posterior dislocations. The radiographic evaluation for acute posterior shoulder dislocations is the same as for anterior shoulder dislocations. A trauma series including at least three views is a prerequisite for evaluation and will again confirm the direction. This series includes an AP view, a scapular lateral view, and an axillary view. If the three views cannot be taken, or are difficult to interpret, then a computed tomographic (CT) scan is recommended.

Radiographic signs of posterior dislocations include: overlap of the humeral head on the posterior rim of the glenoid on the AP view; empty glenoid on the axillary or true lateral view; lesser tuberosity avulsion fracture; and reverse Hill-Sachs lesion of the humeral head (Fig. 8).

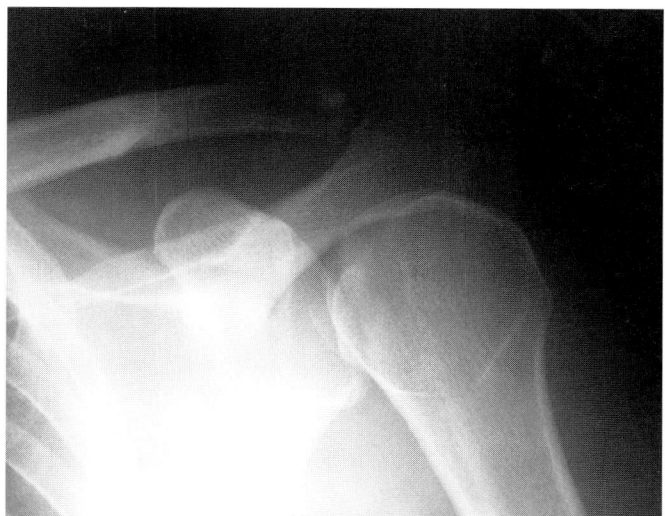 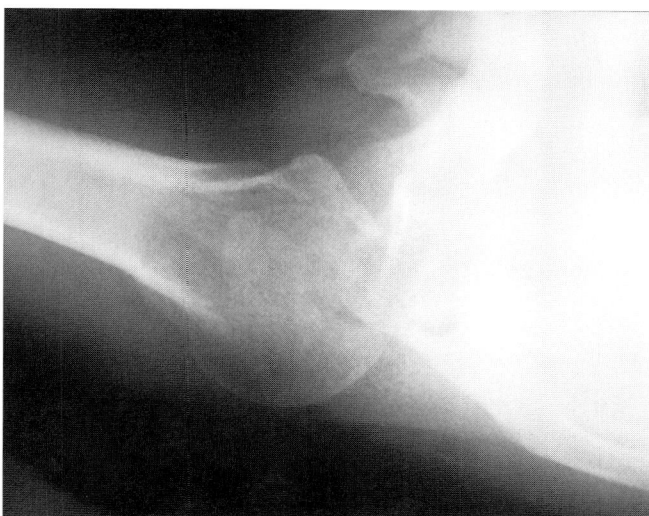

Fig. 8 Left, Anterior radiograph demonstrating overlap of the humeral head on posterior glenoid rim suggestive of posterior dislocation. **Right,** West Point axillary radiograph demonstrating a locked posterior glenohumeral dislocation with a reverse Hill-Sachs lesion involving 40% of the articular surface.

Initial Treatment of Posterior Dislocations

As with anterior dislocations, intravenous narcotics with muscle relaxants or tranquilizers are recommended prior to an attempted closed reduction. Occasionally, general anesthesia will also be necessary. Once the muscle spasm has been eliminated, a closed reduction can usually be obtained. The patient is placed in a supine position while traction is applied to the adducted arm in the line of the deformity. The humeral head is gently lifted back into the glenoid fossa. External rotation is to be avoided during this maneuver because the humeral head may be locked posteriorly on the glenoid rim. A fracture of the humeral head or shaft of the humerus can result if an excessive external rotation force is applied. The addition of lateral traction on the upper arm can help to unlock a humeral head that is locked on the posterior glenoid rim. Likewise, gentle internal rotation of the humerus can facilitate the reduction by stretching the posterior capsule and rotator cuff before the reduction is attempted.

Simple immobilization in a sling and swathe or shoulder immobilizer is indicated if the shoulder is stable after a closed reduction. A shoulder spica cast or a brace orthosis may be required if the shoulder tends to subluxate or redislocate in the adducted, internally rotated position. In this instance, the arm should be positioned in 10° of abduction, 20° external rotation, and 20° of extension to decrease the tension applied to the injured posterior structures. Six weeks of immobilization is recommended for adequate soft-tissue healing. Passive and active assisted range-of-motion exercises are then begun. Once motion has returned to normal, muscle strengthening is initiated. Specific attention is given to the rehabilitation of the external rotators.

Nonsurgical treatment for posterior dislocations appears more successful than nonsurgical treatment of traumatic anterior instability. In a review of 140 shoulders with varying patterns of instability, the investigators found the subgroup with traumatic posterior instability did better with 6 weeks of immobilization and a structured exercise rehabilitation program than the subgroup with anterior instability. Surgery is indicated after an acute traumatic posterior dislocation when there is major displacement of a lesser tuberosity fracture, a major fracture of the posterior glenoid rim involving more than 20% with an irreducible posterior dislocation, an open posterior dislocation, or a markedly unstable reduction.

An open reduction of an acute, locked posterior glenohumeral dislocation can be accomplished via standard anterior approach to the shoulder when a closed reduction is not feasible. The subscapularis tendon or the lesser tuberosity can be transferred to fill the reverse Hill-Sachs lesion if this lesion consists of more than 20% of the humeral head or there is marked instability after reduction. Transferring the lesser tuberosity into the humeral head defect places it in an extra-articular position, improving stability.

Chronic Anterior Shoulder Dislocations

When the glenohumeral joint remains dislocated for several days, a chronic anterior dislocation exists. This type of dislocation is the most difficult to manage. The difficulty of obtaining a reduction is proportional to the chronicity of the dislocation. This rare condition is seen predominantly in the elderly, the unconscious trauma patient with multiple injuries, and with patients whose mental status precludes them from seeking medical attention at the time of the injury.

There are no clear recommendations regarding when to attempt a closed reduction, when to perform an open reduction, or when to leave the shoulder dislocated. If a closed reduction is attempted, total muscle relaxation and general anesthesia are recommended. Traction and leverage should be kept to a minimum to avoid generating further fractures. As time progresses, the Hill-Sachs defect deepens as the humeral head wears from the pressure of the glenoid rim. Successful closed reduction is unlikely after 3 weeks because the soft tissues contract or remain interposed within the joint. MRI may be a useful imaging modality to evaluate any interposed soft tissues and lead to a more effective treatment plan.

An open reduction can be a very difficult procedure because the anatomy is distorted and the neurovascular structures are involved in diffuse scar formation. If function is not significantly limited and symptoms are minimal, as may be the case with more elderly patients, then leaving the dislocation alone may be indicated.

An open reduction is performed through a standard anterior approach to the shoulder. The humeral head can be disengaged from the glenoid rim with a combination of external rotation and lateral traction. Once the head is freed from the glenoid, internal rotation reduces the head. Humeral head defects larger than 40% of the surface usually require a hemiarthroplasty. The rotator cuff and biceps tendons are carefully inspected for injury and addressed appropriately during the procedure.

Recurrent instability is the most common complication of a chronic anterior dislocation. The goal of treatment after reduction is to protect the shoulder from further injury with immobilization that allows the soft tissues to heal. Rehabilitation of the injured muscles (especially the internal rotators) is begun early to minimize the risk of recurrent instability.

The largest series of chronic anterior dislocations included 44 shoulders. The injuries occurred predominantly in the elderly. Half of the dislocations were complicated by fractures of the tuberosities, head or neck of the humerus, coracoid, or glenoid. Neurologic deficits were noted in over one third. Closed reduction was successful in one third of the cases. All but one of the successful closed reductions were performed within 4 weeks of the dislocation. Open reduction was performed in one third of the patients. The remainder were either irreducible or not treated.

A recent series of 17 chronic unreduced anterior dislocations of the shoulder emphasizes that frequently this diagnosis is missed and a delay in diagnosis averaged 2.3 years. It is important to appreciate that in multiple trauma patients or if the history is unobtainable or obscured by alcoholism, coma, and dementia, the diagnosis can be significantly delayed. In this particular series, seven patients were treated without surgery despite severe functional deficits because of reasons of health or motivation. Ten patients were treated with surgery. These authors suggested that if the posterolateral humeral head defect involved less than 40% of the articular surface, and if the dislocation was less than 6 months' duration, articular surfaces may be preserved. It would then be possible to perform an open reduction through an anterior deltopectoral approach. They emphasized that an extensive release of contracted capsule and other soft-tissue distortions must be performed to allow reduction of the humerus. Compression fractures of the anterior glenoid that involve greater than 30% of the glenoid articular surface may require coracoid transfer or bone grafting to restore stability in these cases. One of the patients in this series was treated with open reduction, extensive soft-tissue and capsular release, and coracoid transfer to reestablish stability.

The significant contribution of this series comprised the nine patients treated with shoulder arthroplasty. In these patients the chronicity of dislocation was longer than 6 months and the articular surfaces were destroyed. Humeral impression fractures were often quite large, representing more than 40% of the humeral articular surface, and requiring replacement arthroplasty. In the patients treated with shoulder arthroplasty for chronic anterior dislocation of the shoulder in this series, the results were excellent or satisfactory in all and were clearly superior to those of the nonsurgical group. Shoulder arthroplasty represents another viable and successful treatment option for this complex problem.

Chronic Posterior Dislocations (Locked)

Few reports exist in the literature regarding chronic unreduced posterior dislocations of the shoulder. Hawkins and associates reviewed 41 locked posterior dislocations of the shoulder. The average duration from injury to diagnosis was 1 year. All shoulders had an associated impression fracture of the articular surface of the humeral head. The disabling lack of external rotation and subsequent impairment was related to the size of the impression defect. These patients received a variety of treatment options dependent on activity of the patient and size of the humeral head lesion. Closed reduction was successful in six of 12 shoulders. Transfer of the lesser tuberosity (modified McLaughlin procedure) was successful in four of four shoulders. Transfer of the subscapularis tendon (McLaughlin procedure) was successful in four of nine shoulders. Hemiarthroplasty was successful in six of nine shoulders. Total shoulder arthroplasty was successful in nine of ten shoulders. For seven shoulders, the deformity was accepted. The majority of patients were managed successfully once the diagnosis was established.

These authors recommend treatment based on the needs and condition of the patient, the duration from dislocation to diagnosis, the size of the impression defect, glenoid condition, and surgeon experience. No treatment is recommended if the patient is inactive and a poor surgical risk. Closed reduction followed by 6 weeks of immobilization is recommended if the dislocation is less than 6 weeks old with a small (less than 20%) articular defect on the axillary radiograph. The lesser tuberosity transfer is performed for large defects (20% to 45%) on older and longer standing dislocations (6 weeks to 6 months). Dislocations longer than 6 months or with defects involving greater than 45% of the humeral head may require arthroplasty. A hemiarthroplasty is sufficient with a normal glenoid. Total joint replacement with possible bone grafting of the glenoid is necessary for glenoid destruction and bone loss.

Keppler and associates recently reported on the effectiveness of a rotational osteotomy of the humerus for restoring glenohumeral congruity and functional activity in patients with locked posterior dislocation of the shoulder. This procedure was recommended when the articular cartilage was healthy, the humeral head defect involved less than 40% of the articular surface, and the patient was a good rehabilitation candidate. Six of ten patients had good or excellent results. The remaining four had fair or poor results.

The locked posterior dislocation of the shoulder with humeral head defects involving greater than 40% of the articular surface is difficult to manage. Prosthetic replacement has been preferred for these larger defects. Recently, Gerber and Lambert reported on four patients with very large humeral head defects. These patients were managed with reconstruction of the humeral head with an allograft segment of the femoral head. Stability was restored in all patients. Function was restored to a satisfactory level in three patients. The fourth patient, with unsatisfactory function, developed osteonecrosis of the remaining portion of the humeral head.

Selected Bibliography

Anterior Instability

Arciero RA, Wheeler JH, Ryan JB, et al: Arthroscopic Bankart repair versus non-operative treatment for acute, initial anterior shoulder dislocations. *Am J Sports Med* 1994;22:589-594.

The authors demonstrated a significant improvement in the rate of recurrence with arthroscopic treatment in a young athletic population.

Bigliani LU, Kurzweil PR, Schwartzbach CC, et al: Inferior capsular shift procedure for anterior-inferior shoulder instability in athletes. *Am J Sports Med* 1994;22:578-584.

Burkhead WZ Jr, Rockwood CA Jr: Treatment of instability of the shoulder with an exercise program. *J Bone Joint Surg* 1992;74A:890-896.

This is a noteworthy review detailing the excellent results obtainable with a well thought out rehabilitation program for patients with atraumatic instability. Most patients with traumatic instability require surgery.

Dines DM, Levinson M: The conservative management of the unstable shoulder including rehabilitation. *Clin Sports Med* 1995;14:797-816.

Flatow EL, Miller SR, Neer CS: Chronic anterior dislocation of the shoulder. *J Shoulder Elbow Surg* 1993;2:2-10.

Hawkins RJ, Mohtadi NG: Clinical evaluation of shoulder instability. *Clin J Sports Med* 1991;1:59-64.

The authors provide an excellent review of the mechanism of injury, history, and physical examination of the patient with shoulder instability. A functional classification is also reviewed.

Hovelius L, Malmqvist B, Augustini BG, et al: Abstract: Ten year prognosis of primary anterior dislocation of the shoulder in the young. *Orthop Trans* 1994;18:1066.

The natural history of primary anterior dislocations in 257 young patients followed up for 10 years is presented. The recurrence rate was 48%, the need for surgical stabilization was 23%, and dislocation arthropathy occurred in 20%.

Itoi E, Kuechle DK, Newman SR, et al: Stabilising function of the biceps in stable and unstable shoulders. *J Bone Joint Surg* 1993;75B:546-550.

Jakobsen BW, Sojbjerg JO: Abstract: Primary repair after traumatic anterior dislocation of the shoulder joint. *Orthop Trans* 1995;19:459.

Preliminary results are reported on managing 76 consecutive patients with traumatic anterior dislocations. Patients were randomly assigned to undergo conservative or surgical treatment. The dislocation recurrence rate was significantly reduced in the group that underwent primary repair.

Matthews DE, Roberts T: Intraarticular lidocaine versus intravenous analgesic for reduction of acute anterior shoulder dislocations: A prospective randomized study. *Am J Sports Med* 1995;23:54-58.

This well-designed study found that intra-articular lidocaine provided a cost-effective, efficient means of providing adequate anesthesia for successful closed reduction of acute anterior shoulder dislocations. This method may be especially beneficial when sedation is contraindicated.

Rowe CR: Prognosis in dislocations of the shoulder. *J Bone Joint Surg* 1956;38A:957-977.

This article remains a classic in the area of shoulder instability. The author determined age-related prognosis for recurrence.

Simonet WT, Cofield RH: Prognosis in anterior shoulder dislocation. *Am J Sports Med* 1984;12:19-24.

The authors of this study agree with others in noting the highest recurrence rates in athletes younger than 30 (82%). Symptomatic subluxation was also found to be significant in another 25% of the patients overall. Both age and athletic activity were demonstrated to be important factors for recurrence.

Posterior Instability

Gerber C, Lambert SM: Allograft reconstruction of segmental defects of the humeral head for the treatment of chronic locked posterior dislocation of the shoulder. *J Bone Joint Surg* 1996;78A:376-382.

An allogeneic segment of the femoral head was used to reconstruct the normal shape of the humeral head. This procedure resulted in a stable joint in four of four patients. Three patients considered the functional result satisfactory. The fourth patient developed osteonecrosis of the remaining portion of the humeral head.

Hawkins RJ, Neer CS II, Pianta RM, et al: Locked posterior dislocation of the shoulder. *J Bone Joint Surg* 1987;69A:9-18.

The authors review one of the largest series of locked posterior dislocations. They suggest tailoring the treatment plan to the individual patient's activity demands. The surgical technique indicated is based on the size of the humeral head defect.

Treatment is largely determined by demand of the patient, chronicity of dislocation, and size of the humeral head defect.

Keppler P, Holz U, Thielemann FW, et al: Locked posterior dislocation of the shoulder: Treatment using rotational osteotomy of the humerus. *J Orthop Trauma* 1994;8: 286-292.

This article presents an approach of treating locked posterior shoulder dislocations with rotational osteotomy of the humerus. Six patients had good or excellent results. The other four patients had fair (two) or poor (two) results. The poor results occurred in cases in which articular cartilage damage was advanced. This procedure is recommended only when there is less than 40% involvment of articular surface of the humeral head.

Pollock RG: Posterior instability, in Bigliani LU (ed): *The Unstable Shoulder.* Rosemont, IL, American Academy of Orthopaedic Surgeons, 1996, pp 69-78.

Rockwood CA Jr, Thomas SC, Matsen FA III: Subluxations and dislocations about the glenohumeral joint, in Rockwood CA Jr, Green DP, Bucholz RW (eds): *Rockwood and Green's Fractures in Adults,* ed 3. Philadelphia, PA, JB Lippincott, 1991, pp 1021-1179.

Rowe CR, Zarins B: Chronic unreduced dislocations of the shoulder. *J Bone Joint Surg* 1982:64A:494-505.

Although now slightly dated, this article reviews both anterior and posterior dislocations that remain unreduced and are therefore chronic. The authors review their experience with various treatment options. Treatment is predicated on activity demands of the patient, chronicity of dislocation, and size of the humeral head lesion.

9
Recurrent Anterior Instability

Jon J.P. Warner, MD and Patrick E. Greis, MD

Introduction

Instability of the shoulder has been classified according to four major criteria—frequency, direction, etiology, and degree—so that patients with similar defining features can be grouped together and examined. Unfortunately, as with many problems in medicine, shoulder instability represents a continuous spectrum of pathology that sometimes blurs distinctions between groups of patients, with some patients having characteristics of more than one group. Patients with recurrent anterior instability may have differing etiologies and degrees of instability. Within this group there may be individuals with various degrees of ligamentous laxity, differing events leading to their instability, and different pathologies responsible for their instability.

From a historic view, much of what is written about recurrent anterior shoulder instability pertains to the treatment of this condition following traumatic anterior dislocation of the shoulder, the most common precipitating event. Following this initial event, recurrent episodes of subluxation or dislocation may occur, resulting in pain and disability for the patient. It is this group of patients that is the main focus of this review. This classic pattern of injury, followed by a high rate of recurrent instability, has led many investigators to recommend various treatment regimens as a solution to this problem. As knowledge of both normal anatomy and biomechanics of the shoulder has increased, and as knowledge of the pathoanatomy involved in recurrent anterior instability has become better understood, treatment of this problem has evolved into a more organized anatomic approach.

Evaluation

The evaluation of the patient with recurrent anterior instability begins with a careful history and physical examination. Injury to the extremity typically occurs in the abducted externally rotated position. Recurrent episodes often occur following less dramatic events and may happen with minimal trauma. Patients may complain of recurrent pain in the shoulder with activities with or without an appreciation of subluxation of the joint. In the typical presentation of recurrent anterior instability, the history alone may be sufficient to make the diagnosis. However, many patients present with less than classic histories and require further evaluation in order for a diagnosis to be made. Patients who present with complaints related to recurrent anterior subluxation or dislocation following a minor traumatic event, or those who have not had a traumatic injury and who have significant physiologic laxity of the joints should be considered as a separate group. A multidirectional pattern of instability is common in this patient population. Likewise, overhead athletes with subtle anterior instability associated with activity should also be considered as a separate group. Complaints in these patients may include early fatigue, loss of throwing velocity, and pain in the late cocking and follow-through phases of throwing.

A recent study of patients older than 40 years suffering a first-time dislocation confirmed that this patient population is less likely than younger patients to have problems with recurrent instability. However, patients with continued pain or weakness 3 weeks after their injury were found to have significant associated lesions, including rotator cuff tears and neurologic injury. Of the patients who had minimal symptoms at 3 weeks, few had associated problems at 3 months. The persistence of significant pain or weakness 3 weeks after primary dislocation in this age group was believed to be an indication for further investigation with special attention to rotator cuff pathology.

In patients older than 40 years who experience recurrent instability following a traumatic dislocation, subscapularis injury should be suspected. Subscapularis avulsion may lead to weakness of internal rotation, increased external rotation, and an abnormal lift-off examination. Instability following this injury is not uncommon in the older patient.

The physical examination for patients with suspected anterior instability should include a complete shoulder evaluation. Following traumatic dislocation, evaluation of the neurovascular status of the upper extremity is important and should include assessment of axillary nerve function. Loss of active motion should not be dismissed as being secondary to pain, and a careful evaluation of brachial plexus, rotator cuff, and deltoid function is necessary. Injury to the brachial plexus following anterior dislocation is well documented.

Special provocative tests have been shown to be helpful in evaluating patients with possible anterior instability. The apprehension and relocation test has been shown to be helpful in the diagnosis of anterior instability. However, a recent report has demonstrated that true apprehension for impending dislocation must be present with this test for it to be specific for anterior instability. Pain alone with this maneuver was shown to occur with a variety of shoulder pathologies and was less specific.

In the throwing athlete, posterior shoulder tenderness, impingement signs, and loss of internal rotation secondary to posterior capsular tightness may be associated with anterior instability. In these cases, impingement is often secondary to the instability and treatment is directed at controlling or treating the instability. Increased external rotation with loss of internal rotation is often an adaptive physiologic finding common to overhead athletes. However, excessive posterior capsule tightness and loss of internal rotation may be pathologic and lead to excessive anterior translation of the humeral head.

Although the history and clinical examination remain the most important components of the work-up of a patient with recurrent anterior instability, plain radiographs are a routine part of a proper evaluation. Anteroposterior and axillary views should be performed following dislocation and are needed to document reduction of the joint and to rule out fracture. Special views such as the West Point axillary view for imaging the anterior glenoid, and the Stryker notch view for evaluating posterior humeral head impression fractures (Hill-Sachs lesions), have been advocated. The presence of anterior glenoid fractures must be considered in the treatment of this problem. Osseous defects greater than 3 mm at the glenoid rim were associated with a higher rate of redislocation following a Bankart-type reconstruction in a recent series.

Evaluation of the soft-tissue structures about the shoulder may be accomplished with computed tomography (CT) arthrography, magnetic resonance imaging (MRI), or magnetic resonance arthrography. Recent studies have shown magnetic resonance arthrography to be sensitive at detecting inferior labral ligamentous lesions, which are often associated with anterior instability. A 92% sensitivity and a 92% specificity were reported using this technique. Evaluation of the labrum using magnetic resonance arthrography was found to be superior when compared with plain MRI or CT arthrography for all types of labral pathology. The usefulness of plain MRI in routine cases of anterior instability has been questioned, and its ability to evaluate anterior labral pathology has been shown to be only moderately reliable. In straightforward cases of anterior instability, these tests are rarely necessary in order for the diagnosis to be made and are not routinely ordered.

The examination under anesthesia (EUA) may help confirm or rule out the diagnosis of anterior instability when questions remain despite a thorough work-up. Additionally, it can provide helpful information that may influence surgical technique. The EUA should involve a systematic evaluation of glenohumeral translation in the anterior, inferior, and posterior directions, with a side-to-side comparison between shoulders. The shoulder should be tested in adduction, 45° of abduction, and 90° of abduction, both in internal and external rotation. Recent biomechanical studies have demonstrated the specific roles that the superior, middle, and inferior glenohumeral ligaments (IGHL) play in shoulder stability. These studies suggest that the integrity of the shoulder ligaments can be evaluated by determining shoulder translation in various test positions and that surgical treatment should address each as needed. Generalized ligamentous laxity, or a significant inferior component of laxity demonstrated by an increased sulcus sign in external rotation, indicates the need to address capsular laxity.

In one study using a systematic method of EUA, examination findings were compared with pathology noted at arthroscopic and open surgery. All patients with pathologic evidence of instability (ie, Bankart lesion or excessive capsular laxity) were believed to have an abnormal EUA with increased glenohumeral translation. Only two of 30 patients with no pathologic evidence of instability were believed to have an abnormal EUA. This study confirmed the validity of EUA in the evaluation of the unstable shoulder, and its routine use at the time of surgical stabilization is appropriate. The use of fluoroscopy to aid in the examination under anesthesia has been advocated by some; however, routine use is probably unnecessary.

Arthroscopic Evaluation

The arthroscopic evaluation of the patient with suspected anterior instability can serve as a very useful tool in confirming the diagnosis. The arthroscopic findings of anterior labral detachment (Fig. 1), capsular injury, or damage to the articular cartilage of the posterior humeral head correlate with anterior instability.

This evidence of injury to the IGHL complex at the glenoid insertion is in agreement with the many articles describing the Bankart lesion as the most common pathology in recurrent anterior dislocation. Bankart's original work on recurrent anterior instability described detachment of the labrum from the anterior glenoid rim as the essential lesion in this problem. This conclusion was based on evaluation of pathology found at the time of surgical stabilization. However, many large series have documented cases of traumatic recurrent anterior instability in the absence of a Bankart lesion, citing capsular laxity as a possible etiology. A recent study documented a 17.2% incidence of capsular laxity as the cause of recurrent anterior instability, with 73.5% of patients having a Bankart lesion, and 9.3% having a humeral avulsion of the glenohumeral ligaments as a cause of anterior shoulder instability. The authors stressed the importance of recognizing these various injury patterns arthroscopically to ensure appropriate treatment. Laxity in the IGHL complex from injury either at the glenoid or humeral insertion, from intrasubstance failure, or from a combination of these may result in anterior instability. Biomechanical analysis of failure patterns of bone-ligament-bone specimens support this hypothesis. A recent study has demonstrated that labral detachment alone at the glenoid rim is insufficient injury to allow shoulder disloca-

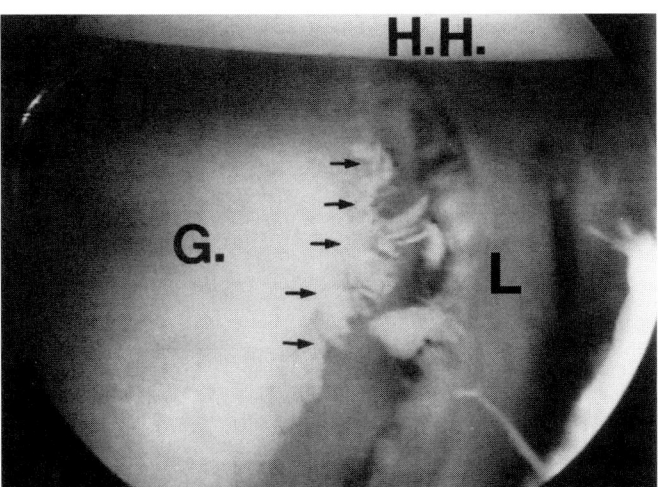

Fig. 1 Anterior labral detachment seen arthroscopically. Arrows indicate cartilage erosion. G = glenoid; HH = humeral head; L = detached labrum.

tion. Capsular injury must occur in conjunction with labral detachment to allow dislocation.

Throwing athletes with subtle anterior subluxation are less likely to have complete detachment of the anterior capsulolabral complex as a cause of their instability. Excessive capsular laxity from repetitive microtrauma has been shown to be a more common cause. Arthroscopic findings of anterior instability in these patients may include posterior labral fraying, posterior articular cartilage wear, a redundant anterior capsule, partial thickness rotator cuff tearing, and superior labral pathology.

The role that proprioception plays in recurrent anterior instability has been recently investigated. Loss of joint position and kinesthesia sense was documented in unstable shoulders using contralateral unaffected shoulders as controls. Improvements in these proprioceptive deficits was found following reconstructive surgery.

Treatment

Treatment for recurrent episodes of anterior instability usually includes a brief period of immobilization for comfort, followed by an active strengthening program to regain muscle strength and range of motion. Motion and strength should be restored prior to resuming full activity following a recurrent episode of instability. Braces, which limit abduction and external rotation, may aid in midseason treatment of some athletes who desire to return to play prior to surgical stabilization.

If no surgical intervention is planned, the patient should be counseled on possible activity restriction and the avoidance of the vulnerable position of abduction and external rotation of the shoulder. In patients unwilling to modify their activity and who do not desire surgical intervention, a discussion concerning the risk of recurrent dislocation is necessary. The risk of progressive damage to the articular structures of the joint as well as risk to neurovascular structures should be discussed.

Indications to proceed with surgical stabilization for patients with recurrent anterior instability should center on the desire to alleviate pain and disability related to recurrent subluxation or dislocation of the shoulder. Numerous open surgical procedures have been described and have been shown to be very successful in preventing the recurrence of dislocation. When redislocation is used as the benchmark for judging success, failure rates of 0 to 6% have been reported for many open procedures. However, as more careful and detailed evaluation of results have been pursued, it has been recognized that the restoration of joint stability cannot be the only criteria for judging a successful reconstruction. Loss of motion and the alteration of normal anatomy may limit the functional capabilities of a patient, particularly in the overhead athlete. Criteria for judging stabilization procedures must include the ability to return to preinjury levels of activity. In throwers and overhead athletes, this requires a near-normal range of motion without loss of external rotation motion or strength. In an analysis of outcome following the Magnusen-Stack, Putti-Platt, and Bristow procedures, loss of external rotation motion and strength were consistent findings, with external rotation motion most limited by the Putti-Platt procedure. This loss of external rotation was found to be significant in another study in that it was associated with severe osteoarthritis of the glenohumeral joint. Long-term results on the Bristow repair have revealed a reliable ability to prevent redislocation (4% failure), with loss of motion of 5° of internal rotation and 9° of external rotation in one study. However, over half of the patients noted a loss of throwing velocity, although all athletes were able to return to throwing sports. Others have reported less encouraging results with this procedure, with only three of 19 (16%) athletes able to return to throwing. In another series, 28% of patients had pain with exertion following a Bristow-type procedure, and complications related to hardware use are well documented.

Recent reports using open techniques now emphasize an anatomic approach to recurrent anterior instability. The key portion of several procedures recently reported on include the repair of the anterior capsulolabral structures back to the glenoid, and retensioning of the anterior capsule. The use of suture anchors to aid in the repair of the Bankart lesion simplifies this type of surgery and was found to be safe and effective in a recent study. Although the exact technique by which capsular tension is restored varies from report to report, the basic principles are the same. This anatomic approach addresses the pathologic findings in patients with recurrent anterior instability and does not distort normal anatomy. In an effort to minimize loss of motion associated with excessive capsular tightening, one author has presented the technique of selective capsular repair in which the inferior and superior portions of the capsule are tensioned with the arm in different positions (Fig. 2). Loss of external rotation in this series was small, with 11 of 18 maintaining symmetric motion and six of 18 having 10° or less loss of motion at 0 and 90° of abduction.

For patients who present with recurrent anterior instability following minimal or no trauma, successful treatment requires capsular plication more in line with the treatment of the multidirectionally unstable patient, despite a predominantly anterior component to their instability. An increased sulcus sign at EUA, generalized ligamentous laxity, and hypermobility of the contralateral shoulder should serve as indicators that surgical stabilization will need to address capsular redundancy and that a Bankart lesion may not be present.

A recent study has addressed the role of the rotator interval in shoulder instability. Isolated closure was successful in a patient population with anterior instability. However, these patients all had increased sulcus signs with no Bankart lesions identified. Many of the patients did not have a traumatic etiology that precipitated their symptoms. This patient population is clearly different from the classic traumatic anterior instability patient.

Arthroscopy has enhanced the ability to assess the intraarticular anatomy and pathology of the shoulder. Its use in the treatment of instability continues to evolve, and arthroscopic stabilization techniques continue to change. The rationale for arthroscopic treatment includes a more precise evaluation of pathoanatomy and the potential for decreased morbidity. A recent comparison between open and arthroscopic Bankart repairs demonstrated shorter surgical time, less blood loss, decreased postoperative narcotic use, a shorter hospital stay, and decreased cost with an arthroscopic technique.

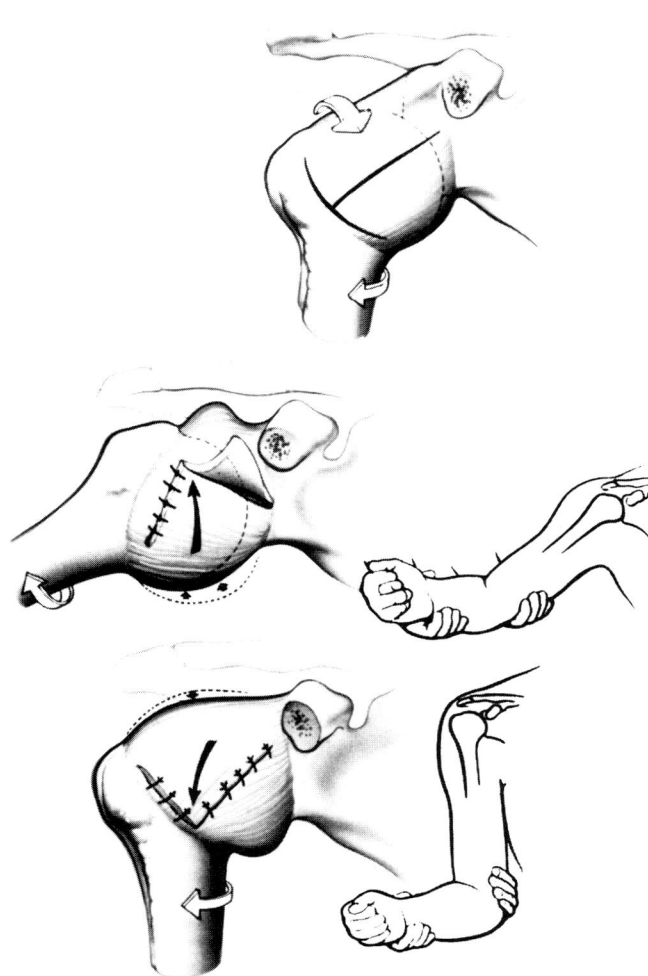

Fig. 2 Selective capsular shift. The inferior limb of the capsule is tensioned with the arm in abduction and external rotation. The superior limb is tensioned with the arm in adduction and external rotation. (Reproduced with permission from Allen AA, Warner JJP: Shoulder instability in the athlete. *Orthop Clin North Am* 1995;26:487-504.)

The earliest attempts at arthroscopic treatment involved staple capsulorrhaphy. Long-term follow-up at several institutions has shown a relatively high rate of recurrence and complications related to the use of metal staples. Staple loosening and migration have been documented, resulting in reoperation to remove loose metal. Damage to the articular surface from staples has also been reported. One study noted a much higher rate of failure when this technique was used in patients who were subluxators (53.8%) versus when used in patients who had recurrent dislocation (14.7%). Because of the high rate of failure and complications, this technique is not recommended.

The transglenoid technique of Bankart repair has been described by several authors. In some series, excellent results have been reported with low complication rates and a low incidence of redislocation. Other series have presented less favorable results, with high redislocation rates (48%) in patients treated for recurrent dislocation. Passage of transosseous sutures does pose a risk to the suprascapular nerve, and injury to this nerve using this technique has been reported.

The use of cannulated bioabsorbable implants to secure the anterior labrum and inferior glenohumeral ligament complex to the anterior glenoid has been investigated (Fig. 3, *left*). A recent report using this device showed a redislocation rate of 7% at 4-year follow-up with a very low complication rate. This rate of recurrence, although higher than what is often quoted for open stabilization procedures, is an improvement when compared with a 20% failure rate reported in another series. Patient selection was believed to be important, with the author recommending its use in the patient with discrete Bankart lesions without evidence of significant capsular injury. Exclusion of patients with hyperlaxity, multidirectional instability, poor capsular tissue, no Bankart lesion, and an atraumatic or voluntary etiology was believed to be important.

A recent report has identified a possible cause of concern with the use of this implant. A 6% incidence of intracapsular synovial reaction with a nonspecific granulomatous inflammatory response thought to be attributable to the implant was seen. All patients responded to arthroscopic lavage, debridement, and injection of an intra-articular steroid. No long-term adverse effects were identified.

Repairs using suture anchors with intra-articular knot-tying techniques are rapidly evolving (Fig. 3, *right*). Large series with long-term follow-up are needed for a more complete evaluation of these procedures, although early reports are encouraging.

Complications

As previously discussed, recurrent dislocation is the most common complication following both nonsurgical and surgical treatment of recurrent anterior instability. Surgical intervention has been shown conclusively to lower the incidence of redislocation; however, failures may occur. An analysis of patients requiring revision surgery for recurrent anterior instability demonstrated that failure to address capsular labral detachment at the glenoid rim was the most common cause of failed open instability surgery. Other causes of recurrent instability were believed to be excessive capsular laxity, technical errors of the original surgical procedure, and severe reinjury.

Other causes of overall failure of surgical treatment include incorrect original diagnosis, severe loss of motion, glenohumeral arthritis associated with loss of motion, continued pain secondary to other causes, loose or painful hardware, and injury to the neurovascular structures at the time of surgery. Many complications are specific to a certain surgical procedure and an awareness of these pitfalls can help minimize their frequency.

A recent report described four cases of subscapularis repair failure following open Bankart repair using a subscapularis incising technique. Evaluation of subscapularis integrity using the lift-off test may aid in the early diagnosis of this complication, and attention to detail in repair of the subscapularis tendon at the end of the procedure was emphasized.

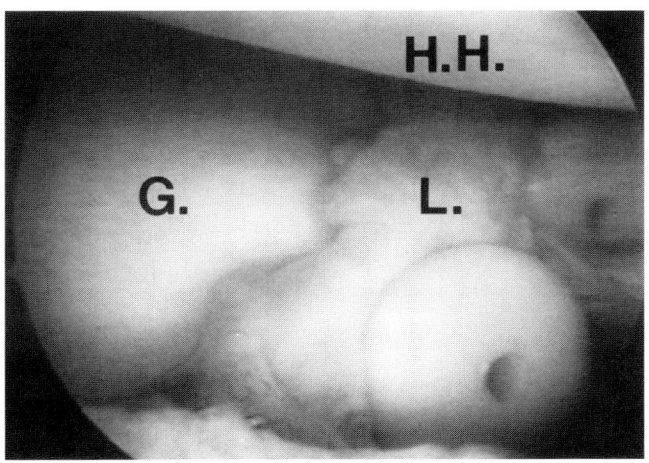 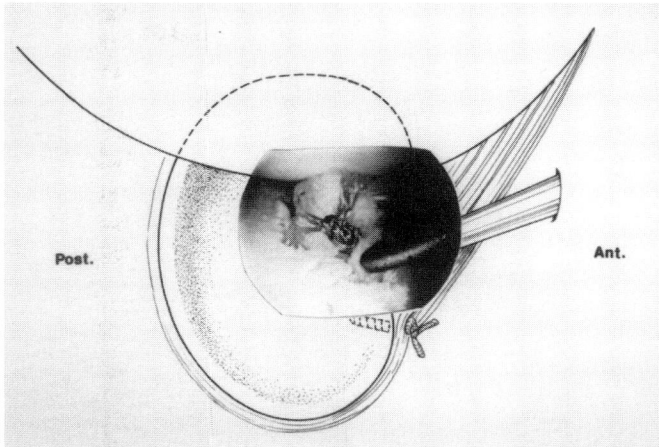

Fig. 3 Left, Repair of Bankart lesion with Suretac (Acufex Microsurgical Inc, Mansfield, MA). G = glenoid; L = labrum; HH = humeral head. **Right,** Arthroscopic repair with suture anchors and arthroscopic knots.

Treatment of the stiff shoulder following open repair has been shown to respond to open or arthroscopic release with improvements in range of motion and pain relief. Failure to address significant internal rotation contractures may result in late arthritis of the glenohumeral joint.

Arthroscopic procedures have some of the same complications as open procedures, as well as some that are unique to these techniques. Failure to eliminate instability symptoms remains the most frequent problem, with recurrence rates exceeding 40% in some series. Traumatic first-time dislocators appear to do well, with arthroscopic techniques providing some justification for early treatment of young athletic individuals who would be at high risk of recurrence. As mentioned previously, intra-articular staples may loosen or break, transosseous sutures may risk injury to the suprascapular nerve, and absorbable implants may be associated with synovial reaction.

Selected Bibliography

Evaluation

Bankart ASB: Recurrent or habitual dislocations of the shoulder joint. *Br Med J* 1973;2:1132-1133.

Bigliani LU, Pollock RG, Soslowsky LJ, et al: Tensile properties of the inferior glenohumeral ligament. *J Orthop Res* 1992;10:187-197.

Cofield RH, Nessler JP, Weinstabl R: Diagnosis of shoulder instability by examination under anesthesia. *Clin Orthop* 1993;291:45-53.

A systematic method of examining the shoulder in an anesthetized patient was described. Using this technique, increased translation on examination under anesthesia (EUA) correlated highly with pathologic evidence of instability. All patients who had pathologic evidence of instability demonstrated increased translocation on EUA.

Green MR, Christensen KP: Magnetic resonance imaging of the glenoid labrum in anterior shoulder instability. *Am J Sports Med* 1994;22:493-498.

In a prospective double-blind study, comparison of magnetic resonance imaging (MRI) with pathology noted at surgery was done in 33 patients. Of 28 surgically confirmed labral lesions, 21 were detected by imaging. Sensitivity was 75% and specificity was 100%, whereas positive and negative predictive values were 100% and 41%, respectively. Overall accuracy was 79%. The authors in this study believed that in only 21% of the patients was MRI precise enough to affect surgical planning. They concluded that for most patients with obvious anterior instability MRI was not useful in the surgical planning.

Hintermann B, Gochter A: Arthroscopic findings after shoulder dislocation. *Am J Sports Med* 1995;23:545-551.

Arthroscopic examination of 212 patients with at least one documented shoulder dislocation demonstrated anterior glenoid labral tears in 87%, capsular insufficiency in 79%, Hill-Sachs compression in 68%, glenohumeral ligament insufficiency in 55%, complete rotator cuff tendon tears in 14%, posterior glenoid labral tears in 12%, and superior labral lesions in 7%. Arthroscopic examination of the shoulder before open surgery was believed to be an important diagnostic tool.

Kvitne RS, Jobe FW: The diagnosis and treatment of anterior instability in the throwing athlete. *Clin Orthop* 1993;291:107-123.

Lephart SM, Warner JJP, Borsa PA, et al: Proprioception of the shoulder joint in healthy, unstable, and surgically repaired shoulders. *J Shoulder Elbow Surg* 1994;3:371-380.

Using a proprioception testing device, differences between healthy and unstable shoulders were identified. These abnormalities diminished following surgical stabilization of the shoulder. The authors thought that a proprioceptive deficit was a possible contributor to shoulder instability.

Speer KP, Deng X, Borrero S, et al: Biomechanical evaluation of a simulated Bankart lesion. *J Bone Joint Surg* 1994;76A:1819-1826.

Ungersbock A, Michel M, Hertel R: Factors influencing the results of a modified Bankart procedure. *J Shoulder Elbow* 1995;4:365-369.

Forty-two shoulders in 40 patients were operated on for anterior instability. Pathoanatomic findings at surgery were a Bankart lesion in 42 shoulders, a Hill-Sachs lesion in 31, and a rounded or defective anterior glenoid rim in 29. An osseous defect of the glenoid rim greater than 3 mm was found in three patients, one of whom had a redislocation after surgery.

Warner JJ, Deng XH, Warren RF, et al: Static capsuloligamentous restraints to superior-inferior translation of the glenohumeral joint. *Am J Sports Med* 1992;20: 675-685.

In a cadaveric study, ligamentous restraints to humeral head translation were tested. The primary restraint to inferior translation of the adducted shoulder was the superior glenohumeral ligament. With progressive abduction, the anterior and posterior portions of the inferior glenohumeral ligament became static stabilizers, resisting inferior translation. The authors believed that these results indicated that the clinical assessment of glenohumeral translation in the superior-inferior plan should be performed in multiple positions of abduction and rotation.

Wolf EM, Cheng JC, Dickson K: Humeral avulsion of glenohumeral ligaments as a cause of anterior shoulder instability. *Arthroscopy* 1995;11:600-607.

A prospective study of 64 shoulders was undertaken to determine intra-articular pathology related to anterior instability. Six patients (9.3%) were found to have a humeral avulsion of the glenohumeral ligaments. Eleven shoulders had generalized capsular laxity (17.2%), and 47 had a Bankart lesion (73.5%). The authors emphasized the need to recognize humeral avulsion of the glenohumeral ligaments as a possible cause of anterior instability. This lesion was readily recognized arthroscopically and appropriate treatment involved repairing the ligaments on the humeral side.

Treatment

Banas MP, Dalldorf PG, Sebastianelli WJ, et al: Long-term follow up of the modified Bristow procedure. *Am J Sports Med* 1993;21:666-671.

Bigliani LU, Kurzweil PR, Schwartzbach CC, et al: Inferior capsular shift procedure for anterior-inferior shoulder instability in athletes. *Am J Sports Med* 1994;22:578-584.

Anatomic repair in 68 shoulders was performed, addressing capsular laxity in patients with anterior inferior instability. Twenty-one of the 68 had a Bankart lesion. Using this approach, 50% of throwing athletes were able to return to prior competitive levels. Loss of external rotation averaged 7°. Redislocation rate after violent falls was 2.9%. The authors recommended this approach to address capsular laxity in patients with anterior inferior instability.

Coughlin L, Rubinovich M, Johansson J, et al: Arthroscopic staple capsulorrhaphy for anterior shoulder instability. *Am J Sports Med* 1992;20:253-256.

Edwards DJ, Hoy G, Saies AD, et al: Adverse reactions to an absorbable shoulder fixation device. *J Shoulder Elbow Surg* 1994;3:230-233.

The authors report on their experience using the Suretac bioabsorbable implant. They reported a 6% incidence of intercapsular synovial reaction that required arthroscopic lavage and debridement. These patients reported increasing pain and loss of shoulder motion after insertion of the bioabsorbable device for treatment of damaged glenoid labrum. Following arthroscopic lavage and debridement, all patients recovered satisfactorily. Histologically, a granulomatous reaction was identified in all cases. No long-term side effects were encountered.

Field LD, Warren RF, O'Brien SJ, et al: Isolated closure of rotator interval defects for shoulder instability. *Am J Sports Med* 1995;23:557-563.

Goldberg BJ, Nirschl RP, McConnell JP, et al: Arthroscopic transglenoid suture capsulolabral repairs: Preliminary results. *Am J Sports Med* 1993;21:656-664.

Grana WA, Buckley PD, Yates CK: Arthroscopic Bankart suture repair. *Am J Sports Med* 1993;21:348-353.

Twenty-seven patients were followed for an average of 36 months after arthroscopic suture stabilization for anterior instability. Results were excellent in ten patients, good in five, and poor in 12. Thirteen of 27 returned to their previous level of activity. Twelve patients were rated as failed, all having recurrent instability of the shoulder. Failures were associated with shorter immobilization periods (less than 3 weeks), and recurrent dislocations. The authors recommended caution in the use of this arthroscopic procedure.

Green MR, Christensen KP: Arthroscopic versus open Bankart procedures: A comparison of early morbidity and complications. *Arthroscopy* 1993;9:371-374.

A retrospective analysis of open versus arthroscopic Bankart repairs was undertaken. Twenty arthroscopic and 18 open Bankart procedures were examined. Using an arthroscopic method, there was a 1.8-fold decrease in surgical time, a tenfold decrease in blood loss, and a 2.5-fold decrease in postoperative narcotic use when compared with the open procedure. Hospital stay averaged 3.1 days with the open procedure compared with 1.1 days with the arthroscopic method. The authors concluded that the arthroscopic Bankart procedure offered significant improvements in surgical time, perioperative morbidity, and complications compared with the open technique.

Hawkins RJ, Angelo RL: Glenohumeral osteoarthritis: A late complication of the Putti-Platt repair. *J Bone Joint Surg* 1990;72A:1193-1197.

Jobe FW, Giangarra CE, Kvitne RS, et al: Anterior capsulolabral reconstruction of the shoulder in athletes in overhand sports. *Am J Sports Med* 1991;19:428-434.

Lane JG, Sachs RA, Riehl B: Arthroscopic staple capsulorrhaphy: A long-term follow-up. *Arthroscopy* 1993;9:190-194.

Fifty-four shoulders with recurrent anterior instability were evaluated following arthroscopic staple capsulorrhaphy. Follow-up averaged 39 months. A 33% rate of postoperative instability was encountered. Ten patients subsequently underwent an open reconstructive procedure. Loose staples were encountered in 15%. The authors believed that caution should be taken when considering arthroscopic staple capsulorrhaphy because of the high recurrence rate and problems with intra-articular staples. Consideration of routine staple removal was suggested.

Levine WN, Richmond JC, Donaldson WR: Use of the suture anchor in open Bankart reconstruction: A follow-up report. *Am J Sports Med* 1994;22:723-726.

The authors reported their experience using suture anchors to perform a modified Bankart repair. They believed that the suture anchor simplified the Bankart reconstruction. In an average follow-up of 3 years, 26 of 32 patients had returned to presurgery levels of activity without recurrent dislocation or subluxation. Four had been lost to follow-up. Ninety-three percent of the patients in the study objectively had excellent or good results. There were two failures with recurrent anterior dislocation. No complications related to the suture anchors were found. The authors stressed careful attention to anchor placement at the junction at the articular cartilage and the glenoid neck to avoid technical failure.

Morgan C: Arthroscopic transglenoid suture repair. *Op Tech Orthop* 1991;1:171-179.

Neviaser RJ, Neviaser TJ: Recurrent instability of the shoulder after age 40. *J Shoulder Elbow Surg* 1995;4:416-418.

Eleven patients with recurrent anterior instability following a traumatic anterior dislocation were studied. All patients had ruptured the subscapularis and anterior capsule from the lesser tuberosity. No Bankart lesions were seen. Stability of the shoulder was restored by repairing the ruptured tendons and capsule to the tuberosities. Recurrent instability of the shoulder in this group was believed to be caused by the injury to the subscapularis and capsular rupture from the tuberosities without additional injury to the ligament labral complex at the glenoid.

Norlin R: Use of Mitek anchoring for Bankart repair: A comparative, randomized prospective study with traditional bone sutures. *J Shoulder Elbow Surg* 1994;3:381-385.

Regan WD Jr, Webster-Bogaert S, Hawkins RJ, et al: Comparative functional analysis of the Bristow, Magnuson-Stack, and Putti-Platt procedures for recurrent dislocation of the shoulder. *Am J Sports Med* 1989;17:42-48.

Warner JJP, Johnson D, Miller M, et al: Technique for selecting capsular tightness in repair of anterior-inferior shoulder instability. *J Shoulder Elbow Surg* 1995;4:352-364.

Warner JJP, Miller MD, Marks P, et al: Arthroscopic Bankart repair with the Suretac device: Part I. Clinical observations. *Arthroscopy* 1995;11:2-13.

The authors report their experience using the bioabsorbable Suretac implant. In patients with anterior instability, a 7% redislocation rate was reported at 4-year follow-up. The authors stressed patient selection when using this device and recommended it for patients with discrete Bankart lesions without evidence of significant capsular injury. Patients with hyperlaxity, multidirectional instability, poor capsular tissue, or atraumatic or voluntary etiology of instability were excluded.

Wirth MA, Blatter G, Rockwood CA Jr: The capsular imbrication procedure for recurrent anterior instability of the shoulder. *J Bone Joint Surg* 1996;78A:246-259.

Wolf EM: Arthroscopic capsulolabral repair using suture anchors. *Orthop Clin North Am* 1993;24:59-69.

Wredmark T, Tornkvist H, Johansson C, et al: Long-term functional results of the modified Bristow procedure for recurrent dislocations of the shoulder. *Am J Sports Med* 1992;20:157-161.

Complications

Greis PE, Dean M, Hawkins RJ: Subscapularis tendon disruption after Bankart reconstruction for anterior instability. *J Shoulder Elbow Surg* 1996;5:219-222.

The authors report their experience with four patients who had subscapularis tendon disruption after open Bankart reconstruction. In patients who had a significant injury in the early postoperative period, a careful evaluation is needed to rule out this injury. Findings of increased external rotation, recurrent instability, loss of internal rotation strength, and an abnormal lift-off examination were consistent with this injury. Prompt treatment including open surgical repair was recommended.

Hawkins RH, Hawkins RJ: Failed anterior reconstruction for shoulder instability. *J Bone Joint Surg* 1985;67B:709-714.

MacDonald PB, Hawkins RJ, Fowler PJ, et al: Release of the subscapularis for internal rotation contracture and pain after anterior repair for recurrent anterior dislocation of the shoulder. *J Bone Joint Surg* 1992;74A:734-737.

Ten patients who had internal rotation contracture and pain after an anterior repair for recurrent dislocation were treated by release of the subscapularis muscle. The release was done at an average of 11 years following the original procedure. Most of the patients had a previous Putti-Platt repair. After open release of the subscapularis, patients had less pain in the shoulder, with an average increase in external rotation of 27°. The authors believed release to be an effective means of alleviating the pain and functional limitations associated with a significant internal rotation contracture.

Norris TR: Complications following anterior instability repairs, in Bigliani LU (ed): *Complications of Shoulder Surgery*. Baltimore, MD, Williams & Wilkins, 1993, pp 98-116.

Rowe CR, Zarins B, Ciullo JV: Recurrent anterior dislocation of the shoulder after surgical repair: Apparent causes of failure and treatment. *J Bone Joint Surg* 1984;66A:159-168.

10

Multidirectional and Posterior Instability of the Shoulder

Roger G. Pollock, MD

Historically, much of the literature on glenohumeral instability had focused on locked anterior dislocations, because these represent the most common type of shoulder instability. Over the past 10 to 20 years, however, it increasingly has been realized that other types of instability, such as subluxation or instabilities in other directions (posterior or multidirectional), are more common than previously had been appreciated. More attention has been given to the importance of correctly diagnosing this type of subtle instability in these less common directions. Basic research has attempted to explain the underlying mechanisms for different types of glenohumeral instability, and clinical studies have suggested more effective means of diagnosis and treatment for these different entities. Understanding of glenohumeral instability remains incomplete, although it continues to advance through further efforts in this field. The etiology, diagnosis, and treatment of multidirectional and posterior instabilities of the glenohumeral joint will be discussed in this chapter.

Multidirectional Instability

Multidirectional instability is best defined as symptomatic glenohumeral instability in all three directions: anterior, posterior, and inferior. This type of instability is to be distinguished from unidirectional instability, in which the shoulder dislocates or subluxates in only one direction, as well as from bidirectional instability, in which dislocation or subluxation occurs in two directions (anteriorly and inferiorly or posteriorly and inferiorly). True multidirectional instability is a global type of instability, which can occur in one of three patterns: anteroinferior dislocation with posterior subluxation, posteroinferior dislocation with anterior subluxation, or dislocation in all three directions. It has been correctly pointed out that there can be a wide range of translations with passive manipulation in normal asymptomatic shoulders, and that normal laxity can be quite variable. However, in multidirectional instability, the excessive translations of the humeral head on the glenoid with use of the arm produce symptoms in the individual. Thus, the definition refers not to the amount of native laxity in the shoulder, but rather to the occurrence of symptoms when the shoulder subluxates or dislocates in the three directions. Excessive symptomatic translations in all three directions are necessary for the diagnosis of multidirectional instability of the shoulder.

Etiology

There is no single etiology for multidirectional instability of the shoulder. A number of etiologic factors may be involved in the production of multidirectional instability: a degree of inherent ligamentous laxity, one or several episodes of major trauma, and repetitive microtrauma to the shoulder over a period of years. Many patients with multidirectional instability of the shoulder will possess generalized ligamentous laxity and fit the classic stereotype for this diagnosis: atraumatic and bilateral involvement of the shoulder with hyperextensibility of other joints. However, there is a significant subset of patients with multidirectional shoulder instability who do not have generalized ligamentous laxity, but only "loose shoulders." Frequently, they are athletes who repetitively stress the shoulder capsule with sports activities such as throwing, gymnastics, or swimming. These patients are thought to stretch out the shoulder ligaments selectively by their overhead sports activities. Finally, even in some patients with a shoulder that is thought to be "at risk" for developing multidirectional instability, a frank instability event will occur only with significant trauma to the shoulder. Thus, there may be an overlap of the three etiologic groups or an interplay between these factors in producing a multidirectionally unstable shoulder. To limit the scope of multidirectional instability to those with atraumatic instability on the basis of generalized ligamentous laxity would omit a significant subset of patients with the problem. In a clinical population, it is precisely this sort of "overlap" patient who may have the instability underdiagnosed and be treated inappropriately with a unidirectional repair for a (missed) multidirectional instability.

In the past decade, a number of biomechanical studies have advanced the understanding of inferior and multidirectional instability. In a selective ligament-sectioning study of the capsuloligamentous restraints to superior-inferior translation of the glenohumeral joint, it was found that the primary restraint to inferior translation of the adducted shoulder was the superior glenohumeral ligament. Progressive abduction of the shoulder resulted in the inferior glenohumeral ligament complex becoming the primary static stabilizer against inferior instability. In another biomechanical study, examining the role of the rotator interval capsule in passive motion and stability of the shoulder, instability occurred inferiorly and posteriorly after sectioning the rotator interval capsule. On the other hand, imbrication of that region of the capsule resulted in decreased translation in the inferior and posterior directions, leading the authors to conclude that imbrication of the rotator interval capsule might help to control inferior and posterior instability.

Scapular inclination has also been implicated as a factor in inferior instability of the shoulder. In an experimental model, increased scapular inclination was found to prevent inferior displacement of the humeral head. The authors concluded that this probably occurs because of a bony cam effect that causes tightening of the superior capsule. Other investigators have also studied the effect of scapular mechanics on involuntary inferior and multidirectional instability. Patients with multidirectional instability were found to have not only excessive excursion and sliding motion at the glenohumeral joint, but also diminished scapular abduction and external rotation with the arm progressively abducted, as compared with normal shoulders. Thus, patients with multidirectional instability may also have an abnormal scapulohumeral rhythm and altered scapular muscle function.

Biochemical abnormalities may play a role in the development of multidirectional instability. Authors of one report compared the total collagen content in "loose shoulders" treated with an inferior capsular shift with that in normal controls. Although there was no significant difference in the total collagen content, the multidirectionally unstable shoulders had capsular collagen with less cross-linking, suggesting that these shoulders produce relatively immature collagen. In another study, no differences were found in the amount of type I and type III collagen between multidirectional instability patients and a normal control group. However, the synthesis of type III collagen in vitro was higher in the skin fibroblasts of the patients in the multidirectional instability group. Thus, some patients with multidirectional instability may have abnormal collagen turnover or an altered biochemical response to repetitive microtrauma.

Diagnosis

Patients with multidirectional instability may present in several ways. Those with extremely hypermobile shoulders may experience episodes of instability wholly atraumatically and subluxation or dislocation may begin merely with the performance of activities of daily living. Another group, in which the instability develops gradually though repetitive use in sports such as swimming or gymnastics, may experience the onset of instability with relatively minor trauma, such as in the performance of their sport. Thus, the shoulder may begin to subluxate or become symptomatic with the performance of high-demand activities, such as throwing or swimming the butterfly stroke. If a dislocation has occurred, the shoulder may have spontaneously reduced or have been self-reduced in the multidirectional instability patients. Finally, a smaller subgroup of these patients will present only after major trauma to the shoulder, such as with a dislocation occurring during a wrestling takedown or a football tackle. This entity is seen in males as frequently as in females, and in athletes as frequently as in sedentary loose-jointed patients. Some of these patients will have a family history of shoulder instability.

The patient's symptoms may suggest the directions of instability involved. Pain while carrying objects, such as suitcases, with the arm at the side is typical of inferior instability. Such activities may also elicit paresthesias in the hand, probably from traction on the brachial plexus. Symptoms with the arm in a flexed, adducted, and internally rotated position, such as with pushing a heavy door open, suggest a component of posterior instability. Similarly, athletes with symptoms during the follow-through phase of a throw or swimming stroke are likely to have an element of posterior instability. Anterior instability is manifested by symptoms that occur when the arm is overhead in an abducted and externally rotated position, such as with sleeping with the arm overhead or tucked behind the head. Athletes with a component of anterior instability will typically have symptoms during the cocking phase of a throw or serve in tennis. These movements may produce frank instability (dislocation or subluxation) or, in more subtle cases, they may produce pain or a "dead arm" sensation.

On physical examination, there may be signs of generalized ligamentous laxity: hyperextension of the elbow, the ability to appose the thumb to the forearm, hyperextension of the metacarpophalangeal joints, and hypermobility of the patella. Some of these patients may additionally have hypermobility of the acromioclavicular and sternoclavicular joints. These regions, in particular the acromioclavicular joint, must be carefully examined, because this joint and not the "loose shoulder" may be responsible for the patient's symptoms. The hallmark of inferior and multidirectional instability is the sulcus sign (Fig. 1). This sign should be tested by pulling down with the arm at the side and then by stressing the shoulder inferiorly with the arm abducted to 90°. Patients with multidirectional instability may have multiple positive findings with provocative stress testing, using the anterior apprehension and posterior stress tests, the relocation maneuver, and anterior and posterior drawer tests. The examiner will measure the translations produced by these tests, but more importantly will ascertain whether these translations correlate with the patient's symptoms.

It can be difficult to determine the primary direction of the instability on physical examination. If there is muscle guarding, it can be difficult to elicit meaningful information from the provocative testing. Examination of the asymptomatic contralateral shoulder can provide some data on the relative degree of shoulder laxity. Care must be taken on examination to distinguish between a maneuver that produces a subluxation and one in which a subluxated humeral head is reduced. Using the coracoid process and the posterolateral corner of the acromion as landmarks can be helpful in making such determinations. In light of the difficulty of the examination, multiple office examinations on sequential visits can be quite valuable in assessing patients with suspected shoulder instability.

A subgroup of patients with multidirectional instability will be able to demonstrate the instability on command by placing the shoulder into a provocative position. For example, by placing the arm into combined flexion, adduction, and internal rotation, the individual can produce a posterior subluxation. These "positional dislocators" must be distinguished from willful voluntary dislocators, whose shoulder instability is a manifestation of an underlying emotional or psychiatric problem. Distinguishing between these two groups often requires several office visits, during which the family dynamics are observed (especially in the case of voluntary dislocators in the adolescent age group). It is crucial to discover and fully characterize voluntary components of instability, because willful voluntary dislocators will frustrate treatment and may require attention beyond the scope of the orthopaedic surgeon.

Plain radiographs of patients with multidirectional instability are usually normal, but occasionally may demonstrate humeral head defects or lesions of the glenoid, such as bony rim avulsions, reactive changes, or erosions from multiple

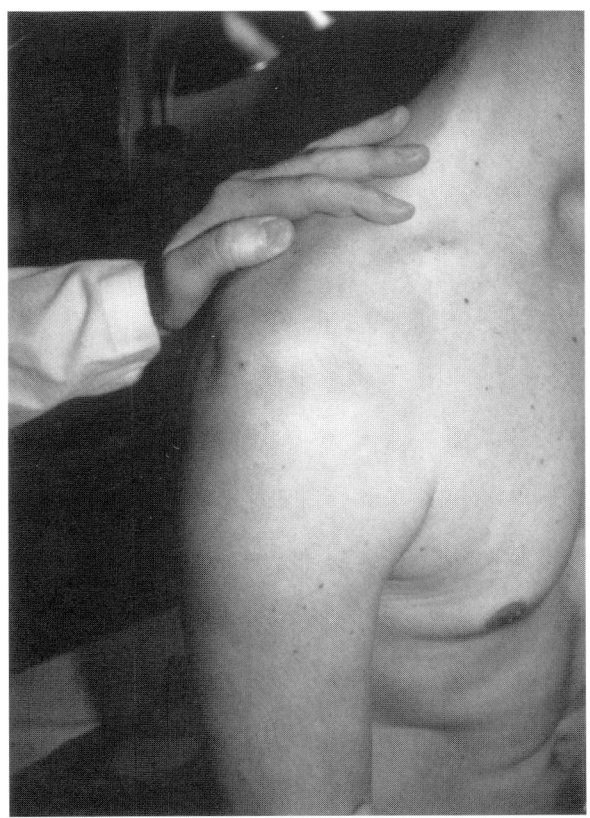

Fig. 1 The sulcus sign is demonstrated here by pulling downward on the neutrally positioned arm. The dimple or sulcus that is seen is a hallmark of inferior and multidirectional instability.

instability events. Computed tomography (CT) arthrograms will demonstrate capsular redundancy and labral detachments (although labral avulsion is less common in this group); however, these studies are not routinely obtained. CT or CT arthrograms are usually reserved for selected cases: when the axillary radiograph suggests bony abnormalities of the glenoid; in litigation cases where additional documentation may later be helpful; and in revision cases to assess the anterior labrum, particularly if a posterior approach is planned. Magnetic resonance imaging is not very useful for showing capsular redundancy and rarely is obtained in the evaluation of patients with suspected multidirectional instability. Stress radiographs and fluoroscopic examination can demonstrate the various directions of the instability and were helpful early on in correlating the examination with quantitative measurements, but generally are no longer used.

Treatment

The initial treatment of multidirectional instability is nonsurgical, combining activity modification (ie, the avoidance of provocative activities) and a prolonged exercise program. The exercises are aimed at strengthening the deltoid and rotator cuff muscles below the horizontal level, as well as the muscles that stabilize the scapula. In one study on the efficacy of treating shoulder instability with an exercise program, it was found that a high percentage of patients with atraumatic subluxation (80%) could be treated successfully with exercises. Moreover, 88% of the shoulders with involuntary multidirectional subluxations on an atraumatic basis had good or excellent results with conservative treatment. Occasionally, patients with multidirectional instability may develop a secondary subacromial inflammation. The patients may benefit from a subacromial cortisone injection, which may reduce their subacromial symptoms and allow them to resume their exercise program.

Surgical treatment is recommended for patients with significant and disabling pain and instability despite a prolonged period of rehabilitative exercises. During the prolonged rehabilitation period, the surgeon is better able to assess the patient's motivation and ability to cooperate with postoperative restrictions and rehabilitation. Patients with suspected willful voluntary instability, in which the shoulder instability is a manifestation of an emotional or psychiatric disorder, are not appropriate surgical candidates because they will find a means of redislocation postoperatively. The difficulty lies in correctly identifying these individuals preoperatively. Similarly, patients who are using the shoulder instability for other means of secondary gain may also be inappropriate candidates. On the other hand, patients with the "positional type" of voluntary instability, who are able to demonstrate their shoulder instability by placing the arm into the provocative position but do not have an underlying agenda, can benefit from surgical reconstruction.

The most widely used surgical repair for multidirectional instability is the inferior capsular shift procedure. In this repair, the capsule is detached from the neck of the humerus and shifted in a superolateral direction. This procedure reduces the inferior capsular redundancy and diminishes the capsular volume on all three sides of the joint (Fig. 2). Because the primary pathology in multidirectional instability is thought to be a loose, redundant capsule, this procedure directly addresses the major pathology. The capsule is overlapped or reinforced on the side of the approach and appropriately tensioned on all three sides of the joint to reestablish a balance of the soft tissues. The side of the approach is chosen, based on the direction of greatest instability. When the shoulder dislocates anteriorly and inferiorly and only subluxates posteriorly or when it dislocates in all three directions, an anterior approach is employed, using a concealed anterior axillary incision. When the shoulder dislocates posteriorly and inferiorly and only subluxates anteriorly, the procedure is performed through a posterior approach.

The inferior capsular shift is a laterally-based or humeral-side capsulorrhaphy. The joint capsule is essentially funnel-shaped with a much broader insertion on the lateral side than on the medial side of the joint; therefore, the lateral side approach is favored for treating multidirectional instability because it allows a greater amount of capsule to be shifted a greater distance as necessary. In this repair, the cleft between the superior and middle glenohumeral ligaments, which often is widened in a multidirectionally unstable shoulder, is closed. The entire superior flap (consisting of the superior and middle glenohumeral ligaments) is then brought in cruciate fashion over the previously shifted inferior flap. If a detachment

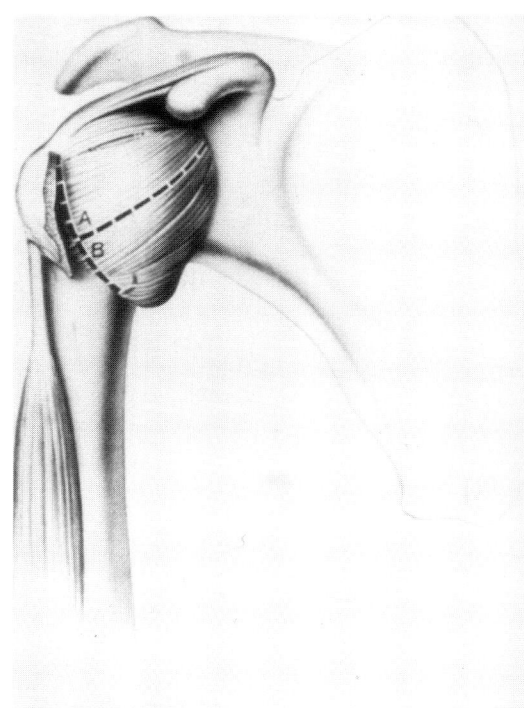 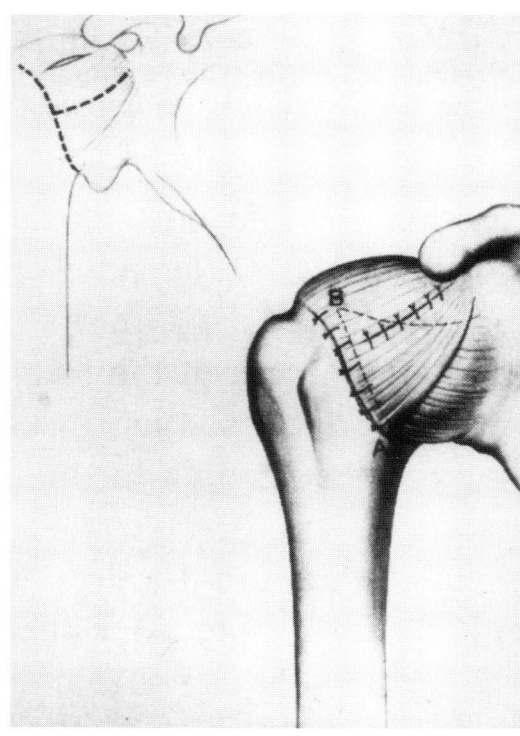

Fig. 2 The inferior capsular shift procedure allows reduction of capsular volume on all three sides of the joint in patients with multidirectional instability. The inferior flap is shifted superiorly and repaired to the lateral cuff of tissue **(left)**. After repair of the superior capsular cleft, the superior flap is then shifted inferiorly and repaired **(right)**. (Reproduced with permission from Neer CS II, Foster CR: Inferior capsular shift for involuntary and multidirectional instability of the shoulder. *J Bone Joint Surg* 1980;62A:897-908.)

of the ligament-labral complex from the rim of the glenoid is encountered, these tissues are repaired back to the glenoid rim with sutures passed through bony tunnels or suture anchor devices, prior to shifting the capsule. Such labral detachments are less common in cases of multidirectional instability than in cases of unidirectional instability, but they occasionally are found. Similarly, if significant deficiency of the glenoid is encountered (> 25% of the articular surface), then the repair may also incorporate a bone graft to the deficient portion of the glenoid (a coracoid transfer may be used if the deficiency is anterior and a scapular graft if it is posterior). Bony deficiency is quite rare in shoulders with multidirectional instability.

Postoperatively, the arm is maintained in an orthosis with the shoulder positioned in essentially neutral flexion/extension, neutral rotation, and slight abduction. This position minimizes stresses on the repair, and the brace supports the weight of the arm, decreasing stresses on the capsule. The arm is immobilized in the brace for 6 weeks, and during this period, only gentle isometric exercises and elbow range-of-motion exercises are allowed. After 6 weeks, the brace is removed and range-of-motion exercises for the shoulder are gradually progressed. Progressive resistive exercises are initiated approximately 8 to 12 weeks postoperatively. Rehabilitation after an inferior capsular shift for multidirectional instability is purposely advanced more slowly than after repairs for unidirectional or even bidirectional instability. The goal is to regain motion gradually over several months, because the likelihood of stretching out the repair with recurrence of the instability is greater than that of stiffness in the multidirectional instability patients. Careful monitoring with frequent follow-up visits is essential in order to assess the postoperative progress and to modulate the rehabilitation (either to accelerate the program if stiffness is a persistent problem or, more commonly, to decelerate it if motion is returning too quickly). Participation in sports is restricted for 9 to 12 months after repair.

Results

In the initial report on the repair of multidirectional instability with an inferior capsular shift, the authors reported that only one shoulder out of 32 had an unsatisfactory result. Ten years later, similar success was reported in another 100 cases treated by this repair. Another group reported on a medial capsulorrhaphy, which they called a T-plasty modification of the Bankart procedure, for treating multidirectional instability of the anterior and inferior types. Out of 40 patients, only four had further episodes of instability (three had posterior instability and one had anterior subluxation) after repair, and 95% were satisfied with the procedure. An anterior labral detachment was seen in 38 shoulders. This group of patients, however, was not reported to have a significant degree of posterior instability preoperatively and might be categorized as having bidirectional rather than multidirectional instability.

More recently, others have reported results using the inferior capsular shift in 43 shoulders, all of which underwent an anterior surgical approach. Four shoulders developed recurrent multidirectional instability, but 39 (91%) had no further instability. In this series, when instability recurred postoperatively, it did so early in the postoperative period, and later deterioration of results was not observed. The inferior capsular shift was successful in eight of a series of ten patients on active duty in the Navy. In both patients who were not improved, previous instability surgery had been performed before the inferior capsular shift.

Another report documents the results with the inferior capsular shift for treating multidirectional instability in young children. Case reports of successful management with the procedure in an 8-year-old and a 4-year-old are presented. The authors recommend performing surgical correction of multidirectional instability in young children only if the instability is severe, compromising their activities of daily living and school attendance, and if the child is able to understand the significance of instability.

An arthroscopic superior medial shift of the capsule for treating multidirectional instability has also been reported. Ten patients were treated with this arthroscopic suture technique, using transglenoid passage of the sutures. All ten patients had a satisfactory result, at 1- to 3-year follow-up. The authors point out that these results are preliminary and need to be reevaluated at an additional period in a large series of patients before a definitive conclusion can be drawn about the efficacy of this procedure.

Complications

Complications of treatment of multidirectional instability can result from failure to fully diagnose and treat the instability, inappropriate selection of patients for surgery, technical surgical errors, and inappropriate rehabilitation and return to high demand activities too quickly. If a multidirectional instability is not suspected and a unidirectional tightening procedure is performed, recurrence of instability may develop because the major pathology of a redundant inferior capsule will not have been adequately addressed. Thus, the shoulder may continue to subluxate inferiorly. Moreover, if the unidirectional procedure overtightens one side of the joint, the humeral head may begin to subluxate in the opposite direction (eg, an anterior tightening can produce posterior subluxation). This problem can result in symptomatic subluxation and alterations in the normal kinematics of the shoulder, which in some cases may lead to the early development of glenohumeral arthritis.

Inappropriate patient selection for surgical repair, such as with willful voluntary dislocators, will yield unsuccessful results. Although it is not always easy to determine which patients fall into this category, an effort should be made in each case, especially when there is any evidence of a voluntary component to the instability. Careful preoperative observation of the patients, particularly adolescents, and of the family dynamics can be helpful in excluding inappropriate candidates for surgery.

Surgical errors and errors of rehabilitation can also result in complications and failed outcomes. The axillary nerve passes close to the inferior aspect of the joint capsule and must be identified and protected during the inferior dissection in order to prevent its injury. In patients with multidirectional instability, the capsular dissection must proceed far enough around the neck of the humerus to allow reduction of the inferior pouch and tensioning of the capsule on the opposite side of the joint. Inadequate capsular mobilization may allow persistent subluxation in the direction not addressed. Finally, progressing rehabilitation too rapidly in the postoperative period may result in stretching out the repair and recurrence of instability. In patients with multidirectional instability, range of motion should be restored more gradually and high-demand activities restricted for a longer period of time than in patients with traumatic unidirectional instability.

Posterior Instability

Recurrent posterior instability of the glenohumeral joint is much less common than anterior instability, although it has been recognized more frequently as understanding of instability has increased. Historically, there had been much confusion over the terminology of instability, with earlier authors combining chronic locked posterior dislocations with recurrent instabilities. Fixed or locked posterior dislocations presently are classified with fracture-dislocations of the proximal humerus (because they represent impression fracture-dislocations), whereas recurrent posterior subluxations/dislocations fall into the spectrum of glenohumeral instability and will be covered in this section. As in the case of anterior instability, recurrent posterior instability can be unidirectional, bidirectional (posterior and inferior), or multidirectional. As in the case of multidirectional instability, a component of volitional control may be seen in recurrent posterior instabilities.

Etiology

Posterior instability may occur with trauma, atraumatically, or with repetitive minor trauma to the glenohumeral joint capsule. Traumatic posterior instability can result from a fall or impact on a flexed, adducted, and internally rotated arm. As previously discussed for multidirectional instability, posterior instability can occur atraumatically in the setting of ligamentous laxity of the shoulder. Finally, repetitive high demand overhead activities, such as pitching a baseball, are also thought to account for some acquired posterior instability through the mechanism of repetitive microtrauma to the capsular ligaments. More than one etiology can contribute to the development of instability in a particular shoulder; a patient with a "loose shoulder" may not develop symptomatic instability until after an episode of significant trauma or until after years of selectively stretching out the posteroinferior capsule through sports activities. Thus, there can be overlap in etiology rather than two or three discrete etiologic groups.

Diagnosis

As with multidirectional instability, the history and physical examination are the keys to diagnosing posterior instability. Typically, patients with posterior instability will complain of pain or a sensation of shoulder subluxation when using the arm in a position of combined flexion, adduction, and internal rotation. Thus, the follow-through phase of throwing or pull-through phase of swimming or rowing strokes may elicit symptoms. Some will complain of symptoms only when participating in high-demand sports activities, while others will have symptoms with less demanding activities, such as pushing open a heavy door or driving (especially with turning the steering wheel away from the involved shoulder). In the most symptomatic patients, even simple activities, such as hair combing and dressing tasks, may be limited by the instability.

Patients with traumatic posterior instability can trace the onset of symptoms to a specific event, although often they cannot recall the exact mechanism of the injury. Typically, in these traumatic cases, the arm is flexed to 90°, adducted, and internally rotated at the time of contact and is driven posteriorly, such as the position of the arm when clutching a steering wheel during a motor vehicle accident or when breaking a fall by diving onto the outstretched arm. The onset of symptoms in the atraumatic group is more insidious. Pain and a sensation of instability may develop gradually, first with higher-demand activities and later even with simple activities of daily living. Dislocations or subluxations in patients with recurrent posterior instability are nearly always spontaneously or self-reduced.

On physical examination, the most useful test for diagnosing posterior instability is the posterior stress test (Fig. 3). In performing this test, the surgeon stabilizes the medial border of the scapula with one hand and with the other applies a posteriorly directed force to the patient's humerus, which is positioned in 90° of flexion with combined adduction and internal rotation. A positive test consists of either subluxation with pain or an uncomfortable sensation, which reproduces the patient's symptoms during an episode of instability. Patients with posterior instability often will have a positive sulcus sign, suggesting that their instability is at least bidirectional (posterior and inferior) or in many cases, multidirectional. Many patients with posterior instability will also have tenderness with palpation at the posterior glenohumeral joint line.

As in multidirectional instability, patients with posterior instability may be able to demonstrate the instability voluntarily for the examiner by placing the arm into the provocative position (combined flexion, adduction, and internal rotation). A subgroup of these patients will perform this maneuver only reluctantly to demonstrate how the shoulder subluxates with activities. These "positional" voluntary dislocators are to be differentiated from the other subgroups with voluntary instability: those with an underlying psychiatric or emotional problem, who use the instability to gain attention or scare their parents, and those with a subconscious muscular tic. As with the multidirectional instability group, it is essential to note and to fully categorize any voluntary elements of instability.

Plain radiographs are usually negative in patients with recurrent posterior instability. Mild reactive changes at the posterior glenoid are seen occasionally, but those changes, as well as an anteromedial impression fracture of the humeral head, are more characteristically seen in patients with a locked posterior fracture-dislocation than in patients with recurrent posterior instability. CT or computed arthrotomography scans can demonstrate capsular redundancy and labral

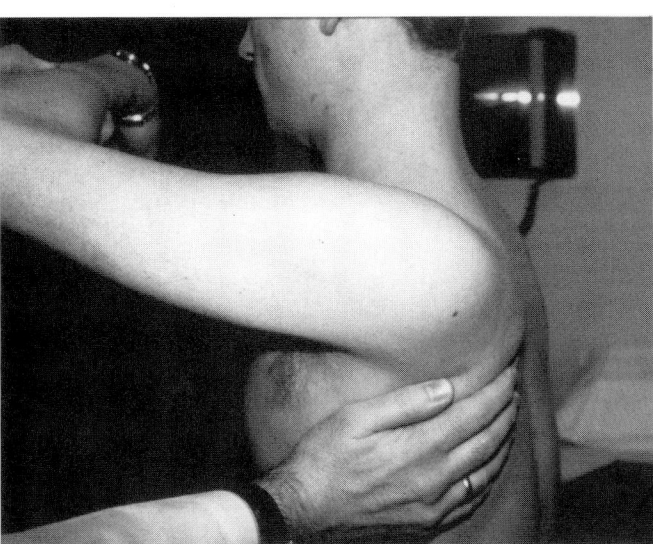

Fig. 3 The posterior stress is a useful test for diagnosing posterior instability. The medial border of the scapula is stabilized with one hand, while applying a posteriorly directed force to the patient's humerus with the other. The arm is flexed to 90°, adducted, and internally rotated.

pathology, but usually are not needed to make the diagnosis. However, when the plain radiographs (especially the axillary view) suggest bony abnormalities, then the CT scan can be helpful in identifying and quantifying unusual problems, such as glenoid bony hypoplasia or severely increased glenoid retroversion.

In selected cases, where posterior instability is suspected but the office examination is limited due to muscle guarding, an examination under anesthesia combined with shoulder arthroscopy can help to confirm the diagnosis and especially the major direction of the instability. As a diagnostic tool, this is necessary only in a small subset of patients with suspected posterior instability. Examination under anesthesia is also performed at the time of surgical repair, if surgery becomes necessary. Although examination under anesthesia rarely contradicts the preoperative history and physical examination, it serves to confirm the major direction of instability, which is particularly important when a posterior approach is considered.

Treatment

Most authors recommend nonsurgical management of posterior glenohumeral instability as the initial treatment. One report on the treatment of subluxation of various types noted that patients with posterior subluxation responded better to exercise than those with anterior subluxation. In another study, the authors reported a higher degree of satisfaction and ability to return to sports in a group treated conservatively than in another group treated surgically. As in the treatment of multidirectional instability, the emphasis in nonsurgical treatment of posterior instability is placed on strengthening the rotator cuff and deltoid, as well as the scapular stabilizers.

Surgical treatment should be considered for patients with recurrent posterior instability, who continue to have disabling pain and limitation of function despite an extensive course of nonsurgical treatment. Patients with voluntary instability must be assessed carefully. Those with the willful type need treatment of the underlying psychological disorder and are not surgical candidates. Patients whose voluntary instability is on the basis of a muscular tic might be treated successfully with a biofeedback program. The "positional type" of voluntary dislocators have responded well to surgical treatment in several series.

There has been no consensus on what procedure to perform when surgery is chosen for patients with posterior instability. A number of pathologic lesions have been cited as the underlying cause for recurrences, including a detachment of the posterior labrum (or reverse Bankart lesion), excessive laxity of the posteroinferior capsule, increased humeral retroversion, and posterior glenoid abnormalities (either hypoplasia or excessive retroversion). Surgical repairs have been designed to address each of these alleged causes of recurrence. The stabilization procedures can be divided into two groups: those that primarily address bony pathology (either deficient or abnormally directed articular surfaces) and those that address the soft-tissue abnormalities (capsular laxity or detachment from the posterior glenoid).

One type of bony stabilization procedure involves the use of a posterior bone block, which is harvested from the scapular spine and affixed to the posterior scapular neck (Fig. 4). The graft projects laterally past the glenoid margin, extracapsularly, and increases the posterior glenoid surface. This procedure can also be combined with a capsulorrhaphy repair. Another bony stabilization procedure involves an opening wedge osteotomy of the posterior glenoid or glenoplasty. In this procedure, the glenoid articular surface is reoriented to decrease its retroversion. An opening wedge osteotomy of the scapular neck is performed, followed by the introduction of a bone graft into the osteotomy site to hold the glenoid fragment rotated forward. This procedure is advocated by those who believe that excessive glenoid retroversion is the underlying cause of posterior instability. A third type of bony stabilization procedure consists of a rotational osteotomy of the humerus, in order to reduce the retroversion of the proximal humerus. The osteotomy is performed close the humeral head in cancellous bone, the humeral head is rotated externally 30°, and the position is held by the use of an AO compression plate and screws.

Soft-tissue repairs for posterior instability aim at correcting pathology involving the posteroinferior capsule and labrum. Labral detachment has been treated surgically by repairing the labrum-capsule complex back to the glenoid rim with sutures or staples. A plication of the posterior capsule with overlapping of the infraspinatus tendon or "reverse Putti-Platt" repair has been used for treating posterior instability. Posterior capsulorrhaphy with an inferior capsular shift performed through a posterior approach has gained favor in the treatment of recurrent posterior instabilities (Fig. 5). Many of these patients have instability in more than one direction (posteroinferior or multidirectional instability); therefore, the posterior inferior capsular shift is advantageous, because it allows reduction of capsular redundancy and capsular tensioning on all three sides of the joint, when necessary. When bony deficiencies of the glenoid are encountered or when the soft tissues are deficient (as in some revision repairs), a posterior bone block can be incorporated into the procedure to augment the capsulorrhaphy. This type of capsulorrhaphy has been reported as a laterally-based (humeral side) and a medially-based (glenoid side) repair, and it has yielded quite satisfactory results in treating posterior instability. After posterior capsulorrhaphy, the arm is immobilized in an orthosis in a position of neutral rotation and slight abduction for 6 weeks to allow for healing of the infraspinatus and inferior capsule. Then, range-of-motion exercises are begun and strengthening is gradually progressed.

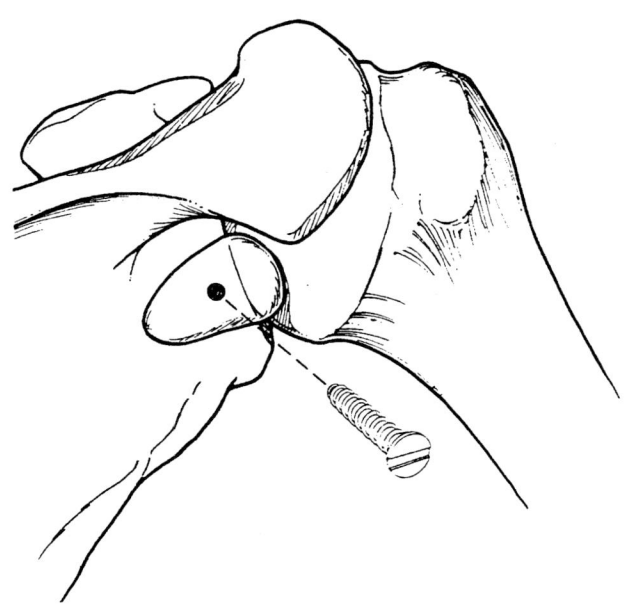

Fig. 4 A posterior bone block increases the posterior glenoid surfaces and thus enhances stability. The graft projects laterally past the glenoid margin, extracapsularly. (Reproduced with permission from Pollock RG, Bigliani LU: Recurrent posterior shoulder instability: Diagnosis and treatment. *Clin Orthop* 1993;291:85-96.)

Results

Historically, surgical repairs for posterior instability had mixed results, with failure rates as high as 50% reported in the literature. In one large series of patients treated with an opening wedge osteotomy of the glenoid, successful stabilization was reported in only ten of 19 shoulders, although results were somewhat better in cases of direct trauma (eight of 12 successfully stabilized). Rotational osteotomy of the humerus resulted in satisfactory results in ten of 12 cases, although many of these patients had significant limitation of external rotation postoperatively, and a second operation was usually necessary for hardware removal. A recent report on glenoid osteotomy for recurrent posterior subluxation questioned the predictability of glenoid osteotomy as a realignment procedure. Despite using a uniform surgical technique for osteotomy, graft size, and graft placement, the authors found

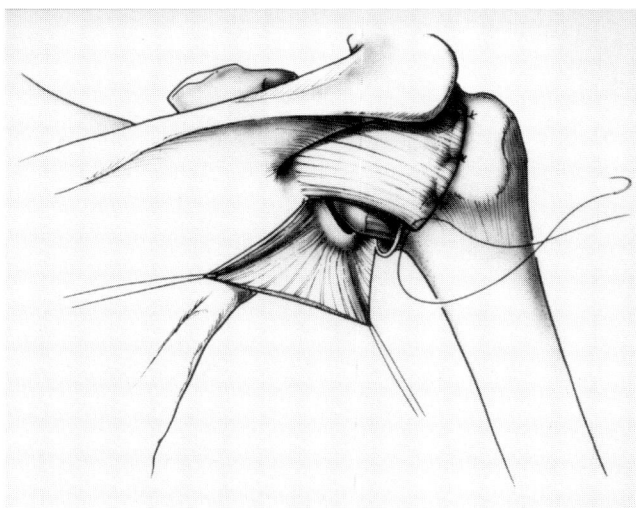 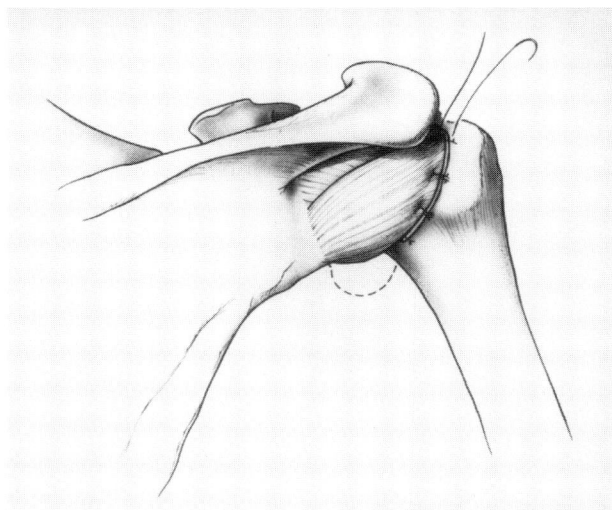

Fig. 5 The inferior capsular shift performed from a posterior approach is an effective procedure for treating recurrent posterior instability. **Left,** After the capsule is split in T-fashion, the superior flap is shifted inferiorly and reattached to the lateral aspect of the humeral neck. **Right,** The inferior flap is shifted superiorly to reduce inferior redundancy and to reinforce the repair. (Reproduced with permission from Bigliani LU, Pollock RG, McIlveen SJ, et al: Shift of the posteroinferior aspect of the capsule for recurrent posterior glenohumeral instability. *J Bone Joint Surg* 1995;77A:1011-1020.)

considerable variability in articular realignment. They concluded that this procedure should be used with caution and that posterior instability was usually a soft-tissue problem rather than one of articular alignment.

Recent results with posterior capsulorrhaphy procedures have been more encouraging. In the initial report on the inferior capsular shift performed through a posterior approach, the authors reported satisfactory results in all 12 patients. In a recent report on the use of this procedure for treating patients with recurrent posterior instability, the authors reported excellent or satisfactory results in 28 of 35 shoulders. Six of the seven unsatisfactory results were seen in shoulders that had undergone previous attempts at stabilization, whereas 23 of 24 shoulders in which this repair represented the initial repair had a successful outcome. Another group achieved satisfactory results with a medially-based capsulorrhaphy (in some cases supplemented with bone graft, if the posterior soft tissues were deficient) in ten of 11 patients. In a recent report on the use of another posterior capsulorrhaphy procedure, the authors reported patient satisfaction in 13 of 14 cases and no cases of recurrent posterior instability. These procedures directly address posteroinferior capsular redundancy and allow precise capsular tightening, perhaps explaining their high rates of clinical success.

Complications

Several complications of posterior instability repair have been reported, some of which are specific to particular surgical procedures. Glenoid osteotomy can result in intra-articular glenoid fracture, osteonecrosis of the glenoid caused by a shallow osteotomy cut, degenerative arthritis of the glenohumeral joint, and symptomatic impingement of the humeral head on the coracoid. Rotational osteotomy of the humerus can result in nonunion of the osteotomy site and significant loss of external rotation. Soft-tissue repairs can fail to appropriately balance the capsule, leading to residual inferior subluxation if only a posterior tightening is performed in a bidirectionally or multidirectionally unstable shoulder or even to persistent anterior subluxation if the posterior capsule is overtightened. Injury to the axillary or suprascapular nerve is possible with errant dissection, especially in revision surgery. Finally, as seen with multidirectional instability, initiation and progression of postoperative exercises too quickly can result in stretching out soft-tissue repairs and resubluxation.

Selected Bibliography

General

Altchek DW, Warren RF, Skyhar MJ, et al: T-plasty modification of the Bankart procedure for multidirectional instability of the anterior and inferior types. *J Bone Joint Surg* 1991;73A:105-112.

Bigliani LU (ed): *The Unstable Shoulder.* Rosemont, IL, American Academy of Orthopaedic Surgeons, 1996.

Fronek J, Warren RF, Bowen M: Posterior subluxation of the glenohumeral joint. *J Bone Joint Surg* 1989;71A:205-216.

Gerber C, Ganz R, Vinh TS: Glenoplasty for recurrent posterior shoulder instability: An anatomic reappraisal. *Clin Orthop* 1987;216:70-79.

Hawkins RJ, Koppert G, Johnston G: Recurrent posterior instability (subluxation) of the shoulder. *J Bone Joint Surg* 1984;66A:169-174.

Mallon WJ, Speer KP: Multidirectional instability: Current concepts. *J Shoulder Elbow Surg* 1995;4:54-64.

Neer CS II: Involuntary inferior and multidirectional instability of the shoulder: Etiology, recognition and treatment, in Stauffer ES (ed): American Academy of Orthopaedic Surgeons *Instructional Course Lectures XXXIV.* St. Louis, MO, CV Mosby, 1985, pp 232-238.

Norwood LA, Terry GC: Shoulder posterior subluxation. *Am J Sports Med* 1984;12:25-30.

Rowe CR, Pierce DS, Clark JG: Voluntary dislocation of the shoulder: A preliminary report on a clinical, electromyographic, and psychiatric study of twenty-six patients. *J Bone Joint Surg* 1973;55A:445-460.

Tibone J, Ting A: Capsulorrhaphy with a staple for recurrent posterior subluxation of the shoulder. *J Bone Joint Surg* 1990;72A:999-1002.

Multidirectional Instability

Cooper RA, Brems JJ: The inferior capsular-shift procedure for multidirectional instability of the shoulder. *J Bone Joint Surg* 1992;74A:1516-1521.

Thirty-eight patients (43 shoulders) with disabling multidirectional instability were treated with an inferior capsular shift through an anterior approach. Four patients had recurrence of symptomatic instability, but 39 (91%) of the shoulders functioned well and were stable. Failures and recurrences occurred early in the postoperative period, and there was no late deterioration of results.

Duncan R, Savoie FH III: Arthroscopic inferior capsular shift for multidirectional instability of the shoulder: A preliminary report. *Arthroscopy* 1993;9:24-27.

Ten consecutive patients with involuntary multidirectional instability who had failed nonsurgical treatment underwent an arthroscopic capsular shift, using a transglenoid suture technique. The average Bankart score was 90 (range, 75 to 95), and all patients had a satisfactory result at a follow-up ranging from 1 to 3 years.

Harryman DT II, Sidles JA, Harris SL, et al: The role of the rotator interval capsule in passive motion and stability of the shoulder. *J Bone Joint Surg* 1992;74A:53-66.

Surgical alteration of the capsular interval was found to affect flexion, extension, external rotation, and adduction. It also affected obligate translation of the humeral head on the glenoid with flexion. Imbrication of the rotator interval increased the resistance to inferior and posterior translation. Thus, the authors conclude that imbrication of this region of the capsule may help to control posterior and inferior instability.

Itoi E, Motzkin NE, Morrey BF, et al: Scapular inclination and inferior stability of the shoulder. *J Shoulder Elbow Surg* 1992;1:131-139.

Eleven fresh frozen cadaver shoulders were studied to examine the influence of scapular inclination on inferior instability of the glenohumeral joint. Scapular inclination was found to contribute significantly to inferior glenohumeral stability. Increased scapular inclination prevented inferior humeral head displacement, probably by a bony cam effect that tightens the superior capsule.

Lebar RD, Alexander AH: Multidirectional shoulder instability: Clinical results of inferior capsular shift in an active-duty population. *Am J Sports Med* 1992;20:193-198.

The results of a capsular shift procedure in ten active-duty patients in the US Navy are reviewed at an average follow-up of 28 months. Eight patients were satisfied with their surgery. Both patients with recurrent instability after surgery had undergone previous instability repairs.

Mizuno K, Itakura Y, Muratsu H: Inferior capsular shift for inferior and multidirectional instability of the shoulder in young children: Report of two cases. *J Shoulder Elbow Surg* 1992;1:200-206.

Two cases of surgical treatment in young children (ages 8 and 4 years) with disabling multidirectional instability were treated successfully with the inferior capsular shift. The authors recommend that surgery be performed on young children with multidirectional instability only if the instability symptoms are severely disabling and if the children are able to understand the significance of instability.

Neer CS II, Foster CR: Inferior capsular shift for involuntary inferior and multidirectional instability of the shoulder: A preliminary report. *J Bone Joint Surg* 1980;62A:897-908.

This is a classic report on the inferior capsular shift for treating involuntary multidirectional instability in 36 patients (40 shoulders). One shoulder had recurrent subluxation postoperatively, but 31 of 32 shoulders followed up for at least 1 year postoperatively had no further instability. This report describes the pathology of multidirectional instability and the surgical technique for treating this difficult problem.

Warner JJ, Deng XH, Warren RF, et al: Static capsuloligamentous restraints to superior-inferior translation of the glenohumeral joint. *Am J Sports Med* 1992;20:675-685.

Eleven cadaveric shoulders were tested to determine the contributions of specific capsuloligamentous structures to superior-inferior stability of the glenohumeral joint. The primary restraint to inferior translation of the adducted shoulder was the superior glenohumeral ligament. The anterior and posterior portions of the inferior glenohumeral ligament became the main static stabilizers with increasing abduction.

Posterior Instability

Bigliani LU, Pollock RG, McIlveen SJ, et al: Shift of the posteroinferior aspect of the capsule for recurrent posterior glenohumeral instability. *J Bone Joint Surg* 1995;77A: 1011-1020.

Thirty-five shoulders (34 patients) were treated with a posterior inferior capsular shift for recurrent posterior instability. At follow-up averaging 5 years, 28 of 35 (80%) had satisfactory results. Six of the seven unsatisfactory results were in shoulders that had undergone previous attempts at stabilization. In primary repairs, 23 of 24 were stabilized successfully using this procedure.

Burkhead WZ Jr, Rockwood CA Jr: Treatment of instability of the shoulder with an exercise program. *J Bone Joint Surg* 1992;74A:890-896.

One hundred forty shoulders with various types of subluxation were treated with a specific set of muscle-strengthening exercises. Only 16% of shoulders with traumatic subluxation had a good or excellent result with exercises, versus 53% with atraumatic subluxation. Patients with posterior instability fared better than those with anterior subluxations in this study.

Hawkins RH: Glenoid osteotomy for recurrent posterior subluxation of the shoulder: Assessment by computed axial tomography. *J Shoulder Elbow Surg* 1996;5:393-400.

Computed tomography was used to measure the change in articular alignment in 12 patients who underwent glenoid osteotomy for recurrent posterior instability. The average correction was 10.8° (range, 1° to 24°). Several complications were encountered, including intra-articular fracture, graft extrusion, and development of osteoarthritis. Because of the unpredictability of correction and the risk of serious complications, the authors urge caution in the use of this repair.

Hawkins RJ, Janda DH: Posterior instability of the glenohumeral joint: A technique of repair. *Am J Sports Med* 1996;24:275-278.

Seventeen patients were treated with a posterior capsulotendinous tensioning procedure for recurrent posterior instability. Fourteen patients were evaluated at an average of 44 months postoperatively. No patients had a recurrence of instability, and 13 of 14 were satisfied with their outcome.

Hurley JA, Anderson TE, Dear W, et al: Posterior shoulder instability: Surgical versus conservative results with evaluation of glenoid version. *Am J Sports Med* 1992;20:396-400.

Twenty-five patients were treated for posterior glenohumeral instability with a specific rehabilitation program, and 25 underwent surgical repair with a reverse Putti-Platt procedure. Recurrence of instability in both groups was very high (72% in the surgically treated group versus 96% in the nonsurgical group). A higher percentage of patients in the nonsurgically treated group (68% versus 50%) felt that their symptoms were improved.

Pollock RG, Bigliani LU: Recurrent posterior shoulder instability: Diagnosis and treatment. *Clin Orthop* 1993;291:85-96.

The authors report that capsular redundancy is the most common pathologic finding in recurrent posterior glenohumeral instability and recommend the use of a posterior inferior capsular shift when surgery is necessary. Augmentation of the repair with a posterior bone block is reserved for unusual cases, such as with glenoid hypoplasia, or in some revision cases in which the soft tissues are deficient.

Surin V, Blader S, Markhede G, et al: Rotational osteotomy of the humerus for posterior instability of the shoulder. *J Bone Joint Surg* 1990;72A:181-186.

Twelve shoulders were treated with external rotational osteotomy of the humerus for recurrent posterior instability. Recurrence of instability postoperatively was seen in one patient with multidirectional instability, and there was one pseudarthrosis in the series. Plate removal was usually performed 1 year after the osteotomy.

11

Arthroscopic Anterior Glenohumeral Reconstruction

Gary M. Gartsman, MD

Introduction

Understanding of the pathophysiology of glenohumeral instability has been improved with advanced surgical techniques and instrumentation. The following is a brief overview of some of these recent advances.

Metallic staples were introduced by Johnson in 1982. The initial recurrence rate of 21% was reduced to 13% if immobilization was extended to 3 to 4 weeks. Other studies describe success rates of 50% to 80%. Disadvantages in using this method include difficulties with capsular transfer, hardware complications, single point fixation, and the high recurrence rate.

The multiple suture technique was first described by Caspari with a 90% success rate. Using the same technique, studies by Youssef, Grana, and Walch had failure rates of 27%, 44%, and 49%, respectively. Advantages of this technique are the ability to place multiple sutures in the glenohumeral ligaments and the ability to shift the capsule to eliminate areas of laxity. Disadvantages include the passage of a drill posteriorly and the tying of sutures over fascia, an action that places the suprascapular nerve at risk and decreases the security of the suture fixation.

Warren introduced the Suretac absorbable anchor to minimize the hardware complications noted with the metallic staple. This device requires good quality ligaments and labrum for successful insertion. Results are usually satisfactory in patients in whom the repair involves simple labrum reattachment, such as that seen in traumatic, initial dislocation, rather than the ligament shifting or reconstruction seen in patients with recurrent dislocation or subluxation. Postoperative immobilization is important because the anchor has 50% initial strength at 4 weeks and a reactive synovitis has been reported. With stringent patient selection, success rates of 80% to 95% are possible.

The use of suture anchors and multiple sutures was initially described by Wolf, who used absorbable sutures. The technique was modified by Snyder, who used permanent sutures. Suture anchors allow the capsule and ligaments to be shifted superiorly and brought to the glenoid rim, and can accommodate the varying quality of the glenohumeral ligaments commonly encountered during surgical repair. In contrast to the Caspari technique, posterior drilling is avoided and soft-tissue fixation strength is improved. The technical difficulty, required instrumentation, and cost of the anchors are disadvantages, however.

Early studies of repair techniques describe nearly 100% excellent results, but later studies report that the incidence of failure has approached 50%. Presently, no single technique is accepted universally; it is more appropriate to discuss the principles of arthroscopic glenohumeral reconstruction rather than to focus on a particular repair method.

Because of the variations in patient selection, surgical technique, postoperative rehabilitation, and outcome ratings, direct comparison among the various studies is limited. However, it is clear that the promising early results have not been substantiated in the more recent literature.

Our understanding of recurrent dislocations has advanced from the essential lesion described by Bankart, Broca, and Perthes to a more complete and complex appreciation of the various factors responsible for this clinical entity. Abnormalities of neuromuscular control, concavity compression, joint adhesion, the suction effect of limited joint volume, and bone and cartilage constraint are all significant factors that are covered elsewhere in this section. The importance of a thorough history, physical examination, radiographic analysis, and preoperative rehabilitation has also been discussed previously.

Other lesions that allow recurrent dislocation may be present. Humeral site anterior inferior glenohumeral ligament avulsion, rotator cuff tears, areas of anterior glenoid bone loss, capsular attenuation, atraumatic instability, and multidirectional instability may all be responsible for recurrent dislocation but at present are being treated on a trial basis.

This discussion will focus on the management of recurrent anterior glenohumeral dislocation. Factors such as traumatic origin, recurrent dislocation, presence of a Bankart lesion, good quality capsular tissues, unidirectional instability, repair site location at the level of the glenoid rim, and multiple suture techniques can favorably affect the outcome of arthroscopic stabilization procedures. Successful arthroscopic stabilization is dependent on patient selection, lesion identification, and precise surgical reconstruction.

Patient Selection

A patient who has had an anterior dislocation as a result of a significant traumatic event with the arm in a position of abduction, external rotation, or extension is an ideal candidate for arthroscopic reconstruction. Radiographic confirmation of the dislocation and reduction performed by medical personnel are good indications of a successful outcome. Episodes of dislocation or instability with the arm in the injury position should be reported. No generalized ligamentous laxity should be noted on physical examination. Examination should confirm that apprehension is present when the arm is placed in the injury position and that the direction of instability is unidirectionally anterior with no significant inferior or posterior component. Radiographs should demonstrate no glenoid bone loss. These elements of the history and physical examination correlate directly with the lesions found at surgery and with the surgeon's ability to reconstruct the shoulder.

Lesion Identification

Arthroscopically, the primary glenohumeral joint lesions involved are separation of the anterior inferior glenoid labrum (Figs. 1 and 2), detachment of the anterior inferior glenohumeral ligament from its glenoid insertion (Fig. 3), and midsubstance plastic deformation (stretching) (Fig. 4) of the anterior inferior glenohumeral ligament; these conditions may occur as isolated lesions or in various combinations. Secondary lesions may include a rotator cuff tear (partial or complete), superior labral anterior posterior (SLAP) lesion, loose bodies, labrum flap tears, and tears of the rotator interval.

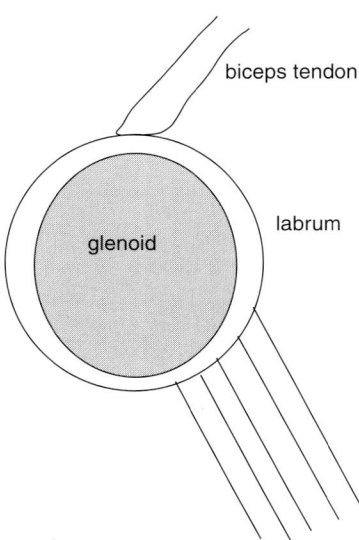

Fig. 1 Normal anatomy of the anterior inferior glenohumeral ligament.

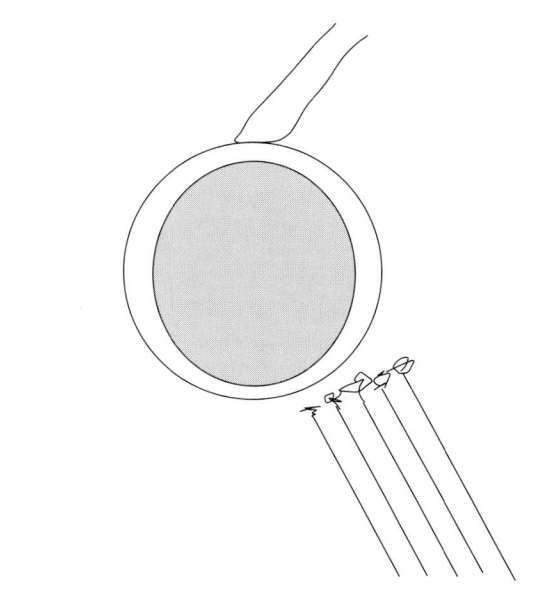

Fig. 3 Ligament detachment.

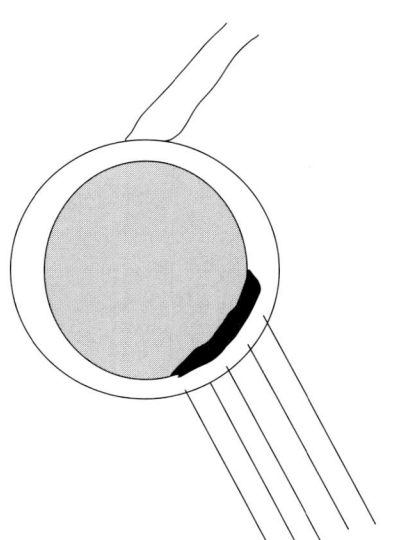

Fig. 2 Labrum separation (Bankart lesion).

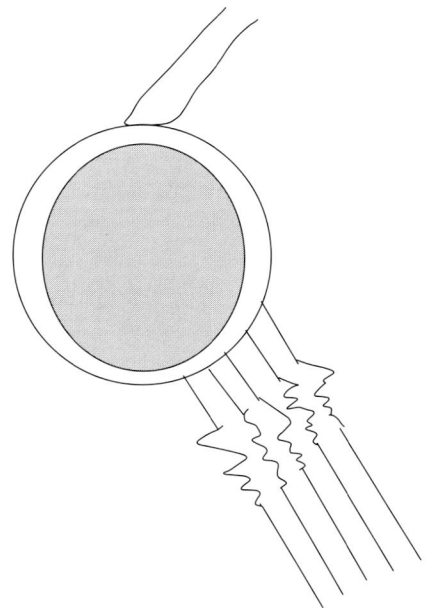

Fig. 4 Midsubstance ligament stretching.

Surgical Reconstruction

The three principles of surgical reconstruction are reattachment of the labrum to the glenoid rim; reattachment of the anterior inferior glenohumeral ligament to the labrum; and reestablishment of tension in the anterior inferior glenohumeral ligament complex. Because the combination of lesions found may vary, the three components of the reconstruction may also be performed alone or in various combinations. Secondary lesions are corrected as needed. Because the etiology of recurrent dislocation involves several factors, the surgical reconstruction necessarily involves many structures. All lesions must be identified and repaired.

Surgical Technique

The arthroscopic reconstruction begins with an examination under anesthesia to document the range of motion and the degree and direction of humeral head translation. The combination of interscalene block (for postoperative pain relief) and general anesthesia is preferred. The patient is in the beach chair position and the arm is supported with a McConnell arm holder. No continuous traction is used.

The arthroscope is inserted posteriorly and a brief diagnostic arthroscopy performed. The anterior inferior portal is created approximately 1 cm lateral to and 5 mm superior to the coracoid. The cannula enters the joint immediately superior to the subscapularis tendon, 1 cm lateral to the glenoid margin. The anterosuperior cannula is inserted through the rotator interval anterior and lateral to the biceps tendon glenoid insertion. The two anterior cannulas must be spaced as far apart as possible. The status of the rotator cuff, rotator interval, superior, middle, and inferior anterior ligaments, glenoid rim, labrum, and inferior recess are evaluated. The arm is placed in the position that produces symptoms and the integrity of the ligaments is reevaluated by both visual inspection and palpation.

The arthroscope is then moved to the anterosuperior portal and the posterior aspect of the joint is examined for posterior lesions, such as a rotator cuff tear or posterolateral capsular rupture. The arthroscope is returned to the posterior cannula.

The labrum should be examined circumferentially around the glenoid for signs of instability such as fraying, tearing, or detachment. The labrum may be absent as a result of repeated trauma or it may be separated from the glenoid and attached to the ligament.

Labrum fraying in the area of clinical instability (anterior-inferior quadrant) or tearing of the labrum substance is commonly indicative of glenohumeral instability. Minimal treatment is required if the labrum is frayed, but flap tears should be debrided, with care taken not to disrupt the labrum-glenoid attachment. Labrum detachment occurs in three forms. (1) The labrum is separated from the glenoid and displaced anteriorly but remains attached to the glenohumeral ligaments (classic Bankart lesion). (2) The labrum may appear well fixed to the glenoid but is actually not well attached. If a probe is inserted between the glenoid and labrum, the labrum peels off the glenoid. (3) The labrum and ligament have torn away from the glenoid and healed in a medial location along the scapular neck.

The insertion of the inferior ligament is assessed next. The anterior inferior glenohumeral ligament may insert directly into the labrum or it may insert medially along the scapular neck. Five types of insertion tears are seen arthroscopically. (1) The labrum has separated from the glenoid but the ligament-labrum complex is intact (classic Bankart lesion). (2) The labrum is attached to the glenoid rim but the ligament has torn from the labrum. The ligament may be found anterior to the glenoid or it may have healed to the glenoid in a medial location. (3) The labrum-ligament complex may appear to be well fixed to the glenoid rim but if a probe is inserted between the labrum and the glenoid, the labrum-ligament complex may be peeled off the scapular neck. (4) The ligament alone or ligament-labrum complex may have healed medially along the scapular neck. (5) The anterior inferior glenohumeral ligament may also insert further superiorly along the glenoid, extending even to the superior pole. A SLAP lesion may be continuous with the anterior inferior glenohumeral ligament. However, this unusual lesion should not be confused with the normal sublabral hole in the anterosuperior quadrant. All five ligament lesions described are consistent with recurrent dislocation, but each requires slight variations in surgical repair.

The substance of the anterior inferior glenohumeral ligament is then assessed. The sling-like nature of the ligament complex must be appreciated. Stretching may have occurred anywhere from the anterior to the posterior band and may extend into the inferior pouch. At this time, assessment of plastic deformation is qualitative, but it is useful to place the arm in the position of clinical instability and determine both visually and by palpation with a probe whether there is adequate tension in the ligaments. If the arm is examined in neutral rotation without abduction, the appearance may be deceptive.

At this point, the surgeon can decide how the elements of ligament insertion disruption, labrum damage, and ligament plastic deformation each contribute to pathology. Repair should be based on restoring each of these elements as necessary.

Labrum Repair

The detached labrum must be repaired to the glenoid rim. This procedure is usually performed in the anterior inferior glenoid quadrant, but the repair may, as noted above, extend superiorly. A SLAP lesion not occurring in direct continuity with the Bankart lesion should be repaired prior to Bankart labrum repair.

If the labrum is only slightly separated it is essentially repaired in situ. If the labrum has healed medially along the scapular neck, it must be dissected free and advanced laterally to the level of the glenoid rim. It is unwise to advance the labrum superiorly because it attaches circumferentially around the glenoid and cannot be advanced in a superior direction. It is the glenohumeral ligament(s) that can be (and usually are) shifted superiorly.

The goal is anatomic positioning of the labrum. If suture anchors are placed along the scapular neck medial to the glenoid rim, the labrum will heal medially and the glenoid deepening and extension effect of the labrum will not be restored. The repair site is abraded with a 4-mm round power bur. The extent of abrasion is usually 5 to 10 mm medial to the rim. Medial abrasion should continue to match the extent of medial dissection of the labrum and may extend up to 2 cm in some cases. Abrasion is also performed 3 mm along the

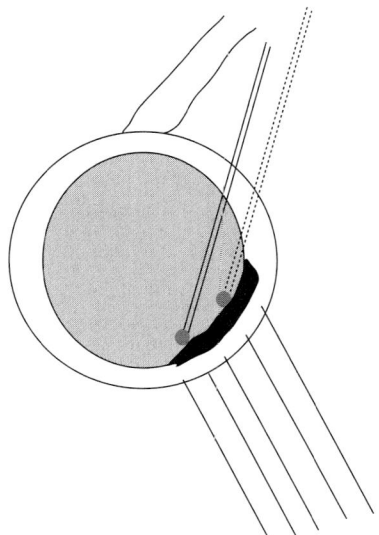

Fig. 5 Anchors are inserted and the labrum is separated.

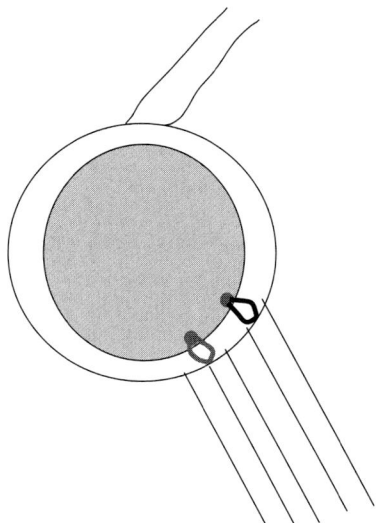

Fig. 7 The ligament is repaired with two suture anchors tied.

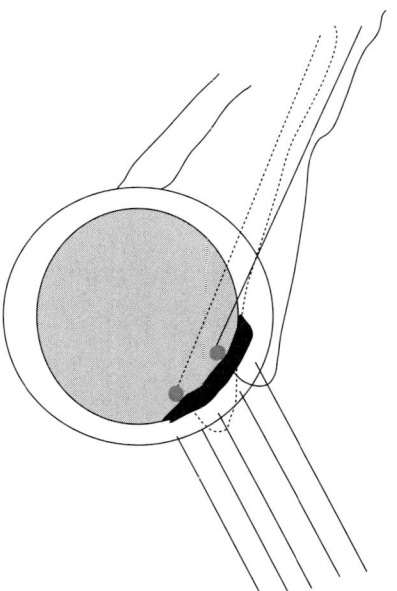

Fig. 6 Anchors are inserted, with sutures through the separated labrum.

glenoid articular surface and requires the sacrifice of a corresponding amount of glenoid cartilage.

Starting holes for the anchor(s) are then made at the level of the rim edge at the most lateral margin of the articular surface. The anchors are placed from inferior to superior. When the labrum suture is tied, approximately one half of the labrum will lie on the articular surface and one half along the scapular neck, thereby recreating the normal anatomy (Figs. 5-7).

Ligament Repair

The anterior inferior glenohumeral ligament is repaired next. With ligament detachment, the normal tension that occurs in the anterior inferior glenohumeral ligament when the arm is taken into abduction and external rotation is absent.

With the upper arm in the scapular plane, the shoulder is positioned in 30° of abduction and 30° of external rotation. A soft-tissue grasper is used to grasp the ligament complex and advance it laterally to the glenoid rim and superiorly as needed to restore ligament tension. The correct tension is qualitative, but as a practical matter, the ligament can be advanced as far laterally and superiorly as possible. If this step is performed with the arm internally rotated, excessive tightening will be created and a significant loss of external rotation results.

The suture-passing instrument is then used to pierce the anterior inferior glenohumeral ligament and advance it superiorly. If the labrum is intact or repaired, the ligament may be sutured directly to the labrum. If the labrum is absent, the ligament(s) is (are) repaired with suture anchors to the glenoid rim. This process is repeated as necessary. The goal is to attach the ligament to the rim through the labrum (Figs. 3, 8, and 9). If the labrum is minimally displaced, labrum repair and ligament repair occur as one step.

Midsubstance Ligamentous Laxity

In most cases of traumatic, unidirectional anterior recurrent dislocation, the superior and lateral advancement of the anterior inferior glenohumeral ligament will correct midsubstance

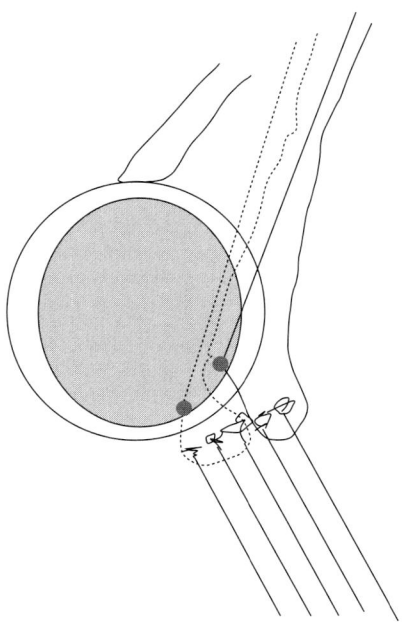

Fig. 8 Anchors are inserted, and the sutures passed through the ligament.

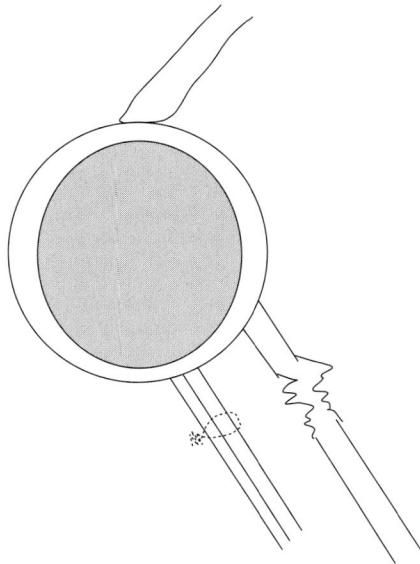

Fig. 10 Capsular stretching is repaired with the suture tied.

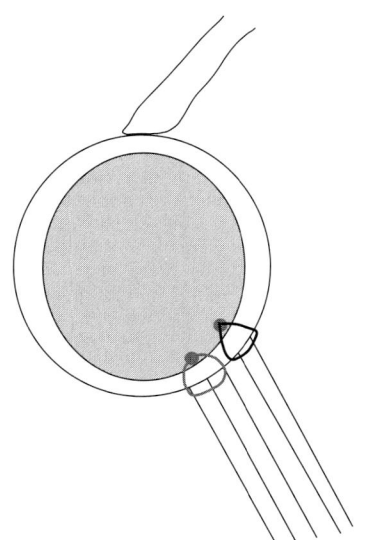

Fig. 9 The Bankart lesion is repaired and the sutures are tied.

laxity. If inadequate tension remains, capsular imbrication is necessary.

The point of the anterior inferior glenohumeral ligament midway between its glenoid and humeral attachments is identified. A suture passer is inserted through the anterior inferior cannula and pierces the ligament at that point. After the tip exits the ligament, the needle pierces the ligament again at a point 5 to 10 mm medially. As the suture is tied, capsular imbrication occurs. This process is repeated as necessary (Figs. 4 and 10).

Postoperative Rehabilitation

Postoperative rehabilitation after arthroscopic repair is identical to that occurring after open repair. If the arthroscopic repair is so poor that prolonged immobilization is required, the advantages of arthroscopic repair will most likely be lost.

Discussion

Arthroscopic management of glenohumeral instability is presently being evaluated. Clear criteria for patient selection and a precise surgical technique with long-term follow-up are critical to the success of an arthroscopic anterior glenohumeral reconstruction.

Selected Bibliography

Arciero RA, Taylor DC, Snyder RJ, et al: Arthroscopic bioabsorbable tack stabilization of initial anterior shoulder dislocations: A preliminary report. *Arthroscopy* 1995;4: 410-417.

This study discusses repair of acute dislocations in cadets. Of 19 patients, 16 had excellent results, two had good results, and one had fair results. There was no recurrent dislocation and one subluxation.

Caspari RB: Arthroscopic shoulder reconstruction. *Orthop Trans* 1989;134:559.

Ellman H, Gartsman GM: *Arthroscopic Shoulder Surgery and Related Procedures.* Philadelphia, PA, Lea & Febiger, 1993, pp 255-316.

This article discussed the advantages and disadvantages of open and arthroscopic techniques.

Grana WA, Buckley PD, Yates CK: Arthroscopic Bankart suture repair. *Am J Sports Med* 1993;21:348-353.

In 27 patients studied, there were 12 failures with recurrent instability.

Green MR, Christensen KP: Arthroscopic Bankart procedure: Two- to five-year follow-up with clinical correlation to severity of glenoid labral lesion. *Am J Sports Med* 1995;23:276-281.

Of 47 patients, there was a 42% failure rate.

Matthews LS, Vetter WL, Oweida SJ, et al: Arthroscopic staple capsulorrhaphy for recurrent anterior shoulder instability. *Arthroscopy* 1988;4:106-111.

Of 23 patients studied, 67% had good or excellent results. Five revision surgeries were performed.

Morgan CD, Bodenstab AB: Arthroscopic Bankart suture repair: Technique and early results. *Arthroscopy* 1987;3: 111-122.

Of 25 patients studied, all had excellent results.

Neviaser TJ: The anterior labroligamentous periosteal sleeve avulsion lesion: A cause of anterior instability of the shoulder. *Arthroscopy* 1993;9:17-21.

This article describes labrum-ligament avulsion and medial displacement.

Pagnani MJ, Deng XH, Warren RF, et al: Effect of lesions of the superior portion of the glenoid labrum on glenohumeral translation. *J Bone Joint Surg* 1995;77A:1003-1010.

This biomechanical study documents increased anteroposterior translation with the superior labral anterior posterior lesion.

Snyder SJ: *Shoulder Arthroscopy.* New York, NY, McGraw-Hill, 1994, pp 179-214.

The author's preferred arthroscopic repair technique is discussed.

Speer KP, Deng X, Borrero S, et al: A biomechanical evaluation of a simulated Bankart lesion. *J Bone Joint Surg* 1994;76A:1819-1826.

This article describes a biomechanical study that shows that the Bankart lesion alone is not responsible for dislocation. Ligament stretching is necessary.

Walch G, Boileau P, Levigne C, et al: Arthroscopic stabilization for recurrent anterior shoulder dislocation: Results of 59 cases. *Arthroscopy* 1995;11:173-179.

Of 59 patients studied, 49% had poor results.

Warner JJ, Miller MD, Marks P, et al: Arthroscopic Bankart repair with the Suretac device. *Arthroscopy* 1995;11:2-22.

This article describes repair with the Suretac anchor.

Youssef JA, Carr CF, Walther CE, et al: Arthroscopic Bankart suture repair for recurrent traumatic unidirectional anterior shoulder dislocations. *Arthroscopy* 1995;11:561-563.

Of 30 patients, results were excellent in 11, good in eight, fair in three, and poor in six. There were six redislocations; the failure rate was 27%.

12
Special Issues in Athletes
George M. McCluskey III, MD and David T. Dellaero, MD

Athletes who participate in overhead sports such as throwing, swimming, tennis, volleyball, and weightlifting subject their shoulders to repetitive stresses when the arm is in extremes of motion. These athletes are vulnerable to injury, and they present with a variety of problems including bursitis, tendinitis, impingement, instability, and nerve injuries. Repetitive overhead stress to the shoulder may cause cumulative injury to the soft-tissue static stabilizers, with recurrent microinjuries to the capsule, glenohumeral ligament, and glenoid labrum.

Traumatic injuries to the glenohumeral and acromioclavicular joints are common and well understood. Most of the literature in the past years has focused on identifying, treating, and rehabilitating these injuries. Recently, surgeons, athletic trainers, and researchers have studied the biomechanics, functional anatomy, and pathophysiology of throwing and other overhead motions. Through their reports, they hope to provide a clearer understanding of the clinical presentation and treatment options that may enable physicians and physical therapists to provide better treatment of these complicated shoulder injuries.

The Instability Complex

The relationship between anterior instability, impingement, and rotator cuff lesions in the throwing athlete is currently being defined. Traditionally, surgeons have believed that shoulder pain and dysfunction in athletes were related to impingement or instability. The distinction between these entities is not always clear. In recent years, clinicians and researchers alike have become interested in clarifying this distinction.

Shoulder pain in athletes can be divided into two general categories based on the patient's age: patients who are older than 35 years of age and patients who are 35 years of age or younger. In the younger population (35 years of age or younger), impingement and instability are not separate entities but represent a spectrum of pathology referred to as the instability complex. In the older athletic population (older than 35 years of age), pure impingement commonly exists without concomitant instability.

Recently, impingement has been divided into outside and inside impingement. Outside impingement is similar to Neer's original description of outlet impingement. Outlet, or outside, impingement involves narrowing of the supraspinatus outlet or the space beneath the coracoacromial area formed by the anterior acromion, coracoacromial ligament, and acromioclavicular joint. Compression of the rotator cuff and subacromial bursa by the coracoacromial arch usually is caused by acromioclavicular arthritis, anterior acromial spurring, or variations in the shape or slope of the acromion. Partial tears of the bursal surface or full-thickness tears of the rotator cuff, as well as fibrosis and adhesions in the subacromial space, are seen. Outside impingement primarily occurs in older athletes who are naturally undergoing the age-related degenerative processes, including thinning of tendons and decreased vascularity, that affect the rotator cuff.

Inside, or internal, impingement associated with recurrent anterior instability is the description Jobe and associates give the type of impingement that occurs in young athletes who participate in overhead activities. Arthroscopic findings reveal a subacromial space that appears normal and that does not fit with the traditional description of outside impingement. Instead, intra-articular findings of labral fraying and tears, chondromalacia of the posterior humeral head, and articular surface tears of the rotator cuff are found. These findings may help explain the poor results of open and arthroscopic acromioplasties in these young athletes.

Shoulder stability depends on a delicate balance between the static and dynamic stabilizers of the glenohumeral joint, especially when the joint is placed under the repetitive stress and strain of throwing. When this balance is disrupted, the resulting instability causes inside impingement between the posterior superior labrum and the articular surface of the rotator cuff. The process of inside impingement begins with hyperangulation of the abducted and externally rotated humerus that abuts the posterior superior labrum during the cocking phase of throwing. This repetitive hyperangulation stretches the anterior static restraints (capsule and ligaments), allowing mild anterior subluxation of the glenohumeral joint. In response to this recurrent subluxation, the dynamic restraints (rotator cuff and scapular stabilizers) work harder to compensate for the instability. Eventually, the muscles fatigue and the anterior subluxation increases, which accentuates and promotes the preexisting posterior superior impingement and hyperangulation. The primary underlying instability, which is often subtle and clinically "silent," may culminate, therefore, in rotator cuff tendinitis or tearing, which has a more dramatic clinical appearance. Thus, the instability complex in throwing athletes may progress along a continuum from anterior subluxation to inside impingement to rotator cuff tendon tearing. Treatment must be directed to the primary instability problem; more than 90% of athletes return to their previous sport following nonsurgical and, occasionally, surgical treatment.

Clinical Diagnosis and Classification of Anterior Shoulder Pain

Diagnosis

The clinical presentation of athletes with shoulder pain is quite varied and may have a special relationship with the specific sporting activity, mechanism of injury, and age of the athlete. This section concentrates on the young throwing athlete who has the typical instability complex and who presents with acquired symptoms that have worsened over time. Plain radiographs of the shoulder generally are not helpful in defining the diagnosis unless they demonstrate a dislocated glenohumeral joint or unless other indications of instability or impingement are present, including a bony Bankart lesion, a Hill-Sachs lesion, tuberosity or glenoid rim fractures, os acromiale, or spur formation involving the anterior acromion or acromioclavicular joint. The most useful diagnostic tools are a careful history and a physical examination. These tools give the clinician enough information to make the correct diagnosis 85% of the time without using additional diagnostic modalities.

Shoulder pain is generally vague and poorly localized. Posterior shoulder pain is more common in athletes with anterior instability. Pain in the subacromial area at the anterolateral acromion and greater tuberosity, as well as referred pain down the biceps tendon and deltoid to its insertion on the humerus, are common in athletes with impingement symptoms. Night pain, rest pain, and pain provoked by repetitive overhead activities are characteristic of rotator cuff lesions. Instability usually causes pain at extremes of motion and at characteristic phases of the particular activity (ie, pain during the late cocking phase of throwing with the anterior instability). The athlete seldom gives a history of the shoulder subluxating or slipping out of place.

A thorough physical examination is necessary to confirm the suspected diagnosis. Both shoulder girdle regions must be visible for comparison, and a complete neurologic and cervical examination must be included. The dominant throwing extremity is often asymmetric when compared with the opposite shoulder and has increased external rotation, particularly at 90° of abduction.

Provocative tests for instability include the apprehension and relocation tests. For the anterior apprehension test, the athlete lies supine with the arm abducted and maximally rotated externally, and the examiner applies an anterior force to the humeral head. Varying degrees of abduction should be used to stress the different glenohumeral ligaments and stabilizing structures. A positive test recreates pain and apprehension that the patient experiences during his or her specific athletic activity. The relocation test complements the apprehension test; the examiner abducts and maximally rotates the arm externally and applies a posterior stress to the humeral head. Relief of pain with relocation of the head is considered a positive test. Apprehension or the feeling of impending subluxation has proven to be a more reliable method of differentiating between anterior instability and impingement than pain produced with these tests.

For the posterior apprehension test, the patient sits or lies supine with the shoulder flexed, internally rotated, and adducted, and the examiner applies a posterior force to the humerus. Reproduction of pain and apprehension with this test is a less reliable method of making the differential diagnosis than reproduction with the anterior apprehension test.

The O'Brien test and glenoid labral compression test demonstrate lesions of the glenoid labrum. O'Brien recommends adducting the patient's arm to 10° across the body with the arm internally rotated and having the patient elevate the arm against resistance in this position. Pain produced by this maneuver but eliminated when the arm is externally rotated in the same position is indicative of a superior labral injury (SLAP lesion).

The two impingement signs described by Neer and by Hawkins and Kennedy demonstrate inflammation of the rotator cuff and subacromial bursa and are generally positive in athletes with shoulder pain. These signs are nonspecific. They must be used in conjunction with other provocative tests and must be considered in the overall clinical picture when making a diagnosis. These impingement signs may be clinically dramatic but may represent secondary impingement or tendinitis rather than the primary problem of instability, acromioclavicular arthritis, osteolysis of the distal clavicle, or cervical abnormalities.

The impingement test is often used to sort out the primary source of pain in a patient with concomitant instability, impingement, rotator cuff, and acromioclavicular joint symptoms. The test involves injecting 10 cc of lidocaine in the subacromial bursa from a posterior approach; repeating range of motion, muscle strength tests, and provocative tests for instability and impingement; and comparing these results with the preinjection findings. For instance, a patient with primary instability and secondary impingement will demonstrate a substantial decrease in pain with impingement signs and improvement in strength of the rotator cuff, but the anterior apprehension and relocation tests remain positive.

The sulcus sign demonstrates inferior capsular laxity and is useful in diagnosing multidirectional and bidirectional glenohumeral instability in the athlete. Hyperlaxity of other joints, including the elbow, knees, and thumb (demonstrated by the ability to touch the thumb to the forearm), should alert the examiner to the possibility of a hyperlaxity problem contributing to shoulder pain in the athlete.

The acromioclavicular joint may also be a primary or secondary cause of shoulder pain in the athlete. Direct palpation over the acromioclavicular joint combined with forceful horizontal and overhead adduction is useful in diagnosing lesions in the acromioclavicular joint.

Classification

Shoulder instability has traditionally been classified according to chronicity, degree, direction, etiology, and volition. The three main causes are traumatic, atraumatic, and acquired instability. Acquired instability results from overuse or repetitive microtrauma to the shoulder and is the primary cause of recurrent anterior and anteroinferior instability in athletes who participate in throwing or overhead sports.

Jobe and associates have further classified anterior shoulder pain in athletes into four groups. Group I patients have primary outlet or outside impingement with no instability component. These individuals are generally older than 35 years of age and have classic impingement signs on examination. Common arthroscopic findings include an inflamed fibrotic subacromial bursa with frequent fraying or partial tearing of the bursal cuff surface. The intra-articular examination is usually benign.

Group II comprises the largest number of athletes. These patients have primary instability from repetitive microtrauma and secondary inside impingement. The clinical examination demonstrates positive impingement signs and positive apprehension and relocation tests. The instability is often subtle and sometimes is not detectable on examination under anesthesia. Arthroscopic findings include anterior and posterior labral fraying and tearing, injury to the capsuloligamentous complex, and subluxation of the humeral head on the glenoid. Other common arthroscopic findings are kiss lesions, which represent contact between the posterior superior labrum and a chondral lesion on the posterior humeral head when the arm is abducted and externally rotated.

Group III comprises athletes with primary instability as a result of ligament hyperlaxity and with secondary inside impingement. These young patients have positive clinical impingement signs and positive apprehension and relocation tests. Both shoulders generally demonstrate increased translation of the humeral head on the glenoid on examination under anesthesia. Arthroscopic findings demonstrate an enlarged patulous capsule and stretching of the inferior glenohumeral ligament complex. Glenoid labral injury and chondromalacia of the humeral head are generally absent.

Group IV patients have traumatic instability without associated impingement. Clinical examination reveals positive apprehension and relocation tests but no impingement signs. Arthroscopic findings include avulsion of the anterior glenoid labrum and a Hill-Sachs lesion. The rotator cuff is generally normal.

Impingement and Rotator Cuff Lesions

The etiology of impingement and rotator cuff lesions in athletes has many factors, with age being a major determinant in the diagnosis and treatment of these lesions. Neer's classification of impingement includes three stages of rotator cuff injury including inflammation and edema (stage I), fibrosis and tendinitis (stage II), and partial or complete tearing of the rotator cuff (stage III). Traditionally, most patients with impingement syndrome that requires surgical intervention fall into the late stage II and the stage III groups with acromioplasty and rotator cuff repair usually performed in patients who are older than 40 years of age. However, physical examination and arthroscopic findings in younger athletes have revealed impingement lesions that do not fit well into this scheme.

Recently, authors have described inside, or internal, impingement in overhead athletes, particularly throwers. Recurrent anterior subluxation of the shoulder in throwers is commonly associated with partial tearing of the supraspinatus and often of the infraspinatus tendons on the articular surface of the rotator cuff. This secondary impingement of the articular surface of the rotator cuff under the posterior superior glenoid rim occurs normally when the arm is hyperangulated in throwers. The pathologic changes described occur with repetitive hard throwing. Another cause of articular tearing of the rotator cuff in young athletes is repetitive microtrauma, which results in eccentric tensile overload failure during deceleration of the arm in the throwing motion.

The etiology of rotator cuff lesions in older athletes is primarily outlet impingement with mechanical attrition and compression of the cuff under the coracoacromial arch. Patients with hooked acromions (type III), acromial spurs, acromioclavicular arthritis with inferior spurring, and os acromiale have an increased incidence of impingement and rotator cuff tearing when participating in athletic activities. This outlet impingement occurs primarily on the bursal surface of the rotator cuff or is intratendinous, and may become a full-thickness tear with time. Other authors have described a primary tendinopathy occurring within the substance of the rotator cuff tendon that causes secondary acromial changes. This age-related degeneration of the rotator cuff as a result of mechanical impingement and ischemic changes places older athletes at increased risk for primary cuff tearing without associated instability.

Most studies that describe the success of arthroscopic or open acromioplasty treatment for impingement involve nonathletic populations, and results are generally satisfactory. In one study of young athletes (under 30 years of age) undergoing open acromioplasty for refractory chronic impingement syndrome, 89% of the athletes were improved but only 43% were able to return to their preinjury level of play. Only four (22%) of 18 throwers achieved a satisfactory result. Thus, return to competitive sports participation was not favorable although pain relief was satisfactory.

One recent report of arthroscopic subacromial decompression in 90 shoulders with an average follow-up of 41 months demonstrated 90% satisfactory results in nonthrowing athletes and only 68% satisfactory results in throwing athletes. Specifically, pitchers had a 50% satisfactory result by Neer's criteria. The differences in treatment results between the patients without a rotator cuff tear and those with a partial rotator cuff tear were not significant.

Reports of several studies comparing open and arthroscopic acromioplasty indicate similar results for both procedures. The surgeon's experience and skill level and other concomitant pathologic lesions should dictate which procedure is used.

Partial rotator cuff tears in the young athlete infrequently require surgical treatment. Participating in a rehabilitation program or having open capsular reconstruction for primary glenohumeral instability generally allows the rotator cuff to heal or makes its extension less likely. Full-thickness tears must be repaired with or without concomitant shoulder reconstruction for instability. In older athletes with partial or full-thickness tears secondary to outlet impingement, rotator cuff repair with acromioplasty and removal of a pathologic bursa is indicated. Studies show that repair of full-thickness tears within 3 to 6 weeks after injury gives better results in athletes who place high demands on shoulder function.

Data on the results of open acromioplasty with rotator cuff repair in athletes are limited. Bigliani reported that 83% of tennis players (average age, 53 years) who had complete rotator cuff tears treated with open repair were able to return to their previous level of participation. Another study reported on 45 young collegiate and professional athletes (average age, 29 years) who had partial and complete cuff tears treated with open acromioplasty and cuff repair. Of these athletes, only 56% returned to their sport at the previous level of competition and 40% returned to throwing. Only 32% of the pitchers returned to competition.

Treatment with arthroscopic acromioplasty and debridement of partial rotator cuff tears achieved satisfactory results in 86% of patients. Debridement should be reserved for partial tears of less than 50% of tendon thickness. Reports of rotator cuff debridement, often in full-thickness tears, have shown unsatisfactory results with long-term follow-up.

Recurrent Anterior Instability

Surgical treatment is recommended to treat recurrent anterior or anteroinferior instability when a well-supervised program of physical therapy and exercise fails. The goals of surgical reconstruction of the athlete's shoulder are to repair or correct the lesions, to reestablish normal motion and function, and to enable the athlete to resume normal sporting activities without pain. Traditional open procedures, including the Bristow, Magnuson-Stack, and Putti-Platt, result in a significant loss of external rotation of the arm and in weakness of the arm, as well as frequent hardware complications. They also fail to address the inferior capsular laxity component of the instability lesion. In one study, only 16% of throwing athletes were able to return to their preinjury level of competition following a Bristow-type procedure.

A recent cadaver study in which glenohumeral ligament bone-tendon-bone specimens were tested to failure showed that 40% of specimens failed at the glenoid, 35% in substance, and 25% at the humeral insertion. A prospective arthroscopic study of 64 shoulders with anterior instability revealed six cases in which the glenohumeral ligaments were avulsed from the humerus. Surgical repair of this lesion restores shoulder stability.

The laterally-based inferior capsular shift is used in patients with traumatic, atraumatic, and acquired instability. Most surgeons now prefer a capsular procedure with a labral repair, if indicated, to treat recurrent anterior instability. Bigliani and associates recommend an inferior capsular shift procedure with the T-plasty based on the humeral side of the joint to treat patients with anteroinferior and multidirectional instability. This approach has proven to be versatile, with the amount of inferior capsule shifted determined by the amount of capsular laxity present. Recently, 68 shoulders in 63 athletes with anteroinferior instability had an inferior capsular shift with 21 also having a repair of a Bankart lesion. Ninety-two percent of the patients returned to their preinjury level of performance. Loss of external rotation was negligible.

The modified anterior capsulolabral reconstruction is another open reconstructive procedure that has been described by Montgomery and Jobe. It employs a horizontal split in the subscapularis instead of detaching the tendon at its humeral insertion. This technique allows for early postoperative mobilization and a shortened period of rehabilitation before returning to sports participation. The procedure is best used in overhead athletes, particularly throwers with recurrent acquired anterior subluxation. The authors report on a minimum 2-year follow-up of 32 athletes treated with the modified anterior capsulolabral reconstruction for recurrent anterior instability. Ninety-seven percent of the patients had satisfactory results, with 81% of patients returning to their sport at the same level of competition and 13% returning at a lower level of competition. Ninety percent of the professional athletes, including 85% of the professional pitchers, were able to return to their sport.

Arthroscopic repair of the unstable shoulder has received mixed reviews in the literature. Most authors have reported an increased failure rate with this procedure when compared with the failure rate of open techniques. Early reports suggest a failure rate of 15% to 35%; however, more recent studies suggest a lower failure rate of 5% to 8%. Most studies recommend that arthroscopic repair be used only in patients with a Bankart lesion. Although these arthroscopic procedures generally can be done on an outpatient basis and with less postoperative pain, the postoperative immobilization time is longer than in open procedures, and the procedure usually is contraindicated in athletes participating in collision sports. Patients with recurrent atraumatic instability are also poor candidates for arthroscopic repair.

The indications for arthroscopic repair in recurrent instability currently are expanding, and the techniques are improving. Surgeons are gaining greater expertise and experience with the arthroscope and will be able to use it more effectively in the future to treat instability problems in athletes.

Injuries to the Acromioclavicular Joint

The acromioclavicular joint is a true diarthrodial joint between the medial facet of the acromion and distal clavicle. A fibrocartilaginous intra-articular disk is present, which may be partial (meniscoid) or complete. The acromioclavicular joint is surrounded by a thin capsule, which is reinforced by the superior, inferior, anterior, and posterior acromioclavicular ligaments. These ligaments provide mostly horizontal stability. The superior ligament is most significant and is reinforced by the attachments of fibers of the deltoid and trapezius muscles. The coracoclavicular ligaments (posteromedial conoid; anterolateral trapezoid) provide vertical stability to the acromioclavicular joint. At increasing loads, the conoid ligament provides the primary restraint to superior displacement. The acromioclavicular ligament provides approximately 90% of the constraint to posterior displacement of the clavicle on the acromion, with both physiologic and pathologic loads.

The coracoclavicular ligaments link the scapula to the clavicle coupling, and glenohumeral elevation to scapular rotation. Through the arc of maximum arm elevation, the clavicle rotates 40° to 50° with only 5° to 8° occurring at the acromioclavicular joint.

Most injuries are the result of a direct impact to the acromion with the arm in adduction. Examination should be performed with the patient seated with both shoulders exposed. This position will reveal asymmetry of the distal end of the clavicle with tenderness and crepitation of the acromioclavicular joint.

Low voltage (50%) anteroposterior view of the acromioclavicular joint (in the plane of the chest) is recommended to evaluate joint displacement. The axillary view is useful for evaluating the anterior-posterior displacement of the distal clavicle, with respect to the acromion.

Rockwood has classified acute traumatic acromioclavicular joint injuries as types I to VI (Fig. 1). Type I injuries

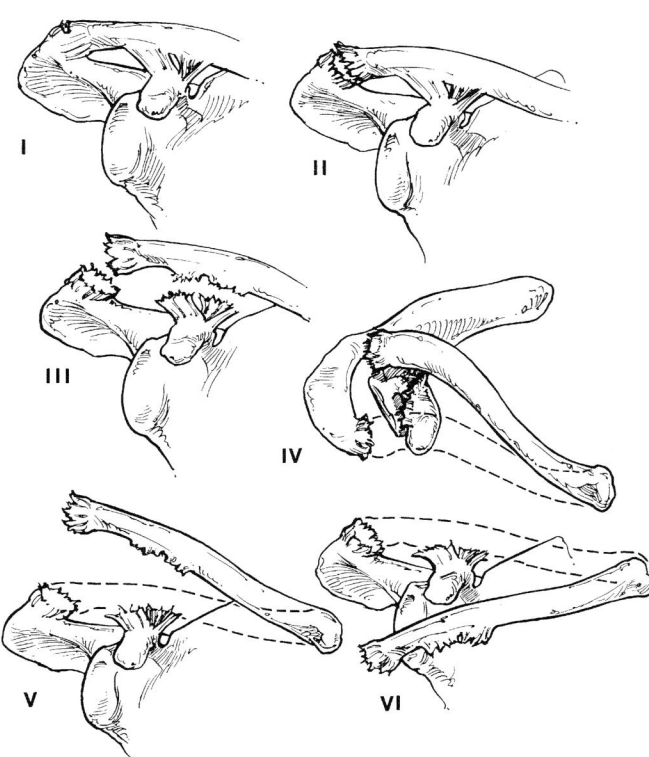

Fig. 1 Rockwood's classification of acromioclavicular joint injuries (six types). (Reproduced with permission from McCluskey GM III, Todd J: Acromioclavicular joint injuries. *South Med J* 1995;4:206-213.)

involve a sprain of the acromioclavicular ligament only. Radiographs are normal. Type II injuries involve disruption of the acromioclavicular ligament and joint capsule. The coracoclavicular ligaments are intact and/or sprained. Radiographs reveal less than 50% vertical subluxation of the clavicle and widening of the acromioclavicular joint. The coracoclavicular distance should be equal to the opposite side. In type III injuries, the acromioclavicular ligament and capsule, as well as the coracoclavicular ligaments, are disrupted. Radiographs reveal 100% displacement with complete loss of contact between the clavicle and the acromion. In the presence of a complete acromioclavicular separation but a normal coracoclavicular distance, a coracoid fracture should be suspected. In type IV injuries, the acromioclavicular ligaments, capsule, and coracoclavicular ligaments are completely disrupted. The clavicle is displaced posteriorly into or through the trapezius muscle. This condition is best confirmed on an axillary lateral view. Type V injuries involve disruption of the acromioclavicular ligament, capsule, coracoclavicular ligaments, and complete detachment of the deltoid and trapezial fascia from the distal clavicle. Radiographs reveal a coracoclavicular distance that is two to three times greater than normal, with marked displacement of the acromioclavicular joint. In the rare type VI injury, the acromioclavicular ligaments, capsule, and coracoclavicular ligaments are disrupted and the clavicle is displaced inferiorly to the acromion and coracoid process. Radiographs reveal decreased and reversed coracoclavicular distance.

Types I and II are treated nonsurgically with ice, analgesics, and use of a sling for a short period. Treatment for type III acromioclavicular injuries and joint dislocations remains controversial. The current literature supports both surgical and nonsurgical treatment. In their study, Tibone and associates evaluated 20 male patients who had type III acromioclavicular joint dislocations and who were treated nonsurgically. The patients performed strengthening exercises in three planes (flexion and extension, internal and external rotation, abduction and adduction at 60° and 100° per second). At an average follow-up of 4.5 years, the study showed no significant difference in strength between the injured and uninjured shoulders, and the patients did not report impairment of daily activities or athletic participation. The authors recommended nonsurgical treatment of grade III injuries. Nevertheless, multiple surgical procedures have been recommended for acromioclavicular dislocations to restore the suspensory function of the acromioclavicular joint and to restore joint alignment. Many authors recommend surgical repair of acute grade III dislocations in young, active individuals, heavy overhead laborers, and noncontact overhead athletes.

There is general agreement that types IV, V, and VI should be treated surgically using open reduction and reconstruction with repair of damaged deltotrapezial fascii. A variety of methods have been described, including augmentation with suture bands, coracoclavicular fixation with transfer of the coracoacromial ligament (Fig. 2), synthetic loop augmentation through drill holes in the base of the coracoid and through the clavicle, use of an acromioclavicular hook plate, and acromioclavicular reconstruction with clavicular corticotomy.

Atraumatic osteolysis of the distal clavicle in athletes is a stress failure syndrome of the distal clavicle. It most commonly appears in weight lifters who use a flat bench press with a straight bar and is bilateral in 20% to 40% of this population. Atraumatic osteolysis of the distal clavicle is also seen in throwing and racket-wielding athletes. The symptoms include insidious onset of pain in the anterior shoulder and acromioclavicular joint. The acromioclavicular joint is usually swollen and slightly tender when palpated. The athlete characteristically describes pain in the acromioclavicular joint when doing bench presses, dips, or push-ups as a part of his or her strength training—a significant aspect of the training regimen. The throwing athlete usually describes increased or more intense pain at the top of the ball release position. The diagnosis is made most often after studying plain radiographs that include special acromioclavicular joint views to demonstrate loss of subchondral bone microcysts in the subcortical area. The radiographs may also show osteoporosis in the lateral third of the clavicle. Joint scintigraphy is used if the clinical suspicion of this problem is high but the radiograph appears negative.

Nonsurgical treatment of atraumatic osteolysis of the distal clavicle should be directed toward eliminating the aspect of the training program that causes the most symptoms. Indications for surgical management are a confirmed diagnosis of traumatic osteolysis of the distal clavicle and an unwillingness of the athlete to accept less exercise or a lower level of performance. The surgical treatment involves resection of the

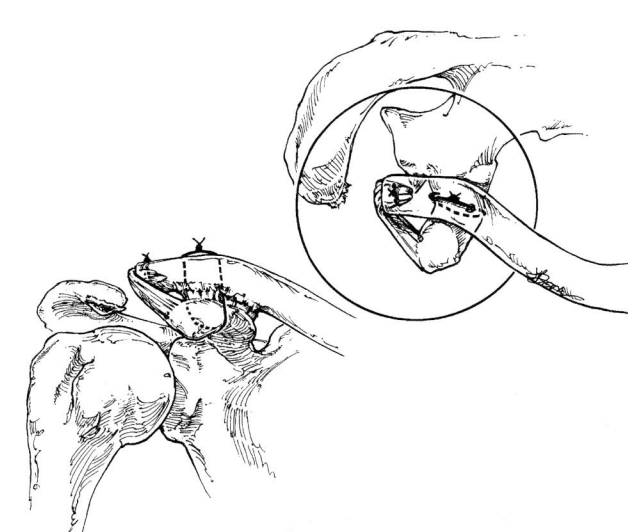

Fig. 2 **Left,** An anterior view of the coracoclavicular repair, augmented with a transfer of the coracoacromial ligament. This procedure is appropriate for acute and chronic acromioclavicular dislocations. **Right,** This superior view demonstrates the line sutures passed through the distal clavicle for fixation of the transferred coracoacromial ligament and the coracoclavicular repair.

distal clavicle. Although open distal clavicle excision or acromioclavicular joint arthroplasty has traditionally been recommended by most authors, arthroscopic resection techniques have been described with results comparable to open techniques and with reduced morbidity. An arthroscopic technique using two superior portals located immediately anterior and posterior to the acromioclavicular joint has been described that can be used in conjunction with a routine arthroscopic decompression procedure or as an isolated procedure for refractory osteolysis of the distal clavicle. A comparison study of 12 patients undergoing six open and six arthroscopic distal clavicle excision procedures demonstrated comparable results regarding bone removal and pain relief, but a lower complication rate and hospital stay in the arthroscopic patients. Also, the arthroscopic group returned to sports in one half the time when compared to the open distal clavicle excision group.

Neurovascular Injuries to the Athlete's Shoulder

Neurovascular injuries in athletes can occur as a result of local trauma or repetitive throwing activities. Acute traction of the brachial plexus is found in athletes who participate in contact sports, such as football and wrestling. Most brachial plexus injuries in sports are low velocity injuries, such as shoulder dislocations, and they have a good prognosis for recovery (neurapraxia or, less commonly, axonotmesis). If, after 4 months of observation, the athlete does not improve and electrical studies show further axonal degeneration, surgical repair with or without cable graft may be indicated.

Burner (stinger) syndrome is an acute upper trunk brachial plexus injury resulting from head, neck, or shoulder contact in football. It is manifested by sharp, burning shoulder pain that radiates to the arm and hand. Pain or weakness that persists for more than 2 weeks indicates more severe brachial plexus injury. The athlete should be restricted from sports participation until strength returns to normal. All patients with bilateral burner syndrome should be treated as though they have a cervical spine injury until the injury can be ruled out.

Thoracic outlet syndrome has also been associated with trauma and the anatomic changes that can occur in the shoulder as a result of throwing mechanics. Injuries to the shoulder musculature can cause additional impairment and secondary compression of the brachial plexus or subclavian vessels in the thoracic outlet. The symptoms usually are associated with specific throwing activities and include coolness and paresthesia of the involved arm. The patients may report that their arm is weak, heavy, or easily fatigued.

Treatment involves using nonsteroidal anti-inflammatory drugs to relieve pain and participating in physical therapy to correct posture and to strengthen shoulder and scapular muscles. Surgical treatment is indicated only if rehabilitation fails, and it is directed toward correcting specific anatomic factors causing the symptoms.

Long Thoracic Nerve

Isolated paralysis of the serratus anterior muscle occurs in a wide variety of sports and is caused by injury to the long thoracic nerve. The superficial course and length of the long thoracic nerve make it vulnerable to injury. Damage may be caused by direct blows to either the shoulder or lateral thorax. Prolonged traction can also cause this injury.

Clinical features include a dull ache or pain around the shoulder girdle, winged scapula, and decreased active shoulder motion. Nonsurgical treatment is prescribed most often and includes physical therapy and rest from the involved sport. The prognosis is generally good unless there has been traumatic high-grade nerve injury.

Suprascapular Nerve Entrapment

Most reports of entrapment neuropathies of the suprascapular nerve have focused on the area of the transverse scapular ligament. The nerve continues around the lateral border of the scapula and through the spinoglenoid notch where a branch innervates the infraspinatus. Entrapment can occur at either of these sites (Fig. 3). The mechanism of entrapment is usually direct trauma but can be traction. Recently, perineural compression has been identified more often. The patient presents with poorly localized shoulder pain, which may be posterolateral, of insidious onset. There is atrophy of the supraspinatus and infraspinatus muscles with associated weakness of abduction and external rotation. Occasionally, compression occurs at the spinoglenoid notch, which results in isolated infraspinatus wasting (Fig. 4). Electromyogram confirms the diagnosis and helps to differentiate suprascapular nerve entrapment from a rotator cuff tear.

A recent study demonstrated the value of magnetic resonance imaging (MRI) in diagnosing 27 perineural masses associated with suprascapular nerve compression. The masses

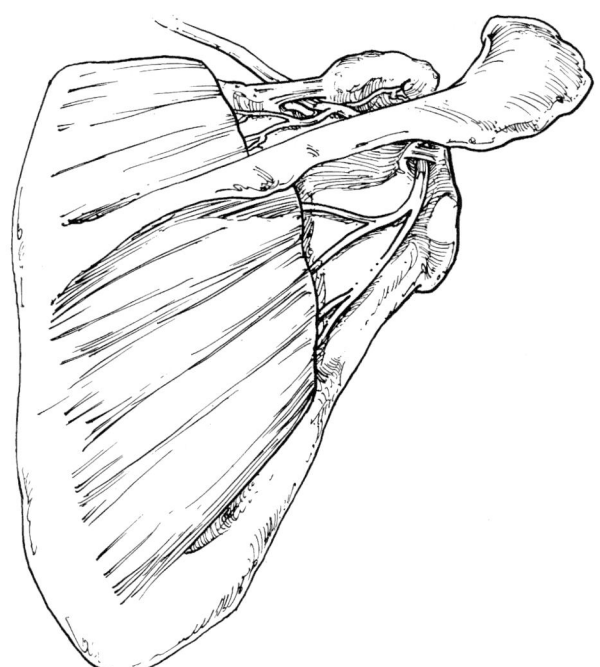

Fig. 3 The course of the suprascapular nerve is demonstrated. The nerve runs under the transverse scapular ligament at the scapular notch and then distal around the lateral border of the scapula. The nerve branches in the infraspinatus fossa after traversing the spinoglenoid notch.

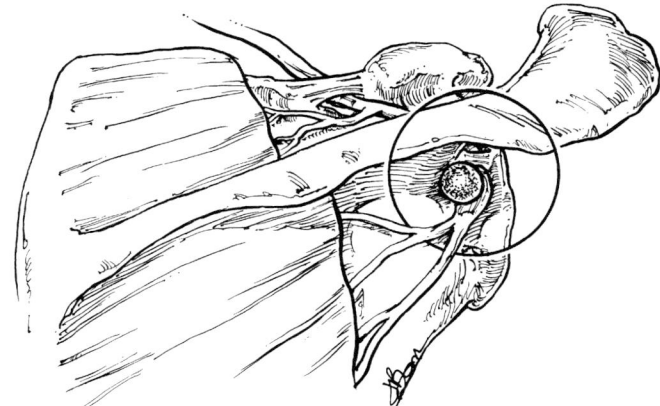

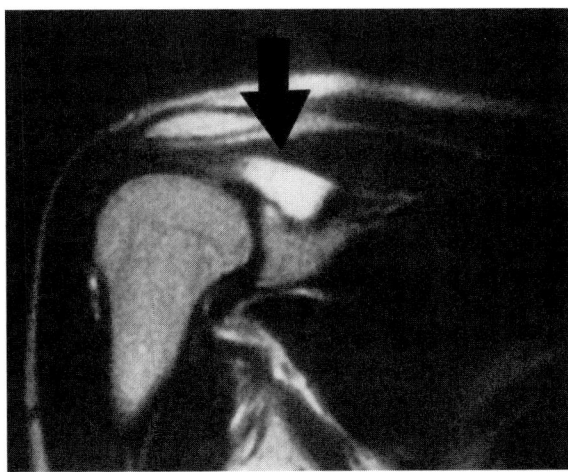

Fig. 4 Top, A ganglion cyst is situated at the spinoglenoid notch with pressure on the suprascapular nerve. The cyst generally originates from the glenohumeral joint. **Bottom,** MRI scan of ganglion cyst. This MRI scan reveals a larger ganglion cyst located posterior to the glenoid and compressing the suprascapular nerve at the spinoglenoid notch (arrow).

included 21 ganglion cysts, two synovial sarcomas, one Ewing sarcoma, one metastatic renal cell carcinoma, one chondrosarcoma, and one hematoma associated with fracture. MRI also correlated atrophy of both the supraspinatus and the infraspinatus nerves with anteriorly located masses and proximal entrapment. Nonsurgical treatment involves rest and nonsteroidal anti-inflammatory drugs. Surgical treatment for refractory cases involves a variety of procedures including release of the transverse scapular ligament, deepening of the spinoglenoid notch, and release of the spinoglenoid ligament.

Using MRI, isolated infraspinatus entrapment was associated with posteriorly located masses and distal entrapment. Treatment includes removal of the cystic mass with decompression of the nerve. The prognosis is variable. Routine arthroscopy of the glenohumeral joint prior to releasing the suprascapular nerve has been suggested; associated intra-articular pathology was noted in more than 50% of cases studied.

Quadrilateral Space Syndrome

The quadrilateral space is bordered spatially by the teres minor muscle, anteriorly by the teres major muscle, medially by the long head of the triceps, and laterally by the shaft of the humerus (Fig. 5, *left*). Quadrilateral space syndrome involves compression of the axillary nerve and the posterior humeral circumflex artery as it courses through this area. The syndrome has been reported in throwing athletes who present with poorly localized shoulder pain and intermittent, nondermatomal paresthesia of the upper arm without associated trauma. The pain can be reproduced by abduction and external rotation of the arm, and it hinders throwing activities.

The diagnosis is confirmed by subclavian arteriogram, which demonstrates occlusion of the posterior humeral circumflex artery when the arm is abducted and externally rotated (Fig. 5, *center* and *right*). Nonsurgical treatment is tried first and involves physical therapy for gentle internal rotation stretching, horizontal stretching in adduction, and rotator cuff strengthening. If this fails, then surgical decompression is used. It involves detaching the insertion of the teres minor and releasing any tethering fibrous bands.

Axillary Artery Occlusion

Transient arterial occlusion caused by pressure from the pectoralis minor muscle has been reported during the cocking

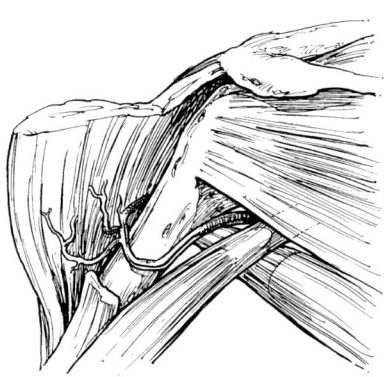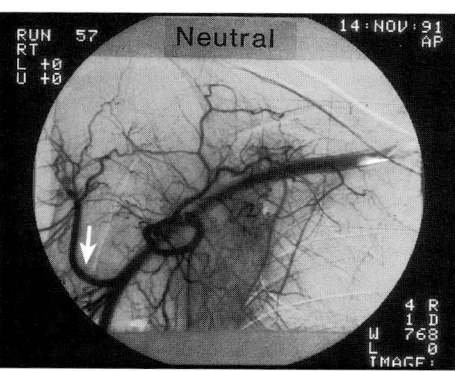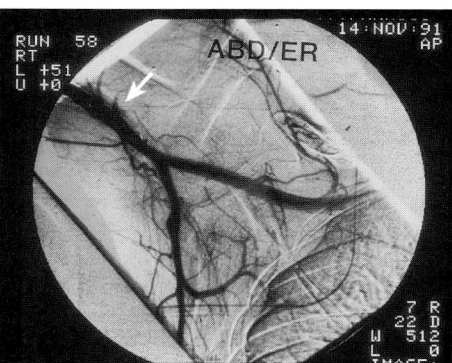

Fig. 5 **Left,** The quadrangular space is bordered by the humeral shaft, teres minor, teres major, and long head of the triceps tendon. The posterior circumflex artery and axillary nerve exit this space from anterior to posterior. Compression of these neurovascular structures may occur in throwing athletes. (Reproduced with permission from Liu SH: Neurovascular compression syndromes about the shoulder, in Baker CL (ed): *The Hughston Clinic Sports Medicine Book.* Baltimore, MD, Williams & Wilkins, 1995, pp 280-284.) **Center,** Arteriogram demonstrating the normal vascular flow in the quadrangular space with an intact posterior humeral circumflex artery (arrow). The arm is in neutral position. **Right,** Arteriogram with the arm in abduction external rotation demonstrating compression/occlusion of the posterior humeral circumflex artery (arrow), which is diagnostic for quadrilateral space syndrome.

phase of throwing in pitchers. Occurrence in other throwing athletes and wind surfers has also been reported. The symptoms include pain, pectoralis minor tenderness, claudication, upper extremity fatigue, diminished pulses, and cyanosis reproduced by hyperabducting and externally rotating the arm. The definitive diagnosis is made by angiographic demonstration of axillary artery occlusion or aneurysmal dilatation. Surgery usually is required for effective treatment. Procedures include thrombectomy, synovectomy, excision and bypass grafting, and angioplasty.

Effort thrombosis is an axillary or subclavian vein thrombosis associated with repetitive, vigorous activities or associated with blunt trauma that results in indirect or direct injury to the vein. Symptoms include aching pain, numbness, and a feeling of heaviness in the arm with associated swollen upper extremity. The neurovascular examination is otherwise normal. The diagnosis is confirmed with venography. Effort thrombosis is treated nonsurgically with elevation and with heparin or warfarin for anticoagulation.

Selected Bibliography

Instability Complex
Kvitne RS, Jobe FW: The diagnosis and treatment of anterior instability in the throwing athlete. *Clin Orthop* 1993;291:107-123.

The mechanism of recurrent anterior instability as it develops in the throwing athlete is discussed with description of both a repetitive microtrauma and posterior-superior glenoid impingement mechanisms. Conservative management is effective in most chronic overuse injuries. Those athletes that fail conservative treatment often require surgical intervention. Capsular redundancy and labral injury are both addressed with the anterior capsulolabral reconstruction. Athletes described include group 1 with primary impingement; group 2 with primary instability from recurrent microtrauma and secondary subacromial impingement; group 3 with primary shoulder instability secondary to generalized ligamentous hyperelasticity and secondary impingement; and group 4 with primary instability without impingement.

Walch G, Boileau P, Noel E, et al: Impingement of the deep surface of the supraspinatus tendon on the posterosuperior glenoid rim: An arthroscopic study. *J Shoulder Elbow Surg* 1992;1:238-245.

Seventeen throwing athletes with shoulder pain were examined arthroscopically and were determined to have primary instability of the shoulder with secondary impingement of the undersurface of the rotator cuff on the posterior-superior glenoid labrum. A partial rotator cuff tear involving the undersurface of the supraspinatus and the infraspinatus tendons were seen in eight patients, with a partial capsulotendinous rupture in nine patients. Twelve patients had additional lesions of the posterior-superior labrum.

Clinical Diagnosis and Classification of Anterior Shoulder Pain
Hawkins RJ, Kennedy JC: Impingement syndrome in athletes. *Am J Sports Med* 1980;8:151-158.

Neer CS II: Impingement lesions. *Clin Orthop* 1983;173: 70-77.

Impingement and Rotator Cuff Lesions

Bigliani LU, Kimmel J, McCann PD, et al: Repair of rotator cuff tears in tennis players. *Am J Sports Med* 1992;20: 112-117.

Twenty-three tennis players with complete rotator cuff tears underwent anterior acromioplasty and rotator cuff repair. Nineteen (83%) were able to return to a pain-free presymptomatic competitive level of tennis. Three (13%) with massive tears had satisfactory results but persistent weakness. One (4%) with a massive tear had an unsatisfactory result and was unable to play tennis.

Roye RP, Grana WA, Yates CK: Arthroscopic subacromial decompression: Two- to seven-year follow-up. *Arthroscopy* 1995;11:301-306.

Eighty-eight patients (90 shoulders) with stage II or early stage III impingement syndrome unresponsive to conservative treatment were studied retrospectively following arthroscopic subacromial decompression. No statistical difference in function was found between the patients without rotator cuff tear (47) and the group with a proximal rotator cuff tear. Satisfactory results were obtained in 68% of throwing athletes and 90% of nonthrowing athletes. Only 50% of competitive baseball and softball pitchers had satisfactory results. Arthroscopic subacromial decompression was determined to be an acceptable alternative to open anterior acromioplasty for the treatment of the impingement lesion.

Tibone JE, Jobe FW, Kerlan RK, et al: Shoulder impingement syndrome in athletes treated by an anterior acromioplasty. *Clin Orthop* 1985;198:134-140.

Tibone JE, Elrod B, Jobe FW, et al: Surgical treatment of tears of the rotator cuff in athletes. *J Bone Joint Surg* 1986;68A:887-891.

Recurrent Anterior Instability

Bigliani LU, Kurzweil PR, Schwartzbach CC, et al: Inferior capsular shift procedure for anterior-inferior shoulder instability in athletes. *Am J Sports Med* 1994;22:578-584.

Sixty-three patients (including 31 throwing athletes) with anterior-inferior glenohumeral instability underwent a laterally based capsular shift procedure, combined with repair of the Bankart lesion when present (31%). Satisfactory results were achieved in 94%, and 92% returned to sports (75% at the same level). The rate of recurrence of instability was 3%.

Bigliani LU, Pollock RG, Soslowsky LJ, et al: Tensile properties of the inferior glenohumeral ligament. *J Orthop Res* 1992;10:187-197.

Structural and mechanical properties of the three regions of the inferior glenohumeral ligament in a cadaver study are reported. The thickness of this ligament decreased significantly from its superior band (average, 2.8 mm) to its posterior axillary pouch (average, 1.7 mm). The ligament failures occurred in both the midsubstance (35%) and at the insertion sites (65%), although significant stretching occurred prior to failure, regardless of the ultimate failure mode.

Montgomery WH III, Jobe FW: Functional outcomes in athletes after modified anterior capsulolabral reconstruction. *Am J Sports Med* 1994;22:352-358.

Thirty-two consecutive athletes underwent anterior capsulolabral reconstruction with a horizontal capsulotomy and fixation with suture anchors. Ninety-seven percent good or excellent results were achieved, and 81% returned to the same sport at the same level of competition, including nine of 13 (69%) baseball pitchers.

Morgan CD: Arthroscopic transglenoid Bankart suture repair. *Op Tech Orthop* 1991;1:171-179.

Wolf EM, Cheng JC, Dickson K: Humeral avulsion of glenohumeral ligaments as a cause of anterior shoulder instability. *Arthroscopy* 1995;11:600-607.

The authors studied 64 shoulders with anterior instability that were prospectively evaluated by arthroscopy. Humeral avulsion of the glenohumeral ligaments (HAGL) was found in six shoulders (9.3%). This lesion was easily seen on arthroscopic examination, but is difficult to see during the open procedure because of the anterior approach to the shoulder. The arthroscopic finding of an exposed subscapularis muscle should alert the surgeon to the possibility of a HAGL lesion as a potential cause for shoulder instability.

Injuries to the Acromioclavicular Joint

Berg EE: A preliminary report of acromioclavicular joint reconstruction with clavicular corticotomy. *J Shoulder Elbow Surg* 1995;4:135-140.

The surgical procedure is described for extra-articular acromioclavicular fixation, coracoclavicular ligament repair, and clavicular corticotomy. At a minimum 2-year follow-up, the coracoclavicular interval was improved an average of 12.5 mm and was restored to within 2 mm of the normal side on stress radiographs.

Cahill BR: Osteolysis of the distal part of the clavicle in male athletes. *J Bone Joint Surg* 1982;64A:1053-1058.

Dumontier C, Sautet A, Man M, et al: Acromioclavicular dislocations: Treatment by coracoacromial ligamentoplasty. *J Shoulder Elbow Surg* 1995;4:130-134.

This is a retrospective review of 32 patients who had undergone acute treatment and 24 patients who had undergone late treatment using ligamentoplasty with the coracoacromial ligament. The surgical technique is described. The authors report satisfactory results in 81% of patients who underwent acute treatment and in 79% of patients who underwent late treatment.

Flatow EL, Cordasco FA, Bigliani LU: Arthroscopic resection of the outer end of the clavicle from a superior approach: A critical, quanitative, radiographic assessment of bone removal. *Arthroscopy* 1992;8:55-64.

Twelve patients with osteolysis of the clavicle were treated with open distal clavicle excision and arthroscopic resection via a superior approach in six patients each. Comparable pain relief and function were achieved in both groups, with pain relief achieved an average of 3.4 months earlier in the arthroscopic group. Morbidity was decreased overall with a lessened hospital stay and fewer complications. Satisfactory bone removal was comprobable to the open distal clavicle excision group.

Morrison DS, Lemos MJ: Acromioclavicular separation: Reconstruction using synthetic loop augmentation. *Am J Sports Med* 1995;23:105-110.

This is a retrospective study of 14 patients who underwent acromioclavicular reconstruction using a synthetic loop passed through drill holes in the base of the coracoid and the anterior third of the clavicle. The surgical technique is described. Twelve of the 14 patients had good to excellent results and returned to normal sport or work activities at 6 months.

Nuber GW, Bowen MK: Acromioclavicular joint injuries and distal clavicle fractures. *J Am Acad Orthop Surg* 1997;5:11-18.

A review of the six types of acromioclavicular sprains and three types of distal clavicle fractures is presented.

Sim E, Schwarz N, Hocker K, et al: Repair of complete acromioclavicular separations using the acromioclavicular-hook plate. *Clin Orthop* 1995;314:134-142.

Tibone J, Sellers R, Tonino P: Strength testing after third-degree acromioclavicular dislocations. *Am J Sports Med* 1992;20:328-331.

Twenty male patients with a grade III acromioclavicular joint dislocation were evaluated more than 2 years after injury and treatment using a Cybex II dynamometer in three planes. There was no significant difference between injured and uninjured shoulders. Subjective complaints were minor, and neither activities of daily living nor athletic participation were impaired.

Weinstein DM, McCann PD, McIlveen SJ, et al: Surgical treatment of complete acromioclavicular dislocations. *Am J Sports Med* 1995;23:324-331.

This retrospective study examines 27 patients who underwent repair for acute grade III acromioclavicular separations and 17 patients who underwent reconstructions for chronic grade III acromioclavicular separations. The average follow-up was 4 years. The technique is described. Coracoclavicular fixation with heavy nonabsorbable sutures was used to correct superior displacement. The coracoacromial ligament was transferred to the distal clavicle in 15 of the early repairs and in all of the late reconstructions. Ninety-six percent of the early repairs and 77% of the late reconstructions achieved satisfactory results. Results of early repair were significantly better than the results of repair more than 3 months after injury.

Neurovascular Injuries

Cahill BR, Palmer RE: Quadrilateral space syndrome. *J Hand Surg* 1983;8A:65-69.

Drez D Jr: Suprascapular neuropathy in the differential diagnosis of rotator cuff injuries. *Am J Sports Med* 1976;4:43-45.

Foo CL, Swann M: Isolated paralysis of the serratus anterior: A report of 20 cases. *J Bone Joint Surg* 1983;65B:552-556.

Fritz RC, Helms CA, Steinbach LS, et al: Suprascapular nerve entrapment: Evaluation with MR imaging. *Radiology* 1992;182:437-444.

Twenty-seven masses were identified adjacent to the suprascapular nerve on magnetic resonance imaging of the shoulder. There were 21 ganglion cysts, two synovial sarcomas, one Ewing sarcoma, one metastatic renal cell carcinoma, one chondrosarcoma, and one hematoma associated with a fracture.

Markey KL, Di Benedetto M, Curl WW: Upper trunk brachial plexopathy: The stinger syndrome. *Am J Sports Med* 1993;21:650-655.

The authors undertook a four-phase study of 261 football players. Electromyograms and nerve conduction studies delineated the lesions in 32 players. Compression of the fixed brachial plexus between the shoulder pad and the superomedial scapula was the most common mechanism of injury.

Meyer SA, Schulte KR, Callaghan JJ, et al: Cervical spinal stenosis and stingers in collegiate football players. *Am J Sports Med* 1994;22:158-166.

Redler MR, Ruland LJ III, McCue FC III: Quadrilateral space syndrome in a throwing athlete. *Am J Sports Med* 1986;14:511-513.

Rohrer MJ, Cardullo PA, Pappas AM, et al: Axillary artery compression and thrombosis in throwing athletes. *J Vasc Surg* 1990;11:761-769.

Speer KP, Bassett FH III: The prolonged burner syndrome. *Am J Sports Med* 1990;18:591-594.

Vastamäki M, Göransson H: Suprascapular nerve entrapment. *Clin Orthop* 1993;297:135-143.

Fifty-four patients were evaluated at an average of 5.6 years after surgical release. Sixteen patients had atrophy of the supraspinatus and 26 of the infraspinatus. The mean time from onset of symptoms to surgery was 2.8 years. Fifty-two patients had surgical treatment at the suprascapular notch. Pain disappeared promptly in 24 cases and markedly diminished in 15 cases. Persistent atrophy was found more often in the infraspinatus. There were ten poor long-term results.

# 13

Complications, Failed Repairs, and Revision Surgery

Christopher T. Behr, MD and David W. Altchek, MD

The study of glenohumeral instability has posed a challenge to shoulder surgeons for some time, first in the understanding of the various types of instability in regard to the particular pathoanatomy, and more recently in terms of choosing the appropriate surgical techniques. The common goal of treatment is elimination of instability; however, there is a delicate balance between leaving the joint loose enough to preserve motion versus tightening the joint enough to prevent recurrence. These two issues account for the majority of failures encountered in instability surgery.

Complications

Complications stemming from the treatment of glenohumeral instability can be divided into two groups: intraoperative and postoperative. There is considerable overlap between these two groups, because many "intraoperative" complications are not recognized until the "postoperative" period; intraoperative complications will include those occurring as a direct result of technique in the operating room that become apparent in the immediate perioperative period. The postoperative group will include those that arise later on during recovery/rehabilitation.

Intraoperative

Intraoperative complications are usually procedure-specific and prevention of these can, for the most part, be accomplished with a thorough knowledge of all potential pitfalls. As with any surgery, proper patient positioning is an important first step in the prevention of complications. Padding of all bony prominences and potential sites of nerve compression (such as the head of the fibula and the contralateral ulnar nerve) reduces the chance of pressure necrosis and nerve injury. Because many shoulder procedures are performed in the beachchair position, securing the patient to the operating room table while maintaining an adequate field of surgical exposure is essential. This is especially important when regional anesthesia is used. Patients under the influence of intravenous sedation have been known to move during the procedure. A deflatable beanbag is very helpful in securing the patient while in the beachchair position. The patient should be comfortable and the head secured, usually with the aid of a headrest. The anesthesiologist should be provided with easy access to the airway. If the lateral decubitus position is used for shoulder arthroscopy, no more than 10 to 15 lb (maximum) of traction should be applied; excessive abduction and extension of the arm can lead to neurapraxia.

Open anterior stabilizations are performed through a deltopectoral approach. Care should be taken to locate the cephalic vein which, along with the coracoid, are landmarks to the interval. Failure to find this internervous plane can lead to a difficult dissection through the deltoid and can lead to denervation of the anterior portion of the deltoid. The musculocutaneous and axillary nerves are at greatest risk during anterior shoulder stabilization procedures. The musculocutaneous nerve enters the coracobrachialis muscle as close as 2.5 cm distal to the tip of the coracoid. Retractors placed under the conjoint tendon can cause neurapraxia; therefore, vigorous retraction must be avoided. The conjoined tendons are left intact as additional protection to the brachial plexus. The axillary nerve courses laterally over the belly of the subscapularis muscle before it dives into the quadrilateral space around the inferior margin of the subscapularis at the muscle-tendon junction. Exposure of the inferior capsule places this nerve at risk, especially if there is scar tissue in this region. It is usually not necessary to expose the nerve. Simple palpation is usually enough; however, if dissection is difficult and the nerve cannot be palpated, exposure of the nerve may be indicated. In most cases, injury to either the axillary or musculocutaneous nerve is caused by traction neurapraxia, with return of full function over time. The vasculature most at risk are the anterior humeral circumflex vessels that course along the inferior border of the subscapularis. The vessels must be carefully avoided or precisely ligated; if transected vessels are allowed to retract medially, hemostasis can be difficult.

The surgeon must decide whether to incise the subscapularis tendon vertically or to perform a horizontal subscapularis muscle-splitting approach. To maximize exposure, a vertical tenotomy is usually preferred for capsular shift procedures. If the tendon is to be taken down, the incision should be approximately 2 cm medial to the lesser tuberosity, with a cuff of tendon left attached to the tuberosity so that a secure repair can be achieved. Postoperative ruptures of the subscapularis are an unfortunate but important complication following anterior stabilization surgery. In addition, great care should be taken to repair the cut ends of the tendon anatomically to avoid tendon shortening, which can lead to a loss of external rotation. A subscapularis muscle-splitting approach is usually preferred in throwing athletes to decrease the risk of muscle shortening and minimize the chance of motion loss. If this procedure is performed, care should be taken to minimize trauma to the muscle with retraction during this exposure.

The Bankart repair can be a technically demanding procedure because most of the work is done medially and obtaining good exposure can be difficult. Although the advent of suture anchors has made glenoid rim suture fixation much easier, new potential complications have been introduced (Fig. 1). Aberrant drilling through glenoid articular cartilage can cause chondral injury. Alternatively, placing the anchors too medial from the glenoid rim is inappropriate, leaving excess medial redundancy in the capsule. Likewise, failure to cinch down knots onto the glenoid rim will leave too much laxity in the repair. When needles are passed through the medial capsule, the course of the axillary nerve should be noted so that injury can be avoided.

Although suture anchors can occasionally be problematic, these devices have fared much better than staples. O'Driscoll and Evans reviewed the long-term results of 204 staple capsulorrhaphies for anterior instability after an average of 10 years; postoperative instability occurred in 22% of shoulders, loosening and migration of the staple occurred in 12%, and approximately half of all patients continued to have pain at follow-up. For these reasons, staple capsulorrhaphy is no longer recommended to treat glenohumeral instability.

As shown by Neer and Foster in 1980, and later by Altchek and associates, traumatic instability as seen in an athletic population can provide a multidirectional component to the instability. In these cases it is important to incorporate a capsular shift with the Bankart repair to eliminate both anterior and inferior/posterior laxity. A recent biomechanical study examining strategies for anterior capsular shift procedures showed that superior shifting of the inferomedial capsule on the glenoid rim significantly decreased both inferior and posterior translation when compared with medial shifting alone.

Because posterior stabilization surgery is less familiar to most surgeons than the anterior deltopectoral approach, intraoperative complications are more likely. The axillary and suprascapular nerves are both at risk. The infraspinatus-splitting approach provides a more equatorial exposure of the posterior capsule than going through the infraspinatus-teres minor interval. The infraspinatus-splitting approach is safe and does not lead to denervation of the muscle. The suprascapular nerve may be as close as 1.5 cm medial to the posterior glenoid margin, and excessive medial retraction should be avoided. Neer has reported an axillary nerve injury following a posterior capsular shift. The surgeon must take care not to injure the axillary nerve when dissecting the inferior portion of the posterior capsule.

Intraoperative complications of arthroscopic stabilizations include those that exist for any arthroscopic procedure. Improper portal placement may lead to neurovascular injury, especially if anterior portals are made medial to the coracoid. Insertion of fixation devices such as metal anchors and tacks can cause injury to the glenoid articular surface with penetration of the drill bit through the subchondral plate. This injury can be avoided through proper selection of the insertion angle, which is made easier by good portal placement. Before selecting the portal site, the drilling angle should first be checked with a spinal needle. Once the proper angle is achieved, the portal can be placed.

Overimpaction of a fixation device, such as staples or tacks, can cause tearing through the soft tissue that it is intended to hold. This is especially true with thin, friable tissue. It is better to leave the device a millimeter or two above the tissue rather than risk amputation of the tissue.

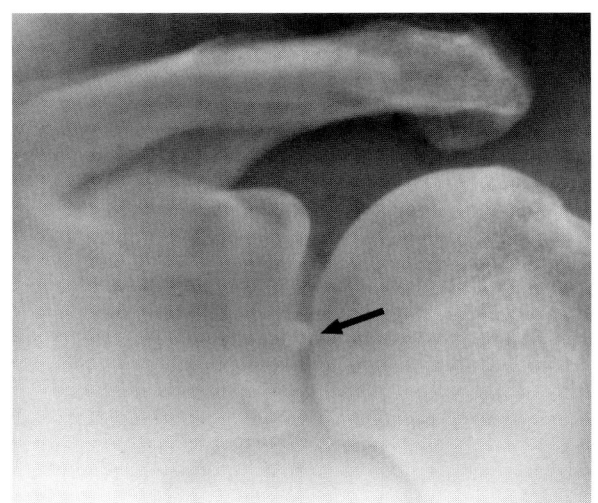

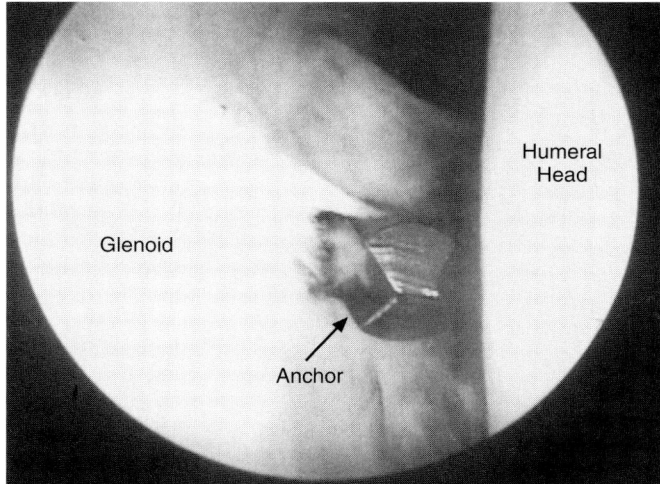

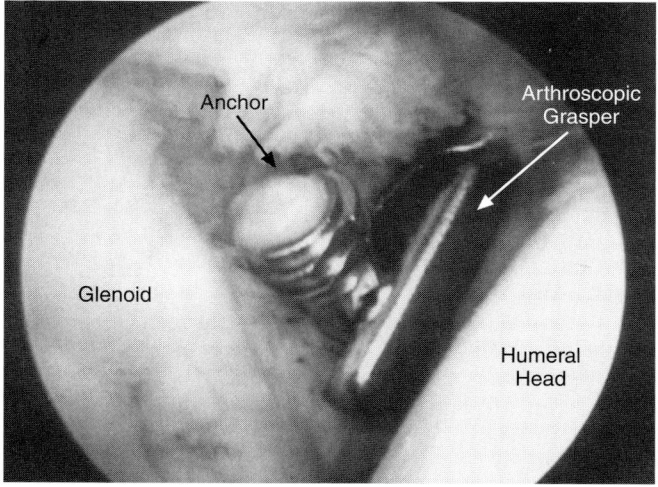

Fig. 1 Migration of a suture anchor to an intra-articular position. **Top,** Plain radiograph that is suspicious for migration of the anchor into the joint (*arrow*). **Center,** Arthroscopic view of the anchor clearly in the joint. **Bottom,** Arthroscopic removal of the hardware.

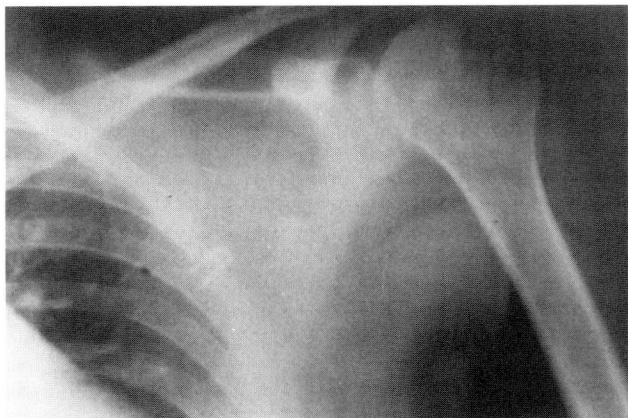 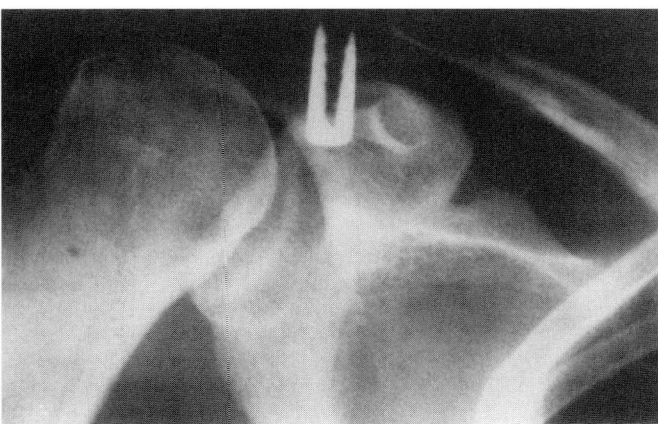

Fig. 2 Loosening and migration of capsular staples. **Left,** Staple has migrated to a position between the scapula and posterior thorax. **Right,** Rotation of a staple 90°, with the tines of the staple now pointed superiorly. (Reproduced with permission from Lane JG, Sachs RA, Riehl B: Arthroscopic staple capsulorrhaphy: A long-term follow-up. *Arthroscopy* 1993;9:190-194.)

Biodegradable tacks avoid the potential complications of metal in the joint because they are gradually reabsorbed over a 6-week period. Arthroscopic staple capsulorrhaphy has been fraught with complications, including humeral head impingement, backing out of the staple into the joint, and loss of fixation (leading to recurrent instability). Migration of staples has also been reported, with their retrieval from such unusual locations as the brachial plexus, subacromial space, and between the scapula and rib cage (Fig. 2). Transglenoid suture techniques also promote injury to the articular surface during drilling, and knots tied posteriorly over the infraspinatus fascia can cause irritation at this site. There is also one report of a patient who developed a synovial cyst that extended posteriorly from the glenoid drill holes along the path of the sutures.

The so-called nonanatomic stabilization procedures, while done extensively in the past, have largely fallen out of favor. Included in this group are the Putti-Platt, Magnusen-Stack, Bristow, bone block procedures, and osteotomies. The most common complication associated with the Putti-Platt procedure is limitation of external rotation by shortening the subscapularis muscle. This is caused by excessive tightening of the subscapularis and capsule. Along with loss of motion, a more disturbing complication of this procedure as reported by Hawkins is chronic posterior subluxation of the humeral head leading to the development of osteoarthrosis (Fig. 3). In the Magnusen-Stack procedure the subscapularis muscle is also functionally shortened as it is transferred from its insertion on the lesser tuberosity to a position lateral to the bicipital groove. Again, loss of external rotation occurs, and the specific capsulolabral pathology is never addressed.

Most complications associated with the Bristow procedure have to do with faulty placement of the coracoid transfer onto the anterior scapular neck (Fig. 4). When the coracoid is misplaced too high, the humeral head can subluxate inferiorly; lateral placement may cause impingement of the humeral head during internal rotation, and medial placement can lead to recurrence of the instability. Nonunion of the bone block has also been reported. Complications of hardware placement can also occur during a Bristow operation. Placement of the screw can injure the suprascapular nerve posteriorly. Fracture of the coracoid bone block can occur, leading to a higher rate of failure. Injury to the musculocutaneous nerve has been reported to be higher during a Bristow than any other stabilization procedure. Young and Rockwood reported a 14% intraoperative complication rate during this procedure.

Bone block procedures and humeral and glenoid osteotomies are now used only rarely in revision surgery, when the anatomy cannot be restored by other means. Complications encountered during these procedures include hardware failure, loss of fixation, and nonunion.

Postoperative

Postoperative complications are the second group of complications encountered with instability surgery. Although many of these complications may not become evident until weeks, months, or even years after surgery, the majority are the result of inadequate preoperative planning, inappropriate procedure selection, poor surgical technique, or inappropriate postoperative care of the patient. History, physical examination, radiologic studies, and examination under anesthesia help provide the information needed for the surgical decision-making process. In addition, the patient's goals, expectations, and level of competition in sports must be carefully addressed to ensure good results and patient satisfaction. For example, limitation of motion in a throwing athlete can be as disabling as recurrent instability.

Limitation of motion and recurrence of instability are the two most common postoperative complications encountered with instability surgery. Historically, the success of this type of surgery was based on the redislocation rate, and a decrease in motion was an expected result to ensure a low recurrence rate. Many of the earlier stabilization procedures

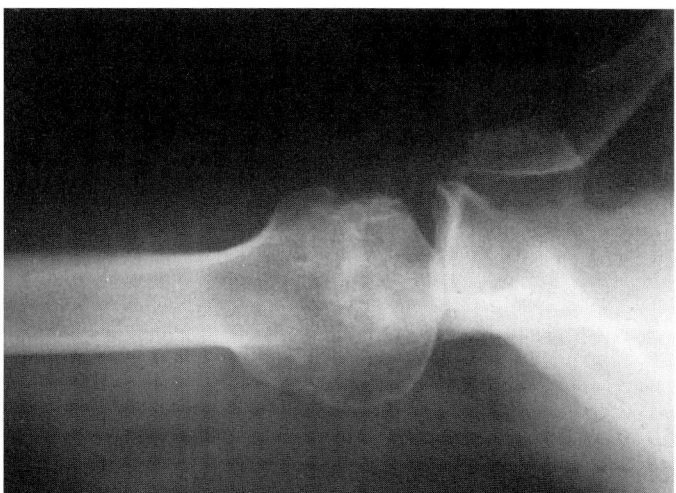 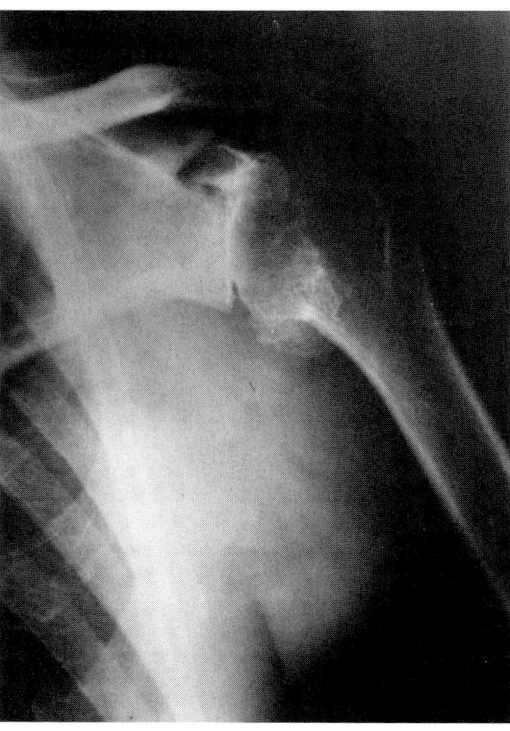

Fig. 3 Development of osteoarthrosis following a Putti-Platt procedure. **Left,** Axillary radiograph revealing posterior subluxation of the humeral head. **Right,** Anteroposterior radiograph showing significant joint space narrowing and a large inferior osteophyte.

were nonanatomic procedures based on altering the anatomy to limit external rotation and/or provide additional static restraints to keep the humeral head located. Anatomic repair of the pathology so that motion is preserved and the patient can return to sports has recently been emphasized. However, the patient must be made aware that a percentage of throwing athletes may not return to their prior competitive levels or regain their prior throwing velocity even when an anatomic repair is performed.

Limitation of external rotation can be one of the most serious postoperative complications that can occur following anterior stabilization surgery. In addition to causing significant functional limitations, restricted external rotation can lead to a number of other problems. A retrospective study analyzed 20 shoulders in 19 patients who had been managed for loss of external rotation after previous anterior capsulorrhaphy; 17 shoulders were painful, seven were either subluxated or dislocated posteriorly, and 16 had some degree of osteoarthrosis. Currently there are no studies that clearly define what degree of loss of external rotation will lead to these significant complications. However, the authors from the above-mentioned study recommend that a minimum of 20° to 25° of passive external rotation must be present at the end of any procedure for instability; patients who are limited to 0° or less of external rotation at 6 months postoperatively should be considered for surgical release, or recession or lengthening of the anterior structures.

An article on techniques for selecting capsular tightness during open repair of anterior-inferior shoulder instability was published recently. The first part of the two-part study consisted of a survey of surgical techniques administered to all members of the American Shoulder and Elbow Surgeons, and the second part is a technique description for tightening of an anterior-inferior capsular shift. Most surgeons agreed that preservation of external rotation was important, and shoulder position during capsular repair probably influences the ultimate range of motion obtained. However, no more than 50% of the respondents agreed on any one position for flexion, abduction, and external rotation. The authors described a technique for selective capsular tightening in which the Bankart repair is done medially to the glenoid without any capsular shortening, followed by a laterally based inferior capsular shift with the shoulder positioned in 60° to 80° of abduction, 45° to 60° of external rotation, and 10° of flexion during tightening. The exact positioning of abduction and external rotation was determined on an individual basis based on patient need, hand dominance, and throwing status. Attention to arm position can be essential in achieving the proper tensioning during capsular repair so that the risk of overtightening resulting in loss of motion is minimized.

Failed Repairs

Recurrence of subluxation or dislocation has long been the criteria for failure following shoulder stabilization procedures. The recurrence rate of anterior instability was 3.5% in

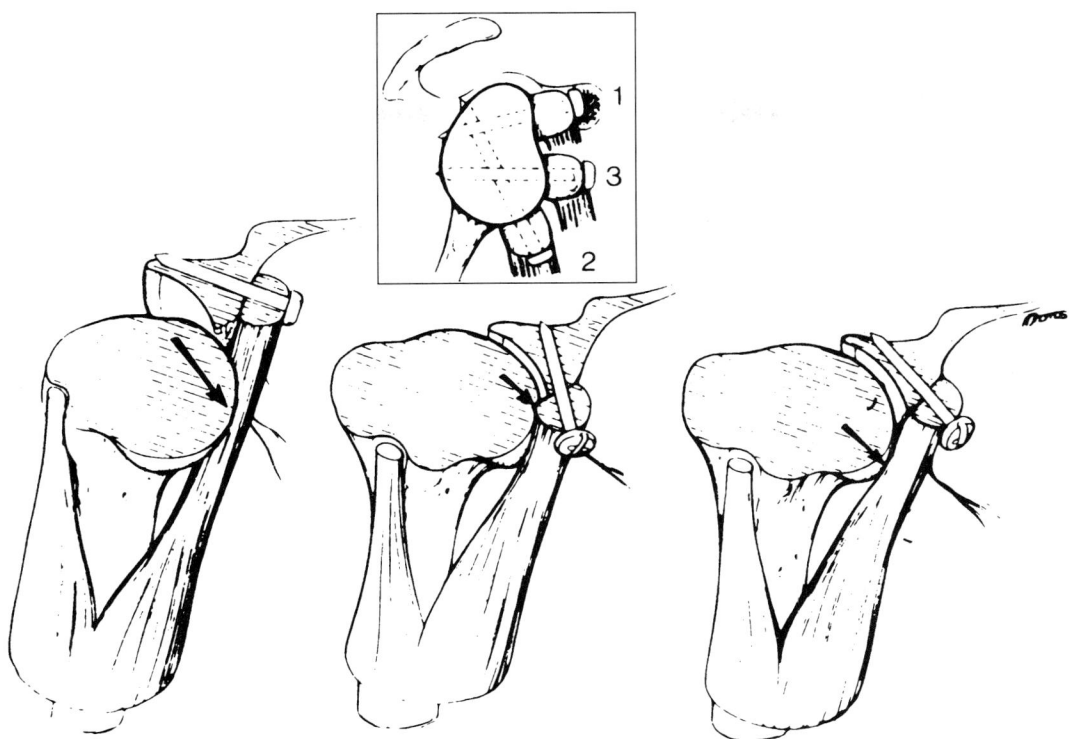

Fig. 4 Errors in placement of the coracoid bone block during Bristow procedures. **Left,** Placement too medial (allows anterior subluxation). **Center,** Placement too lateral (causes humeral head impingement). **Right,** Correct placement helps prevent anterior subluxation. **Top,** Bone placed too high, leading to inferior subluxation (1); Too low (2); Correct placement at approximately 4 o'clock on the glenoid rim (3). (Reproduced with permission from Wall MS, Warren RF: Complications of shoulder instability. *Clin Sports Med* 1995;14:973-1000.)

patients treated with Bankart repair. Patients with multidirectional instability have been treated with a variety of open procedures. The inferior capsular shift procedure has a failure rate of 2.9% to 10% depending on the report. Altchek and associates reported on the results of the T-plasty modification of the Bankart procedure for anterior-inferior multidirectional instability, which failed in four of 42 patients (9.5%) in an athletic population.

In recent years, attempts have been made to match these low failure rates with arthroscopic procedures. A study comparing early morbidity and complications between open and arthroscopic Bankart procedures found a significant reduction in surgery time, estimated blood loss, postoperative narcotic use, duration of hospitalization, and work days missed among the group treated arthroscopically. In addition, it has been suggested that arthroscopic stabilization procedures may lead to an improved postoperative range of motion, a quicker return to competition, and return of preinjury throwing velocity in a higher percentage of throwing athletes. For these reasons, a strong push has been made to develop arthroscopic techniques in which failure rates are decreased to those of open stabilizations.

Initial studies evaluating arthroscopic stabilizations reported on the results of arthroscopic staple capsulorrhaphy, which had evolved from the open duToit capsular stapling procedure. This new arthroscopic stapling technique has had unacceptably high recurrence rates, as much as 25% to 33% in some series. Hardware complications from the intra-articular staple, including painful hardware, loosening, and erosion of the humeral head and subscapularis muscle, are also common. Because of these high failure rates and complications, other fixation techniques including transglenoid sutures, metal rivets, cannulated screws, suture anchors, and biodegradable tacks have been developed. Several authors have reported their results using cannulated screw fixation; again, failure rate was well above that of open techniques (between 15% and 28%), and painful irritation from the hardware occurred in 20% of patients. A minimum 4-year follow-up study of arthroscopic stabilizations using transglenoid suture repair retrospectively reviewed the results in 37 patients; seven patients (19%) developed recurrent instability following the procedure. All recurrences in this series were evident by 2 years after the operation. Absence of a Bankart lesion at operation and participation in contact sports and downhill skiing were associated with the development of postoperative instability. Other factors that have been associated with poor outcomes in terms of postoperative instability include excessive capsular laxity and poorly defined glenohumeral ligaments. Some authors also suggest that arthroscopic stabilizations may require longer periods of immobilization than open surgery in order to prevent postoperative recurrence. This obviates some of the potential advantages of an arthroscopic repair.

Biodegradable fixation devices such as those made of polyglyconate or polylactic acid were developed to avoid complications of metal implants inserted into the glenohumeral joint. Initial 2-year results were very encouraging, with recurrence rates under 10% as reported by Warner and Warren; longer follow-up on this same group of patients at an average of 42 months revealed a failure rate of 21%.

Warner and associates reviewed a group of 96 patients who underwent arthroscopic Bankart repair using a cannulated, absorbable fixation device made of polyglyconate (Suretac; Acufex Microsurgical, Mansfield, MA). A cohort of 15 patients went on to second-look arthroscopy for either pain or recurrent instability; seven of these 15 had developed recurrent instability and at second-look arthroscopy, an inspection of the healing response was performed. Of these seven failed repairs, the Bankart lesion had completely healed in three, partially healed in one, and had recurred in three. In all seven failures, there was evidence of attenuation of the inferior glenohumeral ligament or excessive laxity of the capsule. In two patients, a biopsy specimen was taken from the region where the Suretac device had originally been placed. Histologic section showed a histiocytic infiltrate with foreign body giant cells surrounding amorphous debris, which may indicate that some patients may develop a chronic inflammatory reaction at the repair site; it is unknown how this inflammatory response impacts the healing of the capsulolabral complex to bone.

A biomechanical study evaluating the tensile properties of the inferior glenohumeral ligament in 16 cadaver shoulders was performed by Bigliani and associates. The strain to failure rate averaged 27%, indicating that significant deformation of the ligamentous structures may occur before medial detachment of the glenoid-capsulolabral complex. Speer and associates created a simulated Bankart lesion in nine cadaver shoulders; although this Bankart lesion alone did result in selected increases in anterior translation at all positions of elevation, these increases were very small. The authors concluded that a Bankart lesion alone is not enough to account for the increased translation necessary to produce an anterior dislocation of the shoulder. This further biomechanical evidence suggests that plastic deformation of the capsular ligaments is part of the pathology in recurrent dislocations of the glenohumeral joint.

Several recent studies have examined the initial failure strength of Bankart repairs using many of the more commonly used fixation devices. In a canine shoulder model, the normal intact capsule-to-bone complex fails at 235 N. This failure strength was compared with eight different repair techniques using common commercially available fixation devices. The traditional open Bankart repair failed at 122.1 N (using two sutures) and 74.7 N (one suture). The Acufex TAG rod (Acufex Microsurgical, Mansfield, MA) failed at 143.5 N (two sutures) and 79.8 N (one suture). Transglenoid suture repair using two sutures failed at 166.6 N. Two different suture anchors were tested, each with one suture attached to the anchor: the Mitek GII (Mitek, Norwood, MA) failed at 96.4 N and the Zimmer Statak (Zimmer Inc, Warsaw, IN) at 95.2 N. The Acufex bioabsorbable Suretac (Acufex Microsurgical, Mansfield, MA) failed at 82.2 N. Repair techniques employing one suture were statistically equivalent in strength to one another and to the Suretac device. All types of two-suture repairs were statistically equivalent in strength to one another, but were found to be significantly stronger than one suture repair ($p < 0.01$). The difference between the two groups was in the mode of failure. In the two-suture repair group, failure occurred almost exclusively in the soft tissues around the suture. In the group employing only one suture, approximately half failed because of suture breakage and the other half because of soft-tissue failure around the suture. In no instance did the device break or pull out of bone. The authors concluded that the pullout of suture anchors is rare; two-suture techniques exhibit a stronger initial failure strength than one-suture techniques; suture anchor techniques are equivalent in strength to suture through drill hole techniques; and all repair techniques are initially much weaker than the intact bone-ligament complex. To date no studies have been done to test the strength of repair over time, nor has the strength of a healed Bankart repair been examined.

In summary, when examining the results of stabilization procedures, present data suggests that open procedures for recurrent anterior and anterior-inferior instability have success rates of greater than 90%. Arthroscopic stabilization procedures for traumatic anterior instability have success rates approaching 80%.

Revision Surgery

The approach to revision instability surgery begins with a complete assessment of the patient and obtaining a detailed report of all previous surgeries. It is crucial to identify the reason for failure of the prior surgical procedure(s). The most common reason for a poor outcome in stabilization surgery is the failure to correctly identify and treat the offending pathology. As was emphasized in the section on failed repairs, the most common factor leading to recurrence of instability is inadequate treatment of excessive capsular laxity. Reasons to proceed to revision surgery include recurrence of instability, limitation of external rotation, subscapularis rupture, rotator cuff tears, humeral head impingement, hardware failure, and degenerative joint disease.

The surgical exposure in revision surgery can be complicated by a number of factors. The deltopectoral interval can be difficult to identify because common landmarks are often lost in patients undergoing revision surgery. The cephalic vein may be absent, and if the coracoid has been transferred in a prior procedure, the normal anatomy may be altered. In addition, significant scarring may be encountered, which also makes dissection difficult. Patience and meticulous dissection are essential in revision cases. Neurovascular structures may lie much closer to the surgical field, and a constant awareness, either through palpation or exposure of these structures, will avoid injury.

The primary goal of most revision surgery is to restore normal anatomy. If the subscapularis insertion has been transferred as in a Magnusen-Stack procedure, lateral dissection of the tendon off the capsule is necessary to reattach the tendon to its normal insertion site. If the tendon has been transferred to the greater tuberosity, care must be taken to avoid injuring the biceps tendon during this mobilization. Restoration of subscapularis length is important when revising both failed Putti-Platt and Magnusen-Stack procedures. Passive external rotation of at least 30° is necessary to achieve functional activity. Following a failed Bristow procedure, dense scarring may be encountered in the front of the shoulder where the conjoined tendon has been transferred. If it is possible to free the conjoined tendon and coracoid, they should be transferred back to the base of the coracoid. If this is not possible, then freeing the tethered subscapularis muscle and conjoined tendon from the anterior glenoid and joint capsule is the next best option; this step is followed by restoration of normal subscapularis length (the conjoined tendon can be left attached to the subscapularis muscle belly). When scarring is excessive following a failed Bristow procedure, the musculocutaneous nerve can be protected by not dissecting medial to the transplanted coracoid. In some cases of failed Bristow procedures, there is a bony deficit in the anterior glenoid; repair of the anterior capsule and ligaments to the remaining glenoid rim should be attempted. Finally, all other hardware and fixation devices should be removed and attention should then be directed at restoring the capsular, labral, and ligamentous anatomy of the glenohumeral joint.

A recent study has examined the treatment of loss of external rotation following anterior capsulorrhaphy. It is well accepted that severe loss of external rotation can lead to posterior subluxation or even dislocation, and may ultimately be responsible for osteoarthrosis. It was recommended that anterior soft-tissue release be strongly considered in patients who are limited to 0° of external rotation or less at 6 months after surgery. Nine of 20 shoulders in this study also had significant degenerative changes and were treated by prosthetic arthroplasty as well as soft-tissue release. Significant improvement in external rotation can be achieved.

There remains conflicting information on the results of revision surgery for recurrent instability after previous open repair. Neer and Foster included 11 revision patients in their series on inferior capsular shift and all had a satisfactory outcome. Rowe and associates reported good early results (92% success rate) in a group of patients who had previously undergone revision Bankart repair; however, follow-up was inadequate in 25% of the patients. Steinman and associates reported on 64 patients with 88% elimination of instability. Burkhead and Richie had only one failure in 18 revision surgeries. Young and Rockwood reported satisfactory results in less than 50% of patients overall, and fair or poor results in five of six patients with recurrent multidirectional instability. Recent work by Zabinski and associates reviewed a series of 43 patients who had undergone revision shoulder stabilization at the Hospital for Special Surgery from 1978 to 1992. In patients treated for anterior instability, good or excellent results from the revision surgery were achieved in 78% after a mean follow-up of 77 months. The revision procedure in this group was either Bankart repair or capsular shift. In the group of patients with recurrent multidirectional instability, however, satisfactory results were achieved in only 43%. The patients in this group were treated with either anterior or posterior capsular shift or a combination of the two, graft reconstruction of the capsule and glenohumeral ligaments, or posterior bone block. Use of an Achilles tendon allograft has been successful as a static stabilizer in patients who have recurrent instability following total shoulder arthroplasty and who have deficient tissue needed for the revision stabilization procedure.

Patients with recurrent multidirectional instability in whom multiple attempts at surgical treatment have failed remain a very difficult group to treat. Occasionally, a salvage procedure such as shoulder arthrodesis is the only viable surgical option.

Selected Bibliography

Altchek DW, Warren RF, Skyhar MJ, et al: T-plasty modification of the Bankart procedure for multidirectional instability of the anterior and inferior types. *J Bone Joint Surg* 1991;73A:105-112.

Banas MP, Dalldorf PG, Sebastianelli WJ, et al: Long-term followup of the modified Bristow procedure. *Am J Sports Med* 1993;21:666-671.

Eighty-six procedures with a 2- to 13.7-year follow-up were retrospectively reviewed. Complications included redislocation, coracoid bone block fracture during fixation, painful hardware, broken screw, musculocutaneous nerve paresthesias, wound hematoma, and rotator cuff tendinitis. The group had a 14% reoperation rate (4% repeat stabilization, 10% screw removal).

Bigliani LU, Kurzweil PR, Schwartzbach CC, et al: Inferior capsular shift procedure for anterior-inferior shoulder instability in athletes. *Am J Sports Med* 1994;22:578-584.

In this retrospective review of 68 shoulders in 63 athletes undergoing an inferior capsular shift, there were excellent or good results in 94% and a 3% recurrence rate. Only five of ten elite throwing athletes were able to resume competition and the average loss of external rotation in all patients was 7°.

Bigliani LU, Pollock RG, Soslowsky LJ, et al: Tensile properties of the inferior glenohumeral ligament. *J Orthop Res* 1992;10:187-197.

The tensile properties of the inferior glenohumeral ligament were determined using 16 cadaveric shoulders. The strain to failure for all bone-ligament-bone specimens averaged 27%. The three sites of failure were the glenoid insertion (40%), ligament substance (35%), and humeral insertion (25%).

Cooper RA, Brems JJ: The inferior capsular-shift procedure for multidirectional instability of the shoulder. *J Bone Joint Surg* 1992;74A:1516-1521.

Forty-three shoulders with disabling multidirectional instability were treated with an inferior capsular shift. Ninety-one percent had no recurrence of instability. There were four failures that occurred early in the postoperative period and all were treated with a revision inferior capsular shift. Hemiarthroplasty for degenerative arthritis was eventually required in one of the shoulders in which the procedure failed.

Coughlin L, Rubinovich M, Johansson J, et al: Arthroscopic staple capsulorrhaphy for anterior shoulder instability. *Am J Sports Med* 1992;20:253-256.

This article is a retrospective review of 47 arthroscopic staple capsulorrhaphies with a 4-year follow-up. The recurrence rate was 25% and only 21 of 47 patients were able to resume sporting activities. No loosening of hardware was reported, but three patients required removal of the staple for persistent pain.

Davidson PA, Tibone JE: Anterior-inferior (5 o'clock) portal for shoulder arthroscopy. *Arthroscopy* 1995;11:519-525.

The study describes an anterior-inferior portal technique to facilitate fixation insertion when performing stabilization procedures. Distance of the portal from the musculocutaneous nerve averaged 2.3 cm and from the axillary nerve 2.4 cm.

Duncan R, Savoie FH III: Arthroscopic inferior capsular shift for multidirectional instability of the shoulder: A preliminary report. *Arthroscopy* 1993;9:24-27.

Ten patients were treated with an arthroscopic capsular shift and reexamined at 1 to 3 years with an average Bankart score of 90. No recurrences were reported but only four patients resumed sporting activities. Two patients had pain around the suture knot posteriorly, necessitating removal.

Green MR, Christensen KP: Arthroscopic versus open Bankart procedures: A comparison of early mobidity and complications. *Arthroscopy* 1993;9:371-374.

This article is a retrospective review comparing these two procedures; a reduction in surgery time, blood loss, postoperative narcotic use, duration of hospitalization and work days missed among the arthroscopically stabilized group was noted. The authors alluded to a recurrence of instability in seven of 21 patients treated arthroscopically.

Hawkins RJ, Angelo RL: Glenohumeral osteoarthrosis: A late complication of the Putti-Platt repair. *J Bone Joint Surg* 1990;72A:1193-1197.

Hawkins RH, Hawkins RJ: Failed anterior reconstruction for shoulder instability. *J Bone Joint Surg* 1985;67B:709-714.

Lane JG, Sachs RA, Riehl B: Arthroscopic staple capsulorrhaphy: A long-term follow-up. *Arthroscopy* 1993;9:190-194.

In this retrospective review of 54 shoulders evaluated at an average of 39 months, one third of patients developed recurrent instability and 30% had revision surgery. Loose staples were found in 26% of patients and significant staple migration occurred in several patients.

Lombardo SJ, Kerlan RK, Jobe FW, et al: The modified Bristow procedure for recurrent dislocation of the shoulder. *J Bone Joint Surg* 1976;58A:256-261.

Lusardi DA, Wirth MA, Wurtz D, et al: Loss of external rotation following anterior capsulorrhaphy of the shoulder. *J Bone Joint Surg* 1993;75A:1185-1192.

This article is a retrospective study of 20 shoulders with severe loss of external rotation following previous anterior capsulorrhaphy that were managed successfully with an anterior soft-tissue release alone or a release combined with prosthetic replacement. Average follow-up was 4 years and all patients reported a reduction in pain and improvement in range of motion (average increase, 45°). Patients with severe loss of external rotation following anterior stabilization may be at risk for posterior subluxation of the humeral head (seen in seven shoulders) and the development of glenohumeral osteoarthrosis (16 shoulders).

McEleney ET, Donovan MJ, Shea KP, et al: Initial failure strength of open and arthroscopic Bankart repairs. *Arthroscopy* 1995;11:426-431.

The initial failure strengths of eight currently available Bankart repair techniques were compared in the canine model. The two-suture repairs were statistically equivalent in strength to one another, and they were significantly stronger than the one-suture repairs. Suture anchor techniques are equivalent to the traditional suture through drill hole technique, and the pullout of the anchor from the bone was found to be a rare event.

Neer CS II, Foster CR: Inferior capsular shift for involuntary inferior and multidirectional instability of the shoulder: A preliminary report. *J Bone Joint Surg* 1980;62A:897-908.

Norris TR: Complications following anterior instability repairs, in Bigliani LU (ed): *Complications of Shoulder Surgery.* Baltimore, MD, Williams & Wilkins, 1993, pp 98-116.

O'Driscoll SW, Evans DC: Long-term results of staple capsulorrhaphy for anterior instability of the shoulder. *J Bone Joint Surg* 1993;75A:249-258.

Two hundred four staple capsulorrhaphies were reviewed retrospectively at an average 10-year follow-up. Postoperative instability occurred in 22%, hardware complications in 12%, and approximately half (51%) of the shoulders had pain and half of the patients reported that their quality of life was significantly altered.

Pagnani MJ, Warren RF, Altchek DW, et al: Arthroscopic shoulder stabilization using transglenoid sutures: A four-year minimum followup. *Am J Sports Med* 1996;24:459-467.

In this retrospective study, mean follow-up was 5.6 years after arthroscopic shoulder stabilization using transglenoid suture technique; the procedure failed in 19% of patients and the absence of a Bankart lesion was associated with postoperative instability.

Rockwood CA, Gerber C: Analysis of failed surgical procedures for anterior shoulder instability. *Orthop Trans* 1985;9:48.

Rowe CR, Zarins B, Ciullo JV: Recurrent anterior dislocation of the shoulder after surgical repair: Apparent causes of failure and treatment. *J Bone Joint Surg* 1984;66A:159-168.

Shaffer BS, Conway J, Jobe FW, et al: Infraspinatus muscle-splitting incision in posterior shoulder surgery: An anatomic and electromyographic study. *Am J Sports Med* 1994;22:113-120.

In a combined study, this surgical approach was used in four patients undergoing posterior capsulorrhaphy followed by electromyographic analysis, and in 20 cadavers to demonstrate relevant anatomy. Medial dissection of the interval should be limited to 1.5 cm medial to the posterior glenoid rim to avoid injury to the suprascapular nerve.

Shea KP, O'Keefe RM Jr, Fulkerson JP: Comparison of initial pull-out strength of arthroscopic suture and staple Bankart repair techniques. *Arthroscopy* 1992;8:179-182.

In a canine model, the initial pullout strengths of both the suture repair and staple repair were significantly less than the intact labrum-bone complex, and the suture repair was more than twice as strong as the staple repair.

Small NC: Complications in arthroscopic surgery of the knee and shoulder. *Orthopedics* 1993;16:985-988.

Complications of arthroscopic surgery are reviewed. Complications in shoulder arthroscopy include brachial plexus stretch injuries from traction and fluid extravasation, rotator cuff tears, hardware problems, and bleeding.

Speer KP, Deng X, Borrero S, et al: Biomechanical evaluation of a simulated Bankart lesion. *J Bone Joint Surg* 1994;76A:1819-1826.

Biomechanical analysis was used to determine the effect of sectioning the anterior part of the inferior glenohumeral ligament on glenohumeral translation. Small increases in anterior translation were found but were not enough to allow anterior dislocation of the shoulder; permanent stretching or elongation of the inferior glenohumeral ligament may also be necessary.

Speer KP, Deng X, Torzilli PA, et al: Strategies for an anterior capsular shift of the shoulder: A biomechanical comparison. *Am J Sports Med* 1995;23:264-269.

A biomechanical study was performed on nine shoulders to compare the effect on humeral head translation after a medial capsular shift versus a superior capsular shift. Both superior and medial shifts decreased anterior translation an equivalent amount; however, the superior shift decreased both inferior and posterior translation to a greater extent than the medial shift.

Speer KP, Warren RF, Pagnani M, et al: An arthroscopic technique for anterior stabilization of the shoulder with a bioabsorbable tack. *J Bone Joint Surg* 1996;78A:1801-1807.

In this retrospective review of 52 patients undergoing arthroscopic technique for anterior stabilization using a bioabsorbable tack, instability recurred in 21% (11 patients). Of these 11 failures, four were the result of traumatic reinjury, and seven occurred atraumatically.

Steinmann SR, Flatow EL, Glasgow M, et al: Evaluation and surgical treatment of failed shoulder instability repairs. *Orthop Trans* 1992;16:727.

Warner JJ, Johnson D, Miller M, et al: Technique for selecting capsular tightness in repair of anterior-inferior shoulder instability. *J Shoulder Elbow Surg* 1995;4:352-364.

This study consists of two parts. The first reports on the results of a questionnaire sent to all members of the American Shoulder and Elbow Surgeons, of which 80% responded. All agreed that preservation of external rotation was important and that shoulder position during repair may influence the ultimate range of motion; position of the arm, however, was not agreed upon. Part II is a description of technique for selecting capsular tightness, and the preliminary results in 18 patients.

Warner JJ, Miller MD, Marks P, et al: Arthroscopic Bankart repair with the Suretac device: Part I. Clinical observations. *Arthroscopy* 1995;11:2-13.

A cohort of 15 patients who were experiencing pain (eight patients) or recurrent instability (seven patients) underwent second-look arthroscopy at an average of 9.4 months following the index procedure of arthroscopic Bankart repair using the Suretac device. The purpose of the study was to provide insight into patient selection for the procedure as well as assess healing of the Bankart repair. In the seven patients with instability, three had complete recurrence of the Bankart lesion, and five had poorly developed, attenuated glenohumeral ligaments.

Wirth MA, Butters KP, Rockwood CA Jr: The posterior deltoid-splitting approach to the shoulder. *Clin Orthop* 1993;296:92-98.

A retrospective review is presented of 42 shoulders undergoing a deltoid-splitting approach to avoid the potential complications of detachment of the muscle from the acromion and scapular spine. The approach provided excellent exposure, had no complications of nerve injury, and preserved the strength and function of the deltoid.

Young DC, Rockwood CA Jr: Complications of a failed Bristow procedure and their management. *J Bone Joint Surg* 1991;73A:969-981.

Youssef JA, Carr CF, Walther CE, et al: Arthroscopic Bankart suture repair for recurrent traumatic unidirectional anterior shoulder dislocations. *Arthroscopy* 1995;11: 561-563.

The authors report a 27% failure rate in the repair of Bankart lesions using a transglenoid suture technique. Thirty consecutive patients undergoing this technique were followed an average of 38 months. Of note, redislocation occurred more than 3 years after the stabilization procedure in two patients.

Zarins B, Rowe CR, Stone JW: Shoulder instability: Management of failed reconstructions, in Barr JS Jr (ed): *Instructional Course Lectures XXXVIII.* Park Ridge, IL, American Academy of Orthopaedic Surgeons, 1989, pp 217-230.

Zuckerman JD, Matsen FA III: Complications about the glenohumeral joint related to the use of screws and staples. *J Bone Joint Surg* 1984;66A:175-180.

III
Rotator Cuff Impingement

Joseph P. Iannotti, MD, PhD
Section Editor

14

Anatomy, Function, Pathogenesis, and Natural History of Rotator Cuff Disorders

Jerry S. Sher, MD

Rotator cuff disease has been studied extensively. Increasing information regarding anatomy, pathogenesis, etiology, and natural history has improved understanding of this disorder. Despite the level of interest, several questions regarding the origin of rotator cuff tears remain unanswered. Multiple theories, such as vascular and impingement mechanisms, have been implicated as causative factors, but reports are often conflicting. The belief that rotator cuff lesions are solely a result of intrinsic or extrinsic factors may be an oversimplification of the disease process. More likely, the heterogeneity of the disorder is a reflection of its multifactorial etiology which, in part, may help explain the difference in views regarding the origin of rotator cuff tears.

Normal Anatomy

The shoulder comprises a complex of four articulations that under normal conditions move in synchrony, allowing for smooth, unhindered motion of the arm. An intricate relationship exists between the osseous elements and the surrounding muscles and ligaments. In an attempt to better understand the anatomic arrangement of these structures, an organizational approach to the anatomy of the shoulder has been recently reported. The tissues are grouped into four separate and contiguous layers, and there is alternation between muscular and fibrous elements. The first layer, which is the most superficial level, includes the deltoid and pectoralis major muscles. The second is a continuous fascial layer that extends circumferentially from anterior to posterior and incorporates the clavipectoral and posterior scapular fascia. The third layer, also muscular, includes the rotator cuff, whereas the fourth layer, which is the deepest level, comprises the fibrous capsular elements. This classification helps clarify the shoulder's complex anatomy and can safeguard against deviation from internervous planes during surgical procedures (Fig. 1).

The gross anatomy of the rotator cuff and its relationship to both the glenohumeral joint and capsule has been discussed in the literature. The four rotator cuff muscles act as a functional unit to maintain the humeral head centered within the glenoid during active arm elevation. These muscles are often considered as four distinct, separate musculotendinous units that directly overlie the joint capsule and insert onto the proximal humerus. Recent histologic investigation, however, has better defined the relationships between the rotator cuff tendons and their underlying capsular elements. The fibers of the rotator cuff tendons fuse and form a common insertion on the tuberosities of the humerus. Moreover, fibers from both the subscapularis and infraspinatus were demonstrated to interdigitate with respective fibers of the supraspinatus, and five distinct layers could be identified. These layers also received reinforcement from the coracohumeral ligament and were contiguous with the glenohumeral capsule. This structural architecture may enhance the rotator cuff's resistance to failure with repeated loads as tension generated in any single musculoskeletal unit could be expected to result in a distribution of forces over an expanded area. Moreover, in circumstances in which the rotator cuff does fail, the network of interdigitating fibers contributes to the tissue's structural integrity, allowing for retention of sutures during surgical repair.

The anatomy and function of the coracohumeral ligament, a well-defined structure with a consistent origin at the lateral base of the coracoid process, has also been studied. In one study of gross anatomy, variability was observed at the insertion of this ligament. Seventy-four percent of specimens demonstrated a predominant insertion into the rotator interval; the rest of the specimens had a principal attachment to the supraspinatus tendon. Two of the most notable functions attributed to the coracohumeral ligament are limitation of external rotation in the adducted arm and restraint against inferior translation.

Other anatomic studies have highlighted the course and anatomy of the suprascapular nerve as it enters the posterior aspect of the shoulder. In one investigation, 84% of 31 specimens revealed one or two branches of the nerve to the supraspinatus muscle. Moreover, in 84% of specimens, the first branch originated either under the transverse scapular ligament or 1 mm distal to it. The first motor branch originated proximal to the ligament and passed superficial to it in 3% of the specimens. The infraspinatus muscle demonstrated three to four branches in approximately half of the specimens. Whereas the neurovascular bundle rested an average distance of 2 cm from the posterior rim of the glenoid, variation of this distance has been observed in other studies. These observations emphasize the caution required with such procedures as mobilization of a torn and retracted rotator cuff, arthroscopic portal placement, and neurolysis of an entrapped suprascapular nerve.

The rotator cuff is supplied by multiple arteries. The anterior and posterior humeral circumflex vessels both extend to the superior as well as the anterior and posterior portions of the cuff, respectively. The suprascapular artery also supplies the superior cuff, and in the majority of individuals the acromial branch of the thoracoacromial artery will nourish the supraspinatus. Additional contributions may include branches of the subscapular and suprahumeral branches of the axillary artery. Osseous vessels emanating from the tuberosities of the proximal humerus have also been included in the vascular makeup of the rotator cuff (Fig. 2).

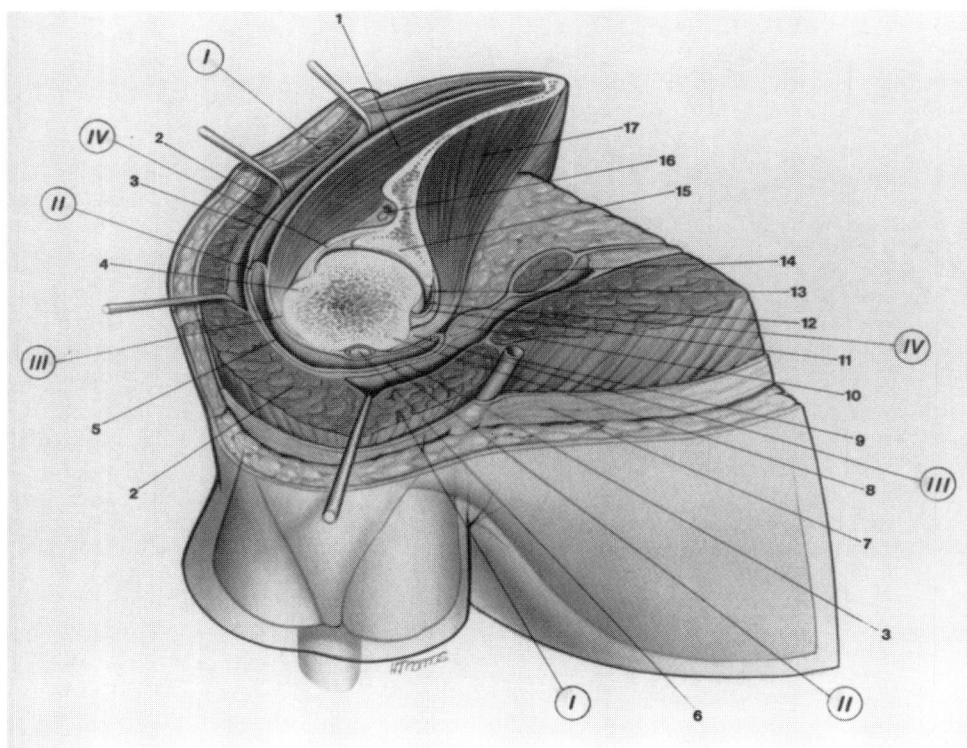

Fig. 1 Supporting layers (Roman numerals) of the glenohumeral joint. Layer 1: deltoid (2) and pectoralis major muscles (12). Layer 2: clavipectoral fascia (3), conjoined tendon (10), coracoacromial ligament and posterior scapular fascia (3), and superficial bursal tissue (5). Layer 3: deep layer of subdeltoid bursa, rotator cuff (1, 17). Layer 4: glenohumeral joint, capsule (11), synovium (13), coracohumeral ligament (3). 4 = greater tuberosity; 6 = biceps long head; 7 = fascia; 8 = lesser tuberosity; 9 = cephalic vein; 11 = joint capsule; 14 = pectoralis minor; 15 = glenoid; 16 = suprascapular neurovascular bundle. (Reproduced with permission from Cooper DE, O'Brien SJ, Warren SF: Supporting layers of the glenohumeral joint: An anatomic study. *Clin Orthop* 1993;289:144-155.)

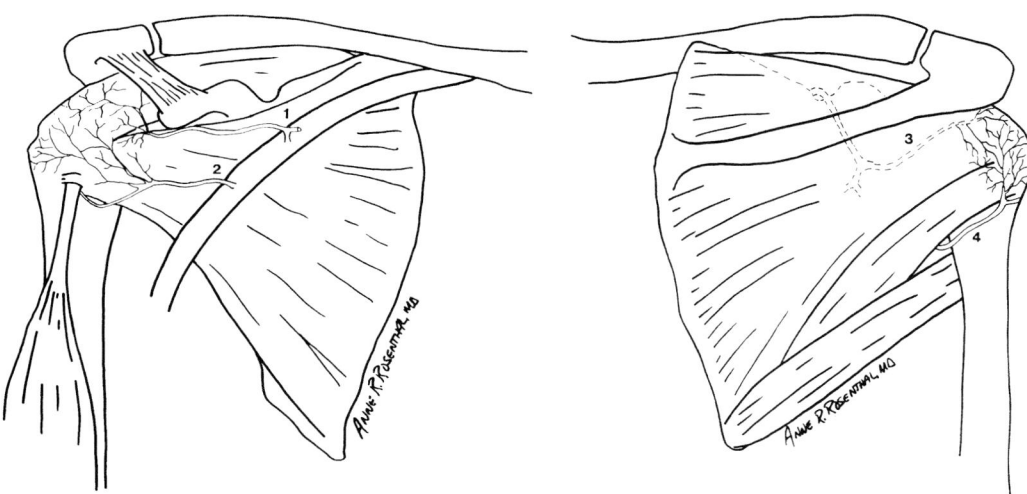

Fig. 2 Vascular supply to the rotator cuff. (Reproduced with permission from Chansky HA, Iannotti JP: The vascularity of the rotator cuff. *Clin Sports Med* 1991;10:807-822.)

Abnormal Anatomy

Rotator cuff tears typically involve the supraspinatus tendon and often include the posterior cuff to a variable degree. The subscapularis tendon may or may not be involved and can be easily overlooked if not considered or tested during diagnostic evaluation.

The torn rotator cuff can demonstrate variably shaped defects, a factor that should be taken into consideration during surgery. A vertical tear in line with the course of the tendon can often be repaired with a side-to-side closure. Horizontal tears run transverse to the normal course of the tendon and will vary in size and in degree of retraction. Typically, closure of such defects requires a transosseous repair to the greater tuberosity. Complex tears containing both horizontal and vertical components also occur and may require a combination of the aforementioned closure techniques.

Tears about the rotator interval, although less common, have recently been described. The rotator interval consists of a fibrous band of tissue which lies between the superior border of the subscapularis and the anterior border of the supraspinatus tendons. The coracohumeral ligament lies along the superficial surface. The biceps tendon, along with the superior glenohumeral ligament, travels deep to this band of tissue. Surgical exploration of this interval in 116 patients with supposed isolated tears of the supraspinatus tendon revealed occult lesions of the coracohumeral ligament, superior glenohumeral ligament, and upper border of the subscapularis in 19. Treatment consisted of a rotator cuff repair and reconstruction of the rotator interval complex. Identification of these lesions can be difficult, and their association with pain or dysfunction and the optimal method of treatment are unknown.

Unfortunately, because a universally accepted classification of rotator cuff disease does not exist, studies evaluating the results of surgical treatment are difficult to compare. However, important parameters to consider when describing rotator cuff lesions include the duration, depth, and size of a tear as well as the condition of the muscle and the tendon. Acute tears are typically associated with a sudden onset of pain and dysfunction after a traumatic event. Chronic tears, which can persist for 3 months or longer, may be associated with a variable degree of weakness and pain. Some patients may have a previously documented chronic rotator cuff tear and develop an acute extension of the lesion after a traumatic insult. The depth of a tear will differentiate partial- from full-thickness lesions. Partial-thickness tears can be present on either the articular or bursal surface or may be intrasubstance. The thickness of the lesion may also vary until it extends through the entire tendon, at which point the subacromial space communicates with the glenohumeral joint. Gradation of partial-thickness lesions has been described in the literature; however, definition and accurate assessment of such lesions are difficult. For example, fraying of the tendon observed during surgery could be considered a partial tear by some surgeons. Moreover, the incidence of such lesions in relation to symptoms and the results of treatment are not easily determined because of variability in imaging capabilities and interpretation skills, and lack of a uniform system of classification.

Full-thickness tears may be described as small (less than 1 cm in diameter), medium (1 to 3 cm), large (3 to 5 cm), or massive (larger than 5 cm). Additionally, a torn rotator cuff may be retracted, deficient, attenuated, or friable at the time of surgical assessment. The muscle can be assessed using magnetic resonance imaging (MRI) or computed tomography (CT) scans, in which cross-sectional area, degree of fatty infiltration, and alterations in overall signal intensity can be determined. The correlation of supraspinatus muscle atrophy with rotator cuff tears and residual function recently has been studied electromyographically. As the supraspinatus became more atrophic, the electromyographic function of the muscle decreased. Although these observations suggest a decrease in function in conjunction with MRI-evident supraspinatus atrophy, the impact of such findings on surgical outcome will require further investigation.

Glenohumeral abnormalities have also been associated with tears of the rotator cuff. A prospective series of 100 patients with full-thickness tears who underwent a diagnostic arthroscopy revealed glenohumeral abnormalities in 74% overall. Common observations included lesions of the anterior labrum in 62%, intra-articular biceps tendon tears in 16%, and articular cartilage abnormalities in 28%. The relevance of such findings in association with full-thickness rotator cuff tears and the effect of treatment on overall results is unknown. Although the role of arthroscopic surgery in the evaluation and treatment of rotator cuff tears continues to be a subject of debate, arthroscopy may be of both prognostic and therapeutic benefit in selected cases.

The Coracoacromial Arch

The coracoacromial arch marks the superior boundary of the subacromial space and is comprised of the coracoid process, the coracoacromial ligament, and the acromion process (Fig. 3). Neer described the role of this structure in the development of impingement syndrome and noted changes in the osseous and soft-tissue morphology in patients with this disorder.

The shape of the acromion varies in each individual. In an anatomic study of 140 cadaveric shoulders, three predominant acromial forms were identified (Fig. 4). A type 1 acromion had a flat undersurface and was present in 17%. A type 2 acromion had a curved undersurface and was found in 43% of specimens. A hooked acromion or type 3, while present in 39% of specimens, was found to exist in 70% of specimens with observed tears of the rotator cuff. Subsequent clinical studies using supraspinatus outlet radiographs to assess acromial morphology and arthrograms to determine rotator cuff integrity have affirmed the association between a type 3 acromion and the presence of rotator cuff tears. However, there is some controversy as to the interobserver reliability of this classification and the absolute definition of each of the three morphologic categories. Moreover, additional acromion shapes have been reported, and similar associations were not demonstrated. Some of these differences may best be explained by the potential for acromion architecture to range from a flat to a hooked configuration, with varying degrees of curvature.

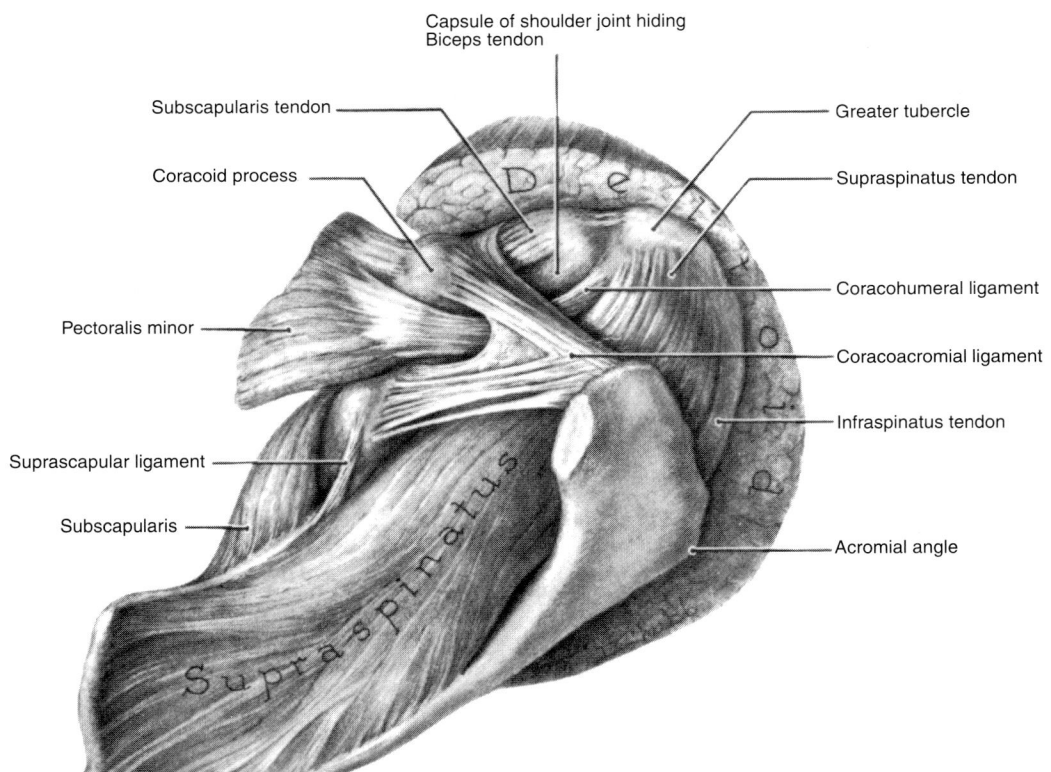

Fig. 3 Anatomy of the coracoacromial arch. Note the "Y" configuration of the coracoacromial ligament. (Reproduced with permission from Moore KL (ed): *Clinically Oriented Anatomy,* ed 2. Baltimore, MD, Williams & Wilkins, 1985.)

Additional studies have highlighted other morphologic characteristics of the acromion that may be associated with disorders of the rotator cuff. Evaluation of scapulae from 200 anatomic specimens demonstrated subacromial spurs and osteophyte formation in 18% overall. Characteristics most commonly associated with these findings included a horizontal lying acromion, an increased acromial length in the anteroposterior plane, and a decreased height of the coracoacromial arch. Although such factors have also been implicated in the pathogenesis of rotator cuff disease, standard acromioplasty may not adequately address these elements in specific cases.

Moreover, standard portal placement for arthroscopic procedures may be difficult and potentially hazardous because of the variability in acromial shapes. In a recent study, the posterior lip of the acromion was observed to project inferiorly overlying the midpoint of the glenohumeral joint in 16% of specimens. Use of the posterior acromion as a sole reference for placement of the arthroscopic cannula may thus result in a portal that is too low, potentially compromising both the axillary nerve and arthroscopic visualization.

Recent interest has focused on the structure and function of the coracoacromial ligament. This structure's configuration is that of an inverted "Y," with its two limbs taking origin from the medial and lateral aspects of the coracoid. The two bands then fuse as they project superiorly to insert onto the undersurface of the acromion (Fig. 3). In contrast to its implicated role in the pathogenesis of impingement syndrome, the coracoacromial ligament has been considered a strut that lends support to the acromion and coracoid during applied loading imposed by the surrounding musculature. Its role as a secondary restraint to anterosuperior migration of the humeral head in patients with severe rotator cuff deficiencies has also been emphasized.

Mechanical forces about the coracoacromial arch, while not fully understood, have been linked to the development of rotator cuff disease. Biomechanical and geometric testing of the coracoacromial ligament demonstrated that the lateral band (that portion of the ligament more likely to impinge on the tendinous cuff) was both shorter in length and smaller in cross-sectional area in shoulders with rotator cuff tears. Although histologically there were no structural differences in the ligament between normal shoulders and those with rotator cuff tears, there was evidence of decreased mechanical properties in the latter. The reduction in mechanical integrity of the ligament was thought to reflect the multiple directional loads imposed on this structure in shoulders with rotator cuff tears. In a study of eight cadaveric shoulders, scanning electron micrographs were used to demonstrate that observed degenerative changes of the rotator cuff were characteristic of alterations secondary to frictional and rubbing mechanisms. Observations support the contention that degenerative changes already present in the cuff, irrespective

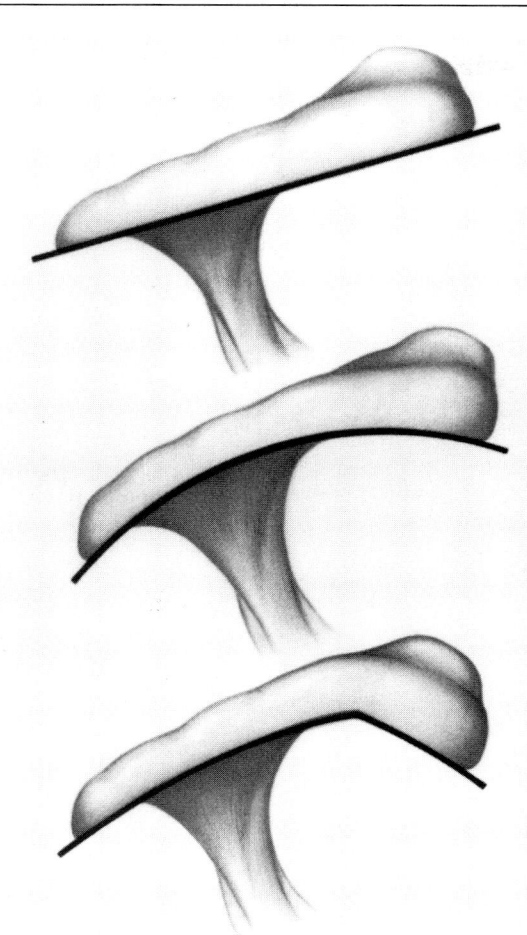

Fig. 4 Acromion morphology. Type 1 **(top)** is flat, type 2 **(center)** is curved, type 3 **(bottom)** is hooked. (Reproduced with permission from Poss R (ed): *Orthopaedic Knowledge Update 3.* Park Ridge, IL, American Academy of Orthopaedic Surgeons, 1990, pp 313-326.)

of etiology, can be aggravated by proposed frictional or abrasive mechanisms.

Other biomechanical studies using stereophotogrammetry to evaluate subacromial contact areas have noted a progressive decrease in the acromiohumeral interval with arm elevation. The humerus and acromion were found to be at closest proximity between 60° and 120° of elevation. Moreover, contact and proximity were observed to begin at the anterolateral aspect of the acromion at 0° of elevation and shift medially with progressive arm elevation. In all cases, only the anterior aspect of the acromion demonstrated potential for subacromial contact. Additionally, acromiohumeral distances were decreased in shoulders with a hooked acromion.

Although such studies have provided quantitative analysis of the coracoacromial arch in relation to shoulder function, additional investigations are needed to further clarify subacromial stresses and contact areas in multiple planes of motion and in different pathologic states. Increased understanding of these issues may enhance the ability to effectively evaluate and treat patients with rotator cuff disease.

Function

Under normal conditions, the rotator cuff plays an important role in providing dynamic stability to the glenohumeral joint. The osseous architecture consists of an apparently flat glenoid as compared to the convex, larger humeral head. Studies have shown, however, that the radius of curvature of the glenoid closely approximates that of the humeral head (conformity), and that the differences observed represent a mismatch in the surface areas of the two articular surfaces (constraint). As a result of the minimal constraint afforded by the articular surfaces, a relative wide arc of motion is present at the glenohumeral articulation. Moreover, there remains a delicate balance between motion and stability of this joint, in which increases in one parameter may occur at the expense of the other. The surrounding soft tissues, which include the rotator cuff as well as the glenoid labrum and glenohumeral ligaments, provide much of the stability required for smooth, unhindered motion of the shoulder.

The rotator cuff comprises a group of muscles that are considerably smaller in size and cross-sectional area when compared to the more superficial structures such as the deltoid, pectoralis major, latissimus dorsi, and trapezius. These muscles, which lie deep in the shoulder and in close proximity to the center of rotation of the glenohumeral joint, are collectively unable to generate the same degree of torque as the larger and more superficial structures. In part, the relatively shorter lever arm, or distance of the muscle from the center of rotation, accounts for observable differences in the generated force. Thus, the anatomic structure of the rotator cuff allows for optimal maintenance of a stable glenohumeral fulcrum during active arm motion.

A normal functioning rotator cuff achieves dynamic stability through multiple mechanisms. It acts through direct joint compression as well as asymmetric contraction and "steering" of the humeral head into the glenoid during active motion. Moreover, it can function as a direct barrier to humeral head translation in the midranges of motion. Recent studies have implicated the rotator cuff's role in "dynamization" of the glenohumeral ligaments. The contiguous or intimate association between the rotator cuff and underlying capsule may allow for asymmetric tensioning of the ligaments in the midranges of motion where previous biomechanical models have shown them to remain lax. Through coordinated muscle contractions, the ligaments can be tensioned to allow further resistance to humeral translation.

The relative contribution of the rotator cuff to strength in abduction of the arm is debatable. In studies that used selective blockade of the suprascapular and axillary nerves, the supraspinatus and deltoid muscles contributed equally to measured torque in abduction. The infraspinatus is also believed to contribute to force in abduction. One investigation employing selective blockade of the infraspinatus muscle indicated a decrease in abduction torque of up to 45%. These findings are in contrast to electromyographic studies, which demonstrated silent electrical activity in the infraspinatus with abduction to 120°.

More recently, however, indirect evidence of the functional relationship of the rotator cuff and deltoid to humeral elevation was determined by calculation of changes in moment arms and measurement of muscular excursion in cadaveric specimens. In this way, both the infraspinatus and subscapularis were shown to contribute to abduction. Changes in rotation further affected the ability of either muscle to augment elevation in the scapular plane. Internal and external rotation enhanced the ability of the upper portions of the infraspinatus and subscapularis, respectively, to abduct the arm. The data help explain, in part, how a supraspinatus defect may not necessarily limit functional abduction of the arm.

Moreover, biomechanical studies have highlighted the role of the infraspinatus and subscapularis in maintenance of normal glenohumeral kinematics. In one cadaveric study, the effect of rotator cuff function on humeral head translation was evaluated. The absence of generated supraspinatus force appeared to have no appreciable difference on humeral head migration when measured radiographically in the anteroposterior plane. However, absence of force generated by the infraspinatus, teres minor, and subscapularis resulted in an increase in superior translation as the deltoid was unopposed. Another study that measured subacromial forces with arm elevation in a dynamic cadaver model demonstrated peak forces when the arm was in abduction. Such findings, in conjunction with stereophotogrammetry data revealing a decrease in the acromiohumeral interval with arm elevation, may parallel some of the pathomechanic mechanisms thought to mediate pain and dysfunction in the shoulder impingement syndrome.

Pathogenesis

The heterogeneity of rotator cuff disease, as well as the notion that the disease may not actually represent a continuum of the same process, but rather a compilation of independent disorders, may in part explain the differing viewpoints regarding its origin. Two contrasting pathogenetic mechanisms, vascular or intrinsic causes and impingement or extrinsic factors, have been extensively described. Other causes, including trauma, congenital or developmental factors, and instability, have also been reported and will be discussed later.

Vascular Factors

The role of the rotator cuff's microvascular blood supply in contributing to attrition of the tendon has remained controversial. Early microinjection studies had demonstrated a region of tendon hypovascularity approximately 1 cm medial to the supraspinatus insertion. This avascular area was subject to ischemia and considered responsible for degeneration of the rotator cuff. This region had been called the "critical zone" and found not to be less vascular, but rather a "watershed" area corresponding to an anastomosis between osseous and tendinous blood vessels. In another microinjection study, there was adequate vascularity within the rotator cuff when injections were performed on the abducted arm, but in the adducted arm the vessels were hypovascular or "wrung out."

It was hypothesized that the critical zone was subject to transient hypovascularity mediated by position of the arm.

A more recent vascular study in 18 anatomic specimens demonstrated differential vascularity between the bursal and articular surfaces of the rotator cuff. The bursal surface was well vascularized, while the articular surface had a sparse arteriolar pattern. These findings may help explain the relative increase in tears to the articular surface of the rotator cuff.

Another study used intraoperative laser Doppler flowtometry to assess tendon vascularity in symptomatic patients. Individuals with tendinitis and intact tendons demonstrated hypervascular changes in the area of greatest mechanical impingement, or the critical zone. Increased vascularity was also observed at the tendon margins of those patients with partial-thickness tears. Individuals with complete tendon tears had variable degrees of vascularity at the tendon edges. Although hypervascular changes have been associated with rotator cuff tears and impingement syndrome, resorption of injured tendon fibers by neovascular tissue was suggested to mediate the progression of rotator cuff disease.

More recently, a postmortem quantitative histologic evaluation of rotator cuff vascularity revealed a decrease in vessel number, size, and percentage of tendon occupied by vessels in both the distal supraspinatus and infraspinatus tendons. Because a hypovascular zone was not isolated to the supraspinatus tendon alone, it was concluded that other factors must be important in the pathogenesis of rotator cuff disease. This theory is further confirmed by the difference in observed frequency of tears of the supraspinatus and infraspinatus tendons.

Despite the findings of many of the earlier microinjection studies, some of the conclusions are limited by inherent shortcomings of the methods used. Postmortem investigations lack the clinical correlation necessary to attribute specific findings to clinical symptoms. Moreover, microinjection studies not using histologic techniques may not afford adequate assessment of tissue vascularity because capillary networks cannot be identified. Employment of either in vivo methods or microscopic tissue evaluation can help overcome some of the deficiencies of earlier reports and allow for a more detailed assessment of tendon vascularity in relation to clinical findings.

Impingement Syndrome

Neer popularized the concept of the impingement syndrome, noting that the rotator cuff was potentially subject to repeated mechanical insult by the overlying coracoacromial arch with elevation of the arm. His observations highlighted the anterior functional arc of shoulder motion with resultant impingement of the rotator cuff by proliferative spurs and excrescences extending from the anterior third of the acromion and coracoacromial ligament, in contrast to impingement by the lateral acromion as had been generally accepted. He subsequently described three stages of impingement as a continuum that ultimately led to tearing of the rotator cuff. Stage 1 was characterized by subacromial edema and hemorrhage and was typical in symptomatic patients under 25 years of age. Stage 2 included fibrosis and tendinitis and was more common in persons 25 to 40 years old. With continued progression, Stage 3 or rotator cuff failure would result and was characterized by partial or complete tendon tears, typically in persons older than 40 years of age. He attributed 95% of all rotator cuff lesions to primary mechanical impingement.

Although multiple studies have demonstrated successful and reproducible outcomes for subacromial decompression in patients with impingement syndrome, they have been unable to sufficiently address the etiology of impingement lesions. Debate continues regarding the origin of rotator cuff tears as it relates to intrinsic factors (eg, degenerative, vascular) or extrinsic causes such as mechanical subacromial impingement.

One histologic evaluation of bursal surface rotator cuff tears revealed tears of variable thickness of the supraspinatus corresponding with areas of impingement of the overlying acromion and coracoacromial ligament. Also observed were avascular regions of the proximal edge of the torn tendon. This combination of findings led to the conclusion that multiple etiologies, including both intrinsic and extrinsic causes, were responsible for the observed abnormalities.

Other sources of impingement have also been implicated in rotator cuff disease. Distally pointing acromioclavicular osteophytes, the coracoid process, and the posterosuperior aspect of the glenoid can contribute to shoulder pain and lesions of the rotator cuff in certain patients. One report noted a strong association between ruptures of the supraspinatus tendon and inferior acromioclavicular joint osteophytes. Although acromial excrescences had also been observed, their frequency in subjects with rotator cuff ruptures was less than that of acromioclavicular bone spurs. Impingement of the rotator cuff between the humeral head and coracoid process can also occur in select patients with forward flexion and internal rotation of the arm. Predisposing factors include traumatic and iatrogenic causes involving the coracoid, glenoid, or humeral head. Idiopathic cases were also described.

More recently, arthroscopic evaluation of throwing athletes with painful arc syndrome has demonstrated impingement of the deep surface of the rotator cuff against the posterosuperior glenoid rim with the arm in 90° to 150° of abduction and external rotation. Associated findings included partial-thickness tearing of the undersurface of the supraspinatus tendon, degenerative lesions of the posterosuperior glenoid labrum, and osteochondral impression fractures of the humeral head. It has been suggested that abduction and external rotation of the arm can entrap a portion of the supraspinatus tendon between the humeral head and glenoid in susceptible individuals. Increased glenohumeral external rotation, scapulothoracic dysfunction, and poor technique in throwing athletes have also been implicated in the development of this disorder. Although these observations help emphasize alternate sources of shoulder impingement, further study is needed to better define this entity and its pathomechanics, and determine optimal treatment.

Etiology

Several etiologic factors associated with the development of rotator cuff disorders, including trauma, glenohumeral instability, scapulothoracic dysfunction, congenital or developmental abnormalities, and degenerative or senescent changes of the cuff, have been described.

In early anatomic investigations, Codman had suggested that degenerative processes within the rotator cuff, in association with trauma, played a role in the genesis of cuff tears. Tears of the supraspinatus tendon were commonly observed approximately 1 cm medial to its insertion on the greater tuberosity. Subsequently, other studies found that degenerative changes about the shoulder and other joints occurred with advancing age.

In one cadaveric study, the relationship between anatomic changes of the acromion undersurface and pathologic findings within the rotator cuff was examined. Histologic and radiographic evaluation demonstrated an association between bursal-side partial rotator cuff tears and pathologic changes of the acromion undersurface. Moreover, the pathologic changes of the acromion correlated with the severity of the tear, and the overall prevalence of rotator cuff disorders increased with advancing age. Interestingly, in shoulders with joint surface partial tears, the acromion undersurface was intact. It was concluded that rotator cuff tears represent an age-associated degenerative process and that abnormalities on the acromion undersurface exemplify secondary changes resulting from a tear on the bursal surface of the cuff. Other cadaveric studies have noted an increase in rotator cuff tears with age, further implicating senescence or degeneration in the development of cuff disorders. Whether precarious tendon vascularity or mechanical insult by the overlying coracoacromial arch also mediate this process remains undetermined; however, it seems conceivable that both factors play a contributing role.

Traumatic events can lead to the development of rotator cuff tears. Ruptures of the rotator cuff have been estimated to occur in up to 80% of persons older than 60 years of age with anterior glenohumeral dislocations. Fractures of the greater tuberosity with or without a glenohumeral dislocation have also been associated with tears of the rotator cuff. Many elderly patients will present with a rotator cuff tear and report some form of earlier trauma. However, it is difficult to determine if trauma was the sole cause of the torn rotator cuff, or if there was a preexisting cuff lesion that increased in size or became symptomatic after the precipitous insult.

Other forms of traumatic rotator cuff lesions include small partial-thickness lesions of the supraspinatus or subscapularis in young athletes who participate in repetitive overhead activities. Tennis, swimming, and baseball are sports that may predispose certain individuals to rotator cuff tears through repeated mechanical stresses. It has been suggested that fatigue of the scapular stabilizers results from repetitive throwing, causing the humeral head and rotator cuff to abut the acromion during arm elevation. The scapula is thought to lag behind the humerus, resulting in insufficient abduction. Other theories describe glenohumeral instability as a mediating factor in such athletes. It has been proposed that observed rotator cuff lesions are the end result of a continuum that progresses from instability, subluxation, impingement, and tension overload of the cuff with resultant tearing.

An association between an unfused acromial epiphysis or os acromiale and tears of the rotator cuff also exists. Abnormal motion at the synostosis or synchondrosis is believed to decrease the volume of the subacromial space and contribute to mechanical insult of the underlying rotator cuff. According to one report, os acromiale may present in up to 6% of people with rotator cuff tears. More recently, a review of 270 cadaveric scapulae demonstrated an 8.2% incidence of os acromiale.

Other abnormalities of the coracoacromial arch linked with the development of rotator cuff disease include congenital subacromial stenosis. A congenitally narrow subacromial space, recently described, may predispose certain patients to impingement and lesions of the rotator cuff. The literature is sparse regarding this entity and further study is required to better define, detect, and treat such patients.

It is apparent that rotator cuff disease represents a heterogeneous disorder with a multifactorial etiology. Vascular factors, impingement syndrome, degenerative processes, and developmental influences all appear to contribute, in some combination, to the formation and progression of rotator cuff lesions.

Natural History

The rotator cuff is subject to substantial forces as it maintains the humeral head within the shallow glenoid. It is situated in a potentially tight subacromial space and undergoes senescent structural changes commonly observed in other joints of the body. When the cuff fails, spontaneous healing of the torn tendon is not expected to occur and multiple factors may be responsible. Its fibers are under tension and typically retract upon tearing. In full-thickness lesions, a defect is created and only bursal or scar tissue may bridge the area of tendon loss. Histologic evaluation of partial tears has demonstrated neovascular tissue at the distal tendon edge and relative avascularity of the proximal stump in surgical specimens. These observations were believed to represent a futile attempt at healing. Other investigators have observed resorption of tendon fibers by neovascular tissue, an occurrence that may potentially weaken surrounding intact fibers placed under increased loads as a result of a tear. As the torn cuff is bathed in synovial fluid, factors responsible for normal healing and formation of fibrin clots may be disrupted. Moreover, tearing may further impair the blood supply to a relatively dysvascular tendon.

The incidence of rotator cuff tears in the general population can be extrapolated from both cadaveric and magnetic resonance studies. The frequency of complete and partial rotator cuff tears ranges from 5% to 39% and 13% to 37%, respectively. Although anatomic studies have reported an increase in pathologic findings about the rotator cuff with increasing age, these findings cannot be sufficiently correlated with symptomatology.

More recently, a prospective study assessing shoulder MRI scans in 96 asymptomatic volunteers demonstrated complete and partial rotator cuff tears in 14% and 20%, respectively. Fifty-four percent of individuals older than 60 years of age had either a full or partial-thickness tear in light of normal function and an absence of symptoms. The results provide in vivo evidence that individuals without a prior history of shoulder complaints can demonstrate normal function regardless of the presence of a rotator cuff tear on MRI. Moreover, they emphasize the dangers of basing surgical decisions on MRI scans alone (Fig. 5).

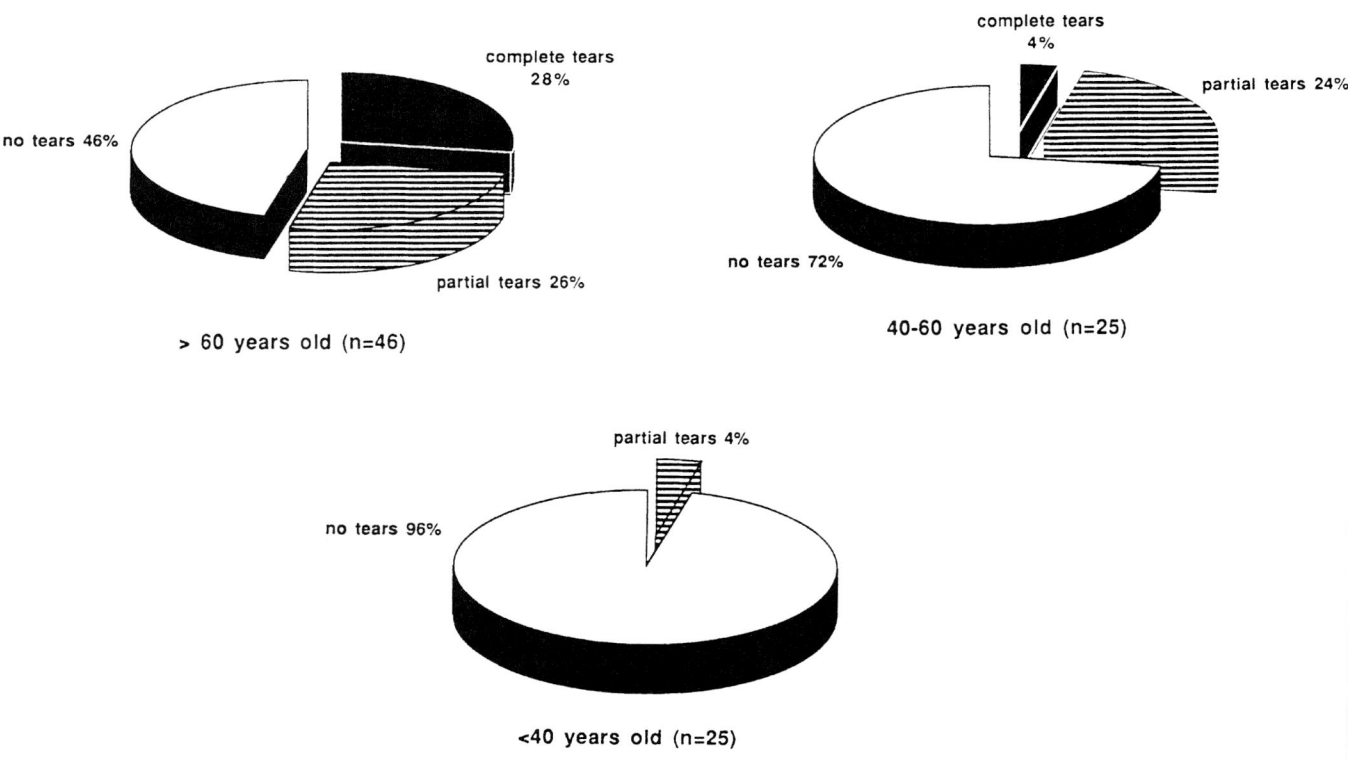

Fig. 5 Prevalence of MRI-evident rotator cuff tears in asymptomatic volunteers older than 60 years of age **(left)**, 40-60 years **(right)**, and younger than 40 years **(bottom)**. (Adapted with permission from Sher JS, Uribe JW, Posada A, et al: Abnormal findings on magnetic resonance images of asymptomatic shoulders. *J Bone Joint Surg* 1995;77A:10-15.)

Both the literature and clinical observation affirm that some patients with rotator cuff tears do not demonstrate significant pain or dysfunction. Clearly, individuals with symptomatic cuff tears may respond well to conservative treatment despite the persistence of a tendon defect. Other reports have documented good short-term functional results in patients who had undergone debridement, rather than repair, of a torn rotator cuff. Because the tendons do not typically heal, it would seem conceivable that factors other than the tendon tear itself must contribute to the generation of symptoms. As of yet, those factors responsible for the development of pain and dysfunction have not been definitively determined. The question of why some patients with rotator cuff tears develop symptoms and others do not remains unanswered. Differences in normal glenohumeral kinematics may play a role, but individual differences in scapular mechanics, compensatory action of surrounding muscles, and variable tolerances to pain may be important factors. One author discussed the role of an anatomically deficient but biomechanically intact rotator cuff. Fluoroscopy was used to assess kinematic patterns of the glenohumeral joint in patients with massive tears of the rotator cuff. Normal kinematic patterns were possible provided sufficient anterior and posterior cuff were present preserving the normal transverse plane force couple. Another biomechanical study evaluating patterns of glenohumeral motion in artificially created tendon defects highlighted the potential for normal kinematics provided only a portion of the cuff was violated. Lesions of the supraspinatus did not alter motion patterns, whereas defects involving both the supraspinatus and infraspinatus demonstrated an increase in humeral cephalad migration.

The heterogeneity, lack of uniform classification, and nonuniformity in treatment strategies of the rotator cuff make it difficult to arrive at conclusions regarding its natural history. The cuff likely has some degree of reserve that provides functional use of the arm in cases of limited tendon deficiencies. Location rather than size of a tear may be more important in the development of symptoms. Moreover, other factors such as synovitis, subacromial bursitis, and intra-articular abnormalities may contribute to pain and dysfunction. Identification of those patients with cuff lesions prone to progression and dysfunction can only be achieved with further study, which would allow for optimal treatment approaches individualized to a given patient's clinical findings.

Selected Bibliography

General

Bigliani LU, Morrison DS, April EW: The morphology of the acromion and rotator cuff impingement. *Orthop Trans* 1986;10:288.

Lohr JF, Uhthoff HK: The microvascular pattern of the supraspinatus tendon. *Clin Orthop* 1990;254:35-38.

Moseley HF, Goldie I: The arterial pattern of the rotator cuff of the shoulder. *J Bone Joint Surg* 1963;45B:780-789.

Mudge MK, Wood VE, Frykman GK: Rotator cuff tears associated with os acromiale. *J Bone Joint Surg* 1984;66A:427-429.

Neer CS: Anterior acromioplasty for the chronic impingement syndrome in the shoulder: A preliminary report. *J Bone Joint Surg* 1972;54A:4150.

Neviaser RJ, Neviaser TJ, Neviaser JS: Concurrent rupture of the rotator cuff and anterior dislocation of the shoulder in the older patient. *J Bone Joint Surg* 1988;70A:1308-1311.

Nicholson GP, Goodman DA, Flatow EL, et al: The acromion: Morphologic condition and age related changes. A study of 420 scapulas. *J Shoulder Elbow Surg* 1996;5:1-11.

An anatomic study of 420 scapulae highlighted differences between acromion morphology and anterior degenerative spur formation. Acromion morphology or type was independent of age and consistent with a primary anatomic rather than developmental characteristic. Anterior acromial spurs were significantly higher in individuals over 50 years of age and consistent with an acquired characteristic. Acromial dimensions were also quantified.

Petersson CJ, Gentz CF: Ruptures of the supraspinatus tendon: The significance of distally pointing acromioclavicular osteophytes. *Clin Orthop* 1983;174:143-148.

Rathbun JB, Macnab I: The microvascular pattern of the rotator cuff. *J Bone Joint Surg* 1970;52B:540-553.

Swiontowski MF, Iannotti JP, Boulas HJ, et al: Intraoperative assessment of rotator cuff vascularity using laser Doppler flowtometry, in Post M, Morrey BF, Hawkins RJ (eds): *Surgery of the Shoulder*. St. Louis, MO, Mosby Year Book, 1990, pp 208-212.

Anatomy

Bigliani LU, Dalsey RM, McCann PD, et al: An anatomical study of the suprascapular nerve. *Arthroscopy* 1990;6:301-305.

Clark JM, Harryman DT II: Tendons, ligaments, and capsule of the rotator cuff: Gross and microscopic anatomy. *J Bone Joint Surg* 1992;74A:713-725.

The gross and microscopic structure of the myotendinous rotator cuff was evaluated. The rotator cuff tendons were found to interdigitate and fuse, forming a common insertion on the humerus. Distinct layers of the tendon were defined histologically.

Cooper DE, O'Brien SJ, Warren RF: Supporting layers of the glenohumeral joint: An anatomic study. *Clin Orthop* 1993;289:144-155.

A description of the anatomy of the shoulder based on anatomic and surgical dissections was presented. Four distinct layers that support the glenohumeral joint were identified. A detailed and organizational review of the pertinent anatomy and relevance to surgical approaches was highlighted.

Iannotti JP, Gabriel JP, Schneck SL, et al: The normal glenohumeral relationships: An anatomical study of one hundred and forty shoulders. *J Bone Joint Surg* 1992;74A:491-500.

Normal anatomic relationships of the glenohumeral articulation in 140 shoulders were evaluated through both anatomic dissection and magnetic resonance imaging. Variability in measured parameters of the humeral head and glenoid were discussed in conjunction with their clinical relevance.

Keyes EL: Anatomical observations on senile changes in the shoulder. *J Bone Joint Surg* 1935;17A:953-960.

Rothman RH, Parke WW: The vascular anatomy of the rotator cuff. *Clin Orthop* 1965;41:176-186.

Walch G, Laurent NJ, Levigne C, et al: Tears of the supraspinatus tendon associated with "hidden" lesions of the rotator interval. *J Shoulder Elbow Surg* 1994;3:353-360.

Surgical exploration of the rotator interval in 116 patients with apparently isolated tears of the supraspinatus tendon revealed occult lesions of the upper subscapularis tendon, superior glenohumeral, and coracohumeral ligaments in 19. Treatment included repair of the rotator cuff and reconstruction of the torn rotator interval complex. The pathologic entity was described along with a detailed review of the pertinent regional anatomy.

Warner JP, Krushell RJ, Masquelet A, et al: Anatomy and relationships of the suprascapular nerve: Anatomical constraints to mobilization of the supraspinatus and infraspinatus muscles in the management of massive rotator cuff tears. *J Bone Joint Surg* 1992;74A:36-45.

Anatomic dissections were performed in 31 cadaveric shoulders to evaluate the neurovascular anatomy of the rotator cuff. The course of the suprascapular nerve was identified in addition to its variational anatomy. Distances between anatomic landmarks and the neural structures were measured and their relationship to clinical issues were discussed.

Coracoacromial Arch
Flatow EL, Soslowsky LJ, Ticker JB, et al: Excursion of the rotator cuff under the acromion: Patterns of subacromial contact. *Am J Sports Med* 1994;22:779-788.

Stereophotogrammetric analysis of nine cadaveric shoulders assessing patterns of subacromial contact revealed a medial progression of contact from the anterolateral acromial edge with arm elevation. The rotator cuff and undersurface of the acromion were noted to be in closest proximity between 60° and 120° of arm elevation. Changes in humeral rotation also affected patterns of contact.

Soslowski LJ, An CH, Johnston SP, et al: Geometric and mechanical properties of the coracoacromial ligament and their relationship to rotator cuff disease. *Clin Orthop* 1994;304:10-17.

Geometric and mechanical analysis of the coracoacromial ligament in 20 specimens revealed decreased mechanical properties of this structure in shoulders with rotator cuff tears. The difference in findings when compared to cadavers with intact rotator cuffs was believed to reflect the multiple directional loads imposed on the ligament in shoulders with cuff defects.

Function
Gerber C, Terrier F, Ganz R: The role of the coracoid process in the chronic impingement syndrome. *J Bone Joint Surg* 1985;67B:703-708.

Harryman DT II, Sidles JA, Harris SL, et al: The role of the rotator interval capsule in passive motion and stability of the shoulder. *J Bone Joint Surg* 1992;74A:53-66.

Howell SM, Imobersteg AM, Seger DH, et al: Clarification of the role of the supraspinatus muscle in shoulder function. *J Bone Joint Surg* 1986;68A:398-404.

Otis JC, Jiang CC, Wickiewicz TL, et al: Changes in the moment arms of the rotator cuff and deltoid muscles with abduction and rotation. *J Bone Joint Surg* 1994;76A:667-676.

Changes in moment arms of the rotator cuff and deltoid with glenohumeral motion were evaluated in a cadaver model. The results demonstrated the potential capacity of both the infraspinatus and subscapularis muscles to contribute to arm elevation in the plane of the scapula.

Poppen NK, Walker PS: Normal and abnormal motion of the shoulder. *J Bone Joint Surg* 1976;58A:195-201.

Sharkey NA, Marder RA: The rotator cuff opposes superior translation of the humeral head. *Am J Sports Med* 1995;23:270-275.

Biomechanical analysis of intact cadaveric shoulders revealed that an absence of simulated force of the supraspinatus alone resulted in no significant change in humeral head position. Absence of force generated by the infraspinatus, teres minor, and subscapularis resulted in an increase in proximal humeral migration. The findings support the importance of the combined and balanced action of the anterior and posterior rotator cuff in maintaining stability of the glenohumeral joint.

Wuelker N, Plitz W, Roetman B: Biomechanical data concerning the shoulder impingement syndrome. *Clin Orthop* 1994;303:242-249.

Evaluation of subacromial forces in a dynamic shoulder model of 10 cadaveric specimens demonstrated peak forces between 85° and 136° of arm elevation. The clinical implications and potential role in the "painful arc sign" were discussed.

Pathogenesis
Brooks CH, Revell WJ, Heatley FW: A quantitative histological study of the vascularity of the rotator cuff tendon. *J Bone Joint Surg* 1992;74B:151-153.

A quantitative histologic vascular analysis of the supraspinatus and infraspinatus tendons revealed a decrease in vessel number, size, and percentage of tendon occupied by vessels at the distal portions of both structures. No significant differences in vascularity were observed between the two tendons. Implications toward the genesis of rotator cuff disease were discussed.

Codman EA, Akerson IB: The pathology associated with rupture of the supraspinatus tendon. *Ann Surg* 1931;93: 348-359.

Fukuda H, Hamada K, Yamanaka K: Pathology and pathogenesis of bursal-side rotator cuff tears viewed from en bloc histological sections. *Clin Orthop* 1990;254:75-80.

Lindblom K: On the pathogenesis of ruptures of the tendon aponeurosis of the shoulder joint. *Acta Radiol* 1939;20: 563-577.

Ozaki J, Fujimoto S, Nakagawa Y, et al: Tears of the rotator cuff of the shoulder associated with pathologic changes in the acromion: A study in cadavera. *J Bone Joint Surg* 1988;70A:1224-1230.

Etiology

Edelson JG, Zuckerman J, Hershkovitz I: Os acomiale: Anatomy and surgical implications. *J Bone Joint Surg* 1993;75B:551-555.

Evaluation of 270 cadaveric scapulae demonstrated an 8.2% incidence of os acromiale. Degenerative changes or osteophytic lipping was present in 56% of the involved specimens.

Walch G, Boileau P, Noel E, et al: Impingement of the deep surface of the supraspinatus tendon on the posterosuperior glenoid rim: An arthroscopic study. *J Shoulder Elbow Surg* 1992;1:238-245.

Arthroscopic evaluation of 17 athletes with unexplained shoulder pain demonstrated findings consistent with impingement of the deep surface of the supraspinatus against the posterosuperior glenoid rim with the arm in maximal external rotation and 90° of abduction. Potential causative factors and findings were described.

Natural History/Clinical Significance

Loehr JF, Helmig P, Sojberg JO, et al: Shoulder instability caused by rotator cuff lesions: An in vitro study. *Clin Orthop* 1994;304:84-90.

Motion patterns of the glenohumeral joint were studied in shoulders with experimentally created rotator cuff tears and intact tendons. Two tendon lesions involving both the supraspinatus and infraspinatus resulted in an increase in cephalad humeral migration not observed in single tendon or isolated supraspinatus defects.

Sher JS, Uribe JW, Posada A, et al: Abnormal findings on magnetic resonance images of asymptomatic shoulders. *J Bone Joint Surg* 1995;77A:10-15.

MRI scans were obtained in 96 normal volunteers without a history of shoulder complaints or evidence of pathology on physical examination. The frequency of positive MR findings increased with age. Complete and partial rotator cuff tears were evident in 14% and 20% of all individuals, respectively. Persons older than 60 years had a 28% and 26% prevalence of complete and partial tears, respectively. The results highlight the potential for normal, painless, functional shoulder activity in light of observed rotator cuff abnormalities on magnetic resonance imaging.

15
Nonsurgical Treatment of Rotator Cuff Tears

Craig D. Tifford, MD and Kevin D. Plancher, MD, MS

Introduction

Rotator cuff injury is common in older patients. In younger individuals, this injury is associated with a sudden, violent, eccentric episode. This chapter will discuss a clinical method to evaluate rotator cuff injuries and explore the benefits of various imaging studies. Nonsurgical treatment and its indications with specific rehabilitation protocols and modalities will also be reviewed.

Patient history and physical examination are of paramount importance in the diagnosis of rotator cuff pathology. The purpose of the history is to help the clinician to perform a directed clinical examination. Likewise, the purpose of the clinical examination is to redirect the clinician to key points of the history that will lead to an appropriate treatment.

History

The overwhelming majority of patients with rotator cuff tears are older than age 40. The incidence of full-thickness cuff tears in patients younger than age 40 is between 2% and 4%. Assuming that most older individuals are less likely to sustain a sudden shoulder injury, it can be theorized that most rotator cuff pathology is a result of repetitive microtrauma. However, in some studies, more than 60% of patients can recall an exact incident after which their shoulder was affected. Teleologically, it makes sense then that rotator cuff tears result from some macrotraumatic event superimposed on age-related microtrauma to the cuff. In fact, patients with cuff tears usually have a history of recurrent episodes of "tendinitis" or "bursitis." These transient episodes usually consist of a period of shoulder soreness that abates following a period of rest, nonsteroidal anti-inflammatory drug administration, and/or steroid injection.

The majority of rotator cuff tears affect the dominant extremity. Hawkins found the dominant extremity to be affected 78% of the time. The symptomatology of rotator cuff pathology is extremely variable. Patients with full-thickness tears may have no signs or symptoms, whereas patients with small tears may have marked weakness and significant loss of motion.

Pain, especially with overhead activity, is a frequent complaint of patients with rotator cuff tears. Patients may complain of pain at night with an inability to sleep on the affected side.

Weakness of the affected shoulder during abduction and external rotation is another frequent complaint. Full-thickness tears may produce crepitus when the supraspinatus is below the acromion, prompting patients to complain of "crackling." Loss of motion is a variable complaint. The ability to assess true loss of motion versus loss of motion secondary to pain is very difficult. This important clinical distinction will be discussed in further detail below.

Physical Examination

The physical examination can be separated into four parts: general inspection, palpation, range of motion/strength testing, and special tests. None of these components are mutually exclusive of one another, so the entire physical examination should flow smoothly.

The astute clinician's examination begins when the patient enters the room. Age, body habitus, and any obvious systemic diseases that may affect the shoulder should carefully be noted. The general "attitude" of the upper extremities should also be noted. Male patients should remove all clothing above the waist whereas female patients may be gowned to a level just proximal to the breasts. This seemingly trivial point is very important in preserving the modesty of the female patient, because a tense, uneasy patient is very difficult to examine. General inspection of the shoulder with a rotator cuff tear may reveal a prominence of the scapular spine—an indication of supraspinatus and/or infraspinatus wasting. Wasting of the infraspinatus is a frequent finding of a chronic massive tear, but may also be seen with a less common suprascapular nerve palsy. Deformity of the biceps muscle usually indicates a rupture of the long head of the biceps tendon. This finding is more pronounced with elbow flexion and is indicative of a biceps rupture, a condition often associated with rotator cuff disease.

Palpation over the greater tuberosity may elicit tenderness. The greater tuberosity is easily palpated with the shoulder extended, allowing it to be free from the cover of the acromion. Tenderness may be present in the bicipital groove when there is associated biceps involvement. Attention should be paid to any tenderness in the region of the acromioclavicular joint because this may help to distinguish cuff pathology from degenerative disease of the acromioclavicular joint.

Patients with full-thickness cuff tears may have a palpable defect posteriorly. In a recent study by Lyons and Tomlinson, rotator cuff tears were divided into four groups according to the estimated size of the tear as determined by clinical examination. At surgery, each tear was measured and the results compared to the preoperative estimate. The investigators concluded that preoperative clinical evaluation of a rotator cuff defect had a sensitivity of 91% and a specificity of 75%.

Range of motion and strength testing may be carried out simultaneously. The current recommendation of the American Shoulder and Elbow Surgeons is that four functionally necessary arcs of motion be recorded: total elevation (forward flexion), external rotation at neutral, external rotation at 90° of abduction, and internal rotation.

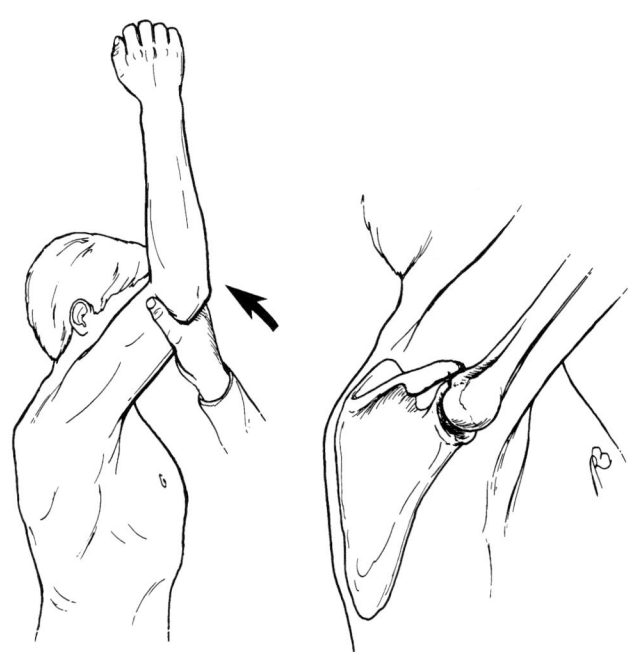

Fig. 1 A demonstration of the Neer impingement sign. (Copyright © 1997 Kevin D. Plancher, MD, Bronx, NY.)

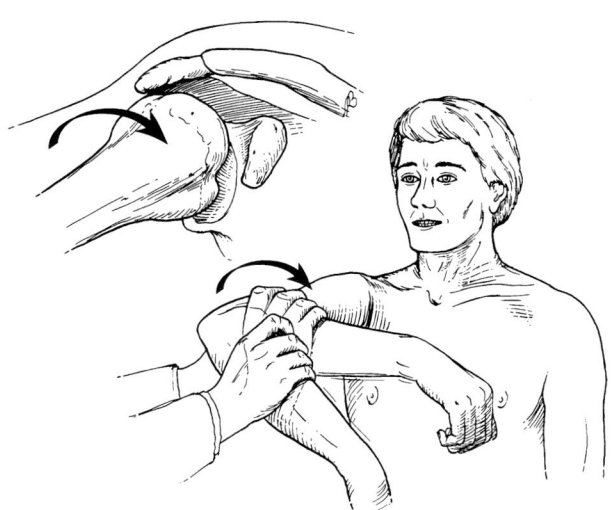

Fig. 2 Hawkins sign demonstrated with internal rotation in an arm elevated 90° and forward flexed. (Copyright © 1997 Kevin D. Plancher, MD, Bronx, NY.)

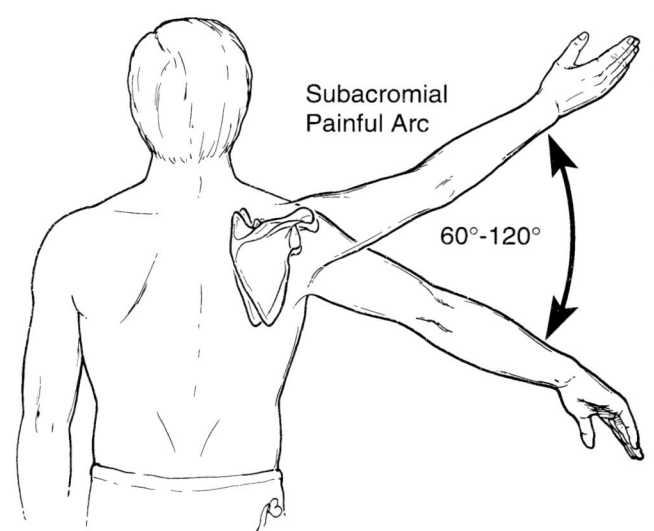

Fig. 3 Diagram showing a painful arc of abduction. (Copyright © 1997 Kevin D. Plancher, MD, Bronx, NY.)

Active and passive motion is assessed in these four planes. The patient is asked to flex the arms in a comfortable plane that is somewhere between the sagittal and coronal planes. After maximal active elevation is achieved, passive range is assessed by stressing the elevated arm into pure forward flexion. The impingement sign as described by Neer is positive if the patient experiences pain with greater than 120° of forward flexion (Fig. 1). The cause of true impingement is a result of the rotator cuff impinging against the anterior edge of the acromion with forced forward flexion. However, many disorders may present with similar findings. Therefore, to delineate isolated subacromial impingement, 10 cc of 1% lidocaine is injected into the subacromial space. The injection may be performed from either anterior or posterior. We prefer an anterior injection with the patient supine. The needle is placed directly into the subacromial space in the area of the pathology. An alternative is to place the needle 1 cm inferior to the posterolateral corner of the acromion, directing the needle toward the coracoid. The impingement test(s) are then repeated. Abatement of pain after injection strongly suggests the diagnosis of subacromial pathology.

Two other impingement tests have also been described. The Hawkins sign is performed with the arm flexed 90° and placed into internal rotation. The rotator cuff impinges on the coracoacromial ligament in this position (Fig. 2). Pain with this maneuver as described by Hawkins is a positive impingement sign. A third impingement sign is the painful arc of motion in the coronal plane with the arms abducted a maximum of 120° (Fig. 3). The pain is often exacerbated with added resistance as the supraspinatus is stressed. When all three signs are positive, the clinician can be certain that a diagnosis of impingement is appropriate.

External rotation is assessed in both neutral and 90° of abduction. The rotator cuff contributes only 30% to 40% of power in forward elevation, but accounts for 80% to 90% of external rotation strength. In a retrospective analysis of 100 patients operated on for full-thickness tears, Hawkins and associates found that shoulder strength in abduction and in external rotation at neutral were the only variables that had a statistically significant correlation with the size of the tear.

Other parameters that were correlated were preoperative pain, motion, and function.

In another recent study by Norwood and associates, 103 patients with known complete rotator cuff tears documented by arthrography were divided into two groups (those with single tendon tears and those with multiple tendon tears) to determine if cuff tear size could be predicted on the basis of history, physical examination, and radiographic findings. The patients with single tendon involvement demonstrated good active abduction and external rotation, measuring 116° and 61°, respectively. The patients with multiple tendon tears had an arc of motion of 52° and 36°, respectively. Furthermore, 75% of patients in the single tendon group could actively abduct the affected shoulder at least 90°, whereas only 16% of the patients with multiple tendon involvement could do the same. The difference in the range of abduction was the only statistically significant parameter between the physical examination of both groups. Neither pain, tenderness, nor weakness were useful in estimating cuff tear size. Nevaiser, in 1980, found the opposite to be true when he reported that middle-aged to elderly patients with chronic symptoms of rotator cuff disease did not have significant loss of motion.

A battery of special clinical tests help in the diagnosis of specific cuff pathology. The impingement signs have already been mentioned. Biceps tendon involvement may be evaluated by the Yergason or Speed tests. Yergason in 1931 described the supination sign, that is, pain localized to the bicipital groove when the examiner resists active supination with the elbow flexed to 90° and the forearm pronated. Yergason thought this pain represented wear and tear of the long head of the biceps. Speed's test is performed with the shoulder flexed, elbow fully extended, and hand supinated. Resistance is applied by the examiner (Fig. 4). Pain in the bicipital groove is suggestive of biceps pathology.

Jobe described the supraspinatus test in which the arms are extended at the elbows, flexed in the scapular plane, and the thumbs point toward the floor. The patient attempts to resist downward pressure applied to the arms by the examiner. Weakness is reported to be specific for evaluating the supraspinatus tendon. In this position, the infraspinatus, subscapularis, and teres minor are electrically silent when compared to the supraspinatus.

Gerber and Krushell described the lift-off test, a physical finding that has been shown to be both sensitive and specific for a subscapularis tendon tear. Patients with subscapularis tears have an increase in passive external rotation and weakness of internal rotation. The original lift-off test was positive if the patient was unable to move his/her hand off the small of the back. In this position, the arm is extended and internally rotated (Fig. 5). Gerber later described the modified lift-off test, reported to be even more sensitive. The upper extremity is placed into the same position as in the originally described test. The examiner passively lifts the hand off the small of the back, placing the arm in maximal internal rotation. The test is positive when the hand falls onto the back because of the inability of the subscapularis to maintain internal rotation. Greis and associates were able to validate the lift-off test with electromyographic testing. They concluded that performing the lift-off test required substantial subscapularis activity and

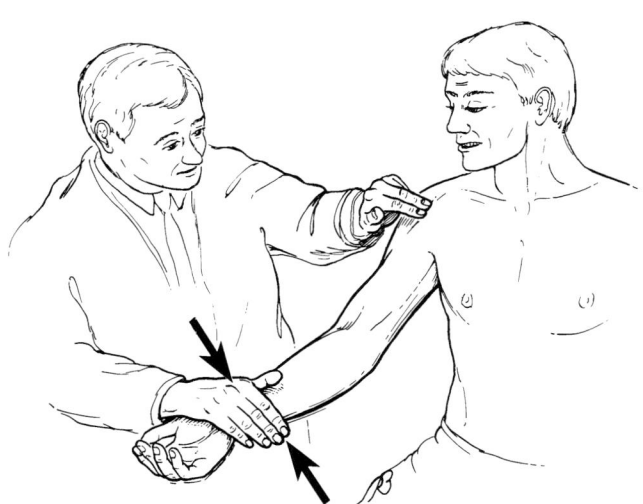

Fig. 4 Speed's test with pain in the bicipital groove. (Copyright © 1997 Kevin D. Plancher, MD, Bronx, NY.)

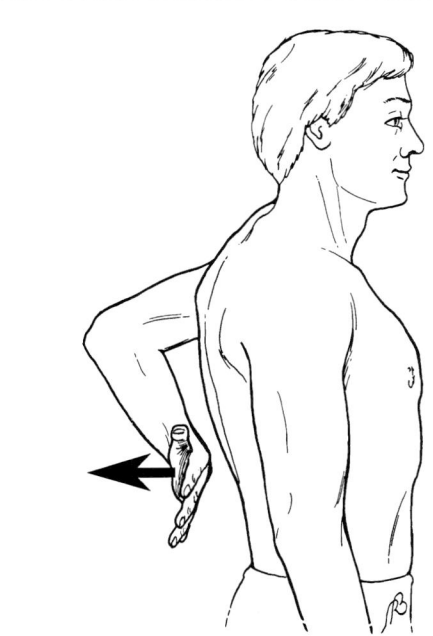

Fig. 5 The lift-off test demonstrated clinically. (Copyright © 1997 Kevin D. Plancher, MD, Bronx, NY.)

was a rigorous challenge to the muscle, requiring approximately 70% of maximal activity to perform.

Recently, Hertel and associates described three new clinical tests to assess the integrity of the rotator cuff. These lag signs include the external rotation lag sign (ERLS), the drop sign, and the internal rotation lag sign (IRLS). The external rotation lag sign is used to assess the supraspinatus and infraspinatus tendons. It is performed by passively flexing the elbow to 90° with the shoulder elevated in the scapular plane 20° and near maximally externally rotated. The examiner then lets go of the wrist while maintaining support of the elbow. The test is positive if the patient cannot maintain position and a drop or lag occurs. The magnitude of the lag is recorded to the nearest 5°. The drop sign, specific for the infraspinatus, is performed as follows: the examiner maintains the affected arm in 90° elevation and in near maximal external rotation with the elbow flexed 90°. Again, elbow support is maintained while the wrist is released. The infraspinatus is mainly responsible for the maintenance of external rotation in this position. Failure to maintain this position is seen as a drop or lag when the wrist is released. The lag should again be recorded to the nearest 5°. The internal rotation lag sign is specific for the subscapularis tendon. The patient's elbow is passively flexed to 90° and the shoulder is held at 20° of elevation and 20° of extension. The hand is then passively lifted off the small of the back, thereby placing the shoulder in near-maximal internal rotation. The wrist is released while supporting the elbow, and any lag is recorded to the nearest 5°. A slight lag is indicative of a partial tear, whereas an obvious drop represents a complete tear of the subscapularis tendon.

The ERLS was found to be less sensitive, but more specific, than the Jobe sign. Similarly, the drop sign had poor sensitivity but high specificity. For evaluation of the subscapularis tendon, the IRLS was more sensitive but as specific as the lift-off sign.

A cursory neurologic assessment is performed as part of our range of motion/strength testing. Gross motor skills and muscle mass are noted. Reflexes of the biceps and brachioradialis may be performed as well as evaluation of any dermatomal sensory changes. Distal pulses are recorded. Cervical spine evaluation should also be recorded for all patients with shoulder pain. Spurling's test is a clinical finding that is useful in distinguishing cervical spine radiculopathy from intrinsic shoulder pathology. The neck is extended and rotated to each side, vertically compressing the skull to the left and right. Pain, and more specifically, radiculopathy down the arm with this maneuver may indicate the need for a more extensive neurologic/cervical spine examination.

Physical findings in rotator cuff disease may be minor with an asymptomatic patient or may be significant with a completely disabled patient. The extent of the tear is often manifested by the extent of findings on physical examination. The presence of a massive tear is frequently confirmed by a physical examination, but subtle pathology requires a more involved diagnostic workup.

Imaging of the Rotator Cuff

Plain Radiographs

In early rotator cuff disease, plain films are usually normal. Calcific deposits in the cuff tendons, bony cysts at the greater tuberosity, concavity of the undersurface of the acromion, or acromial spurs are often found with more advanced disease. Degenerative changes may be present in the greater tuberosity, acromioclavicular joint, or anterior acromion. An acromiohumeral interval of less than 7 mm on a true anteroposterior (AP) plain radiograph of the shoulder is considered abnormal and suggests the presence of a chronic tear (Fig. 6). The shape of the acromion is an important radio-

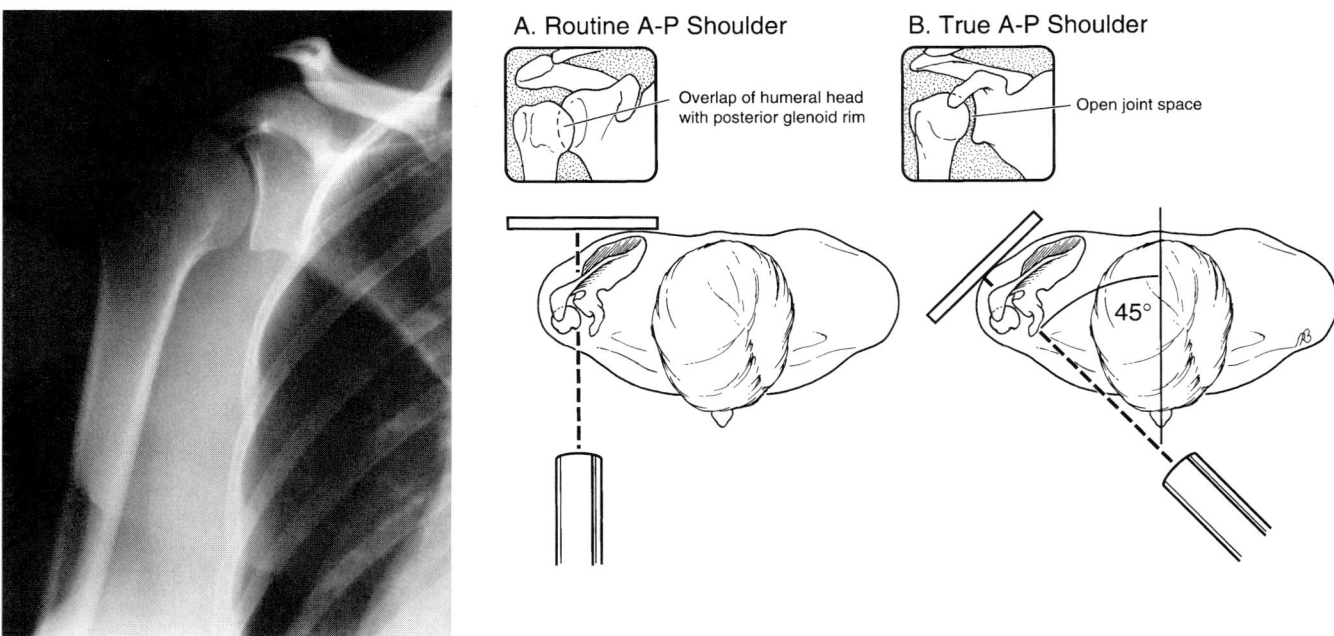

Fig. 6 **Left,** A plain radiograph demonstrating the acromiohumeral interval less than 7 mm on a true anteroposterior (AP) radiograph implying a rotator cuff tear. **Right,** Difference between true AP and routine AP radiographs of the shoulder. (Adapted with permission from Rockwood CA, Szalay EA, Curtis RJ, et al: X-ray evaluation of shoulder problems, in Rockwood, CA, Matsen FA III (eds): *The Shoulder.* Philadelphia, PA, WB Saunders, 1990, p 180.)

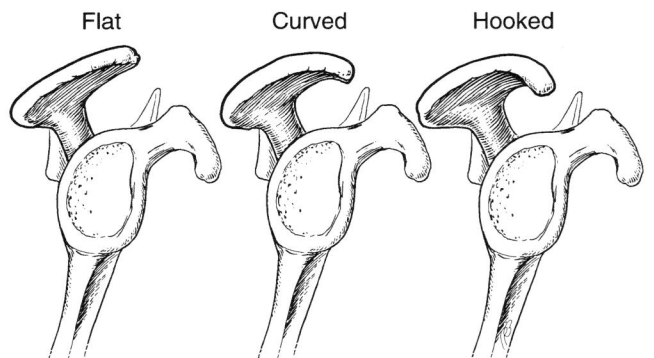

Fig. 7 Diagram of the type III acromion. (Copyright © 1997 Kevin D. Plancher, MD, Bronx, NY.)

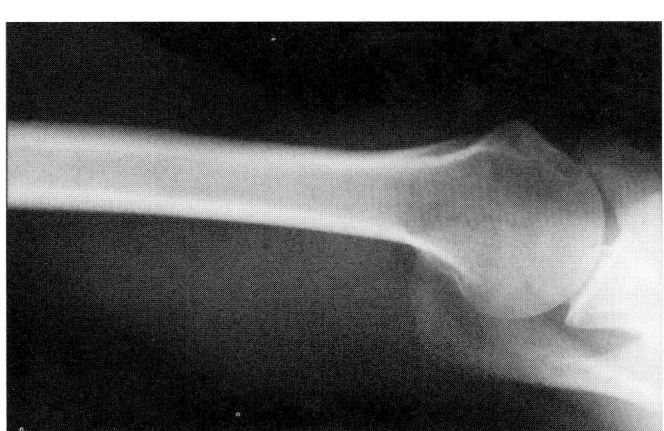

Fig. 8 A normal axillary view of the shoulder.

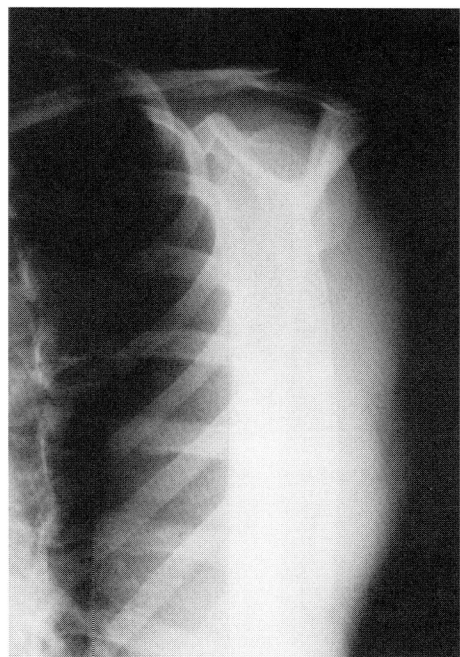

Fig. 9 A scapular outlet view.

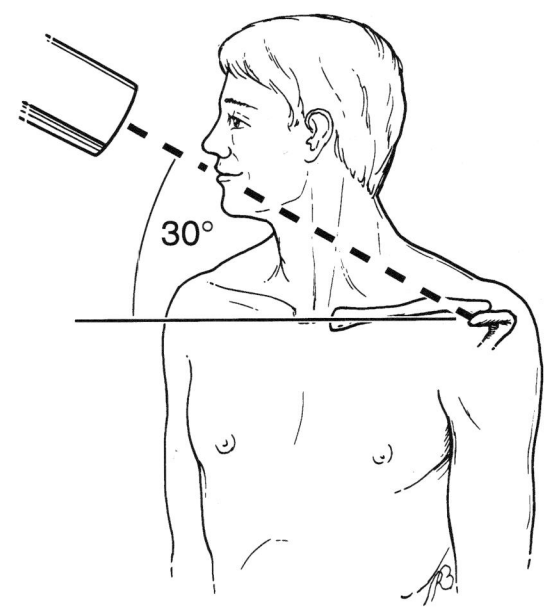

Fig. 10 Diagram of anteroposterior caudal tilt view. (Adapted with permission from Rockwood CA, Szalay EA, Curtis RJ, et al: X-ray evaluation of shoulder problems, in Rockwood CA, Matsen FA III (eds): *The Shoulder*. Philadelphia, PA, WB Saunders, 1990, p 197.)

graphic feature. A majority of rotator cuff tears occur in patients with a hooked (type III) acromion (Fig. 7), an anterior acromial spur, or an os acromiale. The latter finding is best visualized on the axillary view (Fig. 8). In addition to the standard AP, scapulothoracic, and axillary views, there are several other views that help assess the rotator cuff. The scapular outlet view is a true scapulolateral with the x-ray tube angled caudally 5° to 10°. This view will reveal deformities of the anteroinferior acromion (Fig. 9). An AP view of the shoulder with the tube angled 30° caudally (the AP caudal tilt view) also allows demonstration of an anteroinferior acromial spur or coracoacromial ligament calcification (Fig. 10).

Kitay and associates recently examined the interobserver reliability and the correlation of preoperative measurements with surgical findings for four different roentgenographic views. All patients had a diagnosis of impingement and were refractory to nonsurgical treatment. Prior to open acromioplasty, all patients had standard AP and axillary radiographs as well as supraspinatus outlet and 30° caudal tilt views. The 30° caudal tilt view had the highest interobserver reliability; the axillary view had the lowest. The interobserver reliability of the supraspinatus outlet view was found to be less than that of the caudal tilt view but greater than the axillary view. The authors found that the distance from the acromial cortex to the end of the spur, as measured on the 30° caudal tilt view, significantly correlated with intraoperative spur length

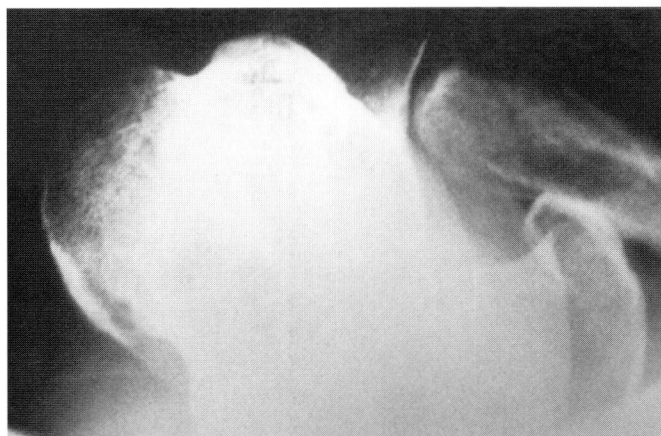

Fig. 11 The Fisk view used to image the bicipital groove.

Outline 1 Radiographic findings

Acromiohumeral interval less than 7 mm
Subacromial calcification
Greater tuberosity sclerosis or irregularity
Cysts at greater tuberosity
Subacromial spur
Concave acromion
Degenerative changes at the acromioclavicular joint
Distally pointing acromioclavicular spur greater than 2 mm in diameter
Degenerative changes at the glenohumeral joint
Exaggerated groove between the greater tuberosity and the humeral articular surface

(Reproduced with permission from Norwood LA, Barrack R, Jacobson KE: Clinical presentation of complete tears of the rotator cuff. *J Bone Joint Surg* 1989;71A:499–505.)

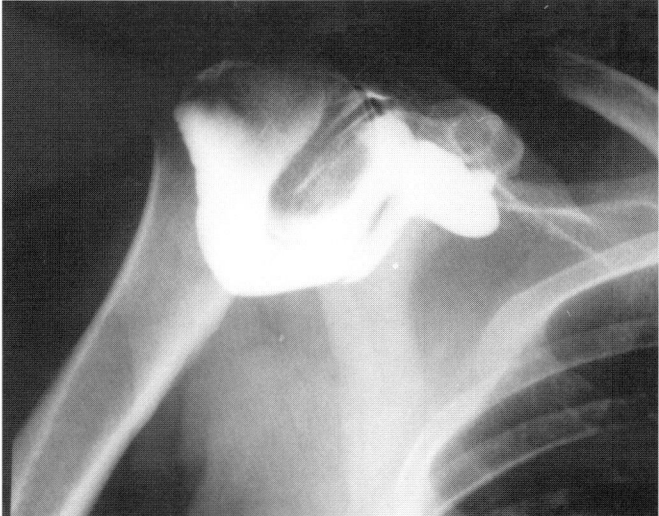

Fig. 12 Normal shoulder arthrogram.

calculation. Additionally, acromial slope, measured on the supraspinatus outlet view, correlated significantly with anterior acromial thickness as measured intraoperatively. The authors therefore concluded that these two views offer distinct information about the morphology of the acromion and anteroinferior spur. We routinely obtain these two views in the evaluation of patients with impingement/rotator cuff symptoms prior to acromioplasty.

The Fisk view is used to image the bicipital groove. In this projection, the x-ray machine is superior to the shoulder. The bicipital groove is projected onto the cassette, which is held by the patient leaning on the table (Fig. 11).

A recent study by Norwood and associates reviewed ten separate plain radiographic findings in patients with a single tendon rotator cuff tear, multiple tendon tears, and patients with symptoms of rotator cuff disease but normal arthrograms. The ten radiographic findings were recorded as being either present or absent (Outline 1). The authors found that a significantly higher number of abnormal findings were present in the multiple tendon group when compared to the control group. However, when the single tendon group was compared to the controls, there were only two abnormal findings that occurred with a significantly higher frequency. When the two tendon tear groups were compared, half of the abnormal radiographic findings showed statistically significant differences. The authors concluded that in the appropriate clinical setting, a patient with five or more plain radiographic findings listed in Outline 1 is more likely to have a tear involving multiple tendons. Patients with three findings or less are likely to have single tendon involvement.

Arthrography

For years, the arthrogram has been considered the gold standard to evaluate full-thickness rotator cuff tears. Known complications such as infection, allergic reaction, and synovial effusions are rare; however, it must be remembered that the arthrogram is an invasive procedure and not without risk. Arthrography exposes the patient to radiation and its usefulness may be limited by the technical skill of both radiologist and technologist. Despite these drawbacks, arthrography remains an excellent imaging modality for full-thickness tears. Double contrast arthrography (using dye and air) or arthrotomography may enhance resolution. The latter technique uses tomograms taken with contrast material in the shoulder.

The fundamental reason that arthrography works is inherent to normal shoulder anatomy. Contrast material injected into the normal glenohumeral joint should only communicate with the subscapularis bursa and biceps sheath as dye extends beneath the transverse humeral ligament. The normal rotator cuff prevents passage of contrast into the subacromial-subdeltoid bursa. In a full-thickness tear, contrast will either fill this bursa or extravasate into the substance of the tendon. AP views in internal and external rotation should be taken after brief exercise to fully evaluate the rotator cuff (Fig. 12). Other views, especially the axillary and Fisk views, may aid

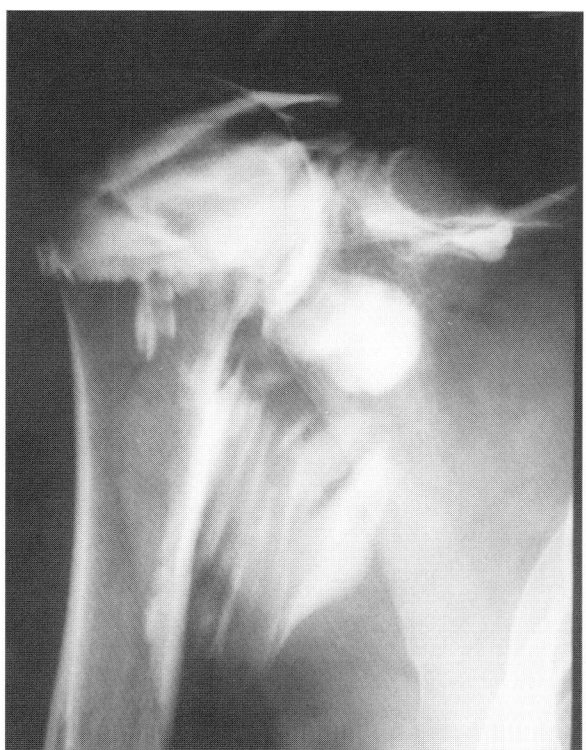

Fig. 13 The geyser sign, which is indicative of a large rotator cuff tear.

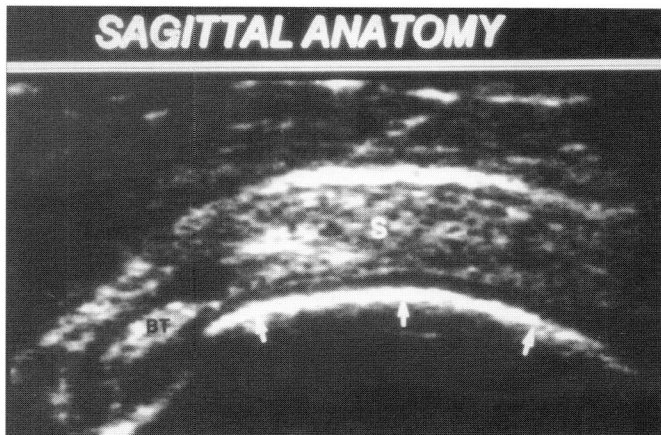

Fig. 14 Sonographic representation of a normal subacromial bursa. BT = biceps tendon; S = supraspinatus.

in evaluating associated pathology of the labrum or long head of the biceps tendon. Dye that is visualized in the acromioclavicular joint has been termed the geyser sign by Craig (Fig. 13). This sign is indicative of a large chronic tear in which contrast material has extravasated from the glenohumeral joint through the torn cuff to fill the acromioclavicular joint.

Arthrography has several limitations. Partial-thickness tears, by definition, will not allow extravasation of dye into the subacromial-subdeltoid bursa. Furthermore, bursal side tears are unable to be visualized with arthrography because there is no tendon discontinuity on the joint surface side to allow for the passage of dye. Arthrography is also unable to identify isolated midsubstance tears. Arthrography in the presence of a partial thickness tear is less accurate than when used to detect a full-thickness tear. The overall incidence of false-negative examinations (those with tears that were missed) in surgically documented tears (full and partial thickness) is between 0 to 8%, depending on which study is referenced.

Ultrasound

Shoulder ultrasonography has been used to diagnose rotator cuff pathology since the early 1980s. It is an inexpensive, noninvasive imaging modality that does not use radiation and is readily available at most centers, with very rapid results. Its main drawback is that ultrasound has been shown to be a tool that is highly technician-dependent.

High resolution, real-time equipment should be used. Most machines today use a 7.5 MHz linear array transducer. To further enhance signal resolution, the shoulder should be examined with the humerus hyperextended; this position allows the cuff to be free from the cover of the acromion.

The outer border of cortical bone covering the humeral head normally appears as a hyperechogenic line. The normal musculotendinous cuff appears homogenous with regard to echogenicity, without any focal changes. The subacromial bursa normally appears as a hypoechogenic focus less than 2 mm thick (Fig. 14). Visualization of the long head of the biceps tendon is made possible with ultrasound. The normal biceps tendon appears echogenic and sits deep in the intertubercular groove.

The most consistent ultrasound findings of a rotator cuff tear are nonvisualization, focal thinning, and discontinuity of the cuff. Hypoechogenic foci within the cuff may represent fluid whereas hyperechogenic foci may represent granulation tissue. These findings are nonspecific and should not be regarded as pathognomonic for a rotator cuff tear. Sonnabend and associates examined 117 patients who underwent shoulder ultrasound followed by surgical intervention for rotator cuff disease. The authors found that preoperative ultrasound assessment of cuff tear size was able to reliably predict full-thickness tears. Their data revealed a positive predictive value of 96%. However, in assessing partial thickness tears, ultrasound failed to detect a significant number of lesions. Diagnosis of subacromial impingement was found to have a positive predictive value of 94% but a negative predictive value of 66%. The authors concluded that ultrasound is reliable in the detection of full-thickness tears, but a negative study in the face of strong clinical findings should prompt further investigation, with methods such as arthrography or magnetic resonance imaging (MRI).

Matsen and associates examined the relationship between the presence of a joint effusion or fluid within the subacromial-subdeltoid bursa and the existence of a rotator cuff tear. A preoperative shoulder sonogram was performed on all patients studied. One hundred sixty-three shoulders were then operated on for a suspected rotator cuff tear. The presence of a joint effusion alone had a sensitivity of 22%, specificity of 79%, and a positive predictive value of 60%. Bursal fluid alone was only seen in ten patients and had a sensitivity of 7%, specificity of 96%, and a positive predictive value of 70%. However, when fluid was seen in both the joint and the bursa, the sensitivity was 22%, specificity 99%, and positive predictive value 95%. The integrity of the rotator cuff tendons was deliberately not assessed. The authors concluded that sonographic evidence of fluid in the subacromial-subdeltoid bursa with or without a joint effusion, is highly specific and has a high positive predictive value for a rotator cuff tear. Although the combined presence of fluid in the joint and the bursae has a low sensitivity, this finding necessitates a careful ultrasound evaluation of the rotator cuff for a tear.

The use of sonography in the postoperative shoulder has also been looked at recently. Because surgical intervention distorts the normal cuff architecture, it is imperative that the sonographer be familiar with normal postoperative changes and the appearance of persistent or newly damaged cuff.

After acromioplasty, sonographic evaluation may reveal distortion of the lateral aspect of the acromial shadow, irregular contour, or medial displacement of the acromial margin. Most commonly, the supraspinatus is reattached at the level of the greater tuberosity via a trough-in-bone procedure, and is sonographically visualized as a linear defect in the humeral head. However, frequently the cuff is retracted medially and mobilization does not permit the repair to take place at the level of the tuberosity. In these instances, the reimplanted tendon and trough are displaced medially, and visualization of the supraspinatus tendon may be difficult. Extension of the arm as well as abduction/adduction may facilitate visualization.

Normally, the postoperative tendon remains thinned and exhibits increased echogenicity. Therefore, unlike preoperative criteria, visualization of a cuff defect is necessary to make the diagnosis of a recurrent rotator cuff tear. If the subdeltoid bursa has been resected, the normal echogenic plane between the supraspinatus tendon and overlying deltoid will be absent. Additionally, sonography may be used postoperatively to diagnose those patients with cuff arthropathy. This is visualized as irregularity of the humeral head with loss of normal overlying hypoechoic cartilage.

In a study by Mack and associates, sonography was used to evaluate 60 symptomatic postoperative shoulders in 53 patients. In ten shoulders that had a previous acromioplasty alone, nine had subsequent surgical intervention; a correct diagnosis of intact rotator cuffs was made in eight of the nine shoulders. Of the 50 shoulders that had previous full-thickness cuff repairs, subsequent surgical procedures were performed on 27. In 26 of these 27, sonography was used to confirm large recurrent tears; the remaining shoulder had an intact cuff. The authors concluded that although the ability of sonography to rule out disease was not adequately tested, ultrasound was an excellent means of assessing the postoperative shoulder. Their results yielded a sensitivity of 100%, specificity of 90%, and overall accuracy of 98% for detecting postoperative rotator cuff tears.

Magnetic Resonance Imaging

The use of MRI represents a major advance in musculoskeletal imaging. Some believe it to be the imaging modality of choice following plain film evaluation of the shoulder. MRI is noninvasive and unlike arthrography does not use ionizing radiation. A significant advantage of MRI is its ability to detect midsubstance and bursal side tears, which allows for detection of cuff pathology earlier in the disease process. These partial thickness tears are very difficult to diagnose using other modalities. MRI is significantly more expensive to use than the previously discussed modalities; this is its major disadvantage. Contraindications to the use of MRI include noncompatible aneurysm clips, cardiac pacers, neurostimulatory devices, and some types of prosthetic heart valves. Morbidly obese patients may not fit into the scanner. With the advent of "open" MRI machines, claustrophobia has become less of a problem and resolution has improved.

MRI changes seen in rotator cuff tendons are the principal means of diagnosing a tear. The grading system of these changes is based on changes in signal intensity and morphology of the cuff tendons. Low signal intensity is black and high signal intensity is white regardless of pulse sequence. A grade 0 tendon has normal signal intensity (low) and normal morphology (Fig. 15, *top left*). Grade 1 is a tendon with diffusely increased signal on short recovery time/echo time (TR/TE) (T1-weighted) and long TR/short TE (proton density-weighted) images but with normal morphology (Fig. 15, *top center* and *top right*). A grade 2 tendon has increased signal intensity on these same pulse sequences but, in addition, has some alteration in tendon morphology, ie, thinning, and/or surface irregularity (Fig. 15, *bottom left*). This group may be further classified into 2A or 2B depending on the degree of morphologic alteration. A grade 3 tendon will exhibit increased signal intensity on T2-weighted images. In this group there is an obvious tendon defect (Fig. 15, *bottom right*) This defect is the most specific finding of a full-thickness tear.

Changes in the subacromial-subdeltoid bursa and peribursal fat plane are clues to presence of a cuff tear. Significant fluid in the bursa, although not pathognomonic, is highly suggestive of a cuff tear. The most commonly offered explanation for this finding is that the complete tear allows the extension of intra-articular fluid into the bursa. This fluid is seen as high signal intensity within the bursa on T2-weighted images. Loss of the normal high signal of the peribursal fat plane is also highly suggestive of a tear. These two findings are present in over 90% of patients with full-thickness tears (Fig. 16).

The bony pathology associated with rotator cuff pathology may also be identified using MRI. The hooked type III acromion is best visualized on the coronal or sagittal oblique cuts. Subacromial spurs are also easily demonstrated. Small spurs (cortical bone) appear black on T2-weighted images. Larger spurs may contain marrow and thus appear as high signal on both T1- and T2-weighted images. Degenerative changes of the acromioclavicular joint may be visualized as hypertrophy of the joint capsule, seen as a medium intensity signal surrounding the acromioclavicular joint on pulse sequences with short TR and short TE (Fig. 17).

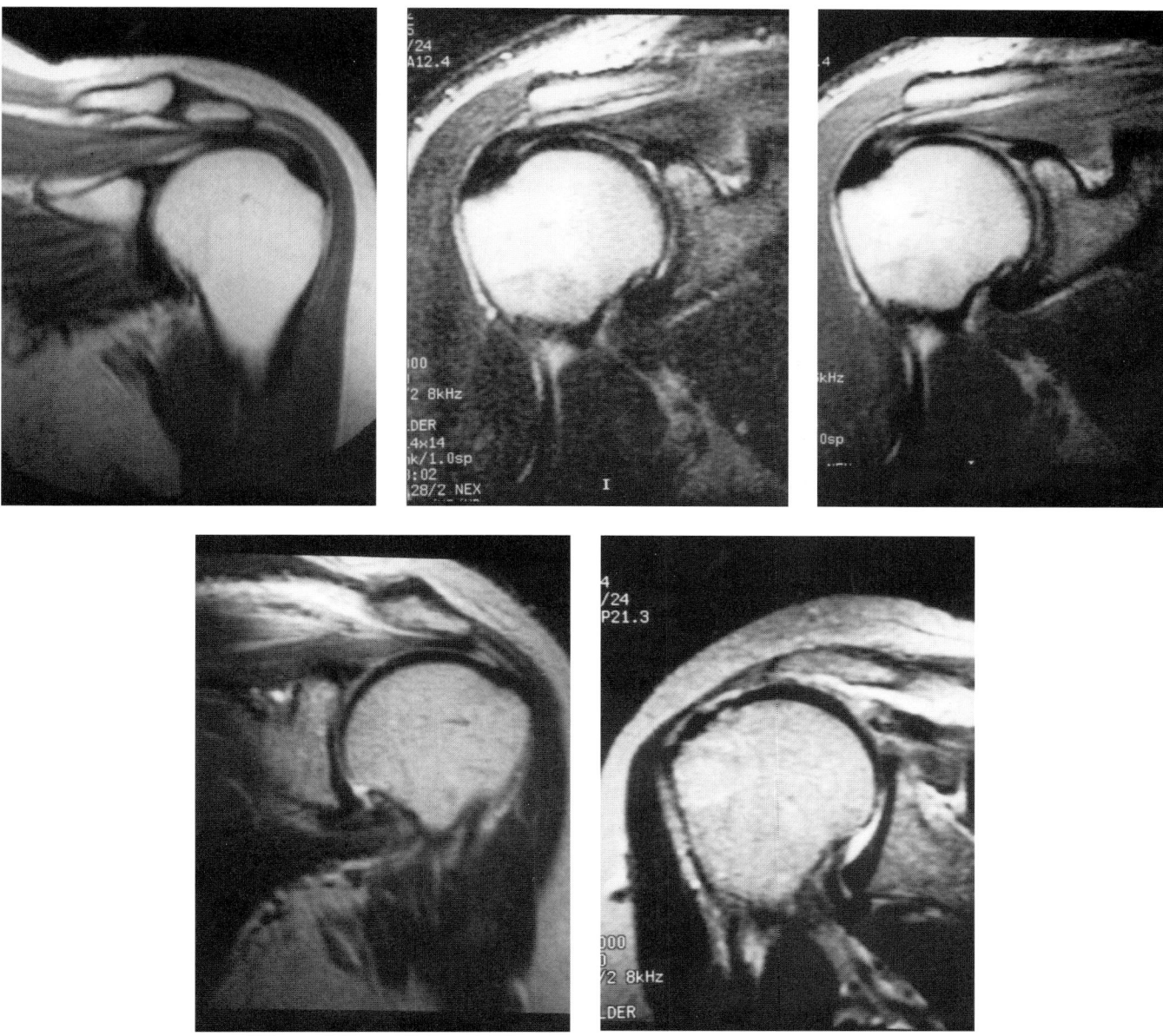

Fig. 15 Top left, A normal supraspinatus tendon grade 0. **Top center,** Grade 1 tendon on T1. **Top right,** Grade 1 tendon on proton density. **Bottom left,** Grade 2 tendon with some alteration of morphology. **Bottom right,** Grade 3 tendon on T2-weighted image.

MRI offers information regarding cuff tear size, specific tendon involvement, and the degree of retraction. It can identify torn tendon edges and frequently delineate whether those edges are frayed to the point of irreparability. By predicting the size of the cuff defect, MRI may aid the surgeon in deciding preoperatively whether to attempt a repair alone, repair with a local tissue transfer, or debridement of the cuff tear.

Iannotti and associates used MRI to preoperatively assess the integrity of the rotator cuff in 91 patients. In 33 patients, the presence of a complete tear of the rotator cuff was confirmed with MRI. The size of the tears was calculated and compared with the findings at operation. Of the 33 complete tears seen at operation, the size of all but two had been correctly assessed by MRI. These two large tears had been incorrectly assessed as being moderate in size. Small tears were those less than 2 cm in diameter, moderately sized tears were 2 to 4 cm, and large tears were 5 cm or larger.

The authors found a correlation between the degree of supraspinatus wasting seen on MRI and the size of the cuff tear at operation. In general, larger tears were seen at surgery in patients whose scans demonstrated a significant amount of supraspinatus wasting on MRI.

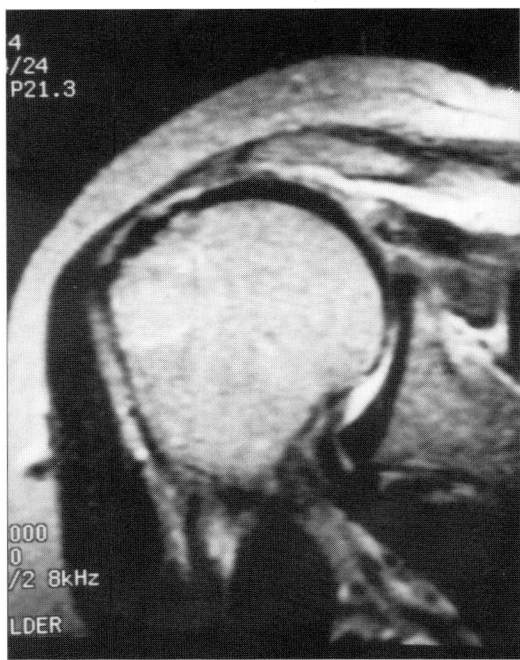

Fig. 16 Fluid in the subacromial bursa and peribursal fat plane on T2-weighted image, which is representative of a full-thickness rotator cuff tear.

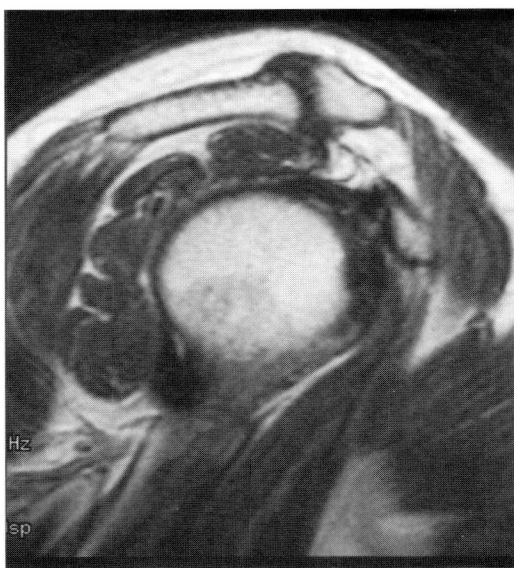

Fig. 17 Degenerative changes of the acromioclavicular joint on a T1-weighted image.

The same authors correlated preoperative MRI assessment with findings seen at open acromioplasty or diagnostic arthroscopy. In 31 shoulders with clinical impingement and radiographically intact tendons, there were four false-positive and three false-negative results. The authors found that in the diagnosis of a complete tear of the rotator cuff, MRI had a sensitivity of 100% and a specificity of 95%. The positive predictive value was 92% and the negative predictive value 100%. The sensitivity and specificity of MRI in differentiating degeneration or partial thickness tears versus tendinitis was found to be 82% and 85%, respectively. The positive and negative predictive values were also 82% and 85%. Finally, with respect to differentiating normal tendon from one affected by tendinitis secondary to impingement, MRI had a sensitivity and specificity of 93% and 87%. Here the positive and negative predictive values were also 93% and 87%.

MRI is best in its ability to detect complete tears of the rotator cuff. However, it is useful in localizing the site of a tear, estimating its size, and differentiating between the various stages of impingement in clinical diagnoses.

The use of MRI in the postoperative shoulder has also been recently studied. As expected, preoperative evaluation is more difficult than the evaluation of a patient who has not had prior surgical intervention. MRI can demonstrate cuff disruption when it is present postoperatively. However, in assessing symptomatic postacromioplasty patients, the criteria for making the diagnosis of a rotator cuff tear needs to be modified. The only consistent findings are definite discontinuity in the cuff with high signal within it on T2-weighted images and nonvisualization of the cuff. The secondary signs discussed above are not useful in assessing the postoperative shoulder.

In a recent study by Owen and associates, MRI was used to assess the postoperative shoulder in 31 patients before repeated surgical intervention. Using the above criteria, a correct diagnosis was made in six of seven patients who had a surgically proven tear. Additionally, MRI was able to rule out the presence of a tear in 22 of 24 patients who had no evidence of a full-thickness tear at surgery. The authors concluded that MRI is a valuable technique in the evaluation of the symptomatic postoperative shoulder. Sensitivity was found to be 86%, specificity 92%, and accuracy 90%. However, these data pertain to full-thickness tears and the appearance of a postoperative tendon-to-tendon repair is indistinguishable from that of a new or recurrent tear. Therefore, MRI is limited in its ability to detect partial or midsubstance tears after primary rotator cuff repair.

Nonsurgical Management

The indications for nonsurgical treatment of a rotator cuff tear are not clearly defined. Each patient needs to be individually assessed with regard to age, occupation, physical demands, size of cuff tear, loss of function, mechanism of injury, and most importantly, pain. Most authors recommend an initial trial of nonsurgical treatment; however, this regimen may not be beneficial to a younger patient who sustains a traumatic tear associated with significant functional impairment and weakness. The length of nonsurgical treatment will vary depending on the degree of cuff involvement and with the patient's response to treatment. If pain persists in the face of an adequate rehabilitation protocol, then surgical intervention should be considered.

Nonsteroidal Anti-Inflammatory Medication

Although there is a paucity of good data to support the fact that nonsteroidal anti-inflammatory drugs are of value in the treatment of impingement and rotator cuff pathology, they remain a mainstay of management. Teleologically, it makes sense that an anti-inflammatory/analgesic medication would work in a setting where the presumed etiology is a spectrum of chronic irritation and inflammation. No data exist that support the benefits of one brand over another, and all patients should be asked about any history of peptic ulcer disease or gastritis prior to initiating therapy.

Corticosteroid Injection

There are few studies in the literature that conclusively show that the subacromial injection of steroids is of any benefit in the treatment of impingement or rotator cuff tears. In a prospective, controlled, randomized, double-blind study, Zuckerman and associates examined the efficacy of subacromial corticosteroid injection. Patients with a diagnosis of impingement without evidence of a rotator cuff tear were randomized to receive a subacromial injection of either 1% lidocaine or 1% lidocaine with 80 mg triamcinolone. Eighty-four percent of patients in the steroid group reported improvement in pain compared to only 36% in the control group. Objectively, active range of motion improved in 74% of the patients who received steroids compared to 36% of the patients in the control group. Finally, 79% of the steroid group patients, compared to 18% of the control group patients, actually had relief of impingement sign on last follow-up examination.

The adverse effects of such injections are well known. Steroid injections in or around the rotator cuff may produce tendon atrophy and can actually impede the repair process. Watson has shown that repeated injections (more than five) have been shown to be associated with poor tissue quality at surgery. However, the use of corticosteroid injections remains widespread. If used, injections should be limited in number, well-spaced out in time, and never administered in the acute phase of injury or directly into the tendons of the rotator cuff.

Ultrasound, Phonophoresis, and Iontophoresis

Ultrasound has been used extensively as a physical therapy modality for over 30 years. Ultrasound waves are sound waves that are above the audible limit (> 20 kHz). The therapeutic effects of ultrasound are a result of both the thermal and nonthermal properties of these high frequency sound waves. The heat induced by ultrasound causes a local hyperemia and is therefore potentially beneficial to the healing process. The nonthermal or mechanical characteristics of ultrasound waves are believed to alter the cell membrane resting potential and thus alter cell permeability.

Phonophoresis is the use of ultrasound to enhance the delivery of topically applied drugs. The most commonly used topical drugs are anesthetics, counterirritants, and anti-inflammatories such as nonsteroidal or steroidal medications. Studies are still lacking that define typical drug doses and duration of sonication. These topically applied drugs avoid the risks and possible complications associated with the use of systemic medications. The first pass effect by the liver is also eliminated by this route of administration. There is less of a chance of underdosing or overdosing the drug.

The mechanism of action is related to the thermal and nonthermal properties of ultrasound waves. Increased heat causes an increase in the kinetic energy of the drug molecules, dilates points of entry in the stratum corneum such as hair follicles and sweat glands, and causes a local increase in blood flow to the sonicated area. At the same time, cell membrane characteristics are altered in such a way that all of these physiologic responses enhance the opportunity for the topically applied drug to traverse the skin. In a study by Griffin and associates, various orthopaedic diagnoses were treated blindly using phonophoresis with either hydrocortisone or placebo. Sixty-eight percent of the patients treated with hydrocortisone with ultrasound had decreased pain and increased range of motion compared to only 28% of those treated with placebo plus ultrasound. A recent study by Kleinkort and Wood revealed that a 10% preparation of hydrocortisone plus ultrasound was more effective than a 1% preparation in reducing the pain associated with a number of inflammatory conditions, including subdeltoid bursitis and epicondylitis.

Like the classic investigations cited above, the more recent literature on the efficacy of phonophoresis appears promising. However, few studies are scientifically sound. Most of the reports lack some element of a fundamentally scientific study such as a control group, small sample size, nonobjective documentation of effectiveness, and nonblinded observers.

Smith and associates compared five modalities for the treatment of shin splints: ice, ice massage, ultrasound, iontophoresis, and phonophoresis. The investigators found no difference among the various treatment groups although all methods decreased pain. In two other recent studies by McElnay and Williams, the authors independently found that phonophoresis had no increased effect on the percutaneous absorption of lidocaine and other topical anesthetics.

Iontophoresis is a process that uses electricity to introduce ions into the skin. It is used by physical therapists to deliver locally higher concentrations of medication while avoiding the potential complications associated with their systemic use. Corticosteroids are the most commonly used drugs with iontophoresis. Several water-soluble preparations are available to enable the drug to dissociate into the negatively charged steroid molecule and therefore move in an electric field. DeLacerda, using iontophoresis with dexamethasone, found rapid improvement in range of motion in patients with myofascial shoulder girdle syndrome when compared to treatment with ultrasound or muscle relaxants. In a group of patients with shoulder tendinitis, Bertolucci found that those treated with dexamethasone and lidocaine iontophoresis had less pain and increased range of motion compared to controls.

The use of iontophoresis has declined; however, this process is occasionally selected by therapists whose patients do not show improvement with more conventional therapy. Fear of chemical skin burns and the paucity of sound scientific data demonstrating the efficacy of this treatment are the reasons why iontophoresis is seldom used.

Exercise

The common denominator in all rehabilitative programs for impingement is adequate resting of acutely inflamed tissues followed by rotator cuff strengthening. One of the functions of the rotator cuff is to serve as a humeral head depressor.

With the rotator cuff strengthened, mechanical impingement and the patient's symptoms are alleviated.

Rockwood has coined the term "orthotherapy" to describe a nonsurgical, rehabilitative program that first focuses on improvement in range of motion and then concentrates on improving shoulder strength. The regimen is designed to permit immediate communication between physician and patient to allow quick adjustments in their rehabilitation protocol. This method facilitates patient compliance and minimizes the chance of a rehabilitation setback.

Orthotherapy should not be used for a select group of patients with injury to the shoulder. The first group is the young or middle-aged patient who, as a result of violent trauma, sustains a rotator cuff tear. The second group of patients are highly competitive athletes, especially those whose sport involves raising the arms overhead, who sustain a rotator cuff tear. It is believed that these patients are best served by early surgical repair.

The rehabilitation of the rotator cuff can be divided into three convenient stages. There should be defined goals for each stage of this process. Criteria must be carefully evaluated before a patient is allowed to progress to the next stage of rehabilitation.

Stage I is aimed at decreasing acute inflammation while maintaining shoulder range of motion. Initially, a short period of rest with avoidance of overhead activity is pursued. A number of adjunctive modalities such as nonsteroidal anti-inflammatory medications, steroid injections, phonophoresis, and iontophoresis may be used. In addition to allowing inflammation to subside, it is equally important to maintain mobility of the glenohumeral as well as the scapulothoracic, acromioclavicular, and sternoclavicular joints. Gentle pendulum exercises are begun and active assisted range of motion exercises are gradually added with the use of a rope and pulley system. This system is set up so that the shoulder is flexed by having the patient grasp one end of the rope with the supinated palm of the affected extremity. The unaffected extremity is used to gently elevate the affected shoulder by pulling downward on the other end of the rope (Fig. 18). Pain should be avoided with all of these exercises.

After achieving full flexion, stick exercise should be performed in flexion and external rotation. In a manner similar to that of the pulley exercises, the contralateral extremity is used to assist the affected shoulder into these positions (Fig. 19). Posterior capsule stretching exercises may be initiated at this point. Posterior glenohumeral capsule tightness has been implicated in the exacerbation of rotator cuff symptomatology. To stretch the posterior capsule, the affected extremity is brought into a position of cross-body adduction and internal rotation with the arm abducted 45° from the body (Fig. 20). After the goals for stage I have been met and there are no inflammatory signs, such as pain with rest or warmth of the affected shoulder, the patient may progress to stage II.

Stage II is characterized by progressive strengthening exercises of the rotator cuff. Strengthening of the deltoid and scapular stabilizers is emphasized. Capsular stretching as described above is continued with increasing degrees of abduction as tolerated. Surgical tubing connected to an eyelet or doorknob makes an inexpensive home gym and allows the patient to progress through the exercises with increasing resis-

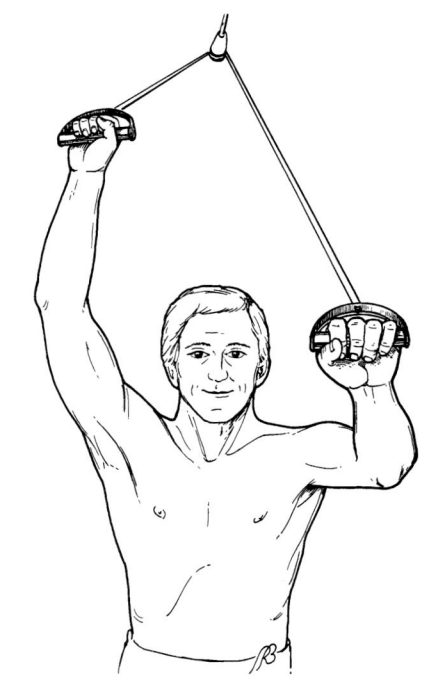

Fig. 18 A patient using a rope and pulley system for stretching of the shoulder capsule. (Copyright © 1997 Kevin D. Plancher, MD, Bronx, NY.)

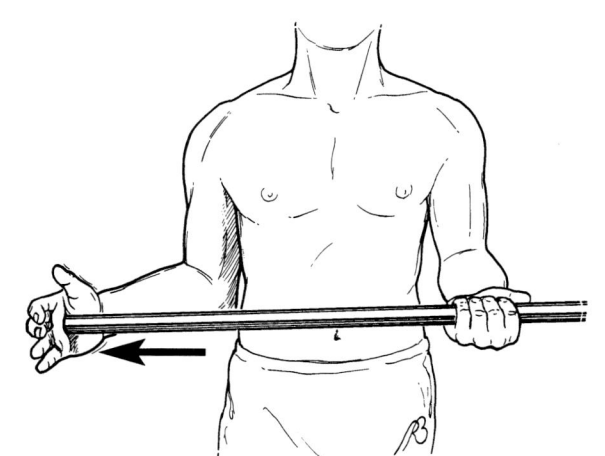

Fig. 19 Stick exercise used to stretch the shoulder in external rotation. (Copyright © 1997 Kevin D. Plancher, MD, Bronx, NY.)

tance as tolerated. There are various companies that make commercially available kits, or a homemade version can be created. The patient should attempt five to ten repetitions each of external rotation, abduction, extension, internal rotation, and flexion. Pain should once again be avoided. Proximal stability of the shoulder girdle is fundamental to the rehabilitation

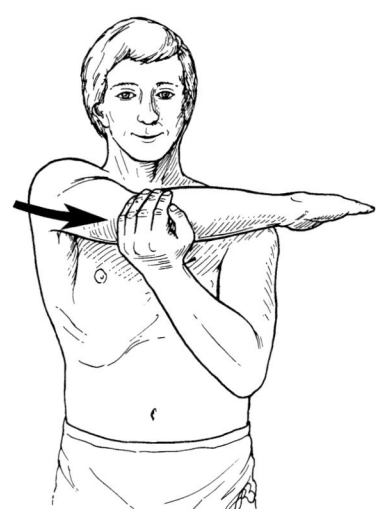

Fig. 20 Posterior capsular stretches in internal rotation and cross-body adduction. (Copyright © 1997 Kevin D. Plancher, MD, Bronx, NY.)

of a rotator cuff tear. Therefore, strengthening of the trapezius, serratus anterior, rhomboids, and levator scapulae is essential for full recovery. Wall push-ups and shoulder shrugs with weights of 15 to 20 lb are employed to isolate these muscles.

When the patient has progressed to the point where symptoms are minimal or absent, range of motion is excellent, and strength is adequate, phase III may be initiated. The goal of phase III is unrestricted symptom-free activity. This goal is accomplished with continued active range of motion and a gradual progression to overhead activities and sports-specific exercises. Early in this phase the sport or activity should be modified to avoid a recurrence of symptoms.

The success of nonsurgical treatment has been reported from less than 50% to greater than 90%. However, most studies to date do not have uniform criteria for nonsurgical management. The large disparity in success rates is in part attributed to the fact that different surgeons have different indications for nonsurgical therapy. Before the advent of MRI, arthrography and clinical examination were largely relied on to establish a diagnosis, and most study groups were heterogenous with results difficult to interpret.

Itoi and Tabata reported the results of 62 shoulders in 54 patients with full-thickness rotator cuff tears treated nonsurgically. Nonsurgical treatment was indicated in middle-aged (30 to 60 years old) and elderly patients (older than 60) who would not require strong muscle power and in those who had mild symptoms. Nonsurgical treatment was also selected for those patients who could not be operated on for medical reasons. The follow-up period averaged 3.4 years. Using a modified version of Wolfgang's criteria, the authors compared subjective findings (function and pain) and objective findings (strength and motion) on both initial and follow-up examinations. Their results showed that 82% of the shoulders had a satisfactory outcome and that scores for pain, motion, and function increased significantly at follow-up examinations. The authors also examined the relationship between length of follow-up and outcome and found that patients followed more than 6 years had significantly lower scores than those patients treated for less than 3 years or from 3 to 6 years. The authors concluded that nonsurgical treatment is effective when applied early during the onset of symptoms and yields satisfactory short-term (1 to 3 years) and midterm (3 to 6 years) results.

In a recent study, Morrison and associates examined the results of 616 patients with isolated subacromial impingement treated nonsurgically with a rotator cuff strengthening program and nonsteroidal anti-inflammatory medication. Sixty-seven percent of these patients had satisfactory results with a mean follow-up of 27 months. Treatment was unsuccessful in 28%, and arthroscopic subacromial decompression was necessary. Conservative treatment failed in an additional 5%, but these patients elected not to have surgery. These authors found that patients older than 60 years of age, those with a type II or III acromion, or those with acromioclavicular joint symptoms fared worse with conservative treatment.

Conclusion

Tears of the rotator cuff are common. A complete history and physical examination will help in the accurate diagnosis of partial and complete rotator cuff injuries. Radiography and its various modalities may be used in clarifying the disease staging process. A complete nonsurgical protocol, including a method to perform a subacromial injection, and rehabilitation protocol are useful. With these techniques, a successful outcome and avoidance of surgical intervention are often possible.

Selected Bibliography

General

Bertolucci LE: Introduction of anti-inflammatory drugs by iontophoresis: Double-blind study. *J Orthop Sports Phys Ther* 1982;4:103-108.

Craig EV: The geyser sign and torn rotator cuff: Clinical significance and pathomechanics. *Clin Orthop* 1984;191: 213-215.

DeLacerda FG: A comparative study of three methods of treatment for shoulder girdle myofascial syndrome. *J Orthop Sports Phys Ther* 1982;4:51-54.

Fisk C: Adaptation of the technique for radiography of the bicipital groove. *Radiol Technol* 1965;37:47-50.

Griffin JE, Echternach JL, Price RE, et al: Patients treated with ultrasonic driven hydrocortisone and with ultrasound alone. *J Phys Ther* 1967;47:594-601.

Hawkins RJ, Misamore GW, Hobeika PE: Surgery for full-thickness rotator-cuff tears. *J Bone Joint Surg* 1985;67A: 1349-1355.

A retrospective review of 100 patients who were surgically treated for a tear of the rotator cuff was performed. One goal of the study was to determine whether the size of the rotator cuff tear could be determined preoperatively by considering the degree of pain, motion, function, and strength. The authors found that the strength of the shoulder in abduction and in external rotation at neutral were the only parameters that had a statistically significant correlation with the size of the tear at operation.

Jobe FW, Jobe CM: Painful athletic injuries of the shoulder. *Clin Orthop* 1983;173:117-124.

Kessel L, Watson M: The painful arc syndrome: Clinical classification as a guide to management. *J Bone Joint Surg* 1977;59B:166-172.

Kleinkort JA, Wood AF: Phonophoresis with 1% versus 10% hydrocortisone. *J Phys Ther* 1975;55:1320-1324.

McElnay JC, Kennedy TA, Harland R: The influence of ultrasound on the percutaneous absorption of fluocinolone acetonide. *Int J Pharm* 1987;40:105-110.

Neviaser RJ: Tears of the rotator cuff. *Orthop Clin North Am* 1980;11:295-306.

Smith W, Winn F, Parette R: Comparative study using four modalities in shin splints treatments. *J Orthop Sports Phys Ther* 1986;8:77-80.

Physical Examination

Boublik M, Hawkins RJ: Clinical examination of the shoulder complex. *J Orthop Sports Phys Ther* 1993;18: 379-385.

This article provides a systematic and thorough approach to the physical examination of the shoulder. Clinical findings important in evaluating the athlete's shoulder and findings related to specific pathologic conditions of the shoulder are emphasized.

Hertel R, Ballmer FT, Lambert SM, et al: Lag signs in the diagnosis of rotator cuff rupture. *J Shoulder Elbow Surg* 1996;5:307-313.

Three newly described clinical signs for the evaluation of the rotator cuff were assessed in 100 patients. The external rotation and internal rotation lag signs independently examine the main components of the rotator cuff. Sensitivity and specificity values were compared to other, more common clinical signs.

Iannotti JP: Full-thickness rotator cuff tears: Factors affecting surgical outcome. *J Am Acad Orthop Surg* 1994;2: 87-95.

The author defines various clinical and radiographic findings that are prognostic of a good outcome in rotator cuff repairs. MRI appears to be useful in evaluating the clinical prognostic factors. Careful clinical examination and preoperative imaging will allow the orthopaedic surgeon to select those patients who are likely to have the best outcomes.

Lyons AR, Tomlinson JE: Clinical diagnosis of tears of the rotator cuff. *J Bone Joint Surg* 1992;74B:414-415.

Clinical examination of the shoulder in 42 patients was carried out to determine the presence and extent of a rotator cuff tear. The preoperative assessment was then compared to findings at operation. The authors found that clinical examination for the presence of a rotator cuff tear had a sensitivity of 91% and specificity of 75%. In 24 of 42 shoulders the type of tear found at operation agreed exactly with that of the preoperative assessment.

Silliman JF, Hawkins RJ: Clinical examination of the shoulder complex, in Andrews JR, Wilk KE (eds): *The Athlete's Shoulder.* New York, NY, Churchill Livingstone, 1994, pp 45-58.

Warner JJP, Allen AA, Gerber C: Diagnosis and management of subscapularis tendon tears. *Tech Orthop* 1994;9:116-125.

Rotator cuff tears that involve the subscapularis tendon are infrequent but not rare. The diagnosis may not always be immediately evident. In order to obtain the correct diagnosis, a careful physical examination is imperative. Even with a correct diagnosis and proper surgical management, these patients have a less favorable prognosis than those patients who undergo a surgical repair of the superior and/or posterior cuff.

Yergason RM: Supination sign. *J Bone Joint Surg* 1931; 13:160.

This case report is the first to describe the findings associated with "wear and tear" of the long head of the biceps tendon.

Imaging of the Rotator Cuff

Ahovuo J: Use of ultrasonography for the diagnosis of shoulder disease, in Vastamaki M, Jalovaara P (eds): *Surgery of the Shoulder.* Amsterdam, The Netherlands, Elsevier Science, 1995, pp 19-23.

The diagnostic performance of ultrasonography in lesions of the shoulder joint, along with the various ultrasound findings seen in the diagnosis of rotator cuff tears, are reviewed. The article concludes that distinctions between tendinitis, cuff degeneration, partial thickness tears, and small full-thickness tears are difficult.

Hollister MS, Mack LA, Patten RP, et al: Association of sonographically detected subacromial/subdeltoid bursal effusion and intraarticular fluid with rotator cuff tear. *Am J Roentgenol* 1995;165:605-608.

A retrospective study of 163 shoulder sonograms in patients who then went on to have surgery found a significant correlation between the presence of fluid in the glenohumeral joint and subacromial-subdeltoid bursa and the existence of a rotator cuff tear. These two findings, when present together, are highly specific for a rotator cuff tear. The specificity was found to be 99% and the positive predictive value was 95%.

Iannotti JP: MR imaging of the shoulder, in Vastamaki M, Jalovaara P (eds): *Surgery of the Shoulder.* Amsterdam, The Netherlands, Elsevier Science, 1995, pp 31-39.

MRI was responsible for major changes in the diagnosis or treatment of common shoulder disorders in approximately 10% of patients from several different studies. MRI was responsible for minor changes in 20% of the cases. The author found the most effective use of MRI to be during the preoperative assessment in the patient with a rotator cuff tear in whom nonsurgical management has failed.

Iannotti JP, Zlatkin MB, Esterhai JL, et al: Magnetic resonance imaging of the shoulder: Sensitivity, specificity, and predictive value. *J Bone Joint Surg* 1991;73A:17-29.

MRI was used to evaluate 91 patients and 15 asymptomatic volunteers. MRI was found to have a sensitivity of 100% and a specificity of 95% in the diagnosis of full-thickness rotator cuff tears. It also consistently predicted the size of the tear. In determining normal tendon from one affected by tendinitis, the sensitivity and specificity were 93% and 87%, respectively.

Jalovaara P, Paivansalo M, Myllyla V: Plain roentgenograms in the diagnosis of shoulder disorders, in Vastamaki M, Jalovaara P (eds): *Surgery of the Shoulder.* Amsterdam, The Netherlands, Elsevier Science, 1995, pp 3-11.

Plain anteroposterior and axillary radiographs are the essential basis for shoulder imaging. Supplementary projections may be implemented to demonstrate specific pathologic conditions about the shoulder complex. These additional views, the nature in which they are obtained, and the information derived from them are emphasized in this article.

Kitay GS, Iannotti JP, Williams GR, et al: Roentgenographic assessment of acromial morphologic condition in rotator cuff impingement syndrome. *J Shoulder Elbow Surg* 1995;4:441-448.

Standard anteroposterior and axillary views as well as supraspinatus outlet and 30° caudal tilt views were obtained preoperatively for patients with isolated impingement. Interobserver reliability and correlation of calculated radiographic measurements with acromial measurements obtained at surgery were highest for the supraspinatus and caudal tilt views.

Mack LA, Nyberg DA, Matsen FR, et al: Sonography of the postoperative shoulder. *Am J Roentgenol* 1988;150:1089-1093.

Sonography was used to assess the rotator cuff in 60 symptomatic shoulders following either acromioplasty alone or in addition to a rotator cuff repair. In patients for whom postoperative follow-up was available, sonography correctly diagnosed a recurrent tear in all 26 shoulders. Likewise, an intact cuff was confirmed in ten of 11 cases.

Norwood LA, Barrack R, Jacobson KE: Clinical presentation of complete tears of the rotator cuff. *J Bone Joint Surg* 1989;71A:499-505.

Data from the histories and physicals of 103 patients with known rotator cuff tears was compared with radiographic and surgical findings to determine if the presence and extent of the tear could be predicted on the basis of history, physical examination, and radiographic findings. When patients with multiple tears were compared to patients with a single tendon tear, it was evident that the multiple tendon group had significantly more findings on their plain radiographs.

Owen RS, Iannotti JP, Kneeland JB, et al: Shoulder after surgery: MR imaging with surgical validation. *Radiology* 1993;186:443-447.

Thirty-one patients with persistent symptoms following shoulder surgery were examined with MRI prior to repeat surgical intervention. In patients examined with MRI, a correct diagnosis was made in six of seven full-thickness rotator cuff tears. However, partial tears were indistinguishable from repaired tendons. The accuracy of diagnosing impingement postoperatively was found to be 74%.

Sonnabend DH, Hughes JS, Giuffre BM, et al: Ultrasound assessment of shoulder pathology, in Vastamaki M, Jalovaara P (eds): *Surgery of the Shoulder.* Amsterdam, The Netherlands, Elsevier Science, 1995, pp 13-17.

In a series of 117 patients who underwent shoulder ultrasound followed by surgical management, ultrasound was found to be very reliable for the detection of full-thickness rotator cuff tears with a positive predictive value of 96%. In the diagnosis of partial thickness tears there were few false-positive studies but a significant number of false-negatives with a negative predictive value of 66%.

Zlatkin MB: Rotator cuff disease, in Zlatkin MB, Iannotti JP, Schnall MD (eds): *MRI of the Shoulder.* New York, NY, Raven Press, 1991, pp 55-97.

Nonsurgical Management

Blair B, Rokito A, Cuomo F, et al: An analysis of the efficacy of corticosteroid injection for subacromial impingement syndrome. Presented at the American Academy of Orthopaedic Surgeons 62nd Annual Meeting, Orlando, FL. Rosemont, IL, American Academy of Orthopaedic Surgeons, 1995, p 354.

A prospective, randomized, controlled, double-blind study was undertaken in 41 patients with impingement. Patients that received 1% lidocaine with 80 mg triamcinolone had significant improvements in pain, range of motion, and relief of impingement sign when compared to patients who received 1% lidocaine alone.

Byl NN: The use of ultrasound as an enhancer for transcutaneous drug delivery: Phonophoresis. *Phys Ther* 1995;75:539-553.

This article reviews the basic principles of phonophoresis, summarizes the anatomy and physiologic principles that are pertinent to phonophoresis, and provides a critical examination of the most recent literature.

Costello CT, Jeski AH: Iontophoresis: Applications in transdermal medication delivery. *Phys Ther* 1995;75:554-563.

This article provides an overview of the literature on iontophoresis and a discussion of the biologic and physical aspects that affect iontophoretic drug transfer. Clinical applications including the use of iontophoresis in the physical therapy of various musculoskeletal disorders are also presented.

Itoi E, Tabata S: Conservative treatment of rotator cuff tears. *Clin Orthop* 1992;275:165-173.

This study examined 62 shoulders in 54 patients with complete rotator cuff tears that were treated nonsurgically over an average period of 3.4 years. According to modified Wolfgang's criteria, the results were satisfactory (excellent or good) in 82% of the patients. Results were less satisfactory in those patients who initially had limited range of motion and decreased strength and in those patients who were followed for more than 6 years.

Seltzer DG, Kechele P, Basamania C, et al: Conservative management of rotator cuff tears, in Burkhead WZ (ed): *Rotator Cuff Disorders.* Baltimore, MD, Williams & Wilkins, 1996, pp 258-267.

16

Surgical Treatment of the Intact Cuff and Repairable Cuff Defect: Arthroscopic and Open Techniques

Joseph P. Iannotti, MD, PhD, R. John Naranja, Jr, MD, and Gary M. Gartsman, MD

Indications

The indications for surgery in patients with chronic impingement syndrome and an intact rotator cuff include pain of sufficient severity to warrant surgical intervention, failure of nonsurgical treatment for at least a 6-month period, and anatomic pathology consistent with supraspinatus outlet narrowing as demonstrated on imaging studies. Patients with an intact rotator cuff may have evidence of intrinsic cuff pathology such as cuff degeneration or a partial thickness tear of the rotator cuff. The indications for surgery in patients with full thickness rotator cuff defects depend on the size of the defect and the mechanism of injury. Early surgical intervention is generally indicated for patients with an acute rotator cuff tear. In patients with chronic cuff tears associated with an insidious onset of clinical symptoms or atraumatic onset of shoulder symptoms, surgery is indicated only after nonsurgical treatment has failed. In the latter clinical situation, chronic cuff defects isolated to the supraspinatus tendon are more responsive to nonsurgical treatment and are more likely to be tolerated by the patient with less functional deficits than by the patient whose cuff tears involve multiple tendons. Other factors that influence the decision and trend toward earlier surgical intervention include younger physiologic age, higher premorbid activity level, and high expectations for future functional activities.

Surgical Techniques for Patients With an Intact Rotator Cuff

Acromioplasty

Decompression of the subacromial space can be performed by either open or arthroscopic techniques, although arthroscopy is generally favored. The goals of surgical technique for either arthroscopic or open acromioplasty are identical. Subacromial decompression should recontour the acromion such that its undersurface is smooth and flat. Acromioplasty does not alter the normal anterior/posterior or medial/lateral dimensions of the acromion. Patients with an acquired bone spur with new bone formation within the coracoacromial ligament generally have extension of bone anterior to the normal extent of the acromion. In these patients, more bone removal is required in order to return the anterior/posterior dimension of the acromion to its original size.

Coracoacromial Ligament Excision

Indications for coracoacromial ligament excision are controversial. Coracoacromial ligament excision without acromioplasty is rarely performed or indicated because of the abnormal shape of the acromion in the majority of patients having subacromial impingement and requiring surgery. However, a recent report by Bigliani has demonstrated satisfactory outcome with isolated excision of the anterolateral band of the coracoacromial ligament in a highly select group of patients with high functional demands of overhead activity with normal acromial morphology.

Acromioclavicular Resection

Open or arthroscopic excision of the distal clavicle is performed and indicated in patients with significant pain localized to the acromioclavicular joint. These patients are identified preoperatively as they exhibit tenderness to palpation to the acromioclavicular joint. This tenderness is often exacerbated by extreme internal rotation or cross-body adduction and is relieved by injection of local anesthetic to the acromioclavicular joint. In the majority of these patients, imaging studies will show significant acromioclavicular degenerative changes. One to 1.5 cm of distal clavicle is excised using either open or arthroscopic techniques. With either technique, the goal of surgery is to completely resect the distal clavicle, leaving a flat and smooth bone surface while preserving the superior and posterior capsular ligaments for stability.

Partial-Thickness Tears

The technique and indications for surgical management of partial-thickness rotator cuff disease remain a controversial issue. Most partial-thickness rotator cuff tears are on the articular surface of the supraspinatus insertion site and are associated with chronic degenerative changes of the tendon. Partial-thickness cuff tears may occur at any age but are often seen in patients older than 50 years, and increase in frequency with advancing age. Most of these partial-thickness cuff defects do not in and of themselves result in significant clinical symptoms of pain or functional limitation. For patients with significant supraspinatus outlet narrowing and partial-thickness rotator cuff tears isolated to the supraspinatus tendon with a defect involving less than 50% of the cuff thickness, subacromial decompression alone with or without arthroscopic debridement of the partial-thickness cuff tear provides good or excellent results in the majority of patients. In younger patients or those with very high functional demands and partial-thickness defects of greater than 50% of the cuff thickness, repair of this defect may be necessary. These patients are generally identified by arthroscopic evaluation of the cuff defect after debridement of the degenerative tissue. These cuff defects may be on either the acromial or articular surface of the rotator cuff. When a deep defect is identified in this particular patient group, the rotator cuff defect is repaired by excision of the remaining tissue, and the full-thickness defect is repaired either by a standard anterior/superior open approach or by a "mini open" lateral deltoid splitting approach. Subacromial decompression may be performed as indicated, based on the morphology of the acromion.

Full-Thickness Tears

The surgical technique for repair of a full-thickness rotator cuff tear requires several steps. The rotator cuff tear margins are identified, and thick bursal tissue that is adherent to and obscures identification of the cuff margins is excised. Traction sutures are placed at the margins of the defect and the rotator cuff tear is mobilized from adherent subacromial scar tissue. Various techniques for mobilization of retracted cuff tendons may be required and are performed as needed in a particular cuff defect. In tendons that have marked retraction, intraarticular release of the glenoid insertion site of the anterior-superior and posterior-superior capsule may be required. If both intracapsular and subacromial release are performed and further cuff mobilization is required in order to bring the cuff tendon edge to the greater tuberosity, then release of the coracohumeral ligament and an incision of the rotator interval capsule may be performed as a rotator interval slide. Following complete cuff mobilization as necessary, the degenerative and mechanically poor tissue at the cuff tendon margins is excised. Most full thickness rotator cuff tears result from avulsion of the cuff tendon from the greater tuberosity, thereby requiring a tendon-to-bone repair. A bone trough is generally recommended for patients with chronic rotator cuff defect. Degenerative tissue from the greater tuberosity is sharply excised and a shallow (2 to 3 mm) bone trough is made over the extent of the greater tuberosity from which the tendon has been torn. Many rotator cuff tears have a component that extends in a lateral to medial direction between the rotator cuff tendons. This portion of the rotator cuff tear is repaired using a tendon-to-tendon suture technique. There have been several suturing techniques described for repair of full thickness rotator cuff tears. A transosseous suture technique is used in the traditional tendon-to-bone repair. Each limb of the suture is passed through an osseous tunnel, and the sutures are tied laterally over a 1-cm cortical bridge of the greater tuberosity. With the recent development of suture anchors, several techniques have been reported for their use in repairing full-thickness cuff defects. Given the osteoporotic nature of the cancellous bone of the greater tuberosity found in the majority of patients having chronic full-thickness cuff defects, these anchors may not provide sufficient fixation. A recent study by Gerber reviewed several mechanical factors that influence suture repair of tendon defects to bone. From this study, it is recommended that a nonabsorbable braided suture of #2 size or greater is placed through the tendon edge using a modified Mason-Allen technique with each limb of the suture passed through a transosseous tunnel. The suture should be placed in the lateral cortical bone at least 1.5 to 2 cm distal to the superior aspect of the tuberosity and each limb of the suture separated by 1 cm of bone. These techniques were demonstrated to provide the optimal fixation of the tendon edge to bone under either single load or cyclic loading conditions.

Coracoacromial Ligament Repair

Coracoacromial ligament resection by either arthroscopic or open techniques in patients with a full-thickness rotator cuff defect is also controversial. The coracoacromial ligament has been shown in biomechanical studies to provide superior restraint and support to the humeral head in shoulders with large, full-thickness rotator cuff defects involving at least two tendons. Preservation and repair of the coracoacromial ligament is even more important in management of the large or massive rotator cuff defect. Clinically, in patients with functional deficits and large rotator cuff defects, the coracoacromial arch helps to prevent anterior/superior subluxation of the humeral head. If acromioplasty is performed in these patients, repair of the coracoacromial ligament to the anterior border of the acromion has been recommended to reestablish an intact coracoacromial arch. The coracoacromial ligament should be incised at the anterior border of the acromion and preserved as a contiguous structure with the deep fascia of the deltoid. The anterior/posterior dimension of the acromion should not be shortened from a normal dimension. Preservation of the coracoacromial ligament is not necessary in patients with an intact rotator cuff or small full-thickness rotator cuff tears that have maintained biomechanical function to maintain the humeral head within the glenoid fossa.

Results and Outcome: Intact Rotator Cuff With Subacromial Decompression

In 1972, Neer first described open anterior acromioplasty. Since that time several series have reviewed the outcome of this procedure with an intact rotator cuff. These series report an average 81% satisfactory result with open acromioplasty; workers' compensation claims generally produce less favorable results. Complications were infrequent and all authors recommended at least 6 to 9 months of nonsurgical treatment as one of the indications for surgical intervention. Arthroscopic subacromial decompression has also been extensively reviewed. On average, these series report 76% of patients having satisfactory results. These series again demonstrate a less favorable outcome with workers' compensation claims and again stress the importance of failure of nonsurgical treatment among the indications for surgical intervention. These reports demonstrate that an equal amount of bone may be removed arthroscopically and in the open procedure. Excellent results may be achieved, comparable to those of open surgical technique.

Recent series comparing arthroscopic and open techniques have demonstrated similar results among variables compared. In these series there was a trend toward better results in the open decompression group but these differences did not reach statistical significance. The arthroscopic acromioplasty group achieved maximal medical improvement in functional outcome in a shorter period of time after surgery.

Results of Open Cuff Repair: Clinical and Anatomic Factors Affecting Outcome

Several series have reported the results of surgical intervention for repair of full-thickness rotator cuff tears. These series describe clinical results that on average support satisfactory (good and excellent) results in 85% to 90% of patients. Clinical factors that affect outcome include adequacy of the acromioplasty, size of the rotator cuff tear, patient age, premorbid activity level, quality of deltoid function, and factors associated with cuff tear size, such as quality of the tissue, degree of cuff retraction, and presence of bicipital tendon rupture. Clinical results are measured by patient satisfaction, subjective pain level, functional activities, and shoulder strength. Clinical results remain stable over long-term follow-up. Analysis of results 7 to 15 years postoperatively has shown that patients who underwent primary repair maintained satisfactory results. There was no significant deterioration of function or recurrence of pain. Patient satisfaction was best correlated with improvement of shoulder pain.

Hawkins' review of 100 patients 4 years postoperatively added to the understanding of the results after rotator cuff repair. After tendon repair and anterior acromioplasty, 86 of the 100 patients had little or no pain. The patients' range of motion improved from 81° preoperatively to 125° postoperatively. Ninety-four patients considered themselves better after surgery. Hawkins concluded that the improvement in the patients' function was related to postoperative relief of pain.

Ellman reviewed the results of 50 of his patients 3.5 years postoperatively. Twenty of 48 patients who had an anterior acromioplasty also had a distal clavicle excision. Acccording to Neer's criteria, 42 (82%) obtained satisfactory results when considering pain, function, and forward flexion strength. Forty-nine patients (98%) were satisfied with postoperative results.

Cofield reviewed the results in 81 of his patients 7.5 years after surgery. Seventy-six patients believed that they were better after surgery. In Cofield's review of the different series of rotator repairs, he reported an overall pain relief in 87% of the patients and patient satisfaction in 77% of the patients. Harryman studied the results of 105 rotator cuff repairs at 5 years postoperatively. He correlated the functional results with the integrity of the cuff as determined by ultrasonography. Most patients were more comfortable and were satisfied with their shoulder postoperatively even if there was a recurrent cuff defect. He did find that the patients with an intact cuff at follow-up had better function and range of motion when compared with patients who had a recurrent defect. Strength measurements also showed that patients with intact cuffs had greater strength in flexion, abduction, and internal rotation. In patients with a recurrent defect, the degree of functional loss was correlated with the size of the tear as measured by ultrasonography. His primary conclusion was that the integrity of the cuff at follow-up best correlated with the outcome of the surgical repair of the cuff.

Selected Bibliography

Adamson GJ, Tibone JE: Ten-year assessment of primary rotator cuff repairs. *J Shoulder Elbow Surg* 1993;2:57-63.

Altchek DW, Warren RF, Wickiewicz TL, et al: Arthroscopic acromioplasty: Technique and results. *J Bone Joint Surg* 1990;72A:1198-1207.

Bayne O, Bateman JE: Long term results of surgical repair of full thickness rotator cuff tears, in Bateman JE, Welsh RP (eds): *Surgery of the Shoulder.* Philadelphia, PA, BC Decker, 1984, pp 167-171.

Bigliani L, Cordasco F, McIlveen S, et al: Operative repair of massive rotator cuff tears: Long term results. *J Shoulder Elbow Surg* 1992;1:120-130.

Bigliani LU, D'Alessandro DF, Duralde XA, et al: Anterior acromioplasty for subacromial impingement in patients younger than 40 years of age. *Clin Orthop* 1989;246:111-116.

Björkenheim JM, Paavolainen P, Ahovuo J, et al: Subacromial impingement decompressed with anterior acromioplasty. *Clin Orthop* 1990;252:150-155.

Björkenheim JM, Paavolainen P, Ahovuo J, et al: Surgical repair of the rotator cuff and surrounding tissues: Factors influencing the results. *Clin Orthop* 1988;236:148-153.

Brems JJ: Digital muscle strength measurement in rotator cuff tears. *Orthop Trans* 1987;11:235.

Cofield RH, Hoffmeyer P, Lanzer WL: Surgical repair of chronic rotator cuff tears. *Orthop Trans* 1990;14:251-252.

Ellman H: Arthroscopic subacromial decompression: Analysis of one- to three-year results. *Arthroscopy* 1987;3:173-181.

Ellman H: Diagnosis and treatment of incomplete rotator cuff tears. *Clin Orthop* 1990;254:64-74.

Ellman H, Hanker G, Bayer M: Repair of the rotator cuff: End-result study of factors influencing reconstruction. *J Bone Joint Surg* 1986;68A:1136-1144.

Ellman H, Kay SP: Arthroscopic subacromial decompression for chronic impingement: Two- to five-year results. *J Bone Joint Surg* 1991;73B:395-398.

Esch JC, Ozerkis LR, Helgager JA, et al: Arthroscopic subacromial decompression: Results according to the degree of rotator cuff tear. *Arthroscopy* 1988;4:241-249.

Frieman BG, Fenlin JM Jr: Anterior acromioplasty: Effect of litigation and workers' compensation. *J Shoulder Elbow Surg* 1995;4:175-181.

Open anterior acromioplasty was performed on 75 shoulders; 97% of patients obtained a good or excellent result according to the American Shoulder and Elbow Surgeons scale. In the workers' compensation group, 97% had either excellent or good results. In the pending litigation group, 96% had excellent or good results. These results indicate no apparent or potential financial gain associated with their impingement syndrome.

Gartsman GM: Arthroscopic acromioplasty for lesions of the rotator cuff. *J Bone Joint Surg* 1990;72A:169-180.

Gartsman GM, Blair ME Jr, Noble PC, et al: Arthroscopic subacromial decompression: An anatomical study. *Am J Sports Med* 1988;16:48-50.

Gazielly DF, Gleyze P, Montagnon C: Functional and anatomical results after rotator cuff repair. *Clin Orthop* 1994;304:43-53.

The anatomic condition of the rotator cuff (measured by ultrasonography) was compared with the functional result (using Constant's functional score) at 4-year follow-up in 100 full-thickness cuff tears treated by repair. The authors found that functional score at follow-up was closely related to anatomic integrity.

Gerber C, Schneeberger AG, Beck M, et al: Mechanical strength of repairs of the rotator cuff. *J Bone Joint Surg* 1994;76B:371-380.

The authors evaluated the mechanical properties of several current techniques of tendon-to-bone suture employed in rotator cuff repair. Nonabsorbable braided polyester and absorbable polyglactin and polyglycolic acid sutures best combined ultimate tensile strength and stiffness. A modified Mason-Allen suture technique was superior with regard to tendon grasping. In cases of osteoporotic bone, the use of a 2-mm thick, plate-like augmentation device will improve failure strength over transosseous sutures.

Gore DR, Murray MP, Sepic SB, et al: Shoulder-muscle strength and range of motion following surgical repair of full thickness rotator-cuff tears. *J Bone Joint Surg* 1986;68A:266-272.

Harryman DT II, Mack LA, Wang KY, et al: Repairs of the rotator cuff: Correlation of functional results with integrity of the cuff. *J Bone Joint Surg* 1991;73A:982-989.

Hawkins RJ, Brock RM, Abrams JS, et al: Acromioplasty for impingement with an intact rotator cuff. *J Bone Joint Surg* 1988;70B:795-797.

Hawkins RJ, Misamore GW, Hobeika PE: Surgery for full-thickness rotator-cuff tears. *J Bone Joint Surg* 1985;67A:1349-1355.

Hawkins R, Saddemi S, Moor J, et al: Arthroscopic subacromial decompression: A 2-year follow-up study. *Arthroscopy* 1992;8:209.

The results of the first 110 consecutive arthroscopic acromioplasties were reviewed at a minimum 2-year follow-up. Only 46% achieved a satisfactory rating, with workers' compensation patients reaching only 32% satisfaction. The authors could not identify any factors that led to the poor result and recommended open decompression for more predictably satisfactory results.

Iannotti JP: Full-thickness rotator cuff tears: Factors affecting surgical outcome. *J Amer Acad Orthop Surg* 1994;2:87-95.

Iannotti J, Bernot M, Kuhlman J, et al: Postoperative assessment of shoulder function: A prospective study of full-thickness rotator cuff tears. *J Shoulder Elbow Surg* 1996;5:449-457.

Forty consecutive patients were prospectively evaluated 2 years after surgery. Results were significantly affected by size of tear, quality of tissue, difficulty of repair, and presence of biceps tendon rupture. Postoperative strength and fatigue were also highly correlated with cuff tear size.

Lazarus MD, Chansky HA, Misra S, et al: Comparison of open and arthroscopic subacromial decompression. *J Shoulder Elbow Surg* 1994;3:1-11.

A comparison of open and arthroscopic acromioplasty performed by one surgeon for chronic impingement syndrome was retrospectively reviewed in 68 patients. There was no statistical difference in mean postoperative shoulder scores between surgical groups at a minimum 12-month follow-up. Arthroscopic acromioplasty, however, was associated with shorter hospital stays and faster achievement of maximal pain relief as compared to open acromioplasty. Also noted was the finding of subacromial calcifications on postoperative radiographs, which is associated with a less favorable result.

Lazarus MD, Yung SW, Sidles JA, et al: Anterosuperior humeral displacement: Limitation by the coracoacromial arch. *American Shoulder and Elbow Surgeons Eleventh Open Meeting.* Rosemont, IL, American Shoulder and Elbow Surgeons, 1995, p 28.

Six cadaver shoulders were analyzed after coracoacromial ligament resection and after anterior acromioplasty followed by humeral head loading. The authors found that the coracoacromial arch provides an important barrier to anterosuperior humeral head displacement. Loss of this barrier may have substantial effects if the normal head centering capacity of the rotator cuff is deficient.

Moorman CT III, Deng XH, Warren RF, et al: The coracoacromial ligament: Is it the appendix of the shoulder? *American Shoulder and Elbow Surgeons Eleventh Open Meeting.* Rosemont, IL, American Shoulder and Elbow Surgeons, 1995, p 33.

Biomechanical testing was performed on 25 cadavers after sequential interventions of capsular venting, release of the rotator interval capsule and coracoacromial ligament (CAL) connection, release of the CAL at the acromion, and after acromioplasty. Superior translation of the humeral head was increased after CAL section and further after acromioplasty. The authors suggested avoidance of CAL release and acromioplasty in two particular clinical situations: cuff deficiency, and patients with high functional demands who poorly tolerate changes in coupled motions (eg, throwing athletes).

Neer CS II: Anterior acromioplasty for the chronic impingement syndrome in the shoulder: A preliminary report. *J Bone Joint Surg* 1972;54A:41-50.

Neer CS II, Flatow EL, Lech O: Tears of the rotator cuff: Long term results of anterior acromioplasty and repair. *Orthop Trans* 1988;12:673-674.

Paulos LE, Franklin JL: Arthroscopic shoulder decompression development and application: A five year experience. *Am J Sports Med* 1990;18:235-244.

Post M, Cohen J: Impingement syndrome: A review of late stage II and early stage III lesions. *Clin Orthop* 1986;207:126-132.

Rockwood CA, Lyons FR: Shoulder impingement syndrome: Diagnosis, radiographic evaluation, and treatment with a modified Neer acromioplasty. *J Bone Joint Surg* 1993;75A:409-424.

The authors describe a modification of the Neer acromioplasty in 71 patients with impingement syndrome. In this "two-step" technique, the portion of the acromion projecting anterior to the anterior border of the clavicle is resected vertically, and then a standard Neer anteroinferior acromioplasty is performed.

Roye RP, Grana WA, Yakes CK: Arthroscopic subacromial decompression: Two- to seven-year follow-up. *Arthroscopy* 1995;11:301-306.

The authors evaluated arthroscopic subacromial decompression in stage II or early stage III impingement syndrome in 90 shoulders. They concluded that arthroscopic subacromial decompression was an acceptable alternative to open acromioplasty with comparable results. There was, however, a significantly less favorable outcome when comparing throwing athletes to nonthrowing athletes.

Thorling J, Bjerneld H, Hallin G, et al: Acromioplasty for impingement syndrome. *Acta Orthop Scand* 1985;56: 147-148.

Tibone JE, Elrod B, Jobe FW, et al: Surgical treatment of tears of the rotator cuff in athletes. *J Bone Joint Surg* 1986;68A:887-891.

Tibone JE, Jobe FW, Kerlan RK, et al: Shoulder impingement syndrome in athletes treated by an anterior acromioplasty. *Clin Orthop* 1985;198:134-140.

Van Holsbeeck E, DeRycke J, Declercq G, et al: Subacromial impingement: Open versus arthroscopic decompression. *Arthroscopy* 1992;8:173-178.

The authors compared the results of 53 patients treated by arthroscopic subacromial decompression with 53 patients treated by open decompression. The results were similar at last follow-up. They recommended arthroscopic decompression for chronic impingement syndrome and reserved open decompression for those cases requiring rotator cuff repair and those with prior failed arthroscopic decompression.

# 17

Complications of Rotator Cuff Surgery

R. John Naranja, Jr, MD, Joseph P. Iannotti, MD, PhD, and Gary M. Gartsman, MD

Introduction

Although the literature has consistently demonstrated the possibility of good results from surgical treatment when conservative measures fail, a more careful analysis demonstrates the pitfalls of poor patient selection, errors in technique, and complications unforeseeable by any measure of preoperative planning. Complications may be divided into those secondary to misdiagnosis, decompression, repair, postoperative rehabilitation, or wound healing difficulties.

Complications Related to Misdiagnosis

The diagnosis of impingement and/or symptomatic rotator cuff tear requires a complete history, physical examination, and appropriate confirmatory tests such as radiographic, electromyographic, and laboratory studies. A diagnosis of impingement is classically confirmed by pain at the anterior aspect of the shoulder that is aggravated by forced forward elevation of the humerus against the acromion (positive impingement sign), and relief of pain after injection of 10 cc of 1% lidocaine in the subacromial space (positive impingement test). Other diagnoses that must be excluded may be classified as those related to referred pain (cervical radiculitis, thoracic outlet syndrome, suprascapular nerve entrapment), intra-articular pathology (glenohumeral instability, labral tears, glenohumeral osteoarthritis, adhesive capsulitis), extra-articular pathology (acromioclavicular joint arthritis, unrecognized or untreated rotator cuff tear), and secondary gain issues (workers' compensation).

Referred pain related to cervical disk disease is a common source of misdiagnosis. Cervical pathology may occur concomitantly with impingement or present alone as a cause of chronic shoulder pain. Patients' response to treatment will depend on the proportion of findings related to cervical pathology versus that attributed to impingement at the coracoacromial arch. Prognosis is more difficult to interpret for those who undergo surgery for impingement in the context of coexisting cervical disk disease.

The suprascapular nerve courses through the confining anatomy of the suprascapular notch and around the spine of the scapula in the spinoglenoid notch. This path makes it susceptible to compression and resulting symptoms that may mimic the findings associated with a rotator cuff tear. The diagnosis must be considered in the young patient with no history of trauma and loss of power associated with vague pain at the posterior aspect of the shoulder. Confirmation with electromyographic examination is essential. Treatment is directed toward the etiology of nerve compression.

Thoracic outlet syndrome as a cause of referred pain to the shoulder is related to compression of the nerves and vessels to the upper limb as they exit the interval between the scalene muscles, travel over the first rib, and course down into the axilla. The history typically includes pain and paresthesias that extend from the neck and shoulder to the medial aspect of the forearm and hand, ending in the small and ring fingers. Exacerbation of symptoms with overhead activity clouds the distinction between impingement and thoracic outlet syndrome. Perhaps the most important physical sign is the ability to reproduce the patient's symptoms by abducting and laterally rotating the arm at the shoulder while palpating the wrist pulses. Loss of pulse is helpful, but not pathognomonic. Rather, reproduction of symptoms confirms the diagnosis.

The most common cause of misdiagnosis as a result of intra-articular pathology comes from glenohumeral instability. Instability tends to occur in young athletic individuals with some element of joint laxity who later develop secondary rotator cuff symptoms. The distinction may be difficult to identify and many series report cases of instability initially diagnosed and treated as impingement syndrome. Clues to the diagnosis include signs of apprehension with provocative positioning and the presence of joint laxity. To optimize outcome, treatment should be directed toward the underlying instability rather than the impingement. Even then, returning this patient population to preinjury competitive levels represents a significant challenge.

Glenohumeral arthritis and labral tears, conditions often encountered during the diagnostic arthroscopy portion of the surgical treatment of impingement syndrome, are also sources of misdiagnosis. Coexisting pathology related to the rotator cuff impingement also hampers its diagnosis. Adhesive capsulitis or primary frozen shoulder may manifest as shoulder pain, but with an additional component of restricted range of motion. Absolute numbers regarding the limitation of motion are variable, but most agree that there is a significant restriction of glenohumeral motion with both active and passive attempts at range of motion. In contrast, impingement syndrome has a relative full range of motion with pain localized anteriorly during the midrange of forward flexion.

Extra-articular pathology as a source of misdiagnosis often includes unrecognized acromioclavicular joint arthritis. This is a very common cause for recurrent impingement and reoperation in patients in whom initial decompression surgery has failed. The dilemma stems from the poor correlation between radiographic findings of acromioclavicular joint degeneration and clinical symptoms. Direct palpation, provocative testing (cross body adduction), and lidocaine injection tests into the acromioclavicular joint help confirm the diagnosis. Distal clavicle resection has been demonstrated to have a positive influence on outcome after unsuccessful initial decompression.

Many investigators have reported successful but less favorable results with debridement of a full-thickness cuff tear combined with decompression. But decompression alone in the context of repairable full-thickness cuff tear can be a source of continued shoulder pain, requiring reoperation for repair of the cuff. As more surgeons use arthroscopy for decompression with visualization of both the articular and bursal sides of the cuff, the incidence of this misdiagnosis will hopefully decrease.

Finally, there are those patients who have undergone surgical management for impingement syndrome whose results may be clouded by factors related to secondary gain or personality. Several reports have documented the less reliable results in those patients who had workers' compensation issues still pending. Others have cited psychiatric disorders in the differential for an unsatisfactory outcome.

Complications Related to Decompression

Deltoid Detachment

Decompression of the subacromial space has been advocated for rotator cuff disorders since Watson-Jones first described complete acromionectomy in the treatment of supraspinatus tendon lesions in 1939. Increasing the space available for the rotator cuff to pass beneath the coracoacromial arch was emphasized. Unfortunately, the early treatment of impingement was based on the idea that shoulder abduction was the primary cause of symptoms. As a result, acromionectomy and lateral acromionectomy were advocated to increase pain-free abduction. Favorable results were possible, but the potential for complications was realized once the anatomy of impingement syndrome was better articulated and forward flexion as the primary plane for functional shoulder motion was recognized. In addition, the complete removal or lateral resection of the acromion was correlated with an increased risk for postoperative detachment of the deltoid origin. In 1981, Neer and Marberry reported on 30 consecutive patients who previously had a radical acromionectomy. All had poor results including persistent pain, marked weakness of the shoulder, and the inability to raise the arm above the horizontal. They concluded that radical acromionectomy weakened the deltoid both by removing its lever arm and by encouraging retraction of the deltoid origin. The implications of disrupting the deltoid attachment may be appreciated by understanding that the deltoid muscle, in concert with the rotator cuff, is responsible for generating synchronized and powerful glenohumeral motion. Loss of deltoid muscle integrity results in significant disability. This disability can outweigh the presence of an isolated rotator cuff tear.

Thus, the risk factors shown to correlate highly with deltoid detachment are complete or lateral acromionectomy, infection/hematoma, postoperative trauma, and/or early aggressive resistive postoperative rehabilitation. Detachment typically occurs in the first 6 weeks postoperatively. In general, any situation that involves detaching a portion of the deltoid for exposure increases the risk for subsequent detachment. This complication has not been reported with arthroscopic techniques of decompression, but could occur if meticulous technique is not followed.

The diagnosis of deltoid detachment is made clinically by observing a defect at the deltoid origin and a bulge in the del-

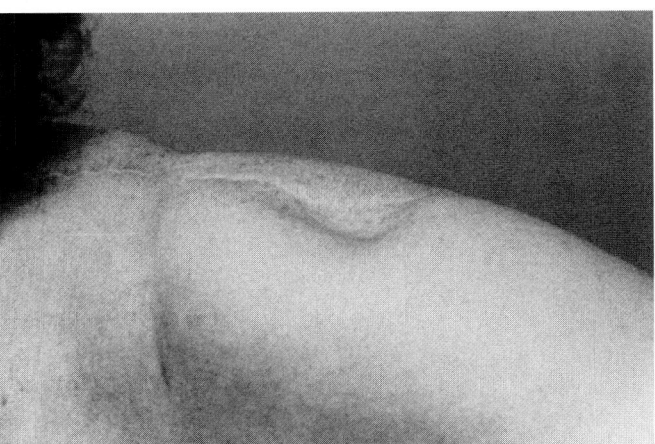

Fig. 1 Clinical appearance of a postoperative deltoid detachment.

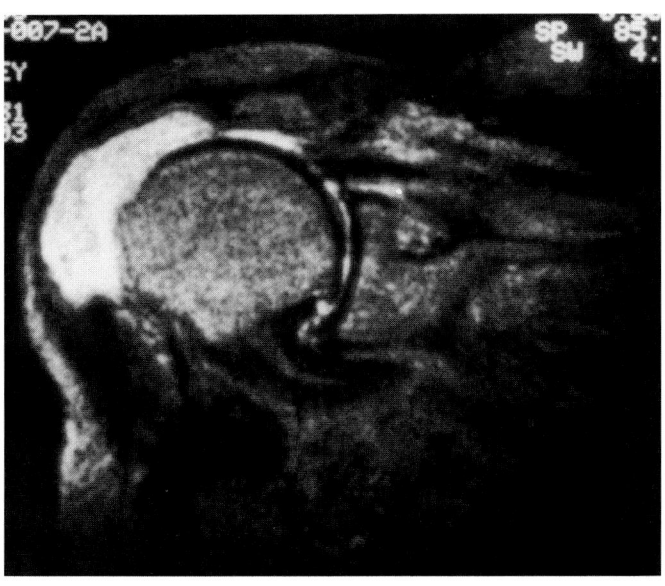

Fig. 2 T2-weighted coronal magnetic resonance imaging scan demonstrating separation of the deltoid from its origin with interposed fluid (high signal).

toid muscle distal to its normal origin (Fig. 1). Less reliable signs include decreased abduction strength, often disabling enough to prevent raising the arm above the horizontal, and/or decreased motion secondary to adherence of the retracted portion of the deltoid to the underlying rotator cuff and humerus. Magnetic resonance imaging may confirm the diagnosis (Fig. 2). Conservative treatment of this complication typically demonstrates poor function. In 1994, Groh reviewed the functional results of 33 patients after deltoid detachment. Twenty-two rated their function as poor, as determined by activities of daily living, and all reported disability. Other treatment options include attempts at deltoid reattachment, rotational deltoidplasty, or salvage with glenohumeral arthrodesis. In 1996, Sher and associates evaluated 24 patients who underwent direct repair or rotational deltoidplasty reconstruction of a detached muscle origin in the setting of prior surgery. At a mean follow-up of 39 months, 67% unsatisfactory results were reported. Poor outcome with deltoid reconstruction was associated with a prior lateral acromionectomy, involvement of the middle deltoid, a concomitant massive rotator cuff tear, and duration of symptoms for longer than 12 months. In both studies, the importance of prevention of this disabling complication is stressed because current nonsurgical and surgical measures to treat deltoid detachment have yielded poor results.

Inadequate Decompression

Neer has been credited with pointing out that the anatomy for impingement includes the anterior edge and undersurface of the anterior third of the acromion, the coracoacromial ligament, and in some cases, the acromioclavicular joint. Inadequate decompression is one of the more common reasons for failure after initial surgical intervention for impingement. It is not surprising to find that in those cases where partial lateral acromionectomy procedures were performed, a high rate of continued impingement occurred because a portion of the impinging anatomy is still left behind. Others have reported attempts to simply divide the coracoacromial ligament. This, too, has resulted in continued pain if a bony spur is present. The role of coracoacromial ligament resection as an isolated procedure in young patients without bone spurs is unclear.

Other cases of inadequate decompression have been related to poor judgment regarding the amount of bone resected with respect to the anterior acromioplasty. In an experimental computer simulation of anterior acromioplasty, the elimination of impingement was specific to an acromioplasty represented by flattening of the acromion from a location extending from the anterior third to the midline. Acromioplasty with flattening of the anterior ridge alone resulted in residual impingement, and a flattening of the entire acromion was excessive.

In summary, decompression of the subacromial space requires a thorough understanding of those anatomic structures that cause impingement combined with an ability to judge the adequacy of the decompression. Preoperative evaluation includes a clinical examination to determine if acromioclavicular symptoms contribute to the impingement syndrome, as well as appropriate radiographic projections. A recent study showed that appropriate radiographic projections for the assessment of acromial morphology have good interobserver reliability and correlation with intraoperative measurements of acromial spur size. Specifically, the supraspinatus outlet and 30° caudal tilt have been shown to accurately evaluate acromial morphology, whereas the axillary view has been less helpful in this regard. Thus, an anteroposterior radiograph in the plane of the scapula, supraspinatus outlet view, 30° caudal tilt, is useful in determining the amount of resection required for an adequate decompression. If confirmed by clinical examination, a 20° cephalic tilt is useful to evaluate the acromioclavicular joint. The results of repeat decompression after failed initial acromioplasty have been relatively good if an inadequate decompression can be confirmed. The results are less favorable in the setting of workers' compensation.

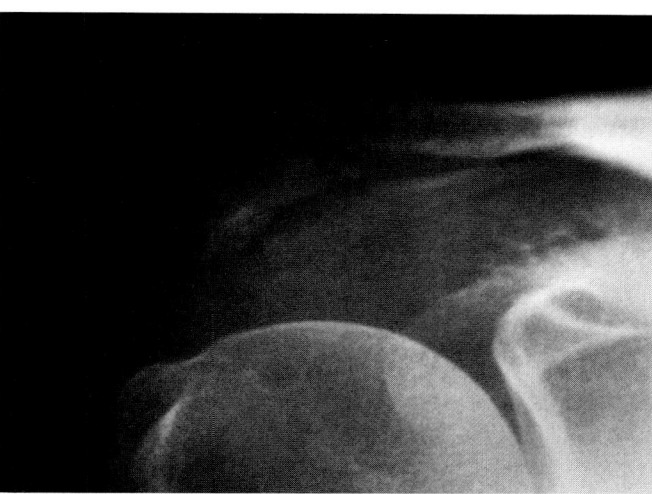

Fig. 3 Oblique plain radiographic view of the acromion demonstrating the complication of acromial fracture.

Acromial Fracture

Acromial fracture, an infrequent complication related to subacromial decompression, has been associated with overaggressive decompression of the acromion, as well as overenthusiastic retraction of the acromion during exposure of the rotator cuff (Fig. 3). In one series of 74 rotator cuff repairs, one patient suffered an acromial fracture that required fixation with a screw. Nine months later, deltoid avulsion was noted and the fragment of acromion and the screw were removed and an attempt was made to resuture the deltoid to the remaining acromion. The long-term outcome was poor.

In another series, an evolving surgical acromioplasty technique was used on 29 consecutive patients for the first group, the surgical technique requiring a partial deltoid origin detachment and anterior acromioplasty with an osteotome. The second technique spared the deltoid detachment but again used an osteotome to perform the acromioplasty. The third technique also spared the deltoid origin, but alternatively used a high-speed bur to perform the acromioplasty. All complications occurred in surgical techniques used in the earliest group. One of these patients suffered an acromion fracture.

The difficulty in healing an acromial fracture may be demonstrated by a case in which union was not achieved after three surgical attempts. The first attempt used a Steinmann pin for fixation, followed by pin fixation and autogenous bone graft. Finally, a plate and screws with iliac crest bone graft was attempted. All failed and the patient complained of persistent pain and severe limitation in motion.

Arthroscopic subacromial decompression has also resulted in acromial fracture. Six patients with this entity reportedly exhibited a poor response to treatment. Risk factors include osteoporotic bone and overzealous bone resection.

Clearly, the potential for healing complications with an acromial fracture and apparent failure to consistently respond to attempts at fixation demand careful attention to surgical technique to avoid this infrequent but significant complication.

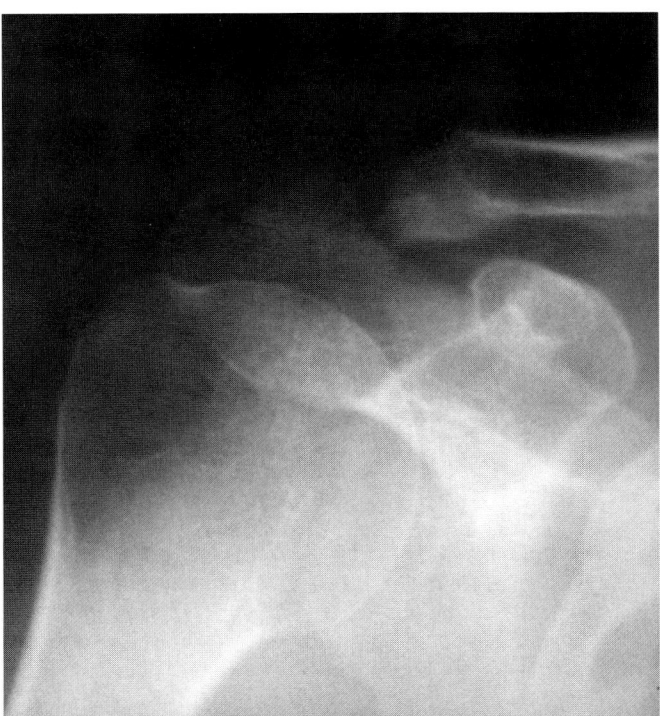

Fig. 4 Anteroposterior radiograph demonstrating heterotopic ossification at the site of a previous distal clavicle resection.

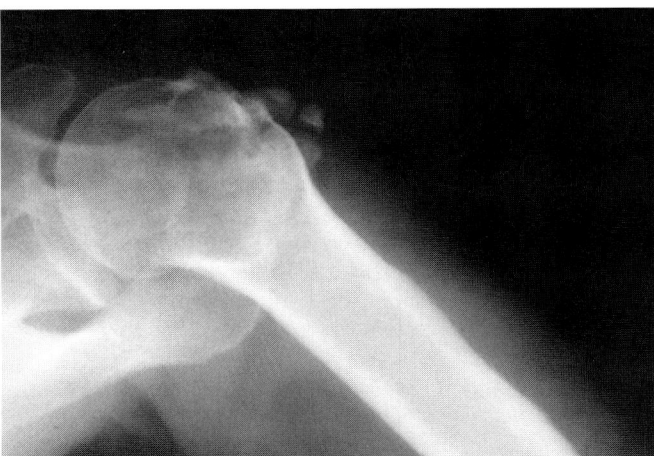

Fig. 5 Axillary view of heterotopic ossification in the region of the lateral acromion.

Heterotopic Ossification

Heterotopic ossification as a complication of rotator cuff surgery was reported as early as 1949. Its occurrence at the site of previous acromionectomy caused recurrent impingement symptoms that required reexcision. Subsequent reports of heterotopic ossification have been variable with regard to the development of recurrent symptoms. The incidence of these symptoms has been thought to relate to bone dust remaining after arthroscopic acromioplasty (Figs. 4 and 5). However, an association with underlying medical disorders has been reported. In one large series of patients, the incidence of heterotopic ossification occurring after distal clavicle excision or subacromial decompression was 3.2%. This complication was disproportionately seen in patients with a history of chronic pulmonary diseases. No correlation between the method of bone resection and incidence of heterotopic ossification was found. Half of the patients, however, required repeat surgery to remove the ossification. The results of surgery after the formation of heterotopic ossification are related to the size, site, and presence of risk factors. Risk factors include a profile of hypertrophic pulmonary osteoarthropathy, active spondylitic arthropathy, and patients with a history of chronic pulmonary disease. It should be understood that bone present on postoperative radiographs may indicate inadequate initial bone resection rather than heterotopic ossification. This matter can be clarified by obtaining radiographs within the first 4 weeks after surgery.

Superior Glenohumeral Instability

The rotator cuff's role in preventing superior migration of the proximal humerus with shoulder abduction and forward flexion is diminished with large full-thickness tears. Later secondary restraint may come from the coracoacromial arch as demonstrated by recent biomechanical studies. In one study, 25 cadavers were evaluated with biomechanical testing after sequential interventions of capsular venting, release of the rotator interval capsule and coracoacromial ligament (CAL) at the coracoid, release of the CAL at the acromion, and after acromioplasty. Superior translation of the humeral head was increased after CAL section and further after acromioplasty. The authors suggested avoidance of CAL release and acromioplasty in two particular clinical situations—cuff deficiency, and in patients with high functional demands who poorly tolerate changes in coupled motions (eg, throwing athletes). As a result, careful consideration must be given to reattaching the coracoacromial ligament in these patients. Further removal of the coracoacromial arch complex is deleterious (Fig. 6). Several reports of superior dislocation/subluxation after acromionectomy with an associated large rotator cuff tear have been described.

Clavicular Instability

In 1988, the results of the Mumford procedure in 23 athletes with a history of grade I or grade II dislocation were analyzed. Ten athletes in the series demonstrated increased horizontal clavicular motion.

In a subsequent evaluation of the results of arthroscopic subacromial decompression where arthroscopic distal clavicle resection was also accomplished, several patients reported instability of the acromioclavicular joint after vigorous weightlifting within the first postoperative week. The symptoms subsided with several weeks of rest.

More recently, in 1993, the complication of a "dropped shoulder" with the clavicle protruding into the trapezius secondary to distal clavicle resection has been reported. Damage

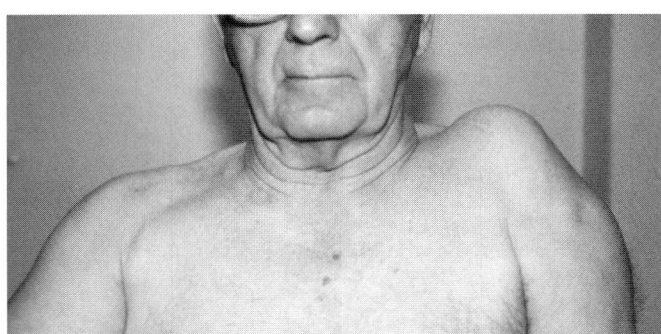

Fig. 6 Clinical example of superior glenohumeral escape following acromioplasty and coracoacromial ligament resection in a patient with a massive rotator cuff tear.

to the superior acromioclavicular capsular ligament was identified as the inciting cause of this instability. It was recommended that only 1 to 1.5 cm of the distal clavicle be resected with a bur in an attempt to preserve the superior acromioclavicular capsular ligament.

Blazar and associates in 1996 reviewed 17 patients who had a distal clavicle resection and correlated anteroposterior instability based on stress radiographs with postoperative pain and functional outcome. They found that increased translation of the distal clavicle after distal clavicle resection was associated with increased postoperative shoulder pain and poor surgical outcome.

Complications Related to Cuff Repair

Recurrent Tear

Tears of the rotator cuff have been classified according to their size: small, less than 1 cm; medium, 1 to 3 cm; large, 3 to 5 cm; and massive, greater than 5 cm. Numerous techniques have been described for rotator cuff repair, particularly for large and massive tears. No technique, however, has been immune from a recurrent tear. Reasons for recurrence have been attributed to quality of the cuff and size of tear at the time of repair, inadequate intraoperative mobilization and exposure of the cuff, failure to remove extrinsic impingement processes, poor fixation techniques, posttraumatic falls or inadequate postoperative protection, and spontaneous rupture.

Recurrent tear from inadequate tendon mobilization and poor exposure of the torn edges of the rotator cuff has been well documented. For example, in 1990, one author reported that at reoperation for failed rotator cuff surgery, thickened hypertrophied bursal tissue was found sutured and closed over a rotator cuff defect. Bursal tissue must be resected if sufficient exposure cannot be obtained to adequately mobilize the underlying cuff. In another series, 25 of 32 patients who underwent postoperative arthrography had a recurrent or persistent tear. Reasons identified included inadequate exposure and/or mobilization of the cuff as determined by review of the surgical notes. Suture type, configuration, and bone quality with regard to strength of repair are also factors.

Decompression of the subacromial space has been recommended as a concomitant procedure with rotator cuff repair. In addition to pain relief, decompression also minimizes the chance for a recurrent tear. In 1984, 27 patients were evaluated after initial failed rotator cuff repair. Inadequate decompression of the coracoacromial arch was a major factor for recurrent tear.

The use of synthetic materials such as carbon, Gore-tex, or Dacron has been attempted to address irreparable massive tears. In 1991, the use of carbon fiber for repair of the rotator cuff in 14 patients was evaluated. One patient was noted to have a recurrent tear by arthrography. Histologic examination 2 years after index repair noted fragmentation of the carbon fibers embedded in a loose connective tissue. Further investigations comparing the mechanical, microangiographic, and histologic results of different synthetic materials in mongrel dogs have confirmed the suggestion that the use of the currently available rotator cuff substitutes cannot be recommended.

Allograft interposition has also been reported to have poor results. In 1988, the results of freeze-dried allografts in rotator cuff repairs was described. This series of seven patients in general did not obtain good functional results. One patient underwent reexploration 9 months after surgery and the allograft was found to be avascular and disrupted.

Other investigators have found that the use of staples to augment rotator cuff repair may be associated with unnecessary complications. In a 1983 study, 63 patients underwent surgical treatment for a chronic rotator cuff tear. Staples were used to augment the repair in four patients. All required later staple removal and none had a good result. Similarly, in another review of complications about the glenohumeral joint related to the use of screws and staples, two in the series who had a rotator cuff repair with the use of staples experienced staple pull-out and migration into the joint. In one patient the staple was removed and the cuff was resutured. The other patient refused further treatment.

Postoperatively, patients require cautious rehabilitation, as postoperative falls and inadequate immobilization have been cited as reasons for recurrent tear. In one series, four cases of traumatic disruption of rotator cuff repair were described. The mechanism was by a fall in each case. In another case of a traumatic recurrent tear, noncompliance with postoperative immobilization resulted in a recurrent tear of a free biceps graft reconstruction. A second repair with free biceps graft was unsuccessful.

There also exist reparable tears that have initially been treated with decompression alone, only to later require repair for continued symptoms. This situation has been illustrated in a recent study of arthroscopic subacromial decompression in three different populations. Group 1 had stage II impingement syndrome, Group 2 had partial tear of the rotator cuff, and Group 3 had a full thickness rotator cuff tear. Seven patients in Group 3 ultimately required an open surgical repair. The result was satisfactory in six of the seven after repair. In another evaluation of the long-term results of 25 patients who underwent arthroscopic subacromial decompression in the treatment of full thickness rotator cuff tears, eight required later rotator cuff repair. In one of the eight, the tear increased in size from large to massive during this interval.

Clearly, meticulous surgical technique and cautious postoperative rehabilitation will minimize the chance for recurrent tears. But the necessity to completely cover the gap occurring at the site of tear has recently been questioned. Initial recommendations for direct repair advocated obtaining a "watertight closure." This concept, however, was disputed in 1986, when the use of arthrography after surgical repair of a torn rotator cuff in 20 patients at an average 30 months postoperation was reported. In 18 of 20 patients, contrast medium leaked into the subacromial bursa, indicating a defect in the cuff. Results, however, did not correlate with this finding because 17 patients no longer complained of pain, and 15 had a full range of shoulder motion. It was concluded that a watertight closure is not essential for a good functional result.

Also in 1986, however, the sensitivity, specificity, and accuracy of postoperative rotator cuff findings at second-look surgery was compared with arthrography and ultrasonography. Arthrography was only 66% sensitive, 50% specific, and 62.5% accurate. In contrast, ultrasonography was 85% sensitive, 100% specific, and 90% accurate. The usefulness of ultrasound was further confirmed in an independent study in which a correct diagnosis of recurrent cuff tears was made in 26 of 26 shoulders, and the presence of an intact cuff was confirmed in ten of 11 cases.

In 1993, magnetic resonance imaging (MRI) was evaluated in patients who had undergone prior shoulder surgery and were experiencing recurrent symptoms of rotator cuff disease. MRI correctly identified six of seven tears found at the time of second surgery for a sensitivity of 86%. In addition, MRI was able to exclude the presence of a tear in 22 of 24 patients in which no full thickness tear was found at surgery, amounting to a specificity of 92%.

Correlation of rotator cuff tear recurrence with results was later analyzed in 1991, when 105 surgical repairs of the rotator cuff were evaluated by ultrasonography and correlated with the functional outcome at follow-up. Twenty percent of those tears that involved the supraspinatus alone originally had a recurrent defect. Of those with tears involving more than the supraspinatus, there was a 50% incidence of recurrent defect. Shoulders with an intact cuff at follow-up had better function and had a satisfactory result in 97% of the cases. In contrast, those with a recurrent defect were satisfied in 87% of cases. There was a high prevalence of bilateral lesions of the rotator cuff (55%).

In 1991, 97 rotator cuff tears were analyzed postoperatively with the use of ultrasonography. Twenty-nine had complete rupture of the cuff. However, a poor correlation between the clinical and ultrasonographic results was reported. One third of the contralateral rotator cuffs were noted to be abnormal. In contrast, as previously described, Gazielly found good correlation between outcome and integrity of cuff at follow-up as determined by ultrasound.

Finally, two separate studies have noted satisfactory results with debridement and decompression alone for massive rotator cuff tears. A "functional cuff tear" then becomes the surgical goal for relief of pain and optimizing function.

Neurologic Injury

Most open anterior surgical approaches for rotator cuff surgery are performed through a limited deltoid muscle split.

The relationship to the axillary nerve may be understood by recalling its anatomy as it arises from the fifth and sixth cervical roots and forms the posterior cord of the brachial plexus. At the inferior border of the subscapularis, it travels posteriorly under the inferior capsule and joins the posterior humeral circumflex artery to exit the quadrangular space. At this point it divides into anterior and posterior trunks. The posterior trunk gives off branches to the teres minor and posterior deltoid and terminates as the superior lateral cutaneous nerve of the arm. The anterior trunk passes anteriorly around the humerus approximately 5 cm distal to the lateral border of the acromion. Tremendous variation in the course and position of the axillary nerve in anatomic studies suggests that this safe zone is only a guideline, and careless, overexuberant retraction must be avoided (Fig. 7). In 1992, a case of deltoid denervation after acromioplasty and rotator cuff repair was reported; the extent of deltoid split was 4 cm. Subsequently, in 1994, two cases of axillary nerve palsy after rotator cuff repair for massive tears were described. Fortunately, these recovered within 3 months. The axillary nerve is also at risk in cases of subscapularis repair and care must be taken during the surgical approach to protect this nerve.

The technique of advancement of the supraspinatus muscle in its fossa through a posterior approach in 23 shoulders was described in 1965. In no case was there evidence of nerve injury by electromyography, but care must be taken in this approach as the suprascapular nerve is in close proximity during this "supraspinatus slide." With respect to a standard anterosuperior approach for cuff repair, Warner, in an anatomic study, demonstrated that the suprascapular neurovascular pedicle only allowed 1 cm of lateral advancement. This represents the actual mobilization of the tendon from its original anatomic position and not the extent of mobilization of retracted tissue. Intuitively, with retracted tissue, the neurovascular pedicle may also be tethered by scar, limiting mobilization even further. Recently, Zanotti reported on a sur-

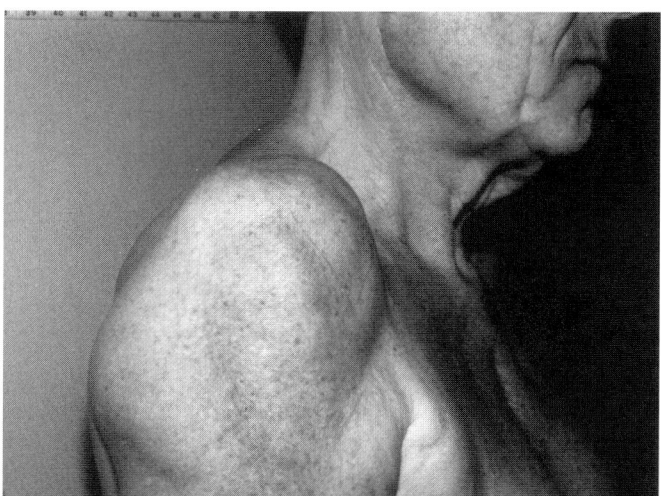

Fig. 7 Clinical example of significant deltoid atrophy following a rotator cuff repair complicated by deltoid denervation.

prisingly low incidence of mobilization of the spinati for repair of massive cuff tears. In only one of ten cases was there electrical evidence of suprascapular nerve injury.

Complications Related to Postoperative Rehabilitation

Postoperative Stiffness

The development of a frozen shoulder after rotator cuff surgery may be associated with prolonged immobilization postoperatively, poor patient compliance, and deltoid detachment. Treatment options include physical therapy, manipulation under anesthesia, and/or open or arthroscopic release of adhesions. Care must be taken during manipulations under anesthesia to avoid excess force and subsequent iatrogenic humeral fracture or retear of the rotator cuff repair. Arthroscopic capsular release is recommended in these cases.

Reflex Sympathetic Dystrophy

Reflex sympathetic dystrophy is a condition characterized by pain, hyperesthesia, vasomotor and sudomotor disturbances, and increased muscular tone, followed by weakness, atrophy, and trophic changes involving the skin, its appendages, muscles, bones, and joints. The etiology is thought to be a result of noxious stimuli (such as surgery) stimulating an aberrant sympathetic response. Its incidence after rotator cuff surgery is extremely low (less than 0.5%). Treatment includes pharmacologic therapy, nerve blocks, and if this is unsuccessful, surgical or chemical sympathectomy. Consultation with a pain management service is helpful in addressing this complication.

Biceps Rupture

The long head of the biceps tendon may be involved in the same degenerative process that occurs with rotator cuff pathology. As a result, the long head of the biceps tendon may become susceptible to rupture following rotator cuff surgery as shown in several reports. Disability after this injury is minimal, and repair is usually not necessary.

Complications Related to Wound Healing

This group of complications includes hematomas, draining sinuses, suture granulomas, superficial infections, and keloids or unsightly scars. The risk factors for these complications are, in general, unpredictable. Early recognition and removal of offending tissues will typically result in resolution. More complex is the issue of deep infection. This situation represents a significant negative impact on the final outcome of surgery. Aggressive debridement and culture-derived parenteral antibiotics are the principles of treatment.

Selected Bibliography

Altchek DW, Warren RF, Wickiewicz TL, et al: Arthroscopic acromioplasty: Technique and results. *J Bone Joint Surg* 1990;72A:1198-1207.

Bakalim G, Pasila M: Surgical treatment of rupture of the rotator cuff tendon. *Acta Orthop Scand* 1975;46:751-757.

Berg EE, Ciullo JV: Heterotopic ossification after acromioplasty and distal clavicle resection. *J Shoulder Elbow Surg* 1995;4:188-193.

This is a retrospective review of 40 cases of postoperative ectopic bone formation after acromioplasty or distal clavicle resection. Bone formation occurred in both open and arthroscopic procedures. Twenty patients required repeat surgery for removal of bone. Patients at increased risk for this complication were noted to have a history of hypertrophic pulmonary osteoarthropathy or active spondylitic arthropathy.

Bigliani LU, Colman WW, Kelkar R, et al: The effect of anterior acromioplasty on rotator cuff contact: An experimental and computer simulation. *American Shoulder and Elbow Surgeons Eleventh Open Meeting*. Rosemont, IL, American Shoulder and Elbow Surgeons, 1995, p 32.

Seven cadaveric shoulders using simulated muscle forces and measurement of subacromial contact patterns were used to determine the optimal location and amount of bone resection for anterior acromioplasty in the treatment of impingement. The authors found that the optimal bone resection was represented by flattening of the acromion extending from the anterior third to the midline. Flattening the anterior ridge alone resulted in continued impingement. Further flattening extending to the posterior aspect of the acromion jeopardizes the deltoid detachment and removes the passive stabilizing effect of the inferior acromion against superior humeral subluxation.

Bigliani LU, Cordasco FA, McIlveen SJ, et al: Operative treatment of failed repairs of the rotator cuff. *J Bone Joint Surg* 1992;74A:1505-1515.

Blazar P, Iannotti J, Williams G: Anteroposterior instability of the clavicle after distal clavicle resection. *American Shoulder and Elbow Surgeons Twelfth Open Meeting*. Rosemont, IL, American Shoulder and Elbow Surgeons, 1996, p 28.

In a review of 17 patients in whom distal clavicle resection was performed, the functional outcome and amount of postoperative shoulder pain with respect to anteroposterior instability of the clavicle were analyzed based on stress radiographs. The authors found that instability and pain were highly correlated with a less favorable outcome.

Burkhart SS: Arthroscopic treatment of massive rotator cuff tears: Clinical results and biomechanical rationale. *Clin Orthop* 1991;267:45-56.

Burkhart SS, Nottage WM, Ogilvie-Harris DJ, et al: Partial repair of irreparable rotator cuff tears. *Arthroscopy* 1994;10:363-370.

In 14 patients with irreparable rotator cuff tears, a technique of partial repair to restore force couples was described. Improvement in function occurred in all 14 patients.

Burkhead WZ Jr, Scheinberg RR, Box G: Surgical anatomy of the axillary nerve. *J Shoulder Elbow Surg* 1992;1:31-36.

The authors describe in detail the tremendous variation from specimen to specimen in the course and position of the axillary nerve. The "safe zone" serves only as a guideline and may be significantly smaller than previously described.

Calvert PT, Packer NP, Stoker DJ, et al: Arthrography of the shoulder after operative repair of the torn rotator cuff. *J Bone Joint Surg* 1986;68B:147-150.

Checchia S, Doneux P: Acromioclavicular resection: Complication in acromioplasty. *J Shoulder Elbow Surg* 1993;2(suppl):S11.

The authors report on 44 acromioclavicular resections in which 86% developed subsequent instability. The authors recommended a modification of the technique in which only 1 to 1.5 cm of the distal clavicle is resected with a bur and the superior acromioclavicular capsular ligaments are left intact.

Crass JR, Craig EV, Feinberg SB: Sonography of the postoperative rotator cuff. *Am J Roentgenol* 1986;146:561-564.

DeOrio JK, Cofield RH: Results of a second attempt at surgical repair of a failed initial rotator-cuff repair. *J Bone Joint Surg* 1984;66A:563-567.

Earnshaw P, Desjardins D, Sarkar K, et al: Rotator cuff tears: The role of surgery. *Can J Surg* 1982;25:60-63.

Ellman H: Diagnosis and treatment of incomplete rotator cuff tears. *Clin Orthop* 1990;254:64-74.

Esch JC: Arthroscopic subacromial decompression and postoperative management. *Orthop Clin North Am* 1993;24:161-171.

Flugstad D, Matsen FA, Larry I, et al: Failed acromioplasty: Etiology and prevention. *Orthop Trans* 1986;10:229.

Gartsman GM: Arthroscopic acromioplasty for lesions of the rotator cuff. *J Bone Joint Surg* 1990;72A:169-180.

Gazielly DF, Gleyze P, Montagnon C: Functional and anatomical results after rotator cuff repair. *Clin Orthop* 1994;304:43-53.

The anatomic condition of the rotator cuff (measured by ultrasonography) was compared with the functional result (using Constant's functional score) at 4-year follow-up in 100 full-thickness cuff tears treated by repair. The authors found that functional score at follow-up was closely related to anatomic integrity.

Gerber C, Hersche O, Farron A: Isolated rupture of the subscapularis tendon. *J Bone Joint Surg* 1996;78A:1015-1023.

Sixteen patients with isolated subscapularis tendon rupture treated by surgical repair were evaluated. Although no reported case of axillary nerve injury was demonstrated, the authors noted the extreme vulnerability of the nerve in the surgical approach to subscapularis repair.

Gerber C, Schneeberger AG, Beck M, et al: Mechanical strength of repairs of the rotator cuff. *J Bone Joint Surg* 1994;76B:371-380.

The authors evaluated the mechanical properties of several current techniques of tendon-to-bone suture employed in rotator cuff repair. Nonabsorbable braided polyester and absorbable polyglactin and polyglycolic acid sutures best combined ultimate tensile strength and stiffness. A modified Mason-Allen suture technique was superior with regard to tendon grasping. In cases of osteoporotic bone, the use of a 2-mm thick, plate-like augmentation device will improve failure strength over transosseous sutures.

Glousman RE: Instability versus impingement syndrome in the throwing athlete. *Orthop Clin North Am* 1993;24:89-99.

Groh GI, Simoni M, Rolla P, et al: Loss of the deltoid after shoulder operations: An operative disaster. *J Shoulder Elbow Surg* 1994;3:243-253.

This series evaluated 36 patients after loss of deltoid function from previous shoulder operations; this loss of function was caused by deltoid detachment in 33 patients and secondary axillary nerve injury in three patients. All patients were significantly disabled. The authors stressed careful attention to surgical technique of deltoid reattachment and protection of the axillary nerve.

Ha'eri GB, Wiley AM: Shoulder impingement syndrome: Results of operative release. *Clin Orthop* 1982;168:128-132.

Hammond G: Complete acromionectomy in the treatment of chronic tendinitis of the shoulder. *J Bone Joint Surg* 1962;44A:494-504.

Harryman DT II, Mack LA, Wang KY, et al: Repairs of the rotator cuff: Correlation of functional results with integrity of the cuff. *J Bone Joint Surg* 1991;73A:982-989.

Hawkins RJ, Brock RM, Abrams JS, et al: Acromioplasty for impingement with an intact rotator cuff. *J Bone Joint Surg* 1988;70B:795-797.

Hawkins RJ, Chris AD, Kiefer GN: Failed anterior acromioplasties. *Orthop Trans* 1987;11:233.

Hawkins RJ, Chris T, Bokor D, et al: Failed anterior acromioplasty: A review of 51 cases. *Clin Orthop* 1989;243:106-111.

Hawkins RJ, Kennedy JC: Impingement syndrome in athletes. *Am J Sports Med* 1980;8:151-158.

Johansson JE, Barrington TW: Coracoacromial ligament division. *Am J Sports Med* 1984;12:138-141.

Kessel L, Watson M: The painful arc syndrome: Clinical classification as a guide to management. *J Bone Joint Surg* 1977;59B:166-172.

Kitay GS, Iannotti JP, Williams GR, et al: Roentgenographic assessment of acromial morphologic condition in rotator cuff impingement syndrome. *J Shoulder Elbow Surg* 1995;4:441-448.

In this prospective study of 23 subjects with isolated impingement syndrome, anteroposterior, axillary, caudal tilt, and supraspinatus outlet views were evaluated with regard to interobserver reliability and correlation with intraoperative measurements of acromial morphology. The authors found the highest reliability for the caudal tilt and lowest for the axillary view. The caudal tilt and supraspinatus outlet views also correlated highly with intraoperative measurements. They continued to recommend both views in the preoperative assessment of the acromial spur for rotator cuff impingement syndrome.

Kujat R: Rotator cuff substitutes: An experimental investigation. *J Shoulder Elbow Surg* 1993;2(suppl):S8.

Dacron, carbon, mersilene net, and Gore-tex patch substitute for rotator cuff repair were evaluated after implantation in 22 mongrel dogs. The implants were examined mechanically, microangiographically, and histologically at 3, 6, or 12 months after reconstruction. It was determined that these substitutes were not optimal for use in humans.

Lazarus MD, Chansky HA, Misra S, et al: Comparison of open and arthroscopic subacromial decompression. *J Shoulder Elbow Surg* 1994;3:1-11.

A comparison of open and arthroscopic acromioplasty performed by one surgeon for chronic impingement syndrome was retrospectively reviewed in 68 patients. There was no statistical difference in mean postoperative shoulder scores between surgical groups at a minimum 12-month follow-up. Arthroscopic acromioplasty, however, was associated with shorter hospital stays and faster achievement of maximal pain relief as compared to open acromioplasty. Also noted was the finding of subacromial calcifications on postoperative radiographs associated with a less favorable result.

Lazarus MD, Yung SW, Sidles JA, et al: Anterosuperior humeral displacement: Limitation by the coracoacromial arch. *American Shoulder and Elbow Surgeons Eleventh Open Meeting.* Rosemont, IL, American Shoulder and Elbow Surgeons, 1995, p 28.

Six cadaver shoulders were analyzed after coracoacromial ligament resection and after anterior acromioplasty followed by humeral head loading. The authors found that the coracoacromial arch provides an important barrier to anterosuperior humeral head displacement. Loss of this barrier may have substantial effects if the normal head centering capacity of the rotator cuff is deficient.

Mack LA, Nyberg DA, Matsen FR III, et al: Sonography of the postoperative shoulder. *Am J Roentgenol* 1988;150:1089-1093.

Matthews LS, Burkhead WZ, Gordon S, et al: Acromial fracture: A complication of arthroscopic subacromial decompression. *J Shoulder Elbow Surg* 1994;3:256-261.

The authors report on six patients who underwent arthroscopic subacromial decompression complicated by acromial fracture. Risk factors for fracture included osteopenia and overaggressive bone resection. They noted that surgical correction may not resolve pain and/or loss of motion, and appropriate preoperative planning and meticulous surgical technique are mandatory to decrease the risk of this complication.

McShane RB, Leinberry CF, Fenlin JM Jr: Conservative open anterior acromioplasty. *Clin Orthop* 1987;223:137-144.

Michelsson JE, Bakalim G: Resection of the acromion in the treatment of persistent rotator cuff syndrome of the shoulder. *Acta Orthop Scand* 1977;48:607-611.

Moorman CT III, Deng XH, Warren RF, et al: The coracoacromial ligament: Is it the appendix of the shoulder? *American Shoulder and Elbow Surgeons Eleventh Open Meeting.* Rosemont, IL, American Shoulder and Elbow Surgeons, 1995, p 33.

Biomechanical testing was performed on 25 cadavers after sequential interventions of capsular venting, release of the rotator interval capsule and coracoacromial ligament (CAL) connection, release of the CAL at the acromion, and after acromioplasty. Superior translation of the humeral head was increased after CAL section and further after acromioplasty. The authors suggested avoidance of CAL release and acromioplasty in two particular clinical situations: cuff deficiency, and in the patient with high functional demands who poorly tolerates changes in coupled motions (eg, throwing athletes).

Nasca RJ: The use of freeze-dried allografts in the management of global rotator cuff tears. *Clin Orthop* 1988;228:218-226.

Neer CS II: Anterior acromioplasty for the chronic impingement syndrome in the shoulder: A preliminary report. *J Bone Joint Surg* 1972;54A:41-50.

Neer CS II, Marberry TA: On the disadvantages of radical acromionectomy. *J Bone Joint Surg* 1981;63A:416-419.

Neviaser JS: Ruptures of the rotator cuff of the shoulder: New concepts in the diagnosis and operative treatment of chronic ruptures. *Arch Surg* 1971;102:483-485.

Neviaser RJ, Neviaser TJ: Reoperation for failed rotator cuff repair: Analysis of fifty cases. *J Shoulder Elbow Surg* 1992;1:283-286.

Reoperation for failure of a previous rotator cuff repair was performed in 50 patients. In a retrospective review, the authors found that the size of the rupture, the number of previous operations, and dysfunction of the biceps did not affect the result. Factors found to be important include adequate decompression, closure of all defects with tendon-to-bone junctures, avoidance of the use of weights during the first 3 months after surgery, and the presence of an intact functioning deltoid.

Neviaser TJ, Neviaser RJ, Neviaser JS, et al: The four-in-one arthroplasty for the painful arc syndrome. *Clin Orthop* 1982;163:107-112.

Nobuhara K, Hata Y, Komai M: Surgical procedure and results of repair of massive tears of the rotator cuff. *Clin Orthop* 1994;304:54-59.

In this series, 187 patients with massive tears of the rotator cuff underwent tendon-to-tendon repair or the McLaughlin procedure. Two patients with axillary nerve palsy recovered in 3 months.

Ogilvie-Harris DJ, Wiley AM, Sattarian J: Failed acromioplasty for impingement syndrome. *J Bone Joint Surg* 1990;72B:1070-1072.

Owen RS, Iannotti JP, Kneeland JB, et al: Shoulder after surgery: MR imaging with surgical validation. *Radiology* 1993;186:443-447.

In 31 patients with recurrent symptoms of rotator cuff disease, magnetic resonance imaging (MRI) was performed prior to undergoing a second surgery. MRI findings regarding cuff integrity were correlated with intraoperative findings. Postoperative MRI findings demonstrated sensitivity of 86%, specificity of 92%, and accuracy of 90%.

Post M: Complications following anterior acromioplasty and rotator cuff repair, in Bigliani LU (ed): *Complications of Shoulder Surgery.* Baltimore, MD, Williams & Wilkins, 1993, pp 34-43.

This review provides an excellent description of the evaluation of complications of anterior acromioplasty and rotator cuff repair.

Post M: Complications of rotator cuff surgery. *Clin Orthop* 1990;254:97-104.

Post M, Silver R, Singh M: Rotator cuff tear: Diagnosis and treatment. *Clin Orthop* 1983;173:78-91.

Rockwood CA Jr, Williams GR Jr, Burkhead WZ Jr: Debridement of degenerative, irreparable lesions of the rotator cuff. *J Bone Joint Surg* 1995;77A:857-866.

Debridement and decompression for irreparable cuff tear was performed in 50 patients. A retrospective evaluation was performed an average of 6.5 years later. Results were satisfactory in 83% and were associated with an intact deltoid and long head of the biceps tendon, and in those in whom acromioplasty had not been previously performed.

Samilson RL, Binder WF: Symptomatic full thickness tears of the rotator cuff: An analysis of 292 shoulders in 276 patients. *Orthop Clin North Am* 1975;6:449-466.

Sher J, Warner J, Groff Y, et al: Treatment of postoperative deltoid origin disruption. *American Shoulder and Elbow Surgeons Twelfth Open Meeting.* Rosemont, IL, American Shoulder and Elbow Surgeons, 1996, p 36.

In 24 patients who underwent direct repair or rotationplasty for deltoid detachment, 67% unsatisfactory results were observed at an average 39-month follow-up. Risk factors for a poor outcome included prior lateral acromionectomy, involvement of the middle deltoid, massive rotator cuff tear, and duration of symptoms for longer than 12 months. Conversely, a satisfactory outcome was associated with acute disruptions isolated to the anterior deltoid, an intact acromion, duration of symptoms for 12 months or less, and evidence of a healed deltoid reconstruction.

Thorling J, Bjerneld H, Hallin G, et al: Acromioplasty for impingement syndrome. *Acta Orthop Scand* 1985;56: 147-148.

Visuri T, Kiviluoto O, Eskelin M: Carbon fiber for repair of the rotator cuff: A 4-year follow-up of 14 cases. *Acta Orthop Scand* 1991;62:356-359.

Warner JP, Krushell RJ, Masquelet A, et al: Anatomy and relationships of the suprascapular nerve: Anatomical constraints to mobilization of the supraspinatus and infraspinatus muscles in the management of massive rotator-cuff tears. *J Bone Joint Surg* 1992;74A:36-45.

This anatomic study of 31 shoulders evaluated the course of the suprascapular nerve with respect to mobilization of the supraspinatus and infraspinatus muscles for repair of massive tears. The authors found that lateral advancement of only 1 cm could be obtained using a standard anterosuperior approach. Using the advancement technique of Debeyre, lateral advancement of as much as 3 cm was obtained.

Wolfgang GL: Rupture of the musculotendinous cuff of the shoulder. *Clin Orthop* 1978;134:230-243.

Wolfgang GL: Surgical repair of tears of the rotator cuff of the shoulder: Factors influencing the result. *J Bone Joint Surg* 1974;56A:14-26.

Wulker N, Melzer C, Wirth CJ: Shoulder surgery for rotator cuff tears: Ultrasonographic 3-year follow-up of 97 cases. *Acta Orthop Scand* 1991;62:142-147.

Zanotti RM, Carpenter JE, Blasier RB, et al: The low incidence of suprascapular nerve injury after primary repair of massive rotator cuff tears. *J Shoulder Elbow Surg* 1997;6:258-265.

Zuckerman JD, Matsen FA III: Complications about the glenohumeral joint related to the use of screws and staples. *J Bone Joint Surg* 1984;66A:175-180.

18

Massive Rotator Cuff Tears

Anthony Miniaci, MD, FRCSC

Rotator cuff tears are common orthopaedic injuries that may result in pain and dysfunction. The diagnosis and management of massive rotator cuff tears is somewhat controversial and perplexing. When the tear is massive, the complexity of the problem is magnified. Discussion of these injuries is difficult because there is no precise definition of what constitutes a massive tear. Full-thickness tears can be classified according to their configuration, dimension in centimeters, number of tendons involved, and tendon retraction. There is a lack of consensus regarding classification of tears of similar dimensions. Cofield has suggested that tears greater than 5 cm should be termed massive, whereas Patte requires a tear diameter of 5 cm in addition to cranial migration and glenohumeral arthrosis to consider the tear as massive. However, the size of the tear is not the only factor to take into account; the mobility or quality of the tendon and subsequently the ease of repair must also be considered. Some 5-cm tears may be relatively easy to mobilize, whereas others are not. For this reason, ease of repair as well as size are factors that have been incorporated into Gerber's classification scheme. Lack of uniformity in classification schemes makes it difficult to perform comparative research, and it is a source of controversy in diagnosis and management of these injuries.

Also, patients present with differing clinical pictures despite having similar-appearing pathology. Individuals with massive tears can have either pain, dysfunction, or both, or sometimes no clinical problems. As a result, recommended management and published results have been quite variable. Finally, there is no uniform agreement about whether the surgical results of patients with massive rotator cuff defects are affected by tear size. Some authors would suggest that results are better with smaller tears, whereas others would argue that tear size is not correlated to the final clinical result. It would appear that surgery for patients with massive tears is better at eliminating pain than restoring function.

Clinical Evaluation

Clinical evaluation of patients with rotator cuff tears is difficult. The extent of the tear, quality of the tendinous tissue, and ease of repair often are not determined until surgery. Many patients have chronic tears that will present with pain and atrophy of the supraspinatus, and often infraspinatus, muscles. Although many patients with an intact biceps tendon, coracoacromial arch, and deltoid will not have significant superior migration and may actually have good function, external rotation tends to be weak.

Diagnostic imaging methods, such as plain radiographs, arthroscopy, ultrasonography, and magnetic resonance imaging (MRI), will help confirm the presence of a rotator cuff tear. Unfortunately, there is no one method that will allow prediction of tissue mobility, ease of repair, and long-term function.

Kaneko has used plain radiographs to screen for massive rotator cuff tears and determined that those patients with superior migration and deformity of the greater tuberosity had massive rotator cuff tears with a sensitivity of 78% and a specificity of 98%. Perhaps the best method that allows prediction of tear size is MRI. Iannotti has demonstrated 100% sensitivity and 95% specificity with the ability to measure tear size and tendon retraction. As discussed previously, the tear size sometimes does not correlate with the ability to repair a tendon defect or with that tendon's ability to restore function. Goutallier and associates have assessed the extent of fatty infiltration of the rotator cuff using computed tomography (CT) and have tried to correlate this with muscle function. MRI has also been used in assessment of fatty infiltration. Nakagaki and associates have demonstrated that linear signals and nonhomogeneity of the supraspinatus muscle were associated with diminished muscle function. In the future, ease of repair and functional outcome for patients may be predictable, but at present they are not.

Surgical Management

The role of surgery in the management of massive rotator cuff tears is not well defined. Two clinical situations usually occur; these should be considered independently. The first is the group of patients who present with massive rotator cuff tears de novo and have not had previous surgery, and the second group are those in whom previous attempts at repair for a massive rotator cuff tear have failed.

Surgical management of primary massive rotator cuff tears includes debridement and decompression with or without limited repair, local repairs, local muscle slides or transfers, distant muscle transfers, autogenous free grafts, fascia lata grafts, freeze-dried grafts, synthetic materials, arthroplasty, or arthrodesis.

Debridement and Decompression

In patients with an irreparable rotator cuff defect, debridement and decompression has been considered the treatment of choice by many authors. The patients who derive the most benefit from this treatment usually have pain as the main presenting complaint, but preoperative function is usually quite good. Burkhart has suggested that if the rotator cuff is balanced and an intact anteroposterior force couple exists, closure of the rotator cuff is not necessary and function will be maintained. In those patients in whom the cable suspension bridge is disrupted, a limited repair may alleviate pain and result in dramatic restoration of function. Rockwood and associates have shown similar improvement in patients with massive rotator cuff tears, especially if patients had an intact biceps tendon and functioning deltoid. Conversely, Apoil and Augereau have abandoned debridement for massive tears, suggesting that after only 5 years, less than 50% of their patients demonstrated significant pain relief with no restoration of function. In addition, at 10 years, progressive cranial migration and cuff arthropathy had developed in more than 25% of their patients. Hawkins also reported poor results despite what was believed to be adequate debridement and decompression.

Recently, Flatow has suggested an important function for the coracoacromial ligament: that it prevents superior migration of the humeral head, especially in the presence of massive rotator cuff deficiencies. In these cases, extensive debridement may exacerbate the propensity to cranial migration and may lead to further difficulties. It appears that in some patients with good function and an intact biceps and deltoid, reasonable success can be achieved with limited debridement. In order to prevent further dysfunction, care should be taken not to disturb the integrity of the coracoacromial arch.

Local Muscle Repairs or Transfer
Many techniques for local rotator cuff repairs or muscle transfer have been described. Depending on the size of the tear and mobility of the muscle, these techniques may or may not be suitable to close rotator cuff defects.

Debeyre described advancement of the supraspinatus on its neurovascular pedicle to close a rotator cuff defect, and Patte demonstrated favorable results when using this procedure for massive defects. Ha'eri and Wiley also noted improved clinical outcomes in 14 of 18 patients treated with this technique for massive rotator cuff tears. Paavolainen and associates have described a way of transferring the infraspinatus by transferring the posterior position of the greater tuberosity with its attached infraspinatus to a more anterior position. In this manner, pain relief was achieved in 29 of 31 patients.

There are some limitations to these approaches. First, the retracted muscle and tendon unit has ceased to be functional and, therefore, advancement of a fibro-fatty muscle may not be an adequate functional reconstruction. In addition, safe advancement of these muscles on the neurovascular pedicles may not be possible. Warner and associates demonstrated by anatomic dissections the location of the suprascapular nerve and its anatomic relationships. They suggested that only 1 cm of lateral advancement of the supraspinatus was possible. By using the technique described by Debeyre, 3 cm of advancement could be achieved; however, the neurovascular pedicle is exposed to significant risk. Assuming an intact and viable supraspinatus at onset, excessive mobilization could cause significant and irreversible damage to the muscle tendon unit.

Cofield has used a rotationplasty of the subscapularis muscle, with good results, in patients with massive defects. Similarly, Neviaser has used the subscapularis and teres minor in massive defects, also with good results. It would appear that in the absence of the supraspinatus or infraspinatus tendons, local rotation of subscapularis with or without rotation of the teres minor is likely the best alternative for local closure of massive rotator cuff defects.

Distant Muscle Transfers
In the absence of local muscle tissue that allows repairs, various techniques have been attempted in which muscles distant to the rotator cuff are transferred to close the defect and perhaps restore some dynamic stability and muscle function to the rotator cuff repair. In 1984, Mikasa reported on a transfer of a flap of trapezius muscle to close the defect in nine patients with global rotator cuff defects, but only six had significant improvement following this procedure. Augereau reported on the use of a section of the anterior fascicle of the middle portion of the deltoid in 22 patients. Overall, 17 (77%) of the patients had a satisfactory result. Augereau suggested that the transplanted muscle acted synergistically with the rotator cuff, maintained a nerve and blood supply so it should remain viable, prevented the migration of the humeral head, and weakened the action of the deltoid, which potentially causes superior migration. Dierickx and Vanhoof performed this procedure in 20 patients, and although they achieved results similar to those of Augereau, they could not demonstrate any superiority in the results of this procedure over open or closed acromioplasty and rotator cuff debridement.

In 1988, Gerber reported encouraging results with the use of a latissimus dorsi muscle transfer for massive rotator cuff defects. Theoretically, the muscle not only acted as a tenodesis to the humeral head, but because of the intact neurovascular pedicle the muscle could potentially be an active humeral head depressor and external rotator, especially as the arm was abducted. Gerber suggested that an intact subscapularis muscle was essential to a good result.

Free Tissue Grafts
Many different types of free grafts have been used in an attempt to close rotator cuff defects. The coracoacromial ligament has reportedly been used as a patch graft. The area of defect was limited to 1×1.5 cm, and this was usually thin tissue. Nasca has used fascia lata grafts with only one good result out of eight patients. Neviaser reported good or excellent results in 14 of 16 patients with massive defects closed with freeze-dried rotator cuff graft. Neviaser has also reported good results with the use of the biceps tendon as a free graft with tenodesis of the remaining tendon. Use of the biceps tendon is somewhat controversial because it has been considered as an important head depressor, especially in the face of rotator cuff deficiency. For this reason, this procedure has not gained wide acceptance or approval. Free grafts in general have only had variable results at best and it is arguable whether a static, nonviable graft is better than a dynamic viable muscle repair or transfer. The use of free grafts, therefore, has not gained wide acceptance.

Synthetic Grafts
Although Ozaki and associates have reported good or excellent results in 25 of 27 patients treated with a Teflon mesh reconstruction, this procedure has not gained wide acceptance for reasons similar to those discussed with free grafts.

Arthrodesis and Arthroplasty
Reconstruction of the rotator cuff may not eliminate end-stage rotator cuff arthropathy and pain. For those patients

with end-stage glenohumeral osteoarthrosis, both hemiarthroplasty and arthrodesis have been considered. Total shoulder arthroplasty is not believed to be a reasonable option. Franklin and associates demonstrated that cuff deficiency will lead to component instability and loosening of the glenoid component. Arntz and associates compared a group of patients with massive cuff defects and cuff arthropathy undergoing either hemiarthroplasty or arthrodesis. They suggested that hemiarthroplasty achieved better results, but they reserved arthrodesis for those patients with irreparable cuff defects and dysfunctional deltoid muscles.

In summary, treatment of primary massive rotator cuff defects remains a difficult decision-making process. In those patients with good function accompanied by pain, there is some evidence to suggest that debridement and decompression may give adequate pain relief. Many surgeons would attempt repair of existing local tissue with transport of the subscapularis or teres minor as necessary. Bigliani and associates have demonstrated that this approach will give good or excellent results in 85% of patients. The surgeon should exercise caution during surgery in those patients with poor function and pain and without enough tissue to perform primary repair. Local transfers of the remaining cuff musculature may disrupt the anteroposterior force couple and could lead to further dysfunction. However, rotation of the subscapularis or teres minor is possible. At this stage, many surgeons would consider the use of distant active muscle transfers to repair the defects and avoid disrupting the anterior and posterior rotator cuff stabilizers.

Failed Massive Rotator Cuff Defects

If the treatment of massive rotator cuff defects is complex, then the further management of patients who have massive rotator cuff defects in whom attempts at repair have failed only increases the complexity of the problem. The causes of failure must be established first; these include inadequate decompression, failure of repair, and deltoid detachment or dysfunction. Despite recognition of these problems, reoperation does not necessarily guarantee success. Cofield and associates suggested that results were considered poor in 58% of patients in whom surgical repair had been attempted a second time. Bigliani and associates reported relief of pain in 81% of patients with the treatment of failed repairs and warned against the expectation of improved function. Neviaser's study demonstrated improved pain relief in 92% with some improvement in motion and function. In patients with deltoid abnormalities, there was no functional improvement after the repeated surgical attempts.

Once it has been established that a repeat surgical attempt is necessary, the choice of procedure becomes similar to that for primary massive rotator cuff defects. Options will include debridement and decompression, local tissue repair, free grafts, distant muscle transfers, arthroplasty, or arthrodesis. Unfortunately, not much evidence exists in the literature to guide the decision-making process. My colleagues and I have reported the use of the latissimus dorsi muscle as an attempt to salvage this difficult clinical problem (Figs. 1 through 4). Review of 12 patients demonstrated

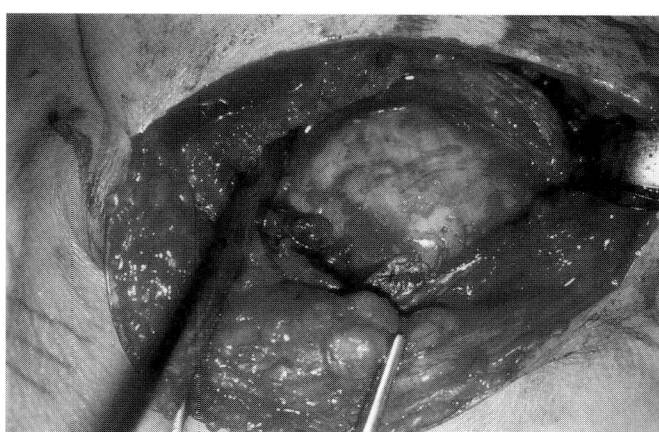

Fig. 1 A symptomatic massive rotator cuff defect in a patient who has had two previous surgical attempts at repair is shown. The subscapularis is intact but the supraspinatus and infraspinatus are retracted and cannot be mobilized for repair.

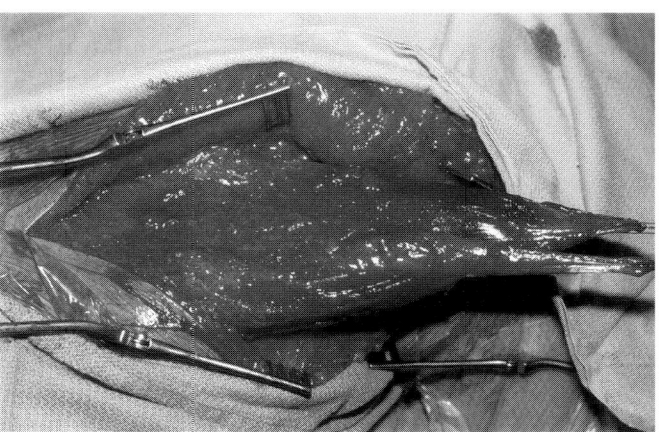

Fig. 2 Through a posterior axillary incision, the latissimus dorsi muscle tendon (inferior) can be mobilized and detached from the humerus. Maximum tendon length can be obtained by visualizing the insertion and abduction and internally rotating the arm to maximize the tendinous portion resected. In this patient, the teres major (superior) has also been mobilized to provide additional tendinous tissue.

good relief of pain in ten patients (83%) and significant improvement in function. Deltoid dysfunction was found in five patients, and these patients benefited greatly from the procedure. According to Gerber, subscapularis integrity seemed to be necessary for a good result; however, in the group reported by my colleagues and me, there was complete absence of the subscapularis in two patients and partial absence in one. Two of these three patients had an improved clinical condition. These results seemed quite promising for this difficult clinical situation.

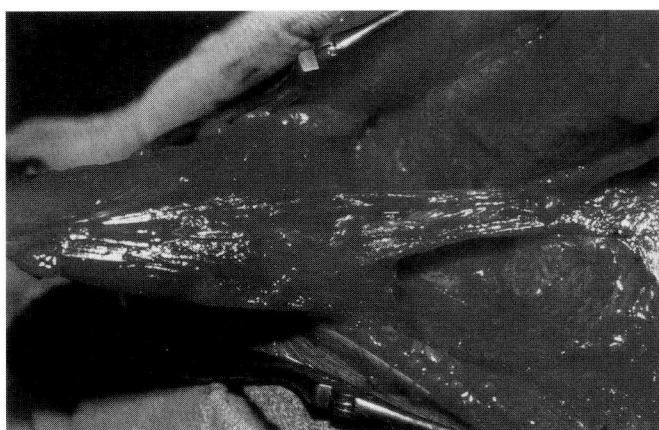

Fig. 3 Great care must be taken to preserve the neurovascular pedicle to the latissimus dorsi to maintain viability and function of the transfer.

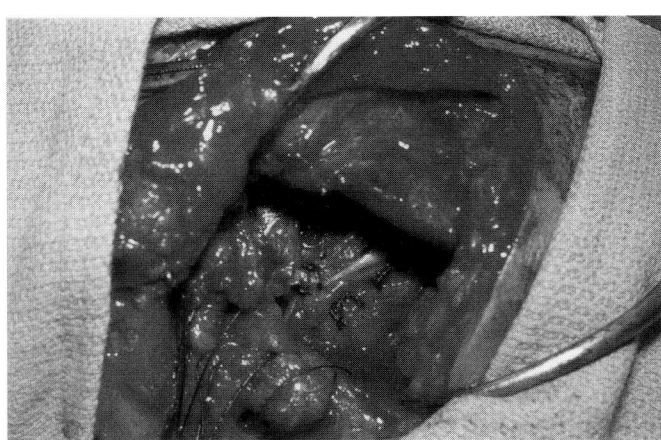

Fig. 4 A completed transfer of latissimus dorsi muscle sutured to intact subscapularis anteriorly and to a bone trough laterally is shown.

Summary

Massive rotator cuff defects can cause patients significant pain and dysfunction. Because a spectrum of clinical presentations is seen, treatment needs to be individualized. The best treatment of primary massive rotator cuff defects is probably repair of local tendinous tissue or rotation of adjacent tissue. In some patients with good function accompanied by pain, debridement and decompression may be sufficient; however, maintaining good results is of some concern. Where no tissue exists for repairs, dynamic, viable tissue transfer is likely preferable to free grafts or synthetics. Finally, revision of these attempts at repair is sometimes necessary and usually is a result of inadequate decompression, deltoid dysfunction, or failure of the previous repair. Treatment in these patients is difficult and published reports are scarce. Latissimus dorsi muscle transfer has been reported as a potential option. Unfortunately, some patients will progress to significant arthropathy and hemiarthroplasty may need to be considered. If the deltoid is dysfunctional in addition to the massive cuff defect, if arthropathy is present and previous attempts at pain relief and return of function have failed, then arthrodesis may be the only option available. Certainly an understanding of the pathology, meticulous attention to surgical detail, and close follow-up of these patients will optimize clinical results.

Selected Bibliography

Apoil A, Augereau B: Anterosuperior arthrolysis of the shoulder for rotator cuff degenerative lesions, in Post M, Morrey BF, Hawkins RJ (eds): *Surgery of the Shoulder.* St. Louis, MO, Mosby-Year Book, 1990, pp 257-260.

Arntz CT, Matsen FA III, Jackins S: Surgical management of complex irreparable rotator cuff deficiency. *J Arthroplasty* 1991;6:363-370.

Augereau B: Reconstruction of massive rotator cuff rupture using a deltoid muscle flap. *Orthopade* 1991;20:315-319.

Twenty-two patients with massive rotator cuff defects who were treated with a section of the anterior deltoid muscle inlay flap were reviewed. Seventeen of the 22 patients had a satisfactory result.

Bakalim G, Pasila M: Surgical treatment of rupture of the rotator cuff tendon. *Acta Orthop Scand* 1975;46:751-757.

Bateman JE (ed): Lesions producing shoulder pain predominantly, in *The Shoulder and Neck*. Philadelphia, PA, WB Saunders, 1972, pp 195-292.

Bigliani LU, Cordasco FA, McIlveen SJ, et al: Operative treatment of failed repairs of the rotator cuff. *J Bone Joint Surg* 1992;74A:1505-1515.

In this review of 31 patients who had a repeat rotator cuff repair following failure of a previous one, repeat repair was successful in only 52%. An intact acromion, deltoid, and good tissue quality were associated with superior results.

Bigliani LU, McIlveen SJ, Cordasco F, et al: Operative repair of massive rotator cuff tears: Long term results. *Orthop Trans* 1990;14:251.

Burkhart SS: Arthroscopic treatment of massive rotator cuff tears: Clinical results and biomechanical rationale. *Clin Orthop* 1991;267:45-56.

    The results of arthroscopic acromioplasty and rotator cuff debridement in ten patients with massive rotator cuff tears are discussed. This technique seems applicable in patients with irreparable tears with good function preoperatively. Biomechanical explanation of intact anteroposterior force couple is important in understanding how some of these patients do well in spite of massive tears.

Burkhart SS, Esch JC, Jolson RS: The rotator crescent and rotator cable: An anatomic description of the shoulder's "suspension bridge". *Arthroplasty* 1993;9:611-616.

Burkhart SS, Nottage WM, Ogilvie-Harris DJ, et al: Partial repair of irreparable rotator cuff tears. *Arthroscopy* 1994;10: 363-370.

Cofield RH: Subscapular muscle transposition for repair of chronic rotator cuff tears. *Surg Gynecol Obstet* 1982;154: 667-672.

Cofield RH, Hoffmeyer P, Lanzer WL: Surgical repair of chronic rotator cuff tears. *Orthop Trans* 1990;14:251-252.

Debeyre J, Patte D, Elmelik E: Repair of ruptures of the rotator cuff of the shoulder: With a note on advancement of the supraspinatus muscle. *J Bone Joint Surg* 1965;47B: 36-42.

DeOrio JK, Cofield RH: Results of a second attempt at surgical repair of a failed initial rotator-cuff repair. *J Bone Joint Surg* 1984;66A:563-567.

Dierickx C, Vanhoof H: Massive rotator cuff tears treated by a deltoid muscular inlay flap. *Acta Orthop Belg* 1994;60: 94-100.

Earnshaw P, Desjardins D, Sarkar K, et al: Rotator cuff tears: The role of surgery. *Can J Surg* 1982;25:60-63.

Ellman H: Arthroscopic subacromial decompression: Analysis of one- to three-year results. *Arthroscopy* 1987;3: 173-181.

Esch JC, Ozerkis LR, Helgager JA, et al: Arthroscopic subacromial decompression: Results according to the degree of rotator cuff tear. *Arthroscopy* 1988;4:241-249.

Flatow EL, Weinstein DM, Duralele XA: Coraco-acromial ligament preservation in rotator cuff surgery. *J Shoulder Elbow Surg* 1994;3(suppl):S73.

    This article describes the potential importance of preserving the coracoacromial ligament when performing rotator cuff surgery. The authors hypothesize that maintenance of the ligament prevents anterosuperior humeral subluxation in patients with massive rotator cuff defects.

Franklin JL, Barrett WP, Jackins SE, et al: Glenoid loosening in total shoulder arthroplasty: Association with rotator cuff deficiency. *J Arthroplasty* 1988;3:39-46.

Gerber C: Latissimus dorsi transfer for the treatment of irreparable tears of the rotator cuff. *Clin Orthop* 1992;275: 152-160.

    This article presents a review of treatment of 16 irreparable primary massive rotator cuff defects with a latissimus dorsi muscle transfer. Pain relief was obtained by 81% on exertion and 94% at rest. The author believed that an intact subscapularis was necessary for the procedure to be useful.

Gerber C, Krushell RJ: Isolated rupture of the tendon of the subscapularis muscle: Clinical features in 16 cases. *J Bone Joint Surg* 1991;73B:389-394.

Godsil RD Jr, Linscheid RL: Intratendinous defects of the rotator cuff. *Clin Orthop* 1970;69:181-188.

Gore DR, Murray MP, Sepic SB, et al: Shoulder-muscle strength and range of motion following surgical repair of full-thickness rotator-cuff tears. *J Bone Joint Surg* 1986;68A:266-272.

Goutallier D, Bernageau J, Patte D: Assessment of the trophicity of the muscles of the ruptured rotator cuff by CT scan, in Post M, Morrey BF, Hawkins RJ (eds): *Surgery of the Shoulder.* St. Louis, MO, Mosby-Year Book, 1990, pp 11-13.

Gschwend N, Ivosevic-Radovanovic D, Patte D: Rotator cuff tear: Relationship between clinical and anatomopathological findings. *Arch Orthop Trauma Surg* 1988;107:7-15.

Gschwend N, Patte D, Grammont P, et al: Die Bedeutung von Schmierz-und funktionsanalysen fur die Diagnostik von Rupturen der Rotatorenmannschette-Ergebnisse einer prospektiven Studie II. *Hefte Unfallheilkunde* 1986;180:47.

Ha'eri GB, Wiley AM: Advancement of the supraspinatus muscle in the repair of ruptures of the rotator cuff. *J Bone Joint Surg* 1981;63A:232-238.

Hawkins RJ, Misamore GW, Hobeika PE: Surgery for full-thickness rotator-cuff tears. *J Bone Joint Surg* 1985;67A: 1349-1355.

    This article is a classic review of surgical treatment of full-thickness rotator cuff tears. Significant improvement in pain and function can be achieved after repair. Patients with massive tears fared better if repair was possible versus decompression and debridement alone.

Lundberg BJ: The correlation of clinical evaluation with operative findings and prognosis in rotator cuff rupture, in Bayley I, Kessel L (eds): *Shoulder Surgery.* Berlin, Germany, Springer-Verlag, 1982, pp 35-38.

McLaughlin HL: Lesions of the musculotendinous cuff of the shoulder: I. The exposure and treatment of tears with retraction. *J Bone Joint Surg* 1944;26:31-51.

Mikasa M: Trapezius transfer for global tear of the rotator cuff, in Bateman JE, Welsh RP (eds): *Surgery of the Shoulder.* Philadelphia, PA, BC Decker, 1984, pp 196-199.

Miniaci A, Dowdy PA, Willits KR, et al: Magnetic resonance imaging evaluation of the rotator cuff tendons in the asymptomatic shoulder. *Am J Sports Med* 1995;23: 142-145.

Nakagaki K, Ozaki J, Tomita Y, et al: Function of supraspinatus muscle with torn cuff evaluated by magnetic resonance imaging. *Clin Orthop* 1995;318:144-151.

Nasca RJ: Rotator cuff grafts. *Orthop Trans* 1985;9:50.

Neer CS II: Cuff tears, biceps lesions, and impingement, in Neer CS II (ed): *Shoulder Reconstruction.* Philadelphia, PA, WB Saunders 1990, pp 41-142.

Neer CS II, Craig EV, Fukuda H: Cuff-tear arthropathy. *J Bone Joint Surg* 1983;65A:1232-1244.

   This classic paper describes and discusses the clinical and pathologic findings in patients with cuff tear arthropathy. Superior migration and instability with massive tears can lead to this condition, which is difficult to treat.

Neer CS II, Flatow EL, Lech O: Tears of the rotator cuff: Long-term results of anterior acromioplasty and repair. *Orthop Trans* 1988;12:735.

Neer CS II, Watson KC, Stanton FJ: Recent experience in total shoulder replacement. *J Bone Joint Surg* 1982;64A:319-337.

Neviaser JS: Ruptures of the rotator cuff of the shoulder: New concepts in the diagnosis and operative treatment of chronic ruptures. *Arch Surg* 1971;102:483-485.

Neviaser JS, Neviaser RJ, Neviaser TJ: The repair of chronic massive ruptures of the rotator cuff of the shoulder by use of a freeze-dried rotator cuff. *J Bone Joint Surg* 1978;60A:681-684.

Neviaser RJ, Neviaser TJ: Transfer of subscapularis and teres minor for massive defects of the rotator cuff, in Bayley I, Kessel L (eds): *Shoulder Surgery*. Berlin, Germany, Springer-Verlag, 1982, pp 60-63.

Neviaser RJ, Neviaser TJ: Reoperation for failed rotator cuff repair: Analysis of fifty cases. *J Shoulder Elbow Surg* 1992;1:283-286.

Ozaki J, Fujimoto S, Masuhara K: Repair of chronic massive rotator cuff tears with synthetic fabrics, in Bateman JE, Welsh RP (eds): *Surgery of the Shoulder*. Philadelphia, PA, BC Decker, 1984, pp 185-191.

Ozaki J, Fujimoto S, Masuhara K, et al: Reconstruction of chronic massive rotator cuff tears with synthetic materials. *Clin Orthop* 1986;202:173-183.

Paavolainen P, Slätis P, Björkenheim JM: Transfer of the tuberculum majus for massive ruptures of the rotator cuff, in Post M, Morrey BF, Hawkins RJ (eds): *Surgery of the Shoulder*. St. Louis, MO, Mosby-Year Book, 1990, pp 252-256.

Patte D, Debeyre J, Goutallier D: Rotator cuff repair by muscle advancement, in Bayley I, Kessel L (eds): *Shoulder Surgery*. Berlin, Germany, Springer-Verlag, 1982, pp 49-59.

Patte D, Goutallier D, Scheffer JC: Large cuff ruptures: Repair results by muscle advancement, in Post M, Morrey BF, Hawkins RJ (eds): *Surgery of the Shoulder*. St. Louis, MO, Mosby-Year Book, 1990, pp 248-251.

Petersson C: Long-term results of rotator cuff repair, in Bayley I, Kessel L (eds): *Shoulder Surgery*. Berlin, Germany, Springer-Verlag, 1982, pp 64-69.

Post M, Silver R, Singh M: Rotator cuff tear: Diagnosis and treatment. *Clin Orthop* 1983;173:78-91.

Rockwood CA Jr, Williams GR Jr, Burkhead WZ Jr: Debridement of degenerative irreparable lesions of the rotator cuff. *J Bone Joint Surg* 1995;77A:857-866.

   This is a retrospective review of 53 shoulders in 50 patients who were treated by acromioplasty and debridement for their massive irreparable rotator cuff tears. Patients with a functioning deltoid, intact biceps tendon, and a good range of motion preoperatively had significant improvement in both pain and function postoperatively.

Tibone JE, Elrod B, Jobe FW, et al: Surgical treatment of tears of the rotator cuff in athletes. *J Bone Joint Surg* 1986;68A:887-891.

Walker SW, Couch WH, Boester GA, et al: Isokinetic strength of the shoulder after repair of a torn rotator cuff. *J Bone Joint Surg* 1987;69A:1041-1044.

Warner JP, Krushell RJ, Masquelet A, et al: Anatomy and relationships of the suprascapular nerve: Anatomical constraints to mobilization of the supraspinatus and infraspinatus muscles in the management of massive rotator-cuff tears. *J Bone Joint Surg* 1992;74A:36-45.

Watson M: Major ruptures of the rotator cuff: The results of surgical repair in 89 patients. *J Bone Joint Surg* 1985;67B:618-624.

Wilson PD: Complete rupture of the supraspinatus tendon. *JAMA* 1931;96:433-439.

19

Cuff Tear Arthropathy

David G. Duckworth, MD and Kevin L. Smith, MD

Introduction

The term "cuff tear arthropathy" was first used by Neer and associates in 1983, to define a problem related to degeneration of the glenohumeral joint in association with massive rotator cuff tears. This condition was described in a group of 26 patients, average age, 69 years; 75% were female. This entity, while similar to other degenerative and destructive processes of the glenohumeral joint, is entirely separate and its diagnosis and treatment remain considerably difficult. It is postulated that approximately 4% of rotator cuff tears will lead to this condition. Its overall pathogenesis has been ill-defined to date, though the condition has been associated with numerous factors.

Etiology

Neer and associates described both mechanical and nutritional factors involved in the evolution of cuff tear arthropathy. Mechanical factors include such problems as overall instability of the glenohumeral joint associated with rotator cuff tear, which results in upward migration of the humeral head with subsequent erosion of the acromion, the acromioclavicular joint, and the clavicle. In addition, it has been proposed that anterior-posterior instability results in some of the glenohumeral deformity seen with cuff tear arthropathy. Stability of the normal shoulder requires that several different mechanisms be intact. These include the overall bony architecture of the glenohumeral joint, the capsuloligamentous complex, a negative intra-articular pressure, and the compressor effect of the rotator cuff. These mechanisms act as the primary stabilizers of the glenohumeral joint. The secondary stabilizers, which act when these primary stabilizers are deficient, include the entire coracoacromial arch. More specifically, the acromion needs to be solid and the coracoacromial ligament intact.

The decrease in motion associated with cuff tear arthropathy causes chronic disuse osteopenia. It is believed that joint narrowing and loss of a well-defined, enclosed joint space results in a decrease in quantity and quality of synovial fluid. These synovial fluid deficiencies may result in an inadequate nutrient diffusion process. Figure 1 summarizes the mechanical and nutritional factors involved in the pathogenesis of cuff tear arthropathy.

Occurring almost simultaneously with the description of cuff tear arthropathy in the orthopaedic literature has been the description of a similar entity, the Milwaukee shoulder. Although the patient group is relatively similar to that with cuff tear arthropathy, the disease process is attributed to the presence of basic calcium phosphate crystals encapsulated into microspheroids without apparent inflammatory cell

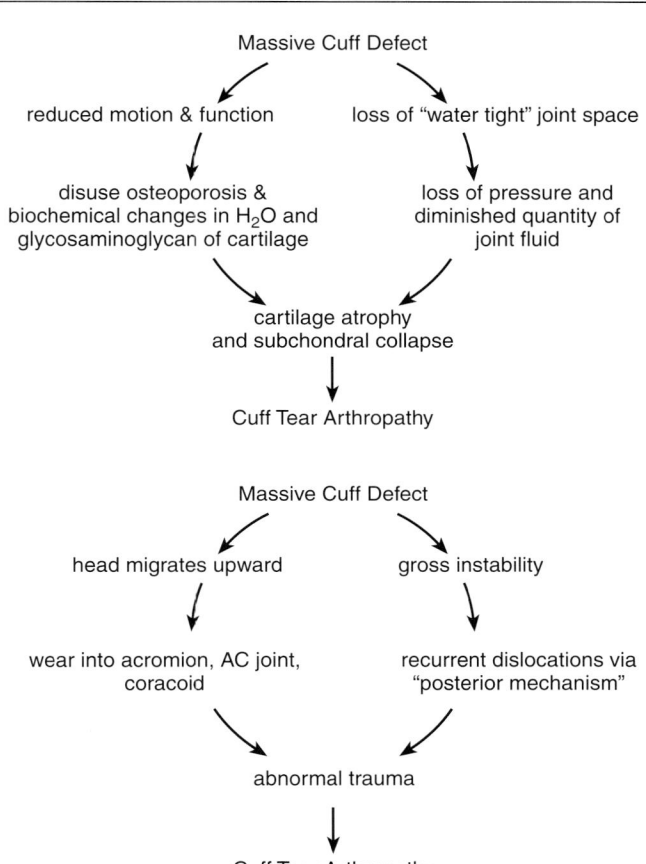

Fig. 1 The nutritional (**top**) and mechanical (**bottom**) factors proposed by Neer and associates to be involved in the genesis of cuff tear arthropathy. (Reproduced with permission from Neer CS III, Craig EV, Fukuda H: Cuff-tear arthropathy. *J Bone Joint Surg* 1983;65A:1232-1244).

responses. Indeed, an altered capsular synovium and degenerate cartilage, possibly with a macrophage response and subsequent release of collagenase and neutral proteases, are associated with this condition, resulting in the attack and subsequent destruction of the glenohumeral joint. Yet another mechanism has been described in which analogous findings of large amounts of calcium apatite crystals seem to result from bone damage. However, joint involvement that differs from that of other reports was found. There remains a question of whether this joint involvement defines the disease process itself or is a final pathway in which the condition evolves. Despite considerable deliberation and discussion regarding the actual cause of this entity, it must be noted that the overall mechanism is presently unknown.

Evaluation

Patients generally present with the predominant finding of pain. This pain occurs with daily activities as well as at night or at rest, and is often accentuated with forward elevation and external rotation. The onset of pain is commonly atraumatic, occurring three times as often in females than in males. In addition, a fluid sign or swelling may be noted; patients demonstrate supraspinatus (and often infraspinatus) atrophy and weakness, long head biceps rupture, and decreased range of motion caused by the joint destruction. Instability may be a feature, in addition to joint tenderness and crepitus.

Radiographic findings include articular collapse with diffuse osteopenia, upward migration of the humeral head relative to the glenoid, and subsequent erosion on the undersurface of the acromion with reactive, sclerotic bone. These findings may progress to involvement of the acromioclavicular joint and the distal clavicle as well. Patients will develop "snow cap" subarticular sclerosis on the superior humeral head, often with cystic changes noted on the greater tuberosity. The greater tuberosity will become progressively rounded, presenting a picture of relative "femoralization" of the humeral head with subsequent "acetabularization" of the coracoacromial arch over time. With further collapse and destruction, the joint space often medializes, abutting and eroding to and beyond the coracoid process. Figure 2 demonstrates the classic radiographic features of cuff tear arthropathy.

Intraoperatively, patients are usually found to have massive rotator cuff tears of a chronic nature that are irreparable. The bone is extremely soft and massive joint destruction is noted.

In evaluating a patient with presumed cuff tear arthropathy, a thorough differential diagnosis must be considered as well. Other entities that present a similar picture include rheumatoid arthritis, infection, posttraumatic arthritis, metabolic disorders including crystalline arthropathies, osteonecrosis, and neuropathic joints associated most commonly with syringomyelia. In working through this differential diagnosis it may be important to obtain other studies, including joint fluid aspiration and culture, magnetic resonance imaging to rule out a syrinx, and other diagnostic tests to determine whether the rotator cuff is intact. As mentioned above, the predominant feature is severe joint destruction in the face of a massive rotator cuff tear. Advanced imaging studies are not necessary for diagnosis of a cuff tear when the humeral head migrates superiorly to the point that the undersurface of the acromion has been eroded.

Treatment

Treatment is aimed mainly at resolution of the patient's pain. Function is almost always improved concomitantly with the relief of pain; nonetheless, functional goals are limited and variable. Possible methods of treatment include glenohumeral arthrodesis, resection arthroplasty, total shoulder arthroplasty using constrained, semiconstrained, or unconstrained components, hemiarthroplasty, and nonsurgical care.

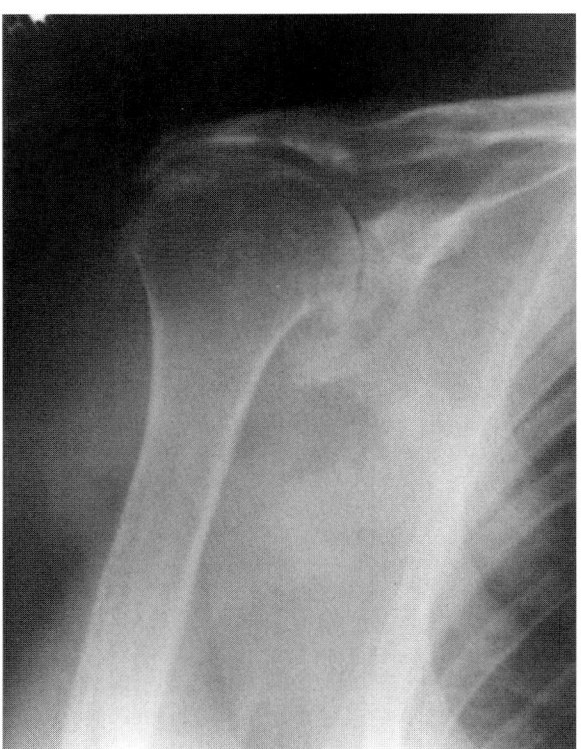

Fig. 2 The radiographic features of cuff tear arthropathy including osteoarthrosis of the glenohumeral joint and upward migration of the humeral head with erosion of the acromion, acromioclavicular joint, and clavicle.

Nonsurgical Treatment

The presence of cuff tear arthropathy on radiographic and clinical examination is not a definite indication for surgical treatment. Despite relatively severe radiographic findings, patients will occasionally have surprisingly good function and minimal pain. In this instance, where pain is not an overwhelming feature, patients may benefit from nonsurgical management, including general strengthening of the anterior deltoid to maximize function. In addition, anti-inflammatory agents are administered to slow or stabilize the problem.

Surgical Debridement and Acromioplasty

By definition, cuff tear arthropathy mandates that the glenohumeral joint be destroyed. In the face of a destroyed glenohumeral joint, it is unlikely that debridement and/or an acromioplasty will result in any long-lasting benefit. Indeed, acromioplasty may result in severe consequences, most importantly, a loss of the secondary stabilizing mechanism of the coracoacromial arch. Therefore, this method is not recommended for patients with definite cuff tear arthropathy.

Glenohumeral Arthrodesis and Resection Arthroplasty

These methods are poorly tolerated in the elderly population; bone stock in these patients is poor, and perioperative immobilization is not handled well. Solid fusion in this group is difficult. Thus, arthrodesis is reserved only for those few with documented deltoid deficiency. The deltoid may be damaged, detached, or denervated as a result of injury or previous surgery; as such, its ability to power any other attempts at joint salvage are diminished significantly, and results are poor. Glenohumeral arthrodesis may indeed be useful for a very small percentage of patients.

Constrained Total Shoulder Arthroplasty
In principle, constrained total shoulder arthroplasty would appear to offer a reliable answer to this difficult problem of joint degeneration. Constrained total shoulder arthroplasty theoretically would result in resurfacing of the destroyed glenohumeral joint and stabilization in the face of absent primary constraints. Nonetheless, as with other constrained arthroplasties, there are considerable problems in the long term, including loosening, implant dissociation, and fracture at the bone-implant interface. Most physicians recommend repair of the stabilizers rather than trying to replace them with a constrained arthroplasty. In addition, revision of a constrained total shoulder arthroplasty to another option is extremely difficult. The constrained arthroplasty has been abandoned in most of North America and Europe.

Semiconstrained Total Shoulder Arthroplasty
Similarly, semiconstrained total shoulder arthroplasty, in theory, is a reasonable option. Many have tried in the past with components using hooded glenoids, for example, to alleviate the lack of inherent stability. However, a considerable increase in stress to the components occurs, often resulting in early loosening. Both semiconstrained and constrained total shoulder arthroplasty attempt to block the superior migration of the humeral head, which occurs because of unbalanced force of the deltoid. These attempts, unfortunately, have been unsuccessful.

Unconstrained Total Shoulder Arthroplasty
Unconstrained total shoulder arthroplasty presents a more reasonable option, yet it has its own set of problems and issues. Unconstrained total shoulder arthroplasties have often been attempted, with variable results. In general, the eccentric forces placed on the glenoid by a high-riding humeral head result in increased stress and uneven wear on the glenoid. This causes a "rocking horse" phenomenon, resulting in early loosening of the glenoid component. Although unconstrained arthroplasty may present a reasonable option in the few patients with minimal or no superior migration of the humeral head, the actual definition of the problem is brought into question. Although this procedure is satisfactory for patients with concomitant rotator cuff deficiency and glenohumeral arthritis, these patients may not have true cuff tear arthropathy.

Bipolar Arthroplasty
Placement of a bipolar prosthesis in the cuff-deficient shoulder has produced some good early results. However, the bipolar head is often quite large, resulting in overstuffing of the glenohumeral joint and subsequent tightness that can cause residual pain and difficulties. Still, bipolar arthroplasty may be a reasonable option in some patients.

Hemiarthroplasty
More recently, the trend in treatment of cuff tear arthropathy has been toward placement of an anatomic hemiarthroplasty. Original series included the use of oversized humeral components to overstuff the glenohumeral joint. However, in doing so, patients were often unhappy with the tightness of their shoulder and the resultant pain. Thus, more recently, placement of a smaller, near-anatomic hemiarthroplasty with normal tensioning of the soft tissues has demonstrated more reliable results. Two principles are extremely important in placing a hemiarthroplasty. The first is maintenance of the secondary stabilizers of the shoulder, that is, the coracoacromial arch, and the second is maintenance of a functioning deltoid. Restoring a smooth joint surface while simultaneously creating a stable fulcrum for the deltoid to work on can lead to improved shoulder function and pain relief. The only controversy concerns whether or not to repair some or all of the rotator cuff tear. Most often in cuff tear arthropathy, the rotator cuff is characterized by chronic tearing of a massive nature that makes rotator cuff repair impossible or implausible. Indeed, complete rotator cuff repair with extensive release has been advocated, as well as muscle transfers and placement of allograft or other constructs. Others, however, maintain that the need for cuff repair is insignificant, and that repair is unreliable and likely to fail shortly thereafter, and therefore is not necessary. Figure 3 is the postoperative radiograph of the shoulder depicted in Figure 2 after an anatomic hemiarthroplasty.

Complications

Complications in treatment of cuff tear arthropathy are related in general to the problem itself. In order for a patient with cuff tear arthropathy to have reasonable function after any surgical intervention, the deltoid must be of good quality. Thus, previous surgery and loss of the deltoid can result in poor functional improvement. The deltoid must be preserved at all costs during any surgical procedures because its acromial attachment and overall structure are of paramount importance.

In the absence of a functional rotator cuff, the secondary restraints of the shoulder become increasingly important. The entire coracoacromial arch indeed becomes the only restraint to anterosuperior escape. Any sacrifice of the coracoacromial arch via acromioplasty and/or coracoacromial ligament resection can result in severe problems. Maintenance of the coracoacromial arch is very important in these patients, both at surgery and in the long term.

Other problems relating to shoulder arthroplasty, including instability, implant loosening, and progressive pain, appear to occur less frequently in this group of patients. In particular, when hemiarthroplasty alone is performed, humeral loosening generally is not found. If the coracoacromial arch is maintained and deltoid force is maximized, with the residual socket providing an adequate fulcrum, instability is not a problem. Any loss of the coracoacromial arch, however, can cause severe problems with anterosuperior escape, usually with no good solution.

Patients with cuff tear arthropathy often present with large sacs of fluid in the subacromial and subdeltoid space. These

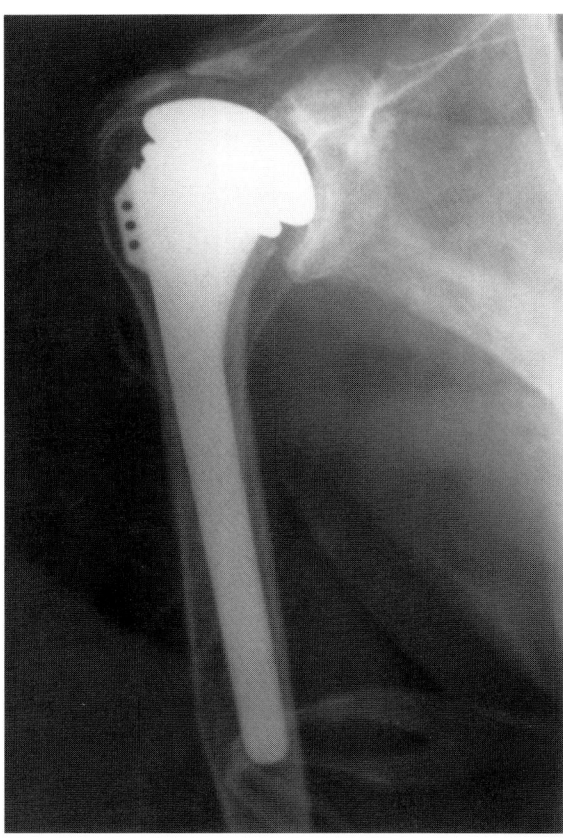

Fig. 3 A postoperative radiograph of a shoulder treated with a modular hemiarthroplasty demonstrating anatomic replacement of the arthritic humeral head.

fluid accumulations appear to be related to the destructive process of the glenohumeral joint. It is imperative that all reactive synovial tissue be adequately debrided and careful hemostasis be obtained.

Persistent migration and/or erosion of the glenohumeral joint after hemiarthroplasty appears to be relatively minimal, because these patients generally place small functional demands on their shoulders. Still, it does present a theoretical problem.

Results

The predominant feature of cuff tear arthropathy is pain, which appears to be the most reliable target of treatment. In particular, problems with pain at night and at rest resolve quite well. Pain associated with functional demands may be minimized, but is often still present.

Function after treatment of cuff tear arthropathy is less reliably improved. Although patients will usually gain forward elevation and external rotation, the force of powering the shoulder is diminished considerably because of the lack of the rotator cuff. Thus, goals of major functional improvement may be unrealistic and are less reliably achieved than those of pain relief.

Following hemiarthroplasty for cuff tear arthropathy, Arntz and associates found an increase in active forward elevation of 66% as well as a subsequent increase in the ability to perform activities of daily living. Nonetheless, there was a 22% revision rate in this group, and only 50% believed that they had achieved even minimal improvement.

In a recent study by Field and associates, 16 patients were evaluated following hemiarthroplasty for cuff tear arthropathy. Of these, ten were rated as successful, and six as unsuccessful. Of these six unsuccessful patients, four had undergone at least one attempt at rotator cuff repair with acromioplasty, four with a hemiarthroplasty. In addition, two of these four patients had resultant deltoid deficiency. Thus, overall results may generally be quite good, albeit with inherent pitfalls.

Recently, the University of Washington sought to document the actual change in self-assessed shoulder function and health status following hemiarthroplasty for rotator cuff tear arthropathy. We analyzed the data of 15 consecutive patients meeting strict diagnostic criteria for rotator cuff tear arthropathy. Prior to treatment, each patient completed a questionnaire pertaining to shoulder function (the Simple Shoulder Test, SST), and one regarding their overall health status (the Health Status Questionnaire Short Form 36, SF 36). These two questionnaires were completed at 6-month intervals after treatment was initiated. One surgeon managed all patients with anatomic humeral head replacement, while carefully preserving the coracoacromial arch and deltoid muscle. The study population consisted of six males and nine females whose average age was 75.8 years (range, 61 to 89 years). The dominant right shoulder was involved in 14. Average length of follow-up was 25 months.

SST data analysis demonstrated an improvement in function in eight of the 12 shoulders following treatment, with function remaining unchanged in one and actually worsening in three. The only significant improvements were in pain with the arm at the side and sleep on the affected side. These improved an average of 27% and 53%, respectively. Analysis of the SF 36 data revealed similar findings, with only two of the eight SF 36 parameters improved, namely comfort and vitality. The remaining six SF 36 scores actually decreased after treatment. Comfort was the only score to improve significantly, with an average mean increase from 25 to 39.

Rotator cuff tear arthropathy often affects patients who are otherwise healthy, without major systemic disease and physical disabilities. Thus, this condition can have a relatively large impact on patients' lives, and its treatment would theoretically make a sizable difference. These data demonstrate that modest gains can be realized in the way of comfort, but activities of daily living and health status in general do not reliably improve following hemiarthroplasty for rotator cuff tear arthropathy. Some, in fact, worsen after treatment. Patients should be counseled regarding the likelihood of improvement in comfort, albeit with minimal functional gains at best. Rotator cuff tear arthropathy remains a difficult, unsolved problem. Future improvements in overall care as well as earlier diagnosis and treatment may improve results.

Summary

Rotator cuff tear arthropathy continues to be rather difficult to understand and treat. Its etiology generally remains unknown. Despite numerous methods of treatment, none has presented the perfect solution. Still, a considerable amount has been learned and current treatment provides a much more reliable result than in past years.

Common pitfalls include disruption of the coracoacromial arch, loss of optimal deltoid function, and placement of a glenoid component in the face of a high-riding humeral head.

Current treatment generally focuses on humeral head replacement alone, attempting to replace that which is removed with a prosthetic humeral head, maintaining soft-tissue balance without overstuffing the joint. Although current treatment provides adequate resolution of overall pain, function may remain limited. Patients should be counseled about this, and surgeons must be aware of the pitfalls associated with treatment.

Selected Bibliography

Arntz CT, Matsen FA III, Jackins S: Surgical management of complex irreparable rotator cuff deficiency. *J Arthroplasty* 1991;6:363-370.

Arntz CT, Jackins S, Matsen FA III: Prosthetic replacement of the shoulder for the treatment of defects in the rotator cuff and the surface of the glenohumeral joint. *J Bone Joint Surg* 1993;75A:485-491.

  This article describes results obtained using anatomic hemiarthroplasty for patients with cuff tear arthropathy. This retrospective review of 18 shoulders in 16 patients documented generally good results in function as well as pain relief and proposed a method for dealing with this challenging condition.

Barrett WP, Franklin JL, Jackins SE, et al: Total shoulder arthroplasty. *J Bone Joint Surg* 1987;69A:865-872.

Cantrell JS, Itamura JM, Burkhead WZ Jr: Rotator cuff tear arthropathy, in Warner JJP, Iannotti JP, Gerber C (eds): *Complex and Revision Problems in Shoulder Surgery.* Philadelphia, PA, Lippincott-Raven, 1997, pp 303-318.

  This article is an excellent review of this problem, and includes an approach to management. The authors advocate the use of a hemiarthroplasty, but propose two separate techniques based on the integrity of the subscapularis.

Collins DN, Harryman DT II: Arthroplasty for arthritis and rotator cuff deficiency. *Orthop Clin North Am* 1997;28:225-239.

  This article presents an extensive review of the condition, its pathogenesis, diagnosis, treatment emphasizing hemiarthroplasty, and potential pitfalls, with a review of published results.

Dieppe PA, Doherty M, Macfarlane DG, et al: Apatite associated destructive arthritis. *Br J Rheumatol* 1984;23:84-91.

Field LD, Dines DM, Zabinski SJ, et al: Hemiarthroplasty of the shoulder for rotator cuff arthropathy. *J Shoulder Elbow Surg* 1997;6:18-23.

  This most recent series in the literature reviews the results of 16 patients treated with a hemiarthroplasty. The problems associated with treatment of previously operated shoulders are documented and the importance of an intact coracoacromial arch is discussed.

Franklin JL, Barrett WP, Jackins SE, et al: Glenoid loosening in total shoulder arthroplasty: Association with rotator cuff deficiency. *J Arthroplasty* 1988;3:39-46.

Garancis JC, Cheung HS, Halverson PB, et al: "Milwaukee shoulder": Association of microspheroids containing hydroxyapatite crystals, active collagenase, and neutral protease with rotator cuff defects. III: Morphologic and biochemical studies of an excised synovium showing chondromatosis. *Arthritis Rheum* 1981;24:484-491.

Halverson PB, Carrera GF, McCarty DJ: Milwaukee shoulder syndrome: Fifteen additional cases and a description of contributing factors. *Arch Intern Med* 1990;150:677-682.

Lohr JF, Cofield RH, Uhthoff HK: Glenoid component loosening in cuff tear arthropathy. *J Bone Joint Surg* 1991;73B(suppl II):106.

Matsen FA III, Arntz CT, Harryman DT II: Rotator cuff tear arthropathy, in Bigliani LU (ed): *Complications of Shoulder Surgery.* Baltimore, MD, Williams & Wilkins, 1993, pp 44-58.

  This article presents a review of cuff tear arthropathy. Challenges associated with its evaluation and management are discussed.

McCarty DJ, Halverson PB, Carrera GF, et al: "Milwaukee shoulder": Association of microspheroids containing hydroxyapatite crystals, active collagenase, and neutral protease with rotator cuff defects. I: Clinical aspects. *Arthritis Rheum* 1981;24:464-473.

McCarty DJ, Lehr JR, Halverson PB: Crystal populations in human synovial fluid: Identification of apatite, octacalcium phosphate, and tricalcium phosphate. *Arthritis Rheum* 1983;26:1220-1224.

McLaughlin HL: Rupture of the rotator cuff. *J Bone Joint Surg* 1962;44A:979-983.

Neer CS III, Craig EV, Fukuda H: Cuff-tear arthropathy. *J Bone Joint Surg* 1983;65A:1232-1244.

Williams GR Jr, Rockwood CA Jr: Massive rotator cuff defects and glenohumeral arthritis, in Friedman RJ (ed): *Arthroplasty of the Shoulder.* New York, NY, Thieme Medical Publishers, 1994, pp 204-214.

  An early summary of the diagnosis and treatment of cuff tear arthropathy is presented.

IV
Trauma/Fracture

Joseph D. Zuckerman, MD
Section Editor

20

Proximal Humerus Fractures

Frances Cuomo, MD

Introduction

Fractures of the proximal humerus account for approximately 5% to 7% of all fractures and can be expected to be more frequent with increasing life expectancies and associated osteoporosis. Most of these injuries are accompanied by no or minimal displacement and are best treated with a short period of immobilization and early passive range of motion exercises. The more serious or displaced injuries will often require surgery for optimal results; identification of these injuries can sometimes be difficult. In addition, the evaluation and treatment of these fractures can be particularly challenging. The complicated anatomy and tendency for bony structures to overlap make complete radiographic evaluation mandatory for each case. Because most of these fractures occur in the older female patient, bone quality is often compromised by age-related osteoporosis. This factor has important implications in the ability to obtain secure internal fixation. The surgeon's technical expertise and the patient's ability to comply with the rigorous postoperative rehabilitation program will weigh heavily in determining outcome. The importance of the surrounding soft tissues cannot be understated and makes treatment outcome dependent on much more than merely restoration of bony anatomy. In both surgical and nonsurgical treatment, the goal is to maximize the function of the entire extremity, which is directly related to the ability to achieve osseous and soft-tissue healing, a stable anatomic reduction, and the institution of early passive range of motion exercises.

Etiology

Proximal humerus fractures result from both indirect and direct mechanisms of injury. The most common mechanism is indirect (a fall onto the outstretched hand). In the younger patient, a similar mechanism may result in dislocation, not fracture, because the strength of the bone is much greater than that of the supporting ligaments. However, in the older patient with osteoporosis, the bone is significantly weaker than the ligament. In addition, a recent study suggested that the increasing number of osteoporosis-related fractures in the elderly population can be attributed to risk factors such as impaired vision and balance, and decreased muscle trophism. However, these authors were unable to find a difference in the healing rates of minimally to moderately displaced fractures in patients with osteoporosis and normal subjects. Although the most common mechanism of injury in the elderly is a fall on the outstretched hand, high velocity injuries are often responsible for the severely displaced fractures encountered in young patients with good bone quality. A second indirect mechanism of injury by which fractures occur is following seizures or electroconvulsive therapy. In these situations, violent contractions of the local musculature of the shoulder girdle often resulted in fractures and fracture-dislocations.

The most commonly described direct mechanism of injury generally consists of a blow to the lateral aspect of the shoulder. This injury may occur as the patient falls and strikes the shoulder against the wall, the floor, or a piece of furniture. This injury usually causes less displacement than that resulting from a fall onto the outstretched hand. The incidence and causes of fractures about the shoulder were examined in a 1-year prospective study in an urban population involving three defined age groups (children, adults, elderly). Differences among the various age groups were identified. In children, the characteristic shoulder injury was the fractured clavicle, which represented 65 of the 75 shoulder injuries seen in this age group. The elderly most often presented with proximal humerus fractures. The significantly higher incidence of these fractures among females was thought to be secondary to osseous fragility. In the adult population, these two injuries occurred with equal frequency, and a 25% incidence of primary glenohumeral or acromioclavicular dislocation was also noted.

Evaluation

Upon clinical presentation, all patients suspected of having fracture or dislocation about the shoulder should submit to a complete neurovascular examination. Early detection is required for adequate treatment. Previous studies report neurologic injury rates between 21% and 36%. In a recent prospective report, 45% of 101 patients with primary glenohumeral dislocations or humeral neck fractures had electrophysiologic evidence of nerve injury. Nerves most commonly involved were the axillary, suprascapular, radial, and musculocutaneous. The elderly population was at higher risk of nerve injury, especially when significant hematomas were identified. Most patients had partial or complete recovery in less than 4 months, but 8% had persistent motor loss. Vascular injuries, most commonly involving the axillary artery, are devastating surgical emergencies that require a high level of suspicion when ischemia is noted despite the presence of distal pulses, which have reportedly been palpable in 27% of patients with major arterial injuries about the shoulder. Rigid fixation of the fracture is believed to be necessary to protect the site of vascular repair, but this point has recently been debated.

An accurate diagnosis is mandatory for successful treatment. The Neer classification of proximal humeral fractures and fracture-dislocations is the most widely accepted. This system is comprehensive and is based on the degree of displacement of the four osseous fragments about the proximal

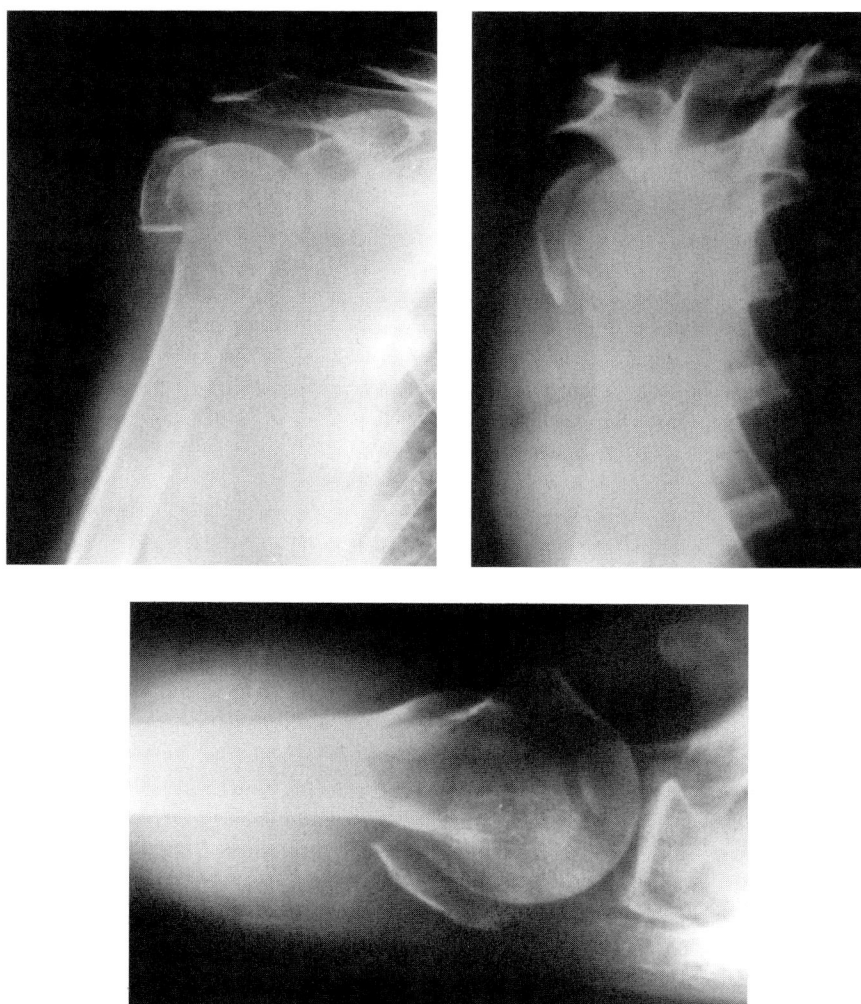

Fig. 1 Trauma series consisting of scapular AP (**top left**), lateral (**top right**), and axillary (**bottom**) views of displaced two-part greater tuberosity fracture. (Reproduced with permission from Flatow EL, Cuomo F, Maday MG, et al: Open reduction and internal fixation of two-part displaced fractures of the greater tuberosity of the proximal part of the humerus. *J Bone Joint Surg* 1991;73A:1213-1218.)

humerus: articular segment, greater tuberosity, lesser tuberosity, and the proximal shaft beginning at the level of the surgical neck. Fragments are considered displaced if they are separated by at least 1.0 cm or angulated greater than 45° from their anatomic position. The displacement of the segments, not the number of fracture lines, is important in this classification. Displacement is the result of the deforming muscle forces of the rotator cuff insertions on the tuberosities and the pectoralis major on the humeral shaft.

Radiographs in three orthogonal planes, consisting of scapular anteroposterior (AP), scapular lateral, and axillary views, represent the trauma series and are the minimum requirement for evaluation and classification of these injuries (Fig. 1). Additional studies, such as computed tomography (CT), aid in the determination of the size of articular surface defects, or can replace the axillary view when pain precludes positioning. Although standard radiographs remain the best method of evaluation and diagnosis of proximal humerus fractures according to the four-segment system, interobserver reliability was found to be fair in a recent 5-year retrospective analysis of 28 fractures with kappa values ranging from 0.37 to 1.00. Surgical neck fractures fared better than tuberosity fractures. The authors admit to basing diagnoses on incomplete trauma series, inclusion criteria of only two radiographs at 90° angles to each other rather than the required three views, and the lack of a standardized radiographic procedure. Despite these conditions, the authors questioned whether the use of plain films is reliable in the classification of complex proximal humerus fractures, suggesting that the addition of routine CT scans may increase the reliability. The crucial need for the axillary view has been emphasized in several studies. Not only does the axillary view define glenohumeral articular surface relationships for dislocations and head defects, but it also helps identify posterior greater tuberosity displacement and medial lesser tuberosity displacement, both of which may not be evident on standard AP films. The axillary view adds significantly more information toward making a definitive diagnosis than the scapular lateral view. Accurate radiographs are required prior to reduction maneuvers because further displacement of neck fractures may be caused iatrogenically. One study reported seven such cases; surgical neck fracture that was unidentified prior to the attempted reduction was apparent in three of these cases. Complete displacement of the head segment occurred in five cases. These authors concluded that surgical neck fractures should be carefully looked for, especially when tuberosity fractures were also identified. It should be noted that only biplanar (scapular AP and lateral) views were used in this series and that perhaps the addition of the axillary view would have increased diagnostic accuracy prior to attempted reduction.

Treatment/Results

Goals of fracture management include restoring anatomy, obtaining soft-tissue and osseous healing, and maximizing the function of the entire upper extremity. Indications for surgical versus nonsurgical management are dictated by a host of factors, including degree of fracture displacement, fracture type, physiologic age, and general medical condition of the patient as well as his/her ability to comply with an intensive rehabilitation program. Bone quality, concomitant medical problems, associated injury, and arm dominance are also important factors to be considered with regard to the patient. The surgeon's level of expertise and knowledge of complex anatomy also plays a role in the management of these injuries.

Although 85% of proximal humerus fractures are minimally displaced, the amount of literature dedicated to this majority is inversely proportional to its incidence. If a fracture fails to meet the above-described criteria according to the Neer classification, it is deemed to be a nondisplaced or minimally displaced fracture. In general, minimally displaced injuries are considered to do well with emphasis placed on functional outcome. A short period of immobilization, usually with a sling and swathe, and early passive range of motion exercises instituted when the fracture fragments are believed to move as a single unit (usually within 14 days) is advised to optimize results. The institution of this exercise program within 14 days has been found to significantly improve postinjury results. Once union has been documented on radiographs, treatment progresses to active range of motion and strengthening with progressive resistant exercises. Overly aggressive passive motion or active motion prior to fracture healing has been correlated with increased rates of nonunion. A detailed functional outcome analysis was performed on 104 nondisplaced or minimally displaced proximal humerus fractures that were treated nonsurgically with immobilization and early passive range of motion exercises. Emphasis was placed on functional recovery and activities of daily living. Good to excellent results were found in 77% of patients; the institution of an early passive range of motion exercise program within 14 days also improved results. Although patients were found to have 94% functional recovery, 44% reported pain of varying degrees and 5% reported a compromised ability to perform activities of daily living.

Unstable displaced fractures are most often not amenable to nonsurgical management and may require surgical intervention by either open reduction and internal fixation or prosthetic replacement. Although some two-part fractures and fracture-dislocations will do well with closed reduction with or without percutaneous pinning, many displaced two- and three-part fractures will require open reduction and internal fixation. Fracture patterns amenable to open reduction and internal fixation include two-part greater and lesser tuberosity fractures, surgical neck fractures in which a closed reduction cannot be obtained or maintained, and some anatomic neck fractures in which there is adequate bone quantity and quality within the humeral head to allow fixation. Surgical neck fracture-dislocations as well as two-part tuberosity fracture-dislocations with persistent tuberosity displacement after glenohumeral joint reduction warrant surgical intervention. Open reduction and internal fixation remains the treatment of choice for most three-part fractures and fracture-dislocations. In the event that the tuberosity and head fragments are too osteoporotic with frail soft-tissue insertions, preventing adequate secure fixation for early passive motion, prosthetic replacement is the better treatment. Prosthetic replacement is also indicated in four-part fractures and fracture-dislocations, head-splitting fractures, and in impression fractures involving greater than 40% of the articular surface.

Techniques of internal fixation are vast and varied. Plate fixation has been popular in the past, but minimal internal fixation techniques have recently been advocated in response to the high morbidity associated with plate fixation, including loss of fixation in osteoporotic bone, plate impingement in the subacromial space, and osteonecrosis from the soft-tissue stripping required for plate application (Fig. 2). Decreased morbidity has been reported with the use of a modified cloverleaf plate. Various other techniques, such as skeletal traction, external fixation, percutaneous pins, staples, and intramedullary nail and wire constructs, have been described. The use of suture or wire tension band fixation, particularly in osteoporotic bone, is reported to have several advantages: (1) Less extensive exposure and soft-tissue stripping may preserve humeral head vascularity. (2) Incorporation of the rotator cuff insertion is often stronger than fixation in osteoporotic bone. (3) When combined in a figure-of-8 tension band fashion with intramedullary nails or rods, this configuration can produce extremely solid fixation, which allows early passive motion critical for successful results.

Management of two-part surgical neck fractures is dependent on the inherent stability of the fracture. Fractures in which stable closed reduction is obtained may be treated as such with or without the addition of percutaneous pin fixation. If a stable reduction cannot be obtained and/or maintained, fixation is warranted. In one series reporting 48 fractures treated with closed reduction and percutaneous pin fixation, the importance of pin placement (at least three 2.5-mm terminally threaded pins are used) is stressed, but open reduction and limited internal fixation is advised for three-part fractures involving the greater tuberosity. Complications of this technique included pin tract infection with fixation loosening, malunion, and humeral shaft fracture at the site of pin insertion after removal of hardware. Eighteen of 29 (62%) two-part surgical neck fractures, all eight three-part

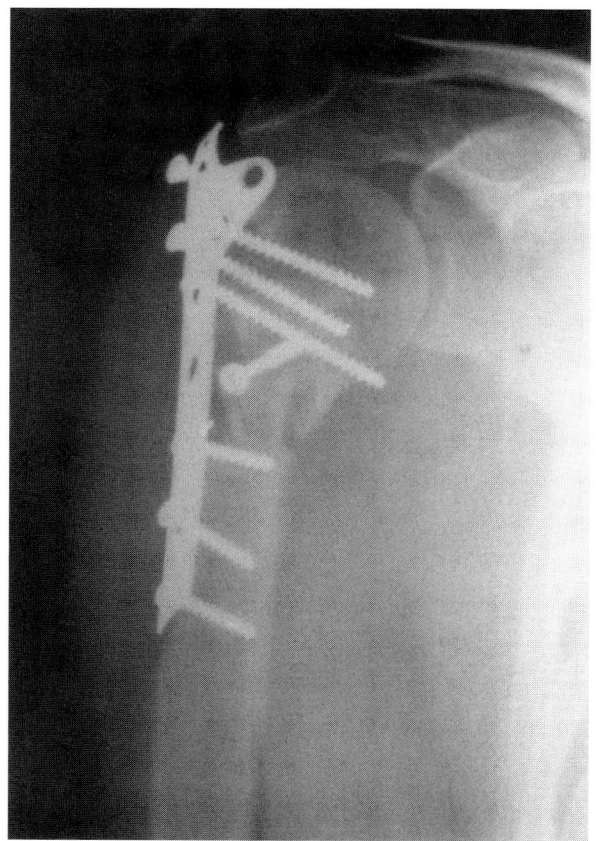

Fig. 2 Loss of plate and screw fixation in osteoporotic bone with subacromial impingement.

fractures, and three of five (60%) four-part fractures had a good or excellent result. Nonunion was noted in two fractures and loss of fixation in four.

Open reduction and internal fixation is indicated for two-part surgical neck fractures in which soft-tissue interposition of the deltoid or biceps tendon precludes obtaining an acceptable closed reduction. Open reduction and internal fixation using plate fixation was compared to Rush pin insertion through the greater tuberosity combined with a tension band wire to the shaft in one series. Plate fixation was found to achieve good functional results for seven of eight patients younger than 50 years of age who sustained injuries from high-velocity trauma. However, injury caused by low energy levels is more common in patients with osteoporosis. Results were unsatisfactory in 12 of 14, with failure usually caused by loss of fixation. The Rush pin technique produced more reliable results in this age group, with satisfactory functional scores obtained in 16 of 23 patients. The authors suggest that the Rush pin technique is preferable to plate fixation in the more common osteoporotic insufficiency fracture in the elderly. Other authors have reported open reduction and internal fixation of two- and three-part surgical neck fractures with heavy nonabsorbable suture or wire that incorporated the rotator cuff tendons, tuberosities, and shaft. In cases with significant surgical neck comminution, curved 3.5-mm Ender nails were inserted antegrade and combined with a tension band construct that provided three-point fixation with additional longitudinal and rotational stability (Fig. 3). Eighteen (82%) of 22 patients had good or excellent results. Results were good to excellent for 71% of two-part and 100% of three-part surgical neck fractures with an average active elevation of 142°, external rotation to 47°, and internal rotation to the 11th thoracic vertebrae. The authors modified the Ender nail procedure by placing an additional hole above the eyelet for passage of the tension band suture, allowing for deeper insertion of the nail well below the surface of the rotator cuff tendon. Subsequent to this modification, no patient required rod removal as a result of prominence with encroachment on the subacromial space. All fractures achieved union. There were no infections, and partial loss of fixation occurred once.

Because of the high incidence of osteonecrosis secondary to the disruption of vascularity to the articular segment, humeral head replacement remains the preferred method of management in two-part anatomic neck fractures. In the young, active patient in whom the articular segment is of adequate size and quality, open reduction and internal fixation or percutaneous pin fixation may be attempted with the understanding that the development of osteonecrosis may necessitate revision surgery.

Two-part tuberosity fractures may occur as isolated injuries or in conjunction with glenohumeral dislocations. Anterior and posterior dislocations are associated with greater and lesser tuberosity fractures, respectively. Fracture-dislocations of this type tend to respond well to closed reduction and subsequent immobilization with early passive motion. Redislocation is rare after fracture healing. Up to 80% of posterior dislocations are still reportedly missed on initial presentation. Complete radiographic evaluation with an axillary view is required to improve diagnostic accuracy. After reduction of the joint, the tuberosity will often return to its cancellous bed in near anatomic position. If there is significant residual displacement, the anatomy should be restored surgically with open reduction and internal fixation in addition to repair of the rotator cuff tear.

Isolated greater tuberosity fractures are pulled superiorly or posteriorly by the rotator cuff insertion. A recent report on open reduction and internal fixation of two-part greater tuberosity fractures indicated that the scapular AP and lateral views failed to demonstrate the precise amount of posterior retraction and overlap of the fragment with the articular surface. The need for surgical intervention was underestimated in four of 16 patients. The authors stress the importance of the axillary view to correctly assess posterior displacement. In the same series, a deltoid-splitting approach combined with heavy nonabsorbable suture fixation of the tuberosity and rotator cuff repair gave good to excellent results in 100% of 12 patients, with active forward elevation to 170°.

Although most often associated with posterior glenohumeral dislocation or with fractures of two or three other segments of the proximal humerus, isolated lesser tuberosity fractures have also been described. The most common mechanism of injury is a forceful external rotation and abduction injury as the tension in the subscapularis is at its maximum in this position. As with greater tuberosity fractures, because of

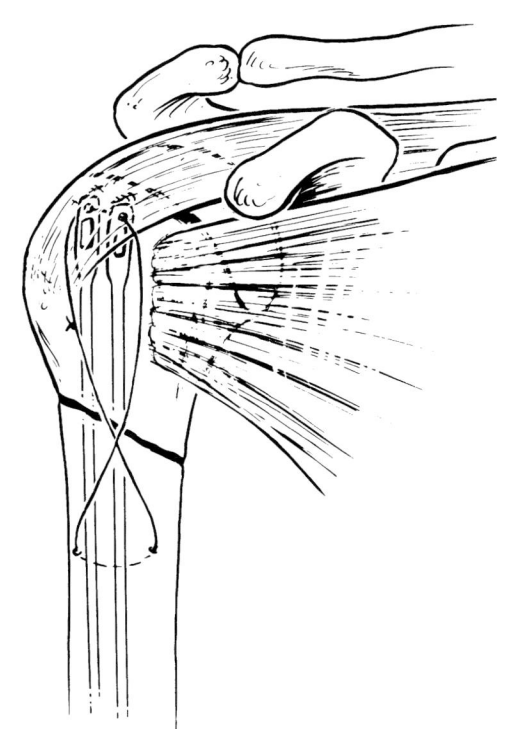

Fig. 3 Figure-of-8 tension band fixation supplemented with Ender nails incorporates strong rotator cuff in repair.

the overlap of the tuberosity fragment with the humeral head on the AP view, this condition may be underdiagnosed unless adequate radiographs are obtained. Specifically, the axillary view identifies medial retraction of the lesser tuberosity. Open reduction and internal fixation is warranted if a significant portion of the articular surface is involved and/or the level of pain or limitation of internal rotation are unacceptable to the patient. Excision of the avulsed lesser tuberosity fragment with repair of the subscapularis and anterior capsule has also been described. One recent study reported on six patients with isolated lesser tuberosity fractures over a 4-year span. Internal and external rotation was impaired in all patients. The diagnosis was missed initially when AP radiographs were used and subsequently confirmed with an axillary view and/or CT scan. Two of the six had concomitant biceps dislocation or rupture. Fractures in five patients were displaced, and reattachment of the lesser tuberosity fragment and the subscapularis tendon improved their condition. The authors recommended obtaining an axillary view to improve diagnostic accuracy in addition to a CT scan to evaluate the size and displacement of the fragment and determine the possibility of an accompanying biceps tendon injury. Treatment recommendations included use of a sling for 3 weeks, which will prevent external rotation and abduction in nondisplaced fractures and promote tuberosity reattachment with rotator cuff repair in displaced injuries.

Three-part fractures and fracture-dislocations are often best managed with open reduction and internal fixation. Techniques similar to those discussed for two-part surgical neck fractures are applicable. Tension band wiring with and without intramedullary nails has yielded excellent results in several reported series. Standard T plate fixation has lost favor because of reported high failure rates related to extensive tissue stripping, inadequate screw fixation, and hardware impingement that required additional surgery for removal. Treatment of three- and four-part fractures with a modified cloverleaf plate in 26 younger patients (19 to 62 years) yielded excellent results in 22, good results in two, and fair results in two. The authors stated that this small, malleable plate, which allows placement of four small cancellous screws into the head and tuberosities, could be placed high on the head without impingement. They suggested that the improved results obtained were related to limited exposure, careful soft-tissue dissection, and stable fixation with less damage to the head fragment than with 6.5-mm cancellous screws used with T plates. Good bone stock in this population was also a factor. In cases in which rigid fixation cannot be obtained to a satisfactory degree, humeral head replacement may be warranted, in order that early passive exercises can be performed.

Immediate humeral head replacement remains the accepted treatment for four-part fractures and fracture-dislocations, although open reduction and internal fixation may be considered in young patients with good bone quality and absence of dislocation. A series of 35 patients with four-part fractures and fracture-dislocations with a mean age of 59 years were treated with Kirschner wires and tension band fixation. Results were satisfactory for 65%, with 35% unsatisfactory and poor results. Nine patients (25%) developed osteonecrosis, and all cases of fracture-dislocation yielded unsatisfactory or poor results with 100% osteonecrosis. These data corroborate results of previous studies that distinguish between four-part valgus impacted fractures and the classic displaced four-part fracture-dislocation. Reconstruction rather than replacement for the valgus impacted humeral head fracture has gained attention in the recent literature because the rate of osteonecrosis has been found to be much lower than in its classic counterpart. Results of repair of this injury were reported in one study in which the medial periosteum and its traversing vascularization to the articular surface were left intact. Open reduction was performed by elevating the impacted humeral head, relocating the tuberosities, and filling the void with cancellous bone chips. Minimal osteosynthesis was employed, with 1.8-mm Kirschner wires used to secure the head to the shaft and numerous sutures used to anchor the tuberosities to each other and to the shaft. With minimum follow-up of 18 months, an osteonecrosis rate of only 9% with positive correlation between the quality of reduction achieved and the functional result was found. Three of 22 patients were found to have mild to moderate arthrosis at follow-up. These authors also suggest that the low incidence of osteonecrosis and the positive results were related to the relatively young patient age (average, 52 years) and the strict inclusion criteria for reconstruction that was based on minimal or no lateral displacement of the shaft in relation to the head, thereby minimizing damage to the medial periosteal vascularity.

The majority of four-part fractures and fracture-dislocations are best managed with humeral head replacement. Technical considerations that have been found to correlate with successful outcome include the restoration of humeral length and retroversion (35° to 45°), secure tuberosity fixation, repair of the rotator cuff, and achievement of anatomic humeral offset. Numerous studies have demonstrated consistently reliable results with respect to pain relief. Outcome after humeral replacement for acute three- and four-part fractures has been reported to be dependent on such factors as age, sex, and fracture type, particularly with respect to active range of motion. Age older than 70 years, four-part fractures, and female sex were factors that correlated with a poor active range of motion (although the female average age was 77 compared to the male average of 68 years). Functional results revealed that pain was minimal, although active motion and function were unpredictably restored as 45% of patients reported difficulty with seven or more of the functional tasks described by the American Shoulder and Elbow Surgeons. These authors report that meticulous tuberosity and rotator cuff repair, appropriate soft-tissue tensioning, and an intensive physician-supervised rehabilitation program are all contributing factors to successful humeral head replacement after fracture.

Articular surface fractures include head-splitting injuries and impression defects that occur as a result of impaction against the glenoid rim. Humeral head replacement is indicated in most head-splitting fractures. Impression fractures most often occur with posterior dislocation; their management is governed by the size of the humeral head defect and the duration of dislocation (Fig. 4). A stable closed reduction can usually be obtained in defects that involve less than 20% of the articular surface and have been present for less than 6 weeks. After reduction, patients are immobilized, with the arm at the side in 10° to 15° of external rotation, for 4 to 6 weeks. If the dislocation is present for more than 6 weeks, open reduction is indicated. Defects involving 20% to 40% of the articular surface that have been present for less than 6 months can be successfully treated with open reduction and transfer of the lesser tuberosity into the defect through an anterior deltopectoral approach. When the defect is greater than 40% of the articular surface or the dislocation has been present for longer than 6 months, humeral head replacement is indicated with decreased retroversion to insure stability. When diagnosis is delayed longer than 6 months, the glenoid may become involved and glenoid resurfacing may be necessary. Acute posterior fracture-dislocations of the shoulder have been treated with Neer's modification of the McLaughlin procedure, described as the transfer of the lesser tuberosity with the subscapularis tendon into the anteromedial impression fracture to enhance stability and prevent the glenoid from falling into the defect. Indications for this procedure included unstable fractures with defects involving 20% to 40% of the articular surface. Fixation was achieved with 6.5-mm cancellous screws sufficient to allow immediate passive and active motion. There were no redislocations and an almost full range of motion was achieved in all patients. Chronic anterior dislocations also present a significant management problem that was discussed in a report of nine patients who were treated with unconstrained replacement arthroplasty. The results were satisfactory or excellent in eight of nine. The authors stressed the need for increased humeral retroversion, glenoid bone grafting when anterior bone loss is

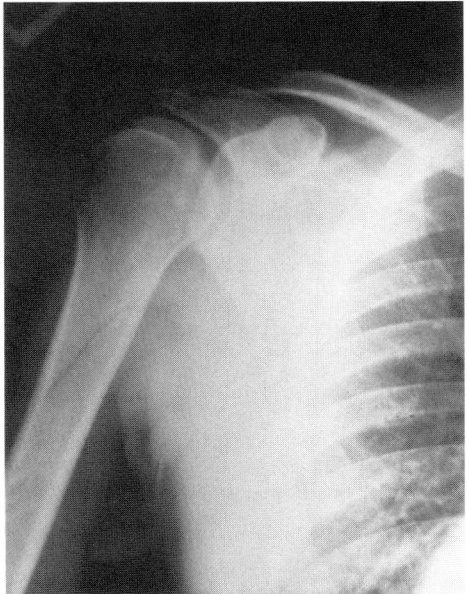

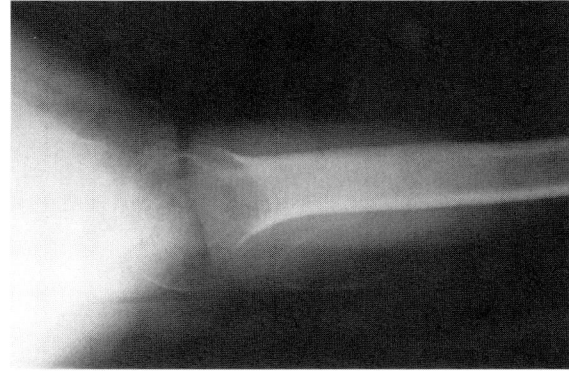

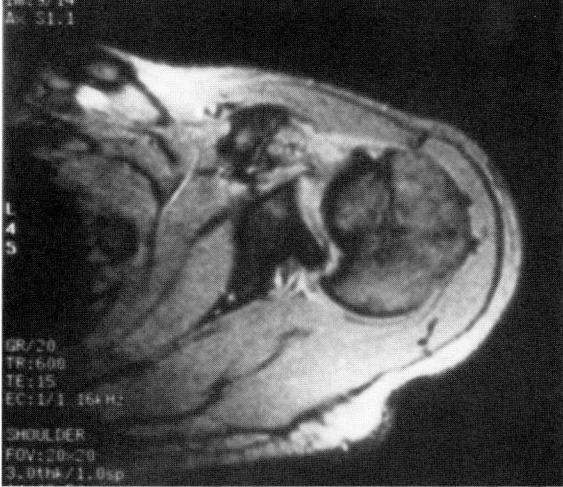

Fig. 4 Scapular AP **(top)**, axillary **(center)**, and MRI **(bottom)** views of locked posterior dislocation.

found to involve 50% of the articular surface, soft-tissue releases, and modified rehabilitation more consistent with an instability repair than with shoulder replacement surgery.

Rehabilitation remains an integral part of the postoperative and postinjury management, with optimum results requiring strict attention to protocols. The most useful protocol consists of three phases. Early passive motion is the initial phase and is imperative after open reduction and internal fixation or humeral head replacement. There should be no active motion for 6 weeks until the fracture or tuberosities have healed. Active and early resistive exercise is then instituted in the second phase after radiographic evidence of healing is apparent. The third phase involves advanced stretching and strengthening exercises with progressive resistance, weights, and bands. Patients often continue to progress over 12 to 18 months. Therefore, to maximize outcomes, the rehabilitation program should persist throughout this time frame.

Complications

Complications following proximal humeral head fracture treatment may be related to the injury itself or to the treatment approach chosen. The most frequently encountered complications include joint stiffness, malunion, nonunion, osteonecrosis, and heterotopic ossification.

Joint stiffness is the most common complication following proximal humeral fractures. The causes of loss of motion are multifactorial and include the severity of the initial injury, prolonged immobilization, noncompliance with a postoperative rehabilitation program, and malunion of the articular surface and/or tuberosities. Management of restricted motion following fracture is dependent on the underlying etiology, with periarticular fibrosis being the most common. This condition may be secondary to the fracture itself or to the soft-tissue changes that occur following open reduction and internal fixation. A structured, comprehensive rehabilitation program will almost always be successful in regaining a functional range of motion as long as significant malunion is not present. At least 6 months of therapy following fracture is required to regain optimal recovery of motion. Closed manipulation is rarely indicated and should be avoided because of the risk of refracture and additional injury. If malunion results in a mechanical block to motion, treatment should be directed toward correction of malunion.

Malunion results from either inadequate reduction of the displaced fragments or loss of fixation following internal fixation. Malunion involving the displaced greater tuberosity often causes pain and restriction of motion. If the direction of displacement of the tuberosity is superior, it will block overhead elevation, whereas posterior displacement limits external rotation. In these situations, osteotomy of the greater tuberosity with lateral advancement and reattachment combined with rotator cuff repair is the preferred treatment. Preoperative CT scanning may help to identify the exact position of the malunited fragment. Two-part surgical neck fractures with residual displacement and angulation of the shaft may also result in restriction of motion; however, this condition is less often associated with pain. The range of motion is often functional and does not require specific treatment. Rarely, significant varus deformity may result in impingement of the undersurface of the acromion in forward elevation and abduction. Acromioplasty may increase the available subacromial space but does not correct the deformity. Corrective osteotomy may be required with realignment of the tuberosity to a more anatomic position. Malunion of three- and four-part fractures is a formidable problem that often requires prosthetic replacement with tuberosity osteotomy and reconstruction.

Nonunions encountered after proximal humerus fractures most often involve the surgical neck. Causes of surgical neck nonunions include overly aggressive early passive range of motion and active exercises prior to radiographic healing. These nonunions are not necessarily painful nor do they always involve functional deficits. Therefore, careful assessment of the disability is necessary. Usually there is a loss of active elevation that may or may not be associated with significant discomfort. If surgical treatment is undertaken secondary to pain and functional disability, treatment options include open reduction and internal fixation with bone grafting or prosthetic replacement. Significant complications and failures from this type of surgery have been reported. Therefore, the indications for surgical management should be carefully considered.

Osteonecrosis is primarily a complication of three- and four-part fracture-dislocations. Several investigators have found that this complication is more common following open reduction and internal fixation with plates and screws than after less extensive or minimal osteosynthesis procedures. The treatment of osteonecrosis of the humeral head is dependent on the extent of symptoms, and its mere presence does not result in pain and loss of motion. When collapse occurs with secondary degenerative changes about the glenoid articular surface, there is often pain and loss of motion. The treatment of choice is then prosthetic replacement with either humeral head replacement or total shoulder replacement based on the condition of the glenoid.

Heterotopic bone formation of different degrees of severity is quite common about the proximal humerus after fracture and fracture-dislocation. The severity of the injury, repeated attempts at closed reduction, and the length of time from injury to the time of surgical intervention are important factors in its development. In most cases, however, heterotopic ossification is not a cause of significant disability. Surgical intervention is rarely warranted. In the unusual case where severe restriction of motion and disability occur, surgical resection can be considered but should not be undertaken until the ossification has completely matured as evidenced by "cold" bone scan.

Selected Bibliography

Cofield RH: Comminuted fractures of the proximal humerus. *Clin Orthop* 1988;230:49-57.

Cuomo F, Flatow EL, Maday MG, et al: Open reduction and internal fixation of two- and three-part displaced surgical neck fractures of the proximal humerus. *J Shoulder Elbow Surg* 1992;1:287-295.

Twenty-two patients with two- and three-part displaced surgical neck fractures were treated with open reduction and limited internal fixation with heavy nonabsorbable sutures incorporating the rotator cuff, tuberosities, and shaft. Humeral Ender nails were incorporated in a tension band fashion to increase rotatory and longitudinal stability. There were 82% good or excellent results, 14% satisfactory, and 4% unsatisfactory results reported. There were no cases of osteonecrosis and only one partial loss of fixation.

de Laat EA, Visser CP, Coene LN, et al: Nerve lesions in primary shoulder dislocations and humeral neck fractures: A prospective clinical and EMG study. *J Bone Joint Surg* 1994;76B:381-383.

Electrophysiologic evidence of nerve injuries was identified in 45% of 101 patients with primary shoulder dislocation or fracture of the humeral neck. Axillary, suprascapular, radial, and musculocutaneous nerves were most often involved. Authors stress early diagnosis to prevent lasting impairment of function.

Esser RD: Treatment of three- and four-part fractures of the proximal humerus with a modified cloverleaf plate. *J Orthop Trauma* 1994;8:15-22.

In 26 young patients who had three- and four-part fractures, open reduction and internal fixation using a modified cloverleaf plate yielded good or excellent results in 24 patients, with no evidence of osteonecrosis. Plate malleability, the use of 4.0-mm rather than 6.5-mm screws in the head region, a low superior plate profile, and a youthful population with good bone stock were believed to be contributing factors to the successful results.

Flatow EL, Cuomo F, Maday MG, et al: Open reduction and internal fixation of two-part displaced fractures of the greater tuberosity of the proximal part of the humerus. *J Bone Joint Surg* 1991;73A:1213-1218.

Twelve patients with two-part greater tuberosity fractures treated with open reduction through a deltoid-splitting approach, internal fixation with heavy nonabsorbable suture, and rotator cuff repair are reviewed. All fractures healed, with six excellent and six good results, and average active forward elevation of 170°.

Goldman RT, Koval KJ, Cuomo F, et al: Functional outcome after humeral head replacement for acute three- and four-part proximal humeral fractures. *J Shoulder Elbow Surg* 1995;4:81-86.

This retrospective review analyzes the results of 26 humeral head replacements for acute three- and four-part fractures identifying factors affecting outcome including humeral offset, age, sex, and fracture type.

Hawkins RJ, Bell RH, Gurr K: The three-part fracture of the proximal part of the humerus: Operative treatment. *J Bone Joint Surg* 1986;68A:1410-1414.

Kristiansen B, Christensen SW: Plate fixation of proximal humeral fractures. *Acta Orthop Scand* 1986;57:320-323.

Hersche O, Gerber C: Iatrogenic displacement of fracture-dislocations of the shoulder: A report of seven cases. *J Bone Joint Surg* 1994;76B:30-33.

This retrospective report discusses seven cases in which open or closed reduction of a shoulder dislocation associated with fracture of the humeral neck led to displacement of the neck fracture. In three of the seven cases the neck fracture was unrecognized with biplanar views (scapular anteroposterior and lateral), reinforcing the need to obtain the axillary view.

Jaberg H, Warner JJ, Jakob RP: Percutaneous stabilization of unstable fractures of the humerus. *J Bone Joint Surg* 1992;74A:508-515.

Closed reduction and percutaneous pinning in 48 patients yielded good to excellent results in 70%, fair to poor results in 30%, loss of fixation in four patients, with complete osteonecrosis in two and subtotal osteonecrosis in eight. Authors suggest that three-part fractures with greater tuberosity displacement and four-part/head-splitting fractures are better suited for open reduction and limited internal fixation and humeral head replacement, respectively.

Neer CS II: Displaced proximal humeral fractures: Part I. Classification and evaluation. *J Bone Joint Surg* 1970;52A:1077-1089.

Neer CS II: Displaced proximal humerus fractures: Part II. Treatment of three-part and four-part displacement. *J Bone Joint Surg* 1970;52A:1090-1103.

Nordqvist A, Petersson CJ: Incidence and causes of shoulder girdle injuries in an urban population. *J Shoulder Elbow Surg* 1995;4:107-112.

This 1-year, prospective, population-based study determines the incidence and causes of major injuries involving fractures and dislocations about the clavicle, scapula, and proximal humerus in children, adults, and the elderly.

Resch H, Beck E, Bayley I: Reconstruction of the valgus-impacted humeral head fracture. *J Shoulder Elbow Surg* 1995;4:73-80.

The authors review results of 22 cases of open reduction and internal fixation of valgus impacted fractures and discuss technical details and diagnostic inclusion criteria.

Sidor ML, Zuckerman JD, Lyon T, et al: Classification of proximal humerus fractures: The contribution of the scapular lateral and axillary radiographs. *J Shoulder Elbow Surg* 1994;3:24-27.

Trauma series radiographs of 50 proximal humerus fractures were used to assess the relative contribution of the scapular lateral and axillary radiographs to fracture classification with the Neer four-segment system. The authors report that when combined with the scapular anteroposterior radiograph, the axillary view makes a more significant contribution to fracture classification than the scapular lateral radiograph.

van Laarhoven HA, te Slaa RL, van Laarhoven EW: Isolated avulsion fracture of the lesser tuberosity of the humerus. *J Trauma* 1995;39:997-999.

Six cases of isolated lesser tuberosity fractures are reviewed with reference to diagnosis and treatment recommendations.

Zuckerman JD, Koval KJ, Powell SE, et al: One-part proximal humerus fractures: A prospective study, in Vastamaki M, Jalovaara P (eds): *Surgery of the Shoulder.* Amsterdam, The Netherlands, Elsevier Science, 1995, pp 423-427.

One hundred four nondisplaced proximal humerus fractures were treated nonsurgically with immobilization and early passive motion. Institution of passive exercises in less than 14 days was found to significantly improve results. The authors stress emphasis on functional outcome and activities of daily living.

21

Clavicle Fractures

Anthony A. Romeo, MD

Introduction

Clavicle fractures represent 10% to 12% of all fractures and are the most common childhood fracture. Two thirds of all shoulder fractures involve the clavicle. Because of its subcutaneous location, clavicle fractures are easily recognized. With few exceptions, clavicle fractures will unite without complications. A variety of successful treatment methods have been used, with the sling or figure-of-8 splint being the most common. Although the majority of clavicle fractures heal, many patients have a residual deformity that is primarily a cosmetic problem. In general, patient satisfaction and return of shoulder function with nonsurgical management is quite favorable.

Anatomy

Ossification of the clavicle usually occurs during the fifth week of gestation. The clavicle is the only long bone in which ossification is intermembranous. The epiphyseal growth plates develop at both the medial and lateral ends of the clavicle; the medial growth plate is responsible for the majority of longitudinal growth. Fusion of the sternal or medial ossification center occurs between 20 and 25 years of age. Injuries to the medial side of the clavicle before fusion of the medial ossification center are actually epiphyseal fractures.

The clavicle connects the shoulder girdle and upper extremity to the axial skeleton through the sternoclavicular joint. The position of the clavicle and the chest wall directly affects scapular motion. If the clavicle is removed, the amount of scapular motion increases substantially and the shoulder is weakened as a result of a loss of trunk-arm linkage.

The shape of the clavicle has important functional implications (Fig. 1). From the anterior view, the clavicle is a relatively straight bone. However, from the superior view, it forms an S-shaped curve. Furthermore, the clavicle is relatively round in its center portion, but on the lateral aspect it widens in its anteroposterior (AP) dimensions and flattens in its superior-inferior dimensions. The middle third of the clavicle is weakest in axial loading and is the location of the majority of clavicle fractures.

The clavicle is the site of numerous muscular attachments, including the trapezius and sternocleidomastoid muscles on its superior surface, the subclavius on the inferior surface, and the deltoid and pectoralis major on its anterior surface. The relationship between the middle third of the clavicle and the neurovascular structures, which lie directly inferior, leads to a small but appreciable level of fracture-associated neurovascular complications. The majority of neurologic injuries associated with clavicle fractures result in deficits of the lower portion of the brachial plexus; ulnar nerve dysfunction is most common. Displaced fractures of the clavicle that heal in a malunited position or develop substantial callus can encroach upon the costoclavicular space and result in compression of the neurovascular bundle as it passes underneath the clavicle.

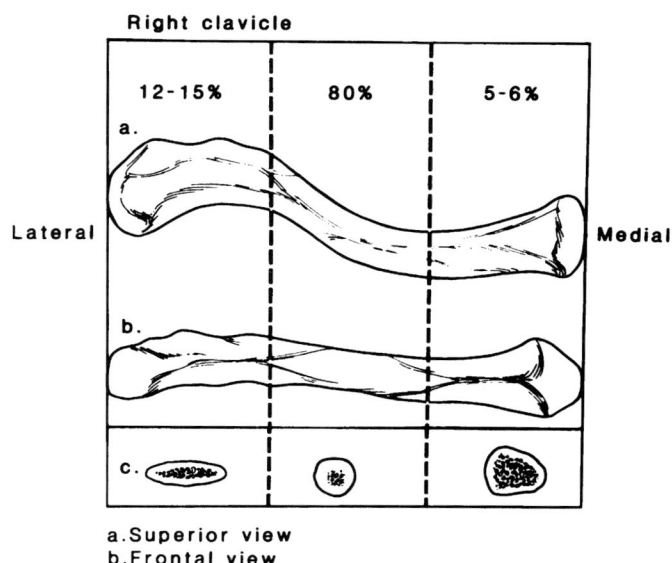

Fig. 1 Anatomy of the clavicle. (Reproduced with permission from Craig E: Fractures of the clavicle, in Rockwood CA Jr, Matsen FA III (eds): *The Shoulder*. Philadelphia, PA, WB Saunders, 1990.)

The motion of the clavicle is complex. When the arm is raised overhead, the clavicle can angle upward approximately 30° and backward an additional 35° based on a fixed sternoclavicular joint axis. The clavicle also rotates approximately 50° on its longitudinal axis. This rotation of the clavicle, particularly at its lateral end, is important for the full elevation of the upper extremity as it is closely integrated with scapular motion. Approximately half of the overall elevation of the scapula is affected by the relationship of the clavicle to the axis of the thorax. Fixation of the clavicle at the sternoclavicular joint or the acromioclavicular joint will result in limitation of overall shoulder motion.

Etiology

Clavicle fractures occur as a result of direct and indirect mechanisms. Recent studies have shown that direct injury is more common and can cause fractures along the entire clavicle. Direct mechanisms include a fall onto the lateral aspect of the shoulder or a direct blow to the clavicle. A fall onto the outstretched hand is the most common indirect cause, resulting in fractures of the middle third of the clavicle. Studies show that clavicle fractures occur more often in patients who participate in sports, and are more common in men than in women.

Clinical Evaluation

The diagnosis of clavicle fractures is easily confirmed with inspection and palpation of the area. Examination usually reveals significant tenderness and swelling with ecchymosis. The degree of deformity depends on the location of the fracture and the degree of displacement. Middle third fractures occur just lateral to the attachment of the sternocleidomastoid muscle. The classic displacement pattern is a superior position of the medial fragment (as a result of the upward pull of the sternocleidomastoid muscle) and inferior position of the lateral fragment (as a result of the weight of the upper extremity). Open clavicle fractures are rare and are easily identified on physical examination. Because of the proximity of the neurovascular structures, a careful neurovascular examination of the upper extremity should be performed.

Three percent of clavicle fractures present with associated injuries, including brachial plexus involvement, vascular injury, and pneumothorax. Rib fractures as well as associated head and neck injuries indicate more severe trauma. A chest radiograph should be obtained in order to rule out associated injuries following a fracture caused by high-energy trauma.

Neurologic injuries occur as a result of the relationship of the clavicle to the brachial plexus. Most brachial plexus injuries represent contusions. Rarely, comminuted clavicle fractures with sharp fragments may be responsible for direct penetrating injury to the brachial plexus or to the underlying subclavian vascular structures. Because the portion of the brachial plexus that forms the ulnar nerve lies adjacent to the middle third of the clavicle, dysfunction of the ulnar nerve is the most common associated neurologic injury.

Acute vascular injuries are rare because the subclavius muscle and the cervical fascia provide soft tissue protection against direct injury. Vascular injuries can include acute compression, laceration, or spasm. The subclavian vein and artery are most commonly injured. The subclavian vein is vulnerable to tearing because of its fixed position beneath the clavicle. If an injury to the major vessels is suspected, an arteriogram and consultation with a vascular surgeon are indicated.

Radiologic Evaluation

Radiologic evaluation is dependent on the location of the fracture. For middle third fractures, the recommended views include an AP projection to evaluate the superior-inferior displacement; a 45° cephalic tilt view to evaluate the anterior-posterior displacement; and a chest radiograph to evaluate evidence of an associated injury, such as pneumothorax.

For lateral one third fractures, an AP view with a 15° cephalic tilt using decreased power (Zanca view) will profile the lateral end of the clavicle away from the scapula, thereby providing enhanced visualization. An axillary lateral view will demonstrate anterior-posterior displacement. Stress views are valuable when an associated ligamentous injury is suspected. Computed tomographic (CT) scans may provide additional information, particularly if extension of the fracture into the articular surface of the acromioclavicular joint is suspected. However, good quality standard radiographs minimize the need for specialized studies such as CT scan or magnetic resonance imaging (MRI).

Fractures of the medial third of the clavicle are best visualized with an AP projection as well as a serendipity view. The serendipity view is obtained with the x-ray beam aimed at a 40° cephalic tilt. Special imaging studies such as a CT scan are more commonly used for medial clavicle fractures because of the difficulty in visualizing this area with standard radiographs. Furthermore, displaced medial clavicle fractures associated with severe direct trauma may result in injuries to the underlying vital structures.

Classification

The classification of clavicle fractures is based primarily on their anatomic location. The three major categories include the middle third, lateral third, and medial third clavicle fractures. These three groups can be further divided into specific fracture patterns.

Middle clavicle fractures represent 80% of all clavicle fractures. The injury generally occurs at the point where the clavicle has no muscular or ligamentous attachments. The description of the fracture is based on long bone fracture patterns (such as oblique or transverse), fracture displacement, and the degree of comminution at the fracture site.

Lateral third clavicle fractures represent 15% of all clavicle fractures and are divided into three types (Fig. 2). Type 1 occurs lateral to the coracoclavicular ligaments but does not involve the acromioclavicular joint. This fracture is stabilized by the coracoclavicular and acromioclavicular ligaments. Type 2 fractures are divided into two subgroups based on the injury to the coracoclavicular ligaments. Type 2A occurs just medial to the conoid and trapezoid ligaments, which remain intact. In type 2B fractures, the conoid ligament is disrupted but the trapezoid ligament remains attached to the lateral fragment. Displaced type 2 fractures have an increased rate of nonunion. The weight of the arm creates a significant inferior force on the lateral fragment, whereas the medial fragment is supported by the pull of the sternocleidomastoid muscle. Type 3 fractures involve an intra-articular extension of the fracture and generally occur on the inferior surface of the lateral aspect of the clavicle.

Because of the late fusion of the lateral clavicle growth plate, injuries to the lateral clavicle in children and young adults may result in an epiphyseal fracture of the lateral clavicle. The term "pseudodislocation" has been used to describe this injury; these fractures have been alternatively classified as type 4 fractures. Type 4 fractures mimic acromioclavicular joint injuries but, in fact, represent epiphyseal fractures. The epiphysis and physes maintain their normal anatomic relationship to the acromion, but the distal metaphyseal section is displaced superiorly. The inferior periosteal sleeve remains anatomic, maintaining its relationship with the coracoclavicular ligaments and acromioclavicular joint.

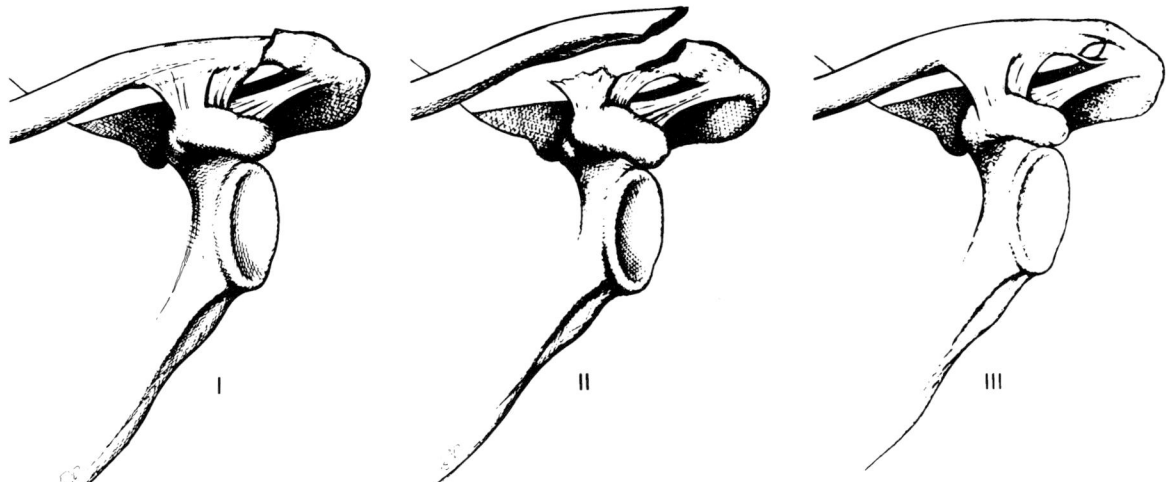

Fig. 2 Distal clavicle fractures. (Reproduced with permission from Neer CS II: Fractures, in Neer CS II (ed): *Shoulder Reconstruction.* Philadelphia, PA, WB Saunders, 1990.)

Fractures of the medial third of the clavicle are uncommon, representing 5% of clavicle fractures. Classification of these fractures is similar to that of lateral clavicle fractures. When these fractures occur in children and younger adults, they are usually epiphyseal injuries.

Treatment

Although a number of methods have been described for the nonsurgical management of clavicular fractures, a sling or a figure-of-8 splint are most common. The figure-of-8 splint may be poorly tolerated by patients because of associated discomfort. Although the sling and the figure-of-8 splint provide minimal immobilization of the fracture fragments, both are associated with a high rate of fracture union and excellent functional outcomes; however, the sling was more comfortable.

Closed Management of Middle Third Clavicle Fractures

There is no consensus regarding the appropriate form of nonsurgical management of middle third clavicle fractures. The sling immobilizes and supports the arm, decreases motion at the fracture site, and is well tolerated; patient compliance is high. The figure-of-8 splint may help the patient maintain better posture, but any benefit to fracture alignment is unclear. The figure-of-8 splint does not support the arm and therefore the lateral fragment may remain depressed. Many patients do not tolerate splinting because of the discomfort involved in maintaining the shoulder in a retracted position. A combination of the sling and the figure-of-8 splint has also been used.

The functional result of nonsurgical management of middle third clavicle fractures is generally acceptable, regardless of the presence of a malunion. Occasionally, a significantly shortened clavicle union may affect shoulder motion, strength, and function.

Open Management of Middle Third Clavicle Fractures

The high rate of union with nonsurgical management and the historical reports of a 10% or more incidence of nonunion with surgical management has clearly discouraged surgical treatment of middle third fractures. Recent reports have demonstrated the efficacy of current techniques of open reduction and internal fixation using either a 3.5-mm pelvic reconstruction plate or a 3.5-mm dynamic compression plate, particularly in the treatment of clavicular nonunions. These reports show faster healing of clavicle fractures and return of full function of the upper extremity.

The indications for open reduction and internal fixation of clavicle fractures include open fracture of the clavicle, associated neurovascular injury with continued neurovascular compromise, associated fracture of the scapular neck, or fracture in conjunction with a scapulothoracic dissociation. Other potential indications include compromise of the skin caused by tenting over the fracture site, multiple trauma requiring early mobilization, and severe displacement of the fracture fragments. Displacement can be distinguished both in terms of separation of the clavicle fractures in the superior-inferior plane as well as the anterior-posterior plane. When greater than 1.5 cm of separation occurs at the fracture site, there may be a higher rate of delayed union and nonunion. In these situations, open reduction and internal fixation may be considered.

The most effective method for open reduction and internal fixation of clavicle fractures is with the use of compression plating techniques as described by the AO/ASIF group (Fig. 3). If adequate compression across the fracture site cannot be achieved, or if more than 30% of bony apposition is compromised by comminution, bone grafting should be performed. For primary clavicle fractures, use of a 3.5-mm pelvic reconstruction plate allows the plate to be contoured in two planes and also provides the opportunity for compression across the fracture site by eccentric drilling of the screw

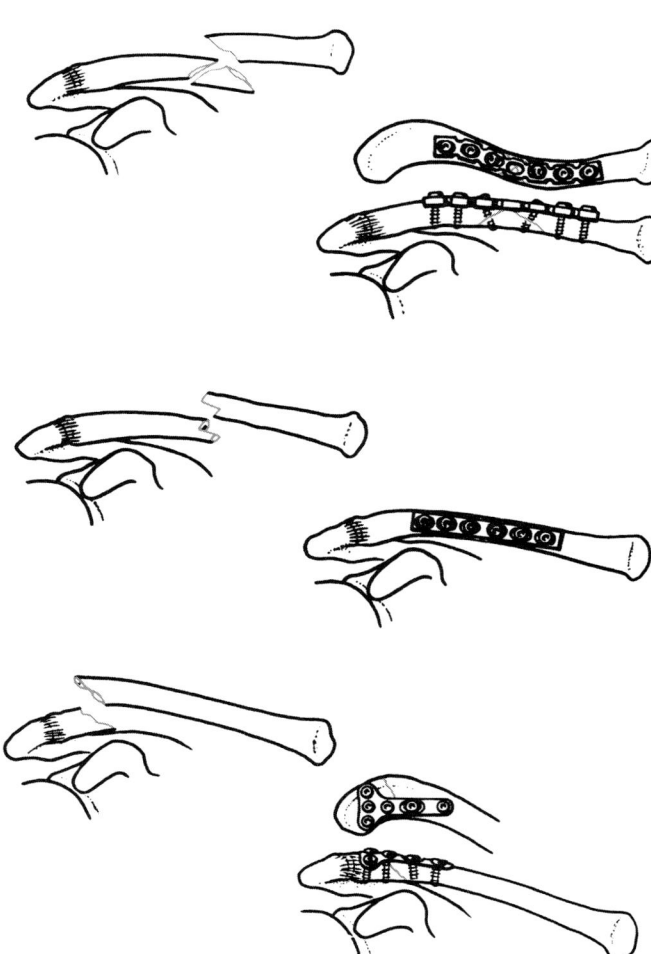

Fig. 3 Fixation of clavicle fractures. **Top,** The 3.5-mm reconstruction plate can be contoured to the shape of the clavicle. The low profile allows for placement on the top or tension side of the clavicle. **Center,** The 3.5-mm dynamic compression plate can be placed on the anterior clavicle, which may allow better soft-tissue coverage. **Bottom,** A small fragment T-plate may be used for fixation of lateral clavicle fractures, allowing placement of multiple screws in the lateral fragment. (Reproduced with permission from Rüedi T, Schweiberer L: Scapula, in Müller ME, Allgöwer M, Schneider R, et al (eds): *Manual of Internal Fixation*. Berlin, Germany, Springer-Verlag, 1991.)

holes. Intrafragmentary compression is preferred because it greatly improves fracture fixation. If the fracture is severely comminuted or if nonunion is present, the stronger 3.5-mm dynamic compression plate is preferred.

Potential technical problems with plate fixation can be overcome with close attention to surgical technique. A cosmetic approach to the fracture includes an oblique incision along Langer's lines over the fracture site. The length of the incision should be equal to the length of the plate. The supraclavicular nerves, which are perpendicular to the clavicle, should be identified and protected. There are generally two or three large branches of the supraclavicular nerves that are within the exposure site of the clavicle fracture. These nerve branches are approximately 2 mm in size. If bone grafting is necessary, it can be obtained from the anterior iliac crest or the distal radius. Using these techniques, very high rates of union have been achieved.

Lateral Third Clavicle Fractures

Type 1 fractures are treated with a sling to immobilize the upper extremity. The arm is rested until symptoms subside, followed by a range of motion program. These fractures usually heal without further intervention and at 6 weeks patients generally have minimal pain and are able to use the arm for everyday activities. By 3 months, most patients have returned to full activities without restrictions. Collision sports should be limited for 6 months after the fracture.

Type 3 fractures are treated in a manner similar to that used for type I fractures. These fractures may result in posttraumatic acromioclavicular joint arthropathy, which can be successfully treated by distal clavicle resection. There is no indication for primary distal clavicle resection.

The treatment of type 2 fractures is controversial. These fractures have a higher rate of nonunion compared to the other types. However, at least 70% of these fractures heal without any further treatment. In addition, fractures that progress to nonunion are often asymptomatic. Activities such as throwing or tennis that involve raising the arm overhead may be substantially limited if nonunion occurs.

The methods for surgical management have been diverse and include suture fixation, wire fixation, taping, coracoclavicular screw fixation, fixation across the acromioclavicular joint, and plate and screw fixation. All of these techniques have been used with satisfactory results. The primary indications for open reduction and fixation of these fractures include wide displacement without bony contact, risk of skin compromise, and open fractures. Other potential indications include young, active patients who require strenuous use of the upper extremity, particularly at shoulder level or above. Open reduction and stable fixation may be associated with a more rapid recovery. Patients are capable of returning to the majority of their activities by 3 months. Heavy labor or contact sports should be restricted until approximately 6 months following this injury.

Nonsurgical management of type 2 lateral clavicle fractures includes sling immobilization for up to 6 weeks, with the understanding that this fracture poses greater risk for delayed union and nonunion. Clinical and radiographic follow-up is performed regularly during the period of immobilization.

One long-term Swedish follow-up study of lateral third clavicle fractures evaluated patients 15 years after injury and included 73 type 1 fractures, 23 type 2 fractures and 14 type 3 fractures. Ninety-five (86%) of the patients were asymptomatic and 15 (14%) of the patients had moderate pain and dysfunction; two of these patients had a nonunion. However, there were eight additional patients with asymptomatic nonunions in this group of 110 patients, for an overall nonunion rate of 9%. Based on this long-term study, nonsurgical management is effective for the treatment of lateral third clavicle fractures.

Medial Third Clavicle Fractures

Nonsurgical management is preferred for medial clavicle fractures, with the use of a sling for immobilization. An early range of motion program is begun as symptoms allow.

Indications for surgical management include open fracture, skin compromise, or neurovascular compromise. These rare situations are generally associated with such severe trauma that the patient has other life-threatening injuries. The recommended surgical technique has been stabilization with heavy, nonabsorbable sutures. The use of pins is avoided because of the possibility of pin migration.

Complications

Malunion

Malunion is common following the nonsurgical management of clavicle fractures. The most frequent deformities are angulation or shortening (with the medial fragment overlying the lateral fragment). Malunion with extensive callus formation produces a cosmetic deformity with minimal functional limitations. Reduction of the prominent area or corrective osteotomy are not indicated.

Nonunion

Nonunion (failure of the fracture to unite within 12 weeks) remains an uncommon complication, with a reported incidence of 1% to 4% for all clavicle fractures. Predisposing factors to nonunion include inadequate immobilization, severity of the initial trauma, and location of the fracture. The severity of the trauma can be determined by the degree of displacement of the fragments, the associated soft-tissue injury, and the degree of comminution at the fracture site. With increased severity of trauma there is a greater likelihood of soft-tissue interposition between the fracture fragments, which interferes with healing. The location of the clavicle fracture, particularly type 2 lateral clavicle fractures, influences the incidence of nonunion. However, the most significant predisposing factor is the degree of initial displacement of the fracture fragments. Other factors suggested as predisposing to the development of nonunions include refracture of a clavicle and primary open reduction and internal fixation using inadequate fixation.

Approximately 25% of all nonunions of the clavicle are asymptomatic and do not require treatment. The most common indication for treatment of a clavicle nonunion is persistent pain at the fracture site. Other indications include impairment of shoulder function, such as weakness or fatigue, as well as persistent neurovascular symptoms. Neurovascular symptoms may include findings consistent with thoracic outlet syndrome as well as ischemia of the upper extremity caused by compression of the vascular structures.

Procedures for surgical management of clavicular nonunions can be divided ino three categories: salvage, reconstruction, or resection. Salvage procedures alleviate the symptoms of the clavicular nonunion by stabilizing the fracture in its position of nonunion. Bone grafting is generally required. Reconstructive procedures reestablish the normal length of the clavicle, eliminating symptoms and providing the potential for return to normal function. Intercalary bone grafting with iliac crest autograft may be necessary if significant shortening is present. Internal fixation with a 3.5-mm dynamic compression plate or 3.5-mm pelvic reconstruction plate has been successful. Resection of the fracture fragment is reserved for lateral or medial clavicular nonunions with small fragments.

Neurovascular Injuries

Neurovascular injuries occurring with acute clavicle fractures are related to the proximity of the brachial plexus and subclavian vessels. However, despite the close location of the neurovascular bundle, trauma to these structures resulting in persistent loss of neurologic function or vascular emergencies is extremely rare.

Late compression of the neurovascular structures is primarily a result of malunion and the formation of significant callus. The area of the brachial plexus most likely to be compressed by bony impingement is the medial cord of the brachial plexus, a complication frequently manifested as dysfunction in the ulnar nerve distribution. The subclavian vein and artery can also be involved. In the setting of neurovascular symptoms secondary to a malunion or callus formation, removal of the callus may decompress the neurovascular structures. However, if the malunion is significant, callus removal and a corrective osteotomy should be performed. The osteotomy site is stabilized using a 3.5-mm pelvic reconstruction plate or 3.5-mm dynamic compression plate, with the addition of bone graft.

Posttraumatic Arthritis

Posttraumatic arthritis may be a sequela of intra-articular fractures at the medial or lateral clavicle. Type 3 fractures affect the articular surface. In addition, at the time of fracture, there may also be injury to the intra-articular cartilaginous disk. Medial clavicle fractures with intra-articular extension predispose to posttraumatic sternoclavicular arthrosis. The treatment for symptomatic arthritis of the acromioclavicular or sternoclavicular joints is activity modification and nonsteroidal anti-inflammatory medication. Steroid injections are often beneficial. In those patients whose symptoms interfere with their everyday activities, partial resection (1.5 cm) of the clavicle with preservation of the ligaments is recommended.

Selected Bibliography

Abbott LC, Lucas DB: The function of the clavicle: Its surgical significance. *Ann Surg* 1954;140:583-599.

Andersen K, Jensen PO, Lauritzen J: Treatment of clavicular fractures: Figure-of-eight bandage versus a simple sling. *Acta Orthop Scand* 1987;58:71-74.

Boehne D, Curtis RJ Jr, DeHaan JT, et al: Non-union fractures of the midshaft of the clavicle: Treatment with a modified Hagie intramedullary pin and autogenous bone grafting. *J Bone Joint Surg* 1991;73A:1219-1226.

Twenty-one patients who demonstrated symptomatic nonunion of the midshaft of the clavicle were treated with open reduction and internal fixation with a modified Hagie intramedullary pin and autogenous bone grafting. At an average duration of 35 months following this surgery, healing occurred in 20 (95%) of the 21 patients. The authors recommend this technique over open reduction and plate fixation because of the limited incision and soft-tissue dissection, the load-sharing properties of an intramedullary device, and the ability to easily remove the intramedullary device.

Capicotto PN, Heiple KG, Wilbur JH: Midshaft clavicle non-unions treated with intramedullary Steinman pin fixation and onlay bone graft. *J Orthop Trauma* 1994;8:88-93.

Craig EV: Fractures of the clavicle, in Rockwood CA Jr, Green DP, Bucholz RW (eds): *Fractures in Adults,* ed 3. Philadephia, PA, JB Lippincott, 1991, vol 2, pp 928-989.

Craig EV: Fractures of the clavicle, in Rockwood CA Jr, Matsen FA III (eds): *The Shoulder.* Philadelphia, PA, WB Saunders, 1990, pp 367-412.

Edwards DJ, Kavanagh TG, Flannery MC: Fractures of the distal clavicle: A case for fixation. *Injury* 1992;23:44-46.

Treatment results of 43 type 2 lateral clavicular fractures were reviewed. Open reduction and internal fixation demonstrated a lower incidence of local complications, shoulder dysfunction, and nonunion when compared to nonsurgical treatment.

Eskola A, Vainionpaa S, Myllynen P, et al: Outcome of clavicular fracture in 89 patients. *Arch Orthop Trauma Surg* 1986;105:337-338.

Eskola A, Vainionpaa S, Patiala H, et al: Outcome of operative treatment in fresh lateral clavicular fracture. *Ann Chir Gynaecol* 1987;76:167-169.

Faithfull DK, Lam P: Dispelling the fears of plating midclavicular fractures. *J Shoulder Elbow Surg* 1993;2:314-316.

Eighteen midclavicular fractures with gross displacement in comminution or shortening of > 15 mm were treated by plate fixation and reevaluated at an average of 39 months following surgery. All fractures united without complications within 4 months of surgery. Modern techniques of internal fixation allow for anatomic reduction and union of the fracture using plate fixation.

Jupiter JB, Leffert RD: Non-union of the clavicle: Associated complications and surgical management. *J Bone Joint Surg* 1987;69A:753-760.

Kay SP, Eckardt JJ: Brachial plexus palsy secondary to clavicular nonunion: Case report and literature survey. *Clin Orthop* 1986;206:219-222.

Manske DJ, Szabo RM: The operative treatment of midshaft clavicular non-unions. *J Bone Joint Surg* 1985;67A:1367-1371.

Mullaji AB, Jupiter JB: Low contact dynamic compression plating of the clavicle. *Injury* 1994;25:41-45.

Natali J, Maraval M, Kieffer E, et al: Fractures of the clavicle and injuries of the sub-clavian artery: Report of 10 cases. *J Cardiovasc Surg* 1975;16:541-547.

Neer CS II: Fractures, in Neer CS II (ed): *Shoulder Reconstruction.* Philadelphia, PA, WB Saunders, 1990, pp 363-420.

Neer CS II: Fracture of the distal clavicle with detachment of the coracoclavicular ligaments in adults. *J Trauma* 1963;3:99-110.

Neer CS II: Fractures of the distal third of the clavicle. *Clin Orthop* 1968;58:43-50.

Neviaser RJ, Neviaser JS, Neviaser TJ: A simple technique for internal fixation of the clavicle: A long term evaluation. *Clin Orthop* 1975;109:103-107.

Eleven patients with clavicle fractures were treated with internal fixation using Knowles threaded pins. Good results were achieved and the threaded pins prevented migration.

Nordqvist A, Petersson C: The incidence of fractures of the clavicle. *Clin Orthop* 1994;300:127-132.

Age- and gender-specific incidences were evaluated in 2,035 clavicle fractures. Clavicle fractures occur more frequently in men, and the incidence of clavicle fractures, both overall and sports-related, has increased over the past 40 years.

Nordqvist A, Petersson C, Redlund-Johnell I: The natural course of lateral clavicle fractures: Fifteen year follow-up of 110 cases. *Acta Orthop Scand* 1993;64:97-91.

One hundred ten patients with lateral clavicle fractures were treated nonsurgically. At an average follow-up of 15 years after the injury, 95 patients (86%) were asymptomatic, including eight patients who experienced nonunion; 15 patients had moderate pain and dysfunction, and two experienced nonunion. The authors conclude that lateral clavicle fractures do not require surgery.

Poigenfurst J, Rappold G, Fischer W: Plating of fresh clavicular fractures: Results of 122 operations. *Injury* 1992;23:237-241.

One hundred thirty-one fractures of the clavicle in 129 patients were treated with open reduction and internal fixation. Four clavicles refractured after plate removal and five operations led to pseudoarthrosis, which was successfully treated with a reoperation.

Post M: Current concepts in the treatment of fractures of the clavicle. *Clin Orthop* 1989;245:89-101.

Riemer BL, Butterfield SL, Daffner RH, et al: The abduction lordotic view of the clavicle: A new technique for radiographic visualization. *J Orthop Trauma* 1991;5: 392-394.

Rüedi T, Schweiberer L: Clavicular fractures (including luxation of adjacent joints), in Müller ME, Allgöwer M, Schneider R, et al (eds): *Manual of Internal Fixation: Techniques Recommended by the AO-ASIF Group,* ed 3. Berlin, Germany, Springer-Verlag, 1991, pp 434-435.

Seiler JG III, Jupiter JB: Intercholary tricortical iliac crest bone grafts for the treatment of chronic clavicular non-union with bony defect. *J Orthop Tech* 1993;1:19-22.

Simpson NS, Jupiter JB: Clavicular nonunion and malunion: Evaluation and surgical management. *J Am Acad Orthop Surg* 1996;4:1-8.

Clavicular nonunions are associated with comminuted and displaced fractures, open injuries, or failed surgical treatment. Reconstruction of the clavicle can gain union and restore clavicular anatomy using modern techniques of plate fixation and autogenous bone grafting. Symptomatic malunited clavicular fractures can be successfuly treated with osteotomy and correction of the deformity.

Stanley D, Trowbridge EA, Norris SH: The mechanism of clavicular fracture: A clinical and biomechanical analysis. *J Bone Joint Surg* 1988;70B:461-464.

Zenni EJ Jr, Krieg JK, Rosen MJ: Open reduction and internal fixation of clavicular fractures. *J Bone Joint Surg* 1981;63A:147-151.

22

Scapular Fractures

Andrew Green, MD

Introduction

Scapular fractures account for less than 1% of all fractures, and therefore have received limited attention in orthopaedic literature. They are usually the result of severe blunt trauma such as occurs in motor vehicle accidents and often present in the context of polytrauma. Scapular fractures are frequently overlooked in the initial evaluation and management of a severely injured patient. Nonetheless, specific injury patterns have been shown to result in significant pain and shoulder girdle disability.

In most cases, nonsurgical treatment results in satisfactory outcomes. Surgical treatment of scapular fractures remains a controversial topic that has been difficult to clarify because of the rarity of these injuries. However, recent additions to the literature have provided some clarity concerning the indications for surgical management.

The following review discusses scapular anatomy, epidemiology, associated injuries, classification, evaluation, and treatment relevant to the management of scapular fractures.

Anatomy

The scapula is a mobile platform upon which the proximal humerus is balanced as the upper extremity moves. When viewed in the frontal plane of the body, the scapula is essentially triangular in shape. The sagittal view demonstrates the relationship of the bony projections of the superolateral aspect. These include the glenoid, acromion, and coracoid process that surround the humeral head. The coracoacromial arch, composed of the coracoid, acromion, and the coracoacromial ligament, forms a roof over the rotator cuff and the proximal humerus. The scapular spine and the borders of the scapular body are the sites of numerous muscle attachments and have cortical thickenings that can provide anchorage for internal fixation. The infraspinatus fossa is paper-thin and makes up the majority of the body of the scapula.

The scapula and the complex of muscles that surround it have a critical role in the mechanics and kinematics of the shoulder girdle. The scapula is held against the chest and moved by the trapezius, levator scapulae, rhomboids, serratus anterior, and pectoralis minor muscles. The scapula is the origin of the rotator cuff and deltoid muscles as well as the long head of the triceps and the long and short heads of the biceps muscles.

The scapula is suspended from the lateral end of the clavicle by the coracoclavicular and acromioclavicular ligaments. These are the only fixed attachments of the scapula to the axial skeleton. Goss has reviewed the variants of injury to the superior shoulder suspensory complex (SSSC) (Fig. 1). The SSSC is a bony/soft-tissue ring at the end of a superior and inferior bony strut. The ring is composed of the glenoid, coracoid process, coracoclavicular ligaments, distal clavicle, acromioclavicular joint, and the acromial process. The superior strut is the middle clavicle and the inferior strut is the lateral scapular body/spine. The complex maintains a normal stable relationship between the scapula/upper extremity and the axial skeleton.

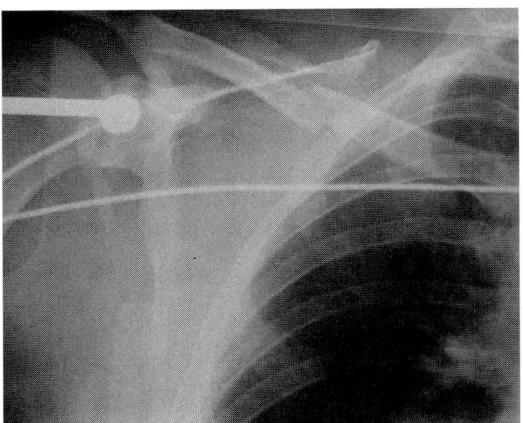 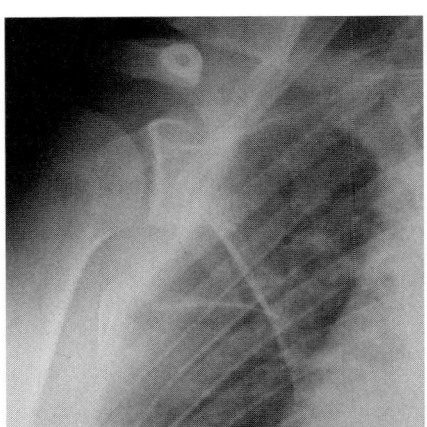 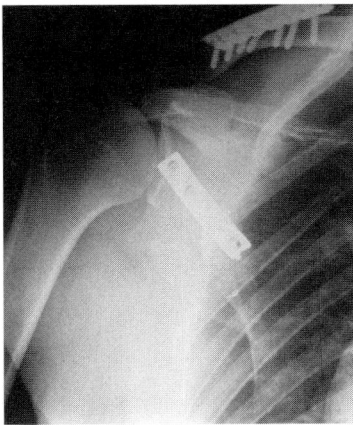

Fig. 1 **Left,** Combined clavicle shaft and scapular neck fracture resulted in significant sagging of the shoulder girdle. **Center,** The glenoid process was completely displaced anterior to the scapula. **Right,** The clavicle shaft and scapular neck were both treated with open reduction and internal fixation. (Copyright © 1997, Andrew Green, MD, Providence, RI.)

Several important neurovascular structures are in close proximity to the shoulder girdle and scapula. The brachial plexus and axillary artery course from the thoracic outlet, past the anterior-inferior aspect of the shoulder girdle, and into the upper extremity. As they pass the shoulder they are tethered by numerous branches. The loose attachment of the scapula to the axial skeleton places the neurovascular structures at risk for significant injury. The axillary and suprascapular nerves are especially vulnerable to injury. Scapular neck fractures can cause direct injury to the suprascapular nerve within the suprascapular notch, or indirect injury as a result of traction because of displacement. Similarly, the axillary nerve can sustain direct or indirect injury with displaced scapular neck fracture.

The features that make the scapula unique—its mobility, shape, and thick muscular envelope—also protect it from injury.

Prevalence and Associated Injuries

Scapular fractures account for 5% or less of shoulder girdle fractures. The majority of scapular fractures are caused by high-velocity blunt trauma. A vehicular accident is a factor in 69% to 84% of cases. A smaller percentage are the result of falls. Most scapular fractures occur in young and middle-aged adults. The average age in most series is about 35 years. More than two thirds of the fractures occur in males.

Scapular fractures frequently occur as part of a constellation of injuries of the ipsilateral thoracic cage that include rib and clavicle fractures and severe pulmonary injury (Fig. 2). The incidence of ipsilateral rib fractures is as high as 40% to 50% in some series and the reported incidence of ipsilateral clavicle fractures is as high as about 25%. Pulmonary contusion, hemopneumothoraces, and closed head injuries are among the life-threatening injuries that are associated with scapular fractures.

Injuries to the brachial plexus and major arteries and veins occur in as many as 12% of cases. The most extreme example is scapulothoracic dissociation, which is the anatomic equivalent of a closed forequarter amputation. This devastating injury is rare.

These associated injuries have far greater significance than the scapula fracture in the initial evaluation and management of these patients.

Classification

Scapular fractures are best described and classified according to the location of the fracture. This approach appears to be the most relevant to treatment and outcome. Included are fractures of the body, neck, glenoid, acromion, and coracoid. Frequently, multiple fracture sites are present. The scapular body is involved in 50% to 60% of cases. Scapular neck fractures occur in about 25% of cases. In the largest series reported,

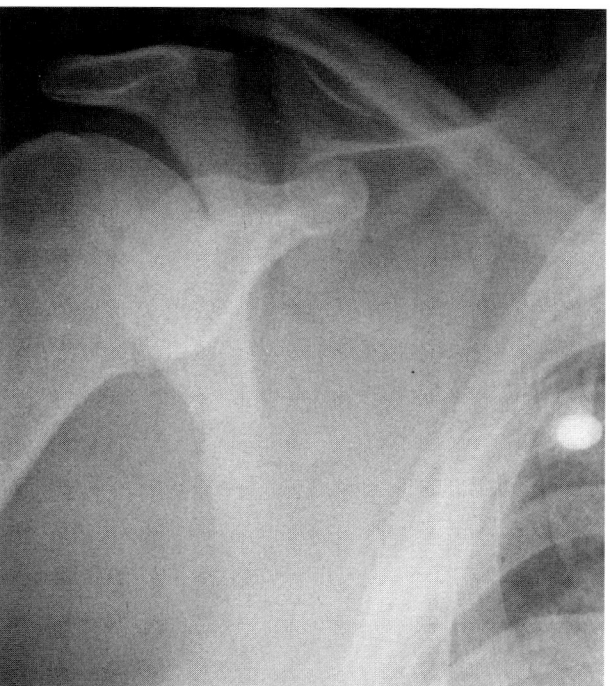
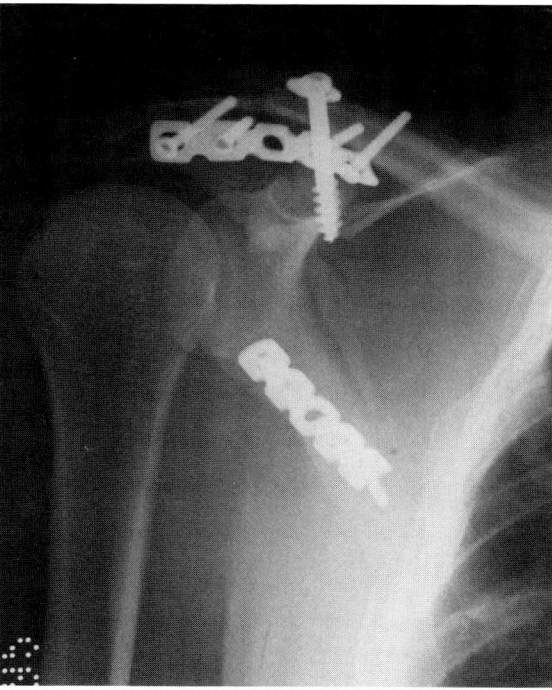

Fig. 2 Left, This complex fracture included a displaced scapular neck fracture that extended from the lateral border of the scapula up through the scapular spine. The superior shoulder suspensory complex was disrupted by the acromioclavicular dislocation. **Right,** Open reduction and internal fixation took advantage of the bone at the superior aspect of the scapular spine and the lateral border of the scapula. (Copyright © 1997, Andrew Green, MD, Providence, RI.)

Ideberg found intra-articular glenoid fractures in 100 out of 338 scapular fractures. Seventeen percent of these were glenoid rim fractures that were caused by glenohumeral dislocation. Acromion and coracoid fractures are much less common.

The Orthopaedic Trauma Association has published the most recent and comprehensive classification of scapula fractures. This scheme is based on the AO/ASIF system of classification. Scapular fractures are grouped either as extra-articular or intra-articular (glenoid fractures). Extra-articular fractures are subgrouped according to whether they involve processes (acromion or coracoid), scapular body, scapular neck, or are complex. Glenoid fractures are subgrouped according to degree of fracturing as either impacted, free, or complex/comminuted. Complex fractures may include multiple fractures and/or scapular fractures with disruption of the SSSC (clavicle fracture or acromioclavicular dislocation).

Ada and Miller reviewed the fracture patterns in 116 scapulae and classified them into four types. Type I involves the acromion, spine, or coracoid; type II, the neck; type III, the glenoid; and type IV, the body.

There are other classifications of specific fracture sites of the scapula. Goss classified glenoid (scapular) neck fractures as either displaced or nondisplaced. Significant displacement is defined as translational displacement greater than or equal to 1 cm or angulatory displacement greater than or equal to 40°. Displacement is especially likely if the SSSC is disrupted.

Eyres and associates classified coracoid fractures according to the degree of extension of the fracture into the base of the coracoid. Types I, II, and III do not involve the base, whereas type IV does and type V includes the glenoid fossa. Types I, II, and III could be treated nonsurgically, whereas surgical treatment was indicated for types IV and V fractures.

Kuhn and associates classified acromial fractures. Type I fractures are nondisplaced. Type II fractures are displaced but do not compromise the subacromial space. Type III fractures cause reduction of the subacromial space. They stressed that nonsurgical treatment of type III fractures has poor results.

Ideberg classified glenoid fractures according to the pattern. Type I fractures are rim fractures whereas types II through V are glenoid fossa fractures. Goss has added a type VI to differentiate severely comminuted glenoid fossa fractures.

Most of the comprehensive classification approaches to scapula fractures have accounted for the anatomic and functional importance of the various parts of the scapula as well as the outcomes of nonsurgical treatment.

Evaluation

The evaluation of shoulder girdle trauma includes assessment of shoulder position and posture, evaluation of the covering soft tissues, and a detailed neurovascular examination. This type of examination is often difficult if not impossible to obtain in the polytrauma patient.

Soft-tissue injury including abrasions, open wounds, closed degloving injuries, and muscular trauma is common. Open wounds that penetrate the dermis must be explored and adequately debrided. Skin surface abrasions lead to bacterial contamination and may delay or preclude surgical intervention.

Deeper soft-tissue injury can lead to wound healing problems after surgery.

Many scapular fractures are initially identified on chest radiographs. Radiographic examination specific to the shoulder and scapula should include the standard shoulder trauma series; anterior-posterior (true AP), axillary, and lateral (Y-views) of the scapula. Greater anatomic detail can be obtained with computed tomography (CT) scanning. CT scanning is especially helpful when considering surgical treatment. In rare, complex cases, three-dimensional CT scanning can provide helpful information.

Complications

Despite the many potential complications considered, there have been few reports that specifically address complications of scapula fractures. Scapulothoracic dissociation is the most devastating injury but it is usually a soft-tissue injury and not associated with scapula fracture.

Late problems, when they occur, are related to malunion of the scapula. Scapulothoracic crepitus can result from malunited scapular body fracture. Malunion of scapular neck fractures is reported to cause rotator cuff dysfunction. Although late glenohumeral arthritis is expected after displaced glenoid fossa fractures, this problem has rarely been discussed. Suprascapular nerve compression has been reported after fractures that extend into the suprascapular notch.

Nonsurgical Treatment and Results

The majority of scapular fractures can be successfully treated nonsurgically with immobilization in a simple sling. In most cases early passive motion exercises can be initiated as soon as comfort allows. Fractures that might be displaced by immediate or early passive motion, such as glenoid fossa, scapular neck, or scapular spine fractures, are immobilized for 2 to 4 weeks to allow early fracture healing. Limited active use is encouraged as soon as immobilization is discontinued. Passive stretching is continued until motion is maximized. Maximal outcome is achieved 6 to 12 months after injury.

Numerous series have documented satisfactory results from nonsurgical treatment. However, most studies have reported only short-term follow-up. The fact that there are few reports of late problems suggests that these results are probably a good representation of outcome.

A few authors have analyzed factors associated with outcome. Wilber and Evans reported that fractures of the spine, neck, and body generally did well. However, more recent studies have contradicted these findings. Ada and Miller found that displaced scapular spine and neck fractures are associated with poor outcomes. Nordqvist and associates found that scapular deformity was associated with pain.

Coracoid fractures that do not extend into the glenoid fossa generally do well with nonsurgical treatment, but these injuries are uncommon. Acromial fractures that are nondisplaced or displaced but do not compromise the subacromial space can also be treated nonsurgically.

Nondisplaced, congruent glenoid fractures also do well with nonsurgical treatment. Displaced glenoid fractures can be problematic. Incongruency can cause posttraumatic arthritis. Glenoid rim fractures can lead to recurrent glenohumeral instability. Goss suggests 5 mm of displacement as the cutoff for glenoid fossa fractures, and 10 mm for rim fractures. Bauer and associates suggest that even as little as 2 mm of articular incongruity can lead to glenohumeral arthritis. However, type VI fractures, with severe comminution, are best treated nonsurgically because of the difficulty of achieving adequate reduction and secure internal fixation.

Surgical Approaches and Technique

Surgical exposure of scapular fractures requires an intimate knowledge and understanding of shoulder girdle anatomy. Most displaced scapular fractures, including glenoid fractures, are exposed through posterior approaches. The posterior approach is tailored to the specific fracture. Most can be reached through a vertical incision and dissection in the intermuscular planes of the external rotators. The Judet approach in which the infraspinatus muscle is elevated off of the scapula body is often described but not usually necessary. Superior extension over the top of the shoulder is occasionally necessary for fixation of the base of the coracoid, superior glenoid, or acromioclavicular joint. Fixation of anterior glenoid fractures is generally via the anterior deltopectoral approach.

The scapular spine, scapular neck, and lateral scapular border provide the best bone for internal fixation, and should be used whenever possible to achieve accurate reduction and stable internal fixation. Fixation of glenoid fossa fractures and posterior rim fractures using a posterior approach can be enhanced by using the lateral scapular border to buttress fracture reduction.

Small fragment AO/ASIF plates and screws are most commonly used; cannulated screws are particularly useful. 3.5-mm dynamic compression plates can provide very stable fixation along the lateral border of the scapula. 3.5-mm reconstruction plates are more easily contoured and are excellent for fixation of the glenoid fragment to the axillary border of the scapula. Reconstruction plates are useful for fixing scapular spine and acromial fractures.

Surgical Treatment and Results

Surgical treatment is appropriate for the minority of scapular fractures. The primary indications for surgical treatment are significant displacement of the scapular neck, spine, or acromion, displaced intra-articular glenoid fractures, and double disruption of the SSSC.

Several groups have reported good results with surgical treatment of a variety of displaced scapular fractures. Bauer and associates had 75% good and very good results in 20 cases of which 19 had no or minimal pain. Hardegger and associates had 79% excellent and good results.

Disruption of the SSSC, which usually consists of combined scapular neck and clavicle fractures, can be treated in two ways. Leung and Lam reported 93% good and excellent results with reduction and fixation of the clavicle and scapular neck fractures (Fig. 1). Rikli and associates only treated the clavicle fractures and reported excellent results in nearly all cases.

Kavanagh and associates reported the greatest detail regarding the results of surgical treatment of displaced glenoid fossa fractures (Fig. 3). Eight of the nine patients available for follow-up had mild or no symptoms and little or no pain.

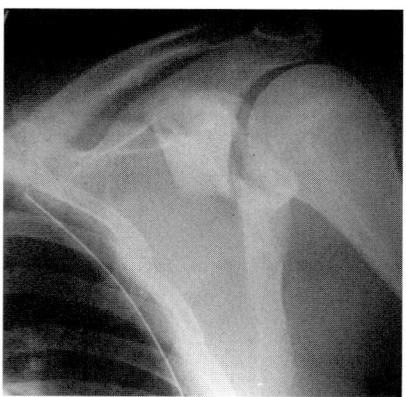
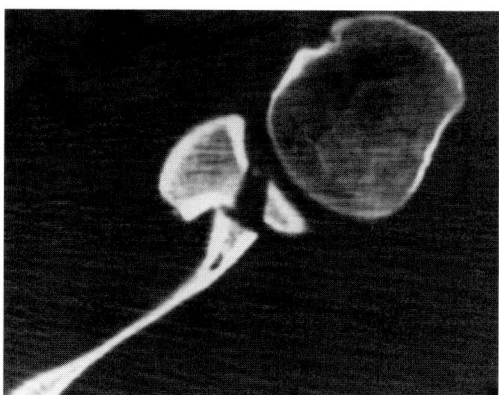
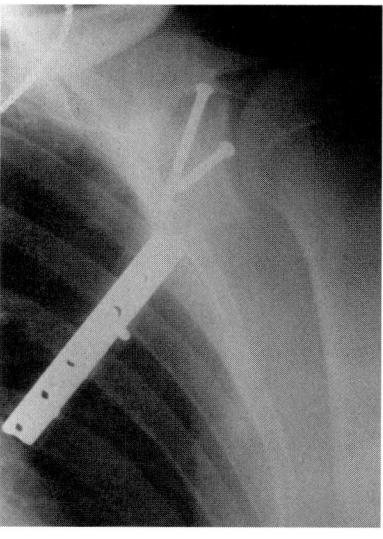

Fig. 3 **Left,** The anteroposterior radiograph suggests that there is a significant intra-articular injury. **Center,** The computed tomographic scan confirms the extent of glenoid articular injury. **Right,** Open reduction and internal fixation was achieved through a posterior spinatus sparing approach. (Copyright © 1997, Andrew Green, MD, Providence, RI.)

Selected Bibliography

Ada JR, Miller ME: Scapular fractures: Analysis of 113 cases. *Clin Orthop* 1991;269:174-180.

This is a large series of fractures. All were treated nonsurgically. Follow-up of 20% of the cases demonstrated significant disability in 50% of patients with displaced scapular spine and neck fractures. Eight subsequent patients with displaced scapular neck fractures were treated with open reduction and internal fixation with satisfactory results.

Armstrong CP, Van der Spuy J: The fractured scapula: Importance and management based on a series of 62 patients. *Injury* 1984;15:324.

Aston JW Jr, Gregory CF: Dislocation of the shoulder with significant fracture of the glenoid. *J Bone Joint Surg* 1973;55A:1531-1533.

Bauer G, Fleischmann W, Dussler E: Displaced scapular fractures: Indication and long-term results of open reduction and internal fixation. *Arch Orthop Trauma Surg* 1995;114:215-219.

This is a relatively large series (25 cases) of displaced scapular fractures treated with open reduction and internal fixation. The majority were either scapular neck fractures (with and without clavicle fracture) or glenoid fractures. Ninety-five percent had no or minimal pain, 75% were rated good or very good. The authors recommended operative treatment for severely displaced acromion and coracoid fractures, displaced anatomic neck fractures, unstable surgical neck fractures, and displaced glenoid fractures.

Butters KP: The scapula, in Rockwood CA, Matsen FA III (eds): *The Shoulder.* Philadelphia, PA, WB Saunders, 1990, pp 335-366.

Ebraheim NA, An HS, Jackson WT, et al: Scapulothoracic dissociation. *J Bone Joint Surg* 1988;70A:428-432.

Edeland HG, Zachrisson BE: Fracture of the scapular notch associated with lesion of the suprascapular nerve. *Acta Orthop Scand* 1975;46:758-763.

Eyres KS, Brooks A, Stanley D: Fractures of the coracoid process. *J Bone Joint Surg* 1995;77B:425-428.

Goss TP: Double disruptions of the superior shoulder suspensory complex. *J Orthop Trauma* 1993;7:99-106.

This article clearly defines the superior suspensory complex of the shoulder and its relevance to scapular fractures. Illustrative cases are used to highlight the injury variants. Surgical treatment is recommended for displaced double disruptions.

Goss TP: Fractures of the glenoid cavity. *J Bone Joint Surg* 1992;74A:299-305.

This review article discusses the epidemiology, classification and treatment options for glenoid fractures. It emphasizes the fact that there is a lack of literature about the outcome of displaced fractures.

Goss TP: Fractures of the glenoid neck. *J Shoulder Elbow Surg* 1994;3:42-52.

Hardegger FH, Simpson LA, Weber BG: The operative treatment of scapular fractures. *J Bone Joint Surg* 1984;66B:725-731.

Thirty-seven fractures, mostly glenoid rim or fossa, were treated with open reduction and internal fixation. Seventy-nine percent had good and excellent results. They recommended open reduction and internal fixation for displaced intra-articular fractures, glenoid rim fractures associated with glenohumeral subluxation, or unstable scapular neck fractures.

Herscovici D Jr, Fiennes AG, Allgöwer M, et al: The floating shoulder: Ipsilateral clavicle and scapular neck fractures. *J Bone Joint Surg* 1992;74B:362-364.

Seven cases of ipsilateral clavicle and scapular neck fracture were successfully treated with open reduction and internal fixation of the clavicle fracture. The extent of scapula neck displacement is not discussed in this article.

Ideberg R, Grevsten S, Larsson S: Epidemiology of scapular fractures: Incidence and classification of 338 fractures. *Acta Orthop Scand* 1995;66:395-397.

This article reviews epidemiologic information about scapular fractures, with particular emphasis on glenoid fractures. The Ideberg classification of intra-articular glenoid fractures is reviewed.

Imatani RJ: Fractures of the scapula: A review of 53 fractures. *J Trauma* 1975;15:473-478.

Kavanagh BF, Bradway JK, Cofield RH: Open reduction and internal fixation of displaced intra-articular fractures of the glenoid fossa. *J Bone Joint Surg* 1993;75A:479-484.

This article is the largest detailed series of open reduction and internal fixation of intra-articular glenoid fractures. The posterior surgical approach is clearly described. The results were uniformly excellent at an average 4-year follow-up.

Kuhn JE, Blasier RB, Carpenter JE: Fractures of the acromion process: A proposed classification system. *J Orthop Trauma* 1994;8:6-13.

This article classifies acromial fractures according to displacement. Type I (minimally displaced) and type II (displaced without compromising subacromial space) do well with nonsurgical treatment. Surgical treatment is recommended for type III (subacromial space compromised) fractures.

Leung KS, Lam TP: Open reduction and internal fixation of ipsilateral fractures of the scapular neck and clavicle. *J Bone Joint Surg* 1993;75A:1015-1018.

This is a relatively large retrospective series of combined scapular neck fracture and clavicle fractures. The authors recommended open reduction and internal fixation of both fractures and report 14 good and excellent results in 15 cases.

Lindholm A, Leven H: Prognosis in fractures of the body and neck of the scapula: A follow-up study. *Acta Chir Scand* 1974;140:33-36.

McGahan JP, Rab GT, Dublin A: Fractures of the scapula. *J Trauma* 1980;20:880-883.

McGinnis M, Denton JR: Fractures of the scapula: A retrospective study of 40 fractured scapulae. *J Trauma* 1989;29:1488-1493.

Miller ME, Ada JR: Injuries to the shoulder girdle, in Browner BD, Jupiter JB, Levine AM, et al (eds): *Skeletal Trauma.* Philadelphia, PA, Saunders, 1992, pp 1291-1310.

This is a well-organized review of scapular injuries. The treatment recommendations are based on the authors' experience.

Nordqvist A, Petersson C: Fracture of the body, neck, or spine of the scapula: A long-term follow-up study. *Clin Orthop* 1992;283:139-144.

This is one of the few studies with long-term outcome of nonsurgical treatment of scapular fractures. Scapular deformity was highly associated with pain.

Nordqvist A, Petersson CJ: Incidence and causes of shoulder girdle injuries in an urban population. *J Shoulder Elbow Surg* 1995;4:107-112.

Norris TR: Fractures of the proximal humerus and dislocations of the shoulder, in Browner BD, Jupiter JB, Levine AM, et al (eds): *Skeletal Trauma.* Philadelphia, PA, WB Saunders, 1992, pp 1201-1290.

Orthopaedic Trauma Association: Fracture and dislocation compendium. *J Orthop Trauma* 1996;10(suppl 1):81-84.

Rikli D, Regazzoni P, Renner N: The unstable shoulder girdle: Early functional treatment utilizing open reduction and internal fixation. *J Orthop Trauma* 1995;9:93-97.

The authors treated double disruptions of the superior shoulder suspensory complex (scapular neck fracture with clavicle fracture) with open reduction and internal fixation of the clavicle. They concluded that the scapular neck fracture is usually reduced indirectly and is sufficiently stable for function after treatment.

Solheim LF, Roaas A: Compression of the suprascapular nerve after fracture of the scapular notch. *Acta Orthop Scand* 1978;49:338-340.

Thompson DA, Flynn TC, Miller PW, et al: The significance of scapular fractures. *J Trauma* 1985;25:974-977.

Wilber MC, Evans EB: Fractures of the scapula: An analysis of forty cases and a review of the literature. *J Bone Joint Surg* 1977;59A:358-362.

Zdravkovic D, Damholt VV: Comminuted and severely displaced fractures of the scapula. *Acta Orthop Scand* 1974;45:60-65.

In contrast to more recent studies, satisfactory outcomes are reported for nonsurgical treatment of displaced scapular neck fractures. Nineteen of 28 patients who were followed up were "completely symptom-free."

Humeral Shaft Fractures

Kenneth J. Koval, MD

Introduction

Humeral shaft fractures are common injuries, accounting for approximately 3% of all fractures; most can be managed nonsurgically with anticipated good to excellent results. Appropriate nonsurgical and surgical treatment of humeral shaft fractures, however, requires an understanding of humeral anatomy, the fracture pattern, and the patient's activity level and expectations.

Etiology

Humeral shaft fractures result from both direct and indirect forces. Common mechanisms for humeral shaft fractures include a fall onto the outstretched hand, injury to the area during a motor vehicle accident, and a direct load to the arm. Extreme muscle traction can also result in a humeral shaft fracture; this injury can occur after throwing a ball or javelin. Fracture patterns are less comminuted in elderly patients who sustain humeral shaft fractures as a result of a fall. Fractures of the humeral shaft have been reproduced experimentally; pure compressive forces result in proximal or distal humerus fractures, bending forces in transverse fractures, and torsional forces in spiral fracture patterns. The combination of bending and torsion usually results in an oblique fracture, with or without an associated butterfly fragment.

Evaluation

Patients with humeral shaft fractures usually present with arm pain, swelling, and deformity. The arm is shortened, and on gentle manipulation gross motion and crepitus will be apparent. In humeral shaft fractures that result from high-energy trauma, other more serious associated injuries should be suspected. Physical examination should include a systematic physical inspection of the entire extremity. Soft-tissue abrasions must be differentiated from open fractures. Intraarticular extension of puncture wounds around the shoulder and elbow can be determined by injecting saline into the joint away from the area of the puncture and noting extravasation of fluid. The neurovascular status of the extremity must be assessed. Doppler pulse and compartment pressure should be determined if indicated.

Imaging

The standard radiographic examination of the humerus includes an anteroposterior and lateral view, taken at 90° to one another. The shoulder and elbow joint should be included on each view. The radiographs are obtained by moving the patient rather than simply rotating the injured extremity. When considering intramedullary nailing, it must be ascertained that the fracture does not extend to the anticipated point of nail entry. In highly comminuted or displaced fractures, traction radiographs may allow better fracture definition. Comparison radiographs of the contralateral humerus are helpful for preoperative planning. Tomograms and computed tomography (CT) scans are rarely indicated.

Nonsurgical Treatment

Most closed humeral shaft fractures can be managed nonsurgically with closed reduction and application of a coaptation splint followed by application of a functional fracture brace 1 to 2 weeks after injury. The coaptation splint is used for initial treatment of humeral shaft fractures. It is preferred over the hanging arm cast because of the support it offers proximal to the fracture site, especially for displaced midshaft humeral shaft fractures with shortening or those fractures with an oblique or spiral pattern. The weight of the splints when the patient is upright has the same function as that of the previously advocated hanging arm cast, without levering or angulation at the fracture site.

A humeral functional brace effects fracture reduction through soft-tissue compression; it consists of an anterior and posterior shell held together with Velcro straps (Fig. 1). Over-the-shoulder extensions are available, but seldom necessary; these extensions restrict shoulder motion and are most often used for comminuted fractures of the proximal humerus. The fracture brace can be applied acutely or following application of a coaptation splint; it is tightened as swelling decreases. Contraindications to use of the functional brace include: (1) massive soft-tissue or bony loss; (2) an unreliable or uncooperative patient; and (3) an inability to obtain or maintain acceptable fracture alignment.

Regardless of the initial fracture treatment, the patient is instructed to sit in a semireclining position and not lean on the elbow for support. The patient is encouraged to perform shoulder pendulum exercises as well as range of motion exercises of the elbow, wrist, and hand. Assisted range of shoulder motion is performed as tolerated.

Surgical Treatment

The indications for surgical management of a humeral shaft fracture are listed in Outline 1. Open humeral fractures require emergent debridement; fracture stabilization after soft-tissue and osseous debridement has been reported to reduce the incidence of infection. The humeral shaft fracture with associated vascular injury is best managed with internal

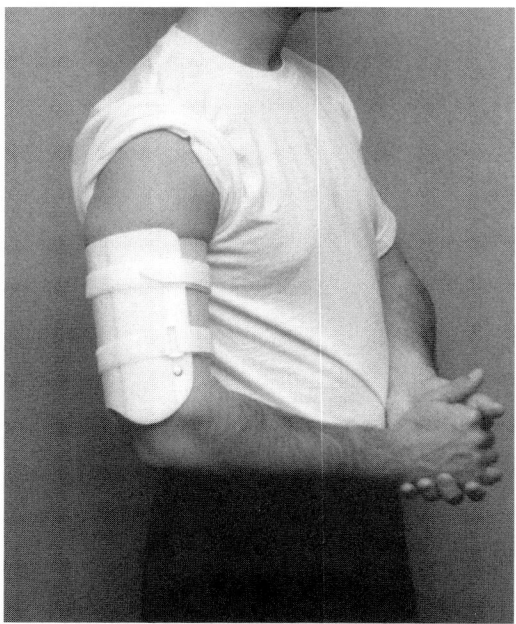

Fig. 1 A humeral functional brace effects fracture reduction through soft-tissue compression; it consists of an anterior and posterior shell held together with Velcro straps.

Outline 1. Indications for surgical management of humeral shaft fractures

Associated vascular injury
Floating elbow
Segmental fracture
Pathologic fracture
Bilateral humeral fractures
Humeral fracture in polytrauma patient
Fractures with unacceptable alignment
Displaced intra-articular fracture extension

or external fixation to protect the vascular repair. The best results after treatment of floating elbow (an ipsilateral fracture of the humerus and radius/ulna) have been reported after internal fixation of fractures of the humerus and radius/ulna followed by early range of elbow motion. Nonsurgical treatment of a segmental humerus fracture is associated with increased risk of nonunion at one or both fracture sites. Internal stabilization of pathologic fractures will maximize patient comfort and upper extremity function. Surgical stabilization of bilateral humerus fractures is necessary to allow patient self-care. The polytrauma patient is often unable to remain in the semisitting position necessary to effect fracture reduction; in addition, surgical stabilization of the humerus maximizes the polytrauma patient's rehabilitation potential. Neurologic loss after a penetrating stab injury is an indication for nerve exploration. The need for surgical intervention secondary to radial nerve dysfunction after fracture manipulation is controversial; there are advocates both for early nerve exploration and for observation. Fractures that cannot be maintained in acceptable alignment should be stabilized with surgery. In the humeral shaft, up to 20° of anterior or posterior angulation, 30° of varus, and 3 cm of shortening is acceptable; less angular deformity may be allowed in thin individuals. Humeral shaft fractures in obese patients and women with large breasts are at increased risk of varus angulation. Malrotation is well tolerated secondary to compensatory shoulder motion. Finally, fractures of the humeral shaft with displaced intra-articular fracture extension require surgical treatment.

Fixation Using Plates and Screws

The best functional results after surgical management of humeral shaft fractures have been reported with the use of plates and screws; these implants allow direct fracture reduction and stable fixation of the humeral shaft without violation of the rotator cuff. Indications for use of plates and screws include humeri with small medullary canals or preexisting deformity, proximal and distal humeral shaft fractures not amenable to intramedullary nailing, humerus fractures with intra-articular extension, humerus fractures that require exploration for evaluation and treatment of an associated neurologic or vascular lesion, and humeral nonunions (Fig. 2).

The surgical approach for plating of the humerus is dependent on the fracture level and the need to visualize the radial nerve. The anterolateral approach is preferred for proximal third fractures; the anterolateral and posterior approaches are both adequate for midshaft and distal third fractures.

During fracture exposure, the surgeon should avoid excessive soft-tissue stripping and take care not to devitalize butterfly fragments. A 4.5-mm broad dynamic compression plate is usually selected for midshaft humerus fractures. In smaller patients, a 4.5-mm narrow dynamic compression plate may be used. Proximal and distal humerus fractures require use of other types of implants (single or double reconstruction plates, T plates). Dependent on the fracture level, a precontoured plate can be used as a reduction aid. If the fracture pattern permits, the plate should be applied in compression. Lag screws should be inserted whenever possible. One should obtain screw fixation in eight to ten cortices (ie, four to five holding screws) proximal and distal to the fracture. Fixation stability should be assessed prior to closure. The need to bone graft is determined by the amount of comminution and soft-tissue stripping.

Intramedullary Fixation

Intramedullary nails offer biologic and mechanical advantages over plates and screws. Intramedullary nails can be inserted without direct fracture exposure, thus minimizing soft-tissue scarring. Because the intramedullary nail is closer to the mechanical axis than the usual plate position on the external surface of the bone, intramedullary nails are subjected to smaller bending loads than plates and are less likely to fail by fatigue. In addition, intramedullary nails can act as load-sharing devices in those fractures that have cortical contact if the nail is not statically locked. Finally, stress shielding with resultant cortical osteopenia, commonly seen with plates and screws, is minimized with intramedullary implants. However, there have been an increasing number of reports of a high incidence of shoulder pain after antegrade humeral nail-

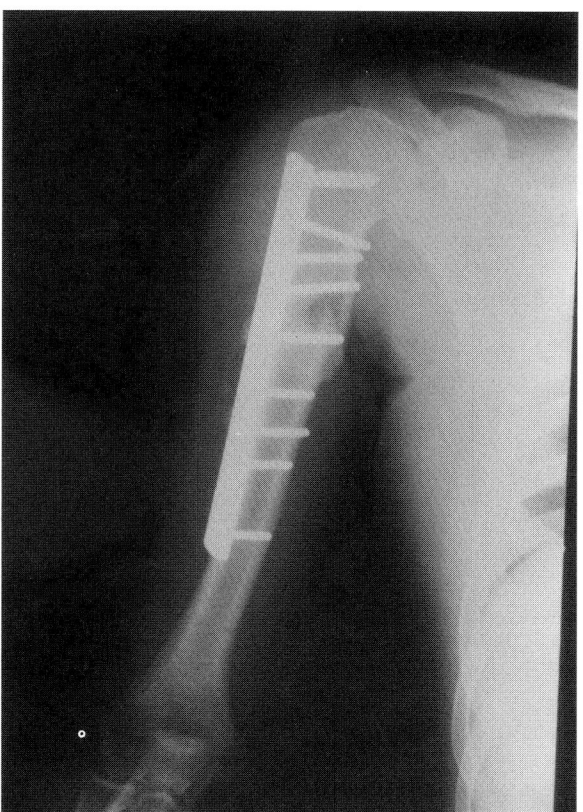

Fig. 2 Proximal humerus fracture stabilized with a compression plate and lag screws.

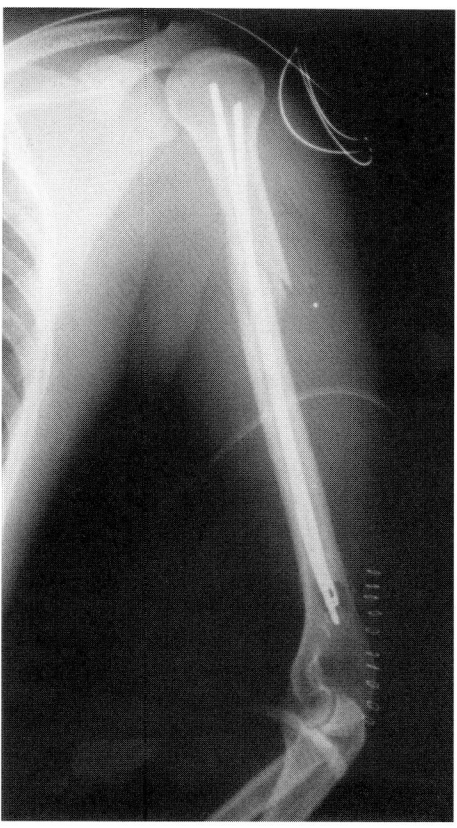

Fig. 3 Retrograde inserted flexible Ender nails used to stabilize a humeral shaft fracture.

ing. Indications for use of intramedullary nails include segmental fractures in which plate placement would require considerable soft-tissue dissection, humerus fractures in osteopenic bone, pathologic humerus fractures, and humeral shaft fractures in polytrauma patients in whom use of the injured arm may be needed for mobilization and ambulation. Two types of intramedullary devices are available for use in the humeral shaft: flexible and interlocked nails. Each will be discussed in turn.

Flexible Nails Flexible intramedullary devices available for use in the management of humerus fractures include Ender nails, Hackethal nails, and Rush rods (Fig. 3). Multiple nails/rods need to be inserted in order to achieve fracture stability. These devices can be inserted retrograde from the distal humerus, or antegrade through the rotator cuff; the best results with use of flexible intramedullary nails have reported using retrograde insertion through an entry portal proximal to the olecranon fossa. Flexible intramedullary nails do not prevent fracture shortening nor do they provide significant rotational control; therefore, they should be reserved for humeral shaft fractures with minimal comminution. Use of a functional fracture brace should be considered after flexible intramedullary nailing of the humerus to prevent fracture displacement.

Interlocked Nails Locked intramedullary nails are able to maintain alignment of unstable fracture patterns and prevent fracture shortening and malrotation (Fig. 4). Interlocked nails can be used to stabilize fractures 2 cm distal to the surgical neck to 3 cm proximal to the olecranon. Most interlocked nails rely on proximal and distal screw fixation to provide stability; these implants can be inserted antegrade through the rotator cuff or retrograde proximal to the olecranon, with or without prior reaming. Reaming increases the length along which the nail contacts the endosteal surface of the intramedullary canal, therefore providing better fracture stability. Reaming also decreases the risk of nail incarceration and permits placement of a larger diameter (and thus stronger) nail. Finally, reaming results in the production of a large quantity of morselized bone chips; these reamings may induce new bone formation and enhance fracture healing. Reaming, however, obliterates the nutrient artery and endosteal blood supply; this blood supply will reconstitute if the nail has channels along its length to permit revascularization. In addition, the cortical thickness of the humerus is much less than that of the femur and tibia; excessive endosteal reaming may thin the humeral cortex and result in increased fracture comminution. With antegrade insertion, the surgeon must bury the humeral nail below the rotator cuff to prevent nail impingement under

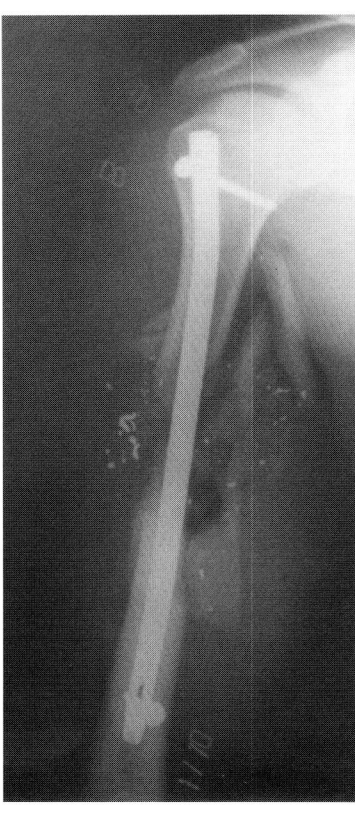

Fig. 4 Locked intramedullary nail used to stabilize a comminuted midshaft humerus fracture with bone loss secondary to a gunshot injury.

the acromion. However, there have been several reports of a high incidence of shoulder pain after antegrade nail insertion despite seating of the nail below the rotator cuff. Oblique proximal locking screws inserted from proximal lateral to distal medial may also result in subacromial impingement if the screws are located proximal to the equator of the humeral head. The axillary nerve is at risk during proximal locking screw insertion. The distal locking screws can be inserted anterior-posterior or posterior-anterior via an open technique.

Complications

Radial Nerve Injury

Up to 18% of humeral shaft fractures have an associated radial nerve injury. Although the Holstein-Lewis fracture (oblique, distal third) is best known for its association with neurologic injury, radial nerve palsy is most commonly associated with middle third humerus fractures. Most nerve injuries are a neurapraxia or axonotmesis; 90% will resolve in 3 to 4 months. Electromyography and nerve conduction studies can help to determine the degree of nerve injury and monitor the rate of nerve regeneration. Indications for early radial nerve exploration are radial nerve palsy associated with an open fracture and penetrating stab wound.

Foster and associates reported 14 patients with an associated radial nerve palsy after open humeral shaft fracture. Patient age averaged 29 years. Nine of 14 patients (64%) had a radial nerve that was either lacerated or interposed between the fracture fragments. There was an equal incidence of radial nerve laceration and entrapment between types I, II, and III open humeral shaft fracture. Epineural radial nerve repair, done primarily or secondarily, provided a satisfactory return of radial nerve function at a minimum of 1-year follow-up. The authors concluded that radial nerve palsy in association with an open humerus fracture should have a nerve exploration at the time of initial fracture surgery.

Management of a radial nerve palsy that develops after manipulation of a closed humeral shaft fracture remains controversial. Historically, this was an indication for surgical fracture treatment with radial nerve exploration because the nerve could be trapped between the fracture fragments. More recently, however, nonsurgical fracture treatment with surgical exploration 3 or 4 months after injury has been recommended if there is no evidence of neurologic recovery. Advantages of late versus early nerve exploration include: (1) enough time will have passed for recovery from neurapraxia or axonotmesis; (2) precise evaluation of a nerve lesion is possible; (3) the associated fracture will have united; and (4) the results of secondary repair are as good as those of primary repair.

Vascular Injury

Although uncommon, laceration or embarrassment of the brachial artery can be associated with fracture of the humeral shaft. Mechanisms of brachial artery injury after humeral shaft fracture include: gunshot wound, stab wound, vessel entrapment between the fracture fragments, and occlusion after hematoma or swelling in a tight retinacular compartment. The brachial artery has the greatest risk for injury in the proximal and distal thirds of the arm. The role of arteriography in evaluation of long bone fractures with associated vascular compromise remains controversial. Unnecessary delays for studies of equivocal value are imprudent in the management of an ischemic limb. Arterial flow should be emergently reestablished in cases approaching an ischemic time of 6 hours. At surgery, the vessel should be explored and repaired and the fracture stabilized. If limb viability is not in jeopardy, one may provide osseous stability prior to vascular repair. If there is significant ischemic time without distal limb perfusion, the vascular surgeon can place a temporary intraluminal vascular shunt and then stabilize the fracture.

Nonunion

The rate of nonunion following humeral shaft fracture ranges from 0% to 15%. The proximal and distal aspects of the humerus are at greatest risk of nonunion. Factors associated with nonunion include a transverse fracture pattern, fracture distraction, soft-tissue interposition, and inadequate immobilization. Limitation of shoulder motion also increases the risk of humeral nonunion. With loss of normal shoulder motion, increased stresses occur at the fracture level. Other factors that may predispose to nonunion include older age, poor nutritional status, osteoporosis, endocrine abnormality affecting calcium balance, use of steroids, anticoagulation, previous radiation, and fractures underlying a burn.

Compression plating is the treatment of choice for established humeral nonunions. The goals of the treatment are to obtain osseous stability, eliminate the nonunion gap, maintain or restore osseous vascularity, and eradicate infection. Two recent series have reported effective treatment of humeral nonunions using compression plating combined with cancellous bone grafting. In one study, successful union was reported in 24 of 25 (96%) aseptic nonunions of the humerus. Rosen reported a 97% healing rate with one surgical procedure in 32 humeral nonunions treated with plates and screws.

Results: Nonsurgical Management

Zagorski and associates reported a series of 233 humeral shaft fractures treated using a prefabricated functional brace. One hundred seventy fractures were available for follow-up, which ranged from 5 weeks to 48 months. Forty-three fractures were open, 127 were closed. One hundred sixty-seven fractures (96%) united; the average time to union for closed fractures was 9.5 weeks and for open fractures it was 13.6 weeks. At follow-up, varus-valgus angulation averaged 5°, anterior-posterior angulation averaged 3°, and shortening averaged 4 mm. One hundred fifty-eight patients had a good to excellent functional result with nearly full range of shoulder and elbow motion.

Sarmiento and associates reported a series of 85 extra-articular comminuted distal third humerus fractures treated with a functional brace. Fifteen percent were open fractures and 18% had initial radial nerve injury. Seventy-two fractures were available for follow-up; 69 fractures (96%) united. There were no infections. All nerve injuries resolved or were improved at the latest examination. At union, 56 fractures had varus deformity which averaged 9°. The most affected shoulder motion was external rotation; 45% of patients lost from 5° to 45°.

Results: Surgical Treatment

Bell reported a series of 39 humeral shaft fractures stabilized with plates and screws. Thirty-three of 34 fractures (97%) available for follow-up united primarily. Shoulder and elbow motion at follow-up was excellent. Complications included one nonunion, one fixation failure, and one infection. There were no instances of permanent nerve damage.

Heim and associates reported a series of 102 humeral shaft fractures stabilized with plates and screws, in patients who had 1 year minimum follow-up. All fractures united; 89 patients (87%) had full functional recovery of their upper extremity. There were two transitory postoperative radial nerve palsies, five early failures of internal fixation because of technical error, two nonunions, and four postoperative infections.

Brumback and associates reported a series of 58 fractures of the humeral shaft stabilized with intramedullary flexible rods or nails. Fifty-five fractures (94%) united at an average of 10.5 weeks after surgery. Both antegrade and retrograde entry portals were used as well as insertion through the distal humeral epicondyles. Antegrade nailing was associated with excellent functional results if the entry portal did not violate the rotator cuff. Symptoms of subacromial impingement required early hardware removal in seven patients. All fractures that had retrograde nail insertion through the epicondyles had a poor result. Retrograde insertion, however, with the entry portal located proximal to the olecranon fossa was associated with excellent results.

Habernek and Orthner reported a series of 19 humeral shaft fractures stabilized using the Seidel interlocking nail. All nails were inserted after reaming. All fractures united at an average of 2 months after surgery. There were no infections or secondary radial nerve injuries. Eighteen of 19 patients regained full shoulder motion by 6 weeks. Time to return to work varied from 4 to 10 weeks.

Ingman and Waters reported a series of 41 humeral shaft fractures stabilized using a modified Grosse-Kempf tibial nail. Eleven nails were inserted antegrade and 30 retrograde. All nails were inserted after reaming. Twenty of 21 acute fractures united. At 6 weeks, significant restriction of active shoulder flexion was apparent in those patients who had antegrade nail insertion.

In a prospective series of 51 consecutive interlocked humeral nailings performed with an interlocked (Russell-Taylor) intramedullary nail, 41 patients were available for 6-month minimum follow-up. Union was achieved in all acute fractures and eight of ten nonunions; all pathologic fractures united or were asymptomatic. Complications included three transient brachial plexus neurapraxias, two infections, three cases of nail impingement, and two intraoperative fractures.

Selected Bibliography

Amillo S, Barrios RH, Martinez-Peric R, et al: Surgical treatment of the radial nerve lesions associated with fractures of the humerus. *J Orthop Trauma* 1993;7:211-215.

Twelve patients had delayed surgical repair of a radial nerve injury associated with a humeral shaft fracture. The mean interval between the injury and surgical repair was 6 months. Perineural fibrosis at the lesion site was observed in four patients. Three nerves were found trapped in the callus. In two cases, the nerve was found to be partially divided, and in three cases, a total section was observed. The techniques employed were microsurgical reconstruction with interfascicular grafting using sural nerve in six patients, neurolysis in five cases, and tendon transfers in one case. Excellent to good results were obtained in 91% of cases. The authors recommend surgical exploration if there are no clinical or electrophysiologic signs of nerve recovery after 3 months.

Bell MJ, Beauchamp CG, Kellam JK, et al: The results of plating humeral shaft fractures in patients with multiple injuries: The Sunnybrook experience. *J Bone Joint Surg* 1985;67B:293-296.

Brumback RJ, Bosse MJ, Poka A, et al: Intramedullary stabilization of humeral shaft fractures in patients with multiple trauma. *J Bone Joint Surg* 1986;68A:960-969.

Catagni MA, Guerreschi F, Probe RA: Treatment of humeral nonunions with the Ilizarov technique. *Bull Hosp Jt Dis* 1991;51:74-83.

Crolla RM, de Vries LS, Clevers GJ: Locked intramedullary nailing of humeral fractures. *Injury* 1993;24:403-406.

A Seidel nail was used to stabilize 30 acute humeral shaft fractures, nine humeral nonunions, and seven pathologic fractures. In the 27 acute fractures available for follow-up, union occurred within 4 months; 18 patients had an excellent functional result, three had a satisfactory result, two had an unsatisfactory result, and four had a poor result (all attributable to a preexisting condition). Union occurred within 6 months in six of nine nonunions. All seven patients who had a pathologic fracture died within 8 months; while alive, however, these patients were pain-free.

Dabezies EJ, Banta CJ II, Murphy CP, et al: Plate fixation of the humeral shaft for acute fractures, with and without radial nerve injuries. *J Orthop Trauma* 1992;6:10-13.

Forty-four humeral shaft fractures were stabilized using plates and screws; 15 had an associated radial nerve injury. Follow-up was available in all patients and averaged 50 months. Forty-three fractures (97%) united at an average of 12 weeks. All 12 anatomically intact radial nerve palsies recovered in an average of 17 weeks after plate fixation. One lacerated radial nerve was repaired with full recovery. One nerve with segmental loss associated with an open fracture was not repaired, as was an avulsed radial nerve associated with a closed fracture. The authors concluded that plate fixation of humeral shaft fractures results in an excellent rate of osseous union. In addition, the dissection required for plate fixation provides information that may be used to determine appropriate treatment of an associated radial nerve injury and the prognosis for spontaneous recovery.

Dalton JE, Salkeld SL, Satterwhite YE, et al: Biomechanical comparison of intramedullary nailing systems for the humerus. *J Orthop Trauma* 1993;7:367-374.

A laboratory study was performed to evaluate three different intramedullary humeral nailing systems. The reamed Russell-Taylor or Seidel humeral nail provided significantly greater torsional resistance than the True-Flex nail, an unreamed nail that relies on cross-sectional geometry for rotational stability. The Russell-Taylor or Seidel humeral nail also provided significantly greater bending resistance than the True-Flex nail in anterior-posterior and medial-lateral bending.

Flemming JE, Beals RK: Pathologic fracture of the humerus. *Clin Orthop* 1986;203:258-260.

Foster RJ, Swiontkowski MF, Bach AW, et al: Radial nerve palsy caused by open humeral shaft fractures. *J Hand Surg* 1993;18A:121-124.

The authors report 14 open humeral shaft fractures with an associated radial nerve injury. In nine of 14 patients (64%), the radial nerve was either lacerated or interposed between the fracture fragments. There was an equal incidence of radial nerve laceration versus entrapment regardless of the degree of soft tissue injury (grade 1, 2, or 3). Epineural radial nerve repair, performed primarily or secondarily, provided satisfactory return of radial nerve function at a minimum of 1 year follow-up. The authors concluded that radial nerve palsy in association with an open humerus fracture should have a nerve exploration at the time of initial fracture surgery.

Habernek H, Orthner E: A locking nail for fractures of the humerus. *J Bone Joint Surg* 1991;73B:651-653.

Hall RF Jr, Pankovich AM: Ender nailing of acute fractures of the humerus: A study of closed fixation by intramedullary nails without reaming. *J Bone Joint Surg* 1987;69A:558-567.

Healy WL, White GM, Mick CA, et al: Nonunion of the humeral shaft. *Clin Orthop* 1987;219:206-213.

Heim D, Herkert F, Hess P, et al: Surgical treatment of humeral shaft fractures: The Basel experience. *J Trauma* 1993;35:226-232.

The authors report 127 patients with humeral shaft fractures stabilized using plates and screws. One hundred two patients in whom fracture union had occurred were available for 1 year follow-up. Eighty-nine patients (87%) had full functional recovery of their upper extremity. Two patients had a transient postoperative radial nerve palsy, four had a postoperative infection, five were considered fixation failures, and two developed a nonunion.

Henley MB, Chapman JR, Claudi BF: Closed retrograde Hackethal nail stabilization of humeral shaft fractures. *J Orthop Trauma* 1992;6:18-24.

This is a retrospective review of 48 consecutive humeral shaft fractures treated with retrograde inserted stacked Hackethal intramedullary nails. Thirty-three patients were available for follow-up; in 32, (97%) fracture union occurred at an average of 7.5 weeks. No angular malunions greater than 10° in either the coronal or sagittal planes were identified. There were no iatrogenic nerve palsies. Loss of elbow extension averaged 5°; elbow flexion averaged 145°. One patient had proximal nail penetration through the humeral head and two patients had distal nail migration that required removal.

Holstein A, Lewis GB: Fractures of the humerus with radial-nerve paralysis. *J Bone Joint Surg* 1963;45A:1382-1388.

Ingman AM, Waters DA: Locked intramedullary nailing of humeral shaft fractures: Implant design, surgical technique, and clinical results. *J Bone Joint Surg* 1994;76B:23-29.

Forty-one humeral shaft fractures were stabilized using a modified 9-mm Grosse-Kempf reamed interlocked tibial nail. The first 11 nails were inserted antegrade through the rotator cuff; the remainder were inserted retrograde through a portal proximal to the olecranon fossa. Union occurred in 95% of acute fractures and 80% of nonunions, and in all seven pathologic fractures available for 3-month follow-up. At 6-week follow-up, all patients who underwent antegrade insertion had significant restriction of active shoulder elevation. The authors concluded that (1) closed, locked intramedullary humeral nailing can reliably provide secure fixation and acceptable clinical results; (2) locked intramedullary humeral nailing is the method of choice for internal fixation of osteoporotic and pathologic fractures; and (3) the nail should be inserted retrograde from the olecranon fossa for most humeral shaft fractures.

Jupiter JB: Complex non-union of the humeral diaphysis: Treatment with medial approach, an anterior plate and a vascularized fibular graft. *J Bone Joint Surg* 1990;72A: 701-707.

Lewallen RP, Pritchard DJ, Sim FH: Treatment of pathologic fractures or impending fractures of the humerus with Rush rods and methylmethacrylate: Experience with 55 cases in 54 patients, 1968-1977. *Clin Orthop* 1982;166:193-198.

Pollock FH, Drake D, Bovill EG, et al: Treatment of radial neuropathy associated with fractures of the humerus. *J Bone Joint Surg* 1981;63A:239-243.

Postacchini F, Morace GB: Fractures of the humerus associated with paralysis of the radial nerve. *Ital J Orthop Traumatol* 1988;14:455-464.

Riemer BL, D'Ambrosia R: The risk of injury to the axillary nerve, artery, and vein from proximal locking screws of humeral intramedullary nails. *Orthopedics* 1992;15:697-699.

A cadaveric dissection was performed to determine the risk of neurologic and vascular injury from locking screws of humeral intramedullary nails. The main trunk of the axillary nerve was found to be at risk with any penetration from anterior to posterior and any screw penetration beyond the medial cortex with internal rotation. The axillary artery and vein were at risk with penetration over 3 cm regardless of transverse or oblique screw orientation. Transverse screws directed from lateral to medial can injure a small branch of the axillary nerve laterally.

Robinson CM, Bell KM, Court-Brown CM, et al: Locked nailing of humeral shaft fractures: Experience in Edinburgh over a two-year period. *J Bone Joint Surg* 1992;74B: 558-562.

The authors report their experiences using a locked Seidel nail for stabilization of 30 humeral shaft fractures. There were frequent technical difficulties encountered at surgery, particularly involving the locking mechanism. Nail protrusion above the greater tuberosity occurred in 12 cases, usually the result of inadequate locking, and resulted in shoulder pain and poor shoulder function. An additional five patients without evidence of nail protrusion had poor shoulder function, which was attributed to local rotator cuff damage during nail insertion.

Rodriques-Merchan EC: Compression plating versus Hackethal nailing in closed humeral shaft fractures failing nonoperative reduction. *J Orthop Trauma* 1995;9:194-197.

A prospective study was performed in 40 patients comparing compression plating to retrograde Hackethal nailing for stabilization of humeral shaft fractures. Union occurred in 19 of 20 patients who had either intramedullary fixation or compression plating. Patients who had intramedullary fixation, however, required prolonged fracture bracing; in addition, 19 of 20 patients who had intramedullary fixation required removal of hardware secondary to nail prominence. There was no difference in functional outcome at latest follow-up between the two groups of patients.

Rommens PM, Verbruggen J, Broos PL: Retrograde locked nailing of humeral shaft fractures: A review of 39 patients. *J Bone Joint Surg* 1995;77B:84-89.

Thirty-nine humeral shaft fractures were stabilized with closed retrograde insertion of a locked Russell-Taylor humeral nail. All fractures united at an average of 13.7 weeks. At latest follow-up, 92.3% of patients had excellent shoulder function and 87.2% had excellent elbow function. One patient had a postoperative radial nerve palsy that recovered spontaneously within 3 months.

Rosen H: The treatment of nonunions and pseudarthroses of the humeral shaft. *Orthop Clin North Am* 1990;21:725-742.

Sarmiento A, Horowitch A, Aboulafia A, et al: Functional bracing for comminuted extra-articular fractures of the distal third of the humerus. *J Bone Joint Surg* 1990;72B:283-287.

Sarmiento A, Kinman PB, Galvin EG, et al: Functional bracing of fractures of the shaft of the humerus. *J Bone Joint Surg* 1977;59A:596-601.

Stern PJ, Mattingly DA, Pomeroy DL, et al: Intramedullary fixation of humeral shaft fractures. *J Bone Joint Surg* 1984;66A:639-646.

Wu CC, Shih CH: Treatment for nonunion of the shaft of the humerus: Comparison of plates and Seidel interlocking nails. *Can J Surg* 1992;35:661-665.

The authors report a series of 35 nonunions of the humeral shaft treated with either a plate and screws (19 patients) or an antegrade inserted interlocked nail (16 patients). Follow-up ranged from 12 to 52 months. Plate fixation resulted in a 89.5% union rate at an average of 4.5 months; antegrade nailing resulted in an 87.5% union rate at an average of 4.4 months. Patients who had plate fixation had more complications than those managed with interlocked nailing (21% versus 12%). The authors concluded that interlocked nailing is comparable to plating for the treatment of humeral shaft nonunions, but may be associated with fewer complications.

Zagorski JB, Latta LL, Zych GA, et al: Diaphyseal fractures of the humerus: Treatment with prefabricated braces. *J Bone Joint Surg* 1988;70A:607-610.

V
Arthritis/Arthroplasty

John J. Brems, MD
Section Editor

24

Inflammatory Arthritis of the Shoulder

Patrick M. Connor, MD and Donald F. D'Alessandro, MD

Introduction

The shoulder is commonly symptomatic in patients with inflammatory arthritis. Although shoulder problems may not be the first manifestation of disease, patients often present to their internist, rheumatologist, or orthopaedic surgeon with shoulder pain caused by acromioclavicular arthritis, acute or chronic bursitis, rotator cuff disease, and glenohumeral synovitis or arthritis. In a review of more than 100 patients with rheumatoid arthritis, 91% reported shoulder pain or functional limitations referable to the shoulder, with approximately 33% of patients having severe complaints. In addition, this same report showed that initiation of the destructive process of the rheumatoid shoulder inevitably leads to painful restriction of shoulder motion and progressive loss of function.

Rheumatoid arthritis is the most common of the inflammatory arthritides. Although other inflammatory disease processes may affect the shoulder (eg, systemic lupus erythematosus, ankylosing spondylitis, gouty arthritis, pseudogout, psoriatic arthritis), the pathologic and clinical manifestations are similar to those of rheumatoid arthritis. Moreover, the management principles are the same. Although this chapter primarily addresses the symptomatic rheumatoid shoulder, the clinical concepts and principles of treatment presented can be applied to other inflammatory etiologies as well.

Pathophysiology

Initially, the rheumatoid shoulder usually presents with an intense glenohumeral synovitis and painful distention of the joint capsule, resulting in marked restriction of motion. Theoretically, this lack of motion diminishes the production and circulation of synovial fluid, compromising articular cartilage nutrition. In addition, there is direct destruction of the hyaline cartilage caused by the effect of proteases and collagenases present in the inflamed synovium and pannus. As a patient splints the painful shoulder and avoids extreme ranges of motion, the humeral head maintains a relatively central position in the glenoid, predisposing to selective central glenoid "wear" or "erosion" of the unhealthy cartilage. Ultimately, the hyaline cartilage is lost, cystic formation occurs, and small bony excrescences appear along the margins of the joint. It is unusual to have asymmetric capsular contractures in rheumatoid arthritis, which also contributes to the characteristic central wear, as opposed to the selective posterior glenoid wear seen most commonly in osteoarthritis. Cartilage destruction continues through this inflammatory process, peripheral bony erosions occur from pannus destruction, and the end result is glenohumeral incongruity and painful arthritis (Fig. 1).

Neer has described three types of involvement in the rheumatoid shoulder: dry, wet, and resorptive. In the dry form, there is loss of joint space with sclerosis and few cystic lesions in the bone, and a marked tendency for stiffness. Minimal erosions are seen and eventual marginal osteophytes may form, although usually smaller than those in osteoarthritis. Clinically, these patients have much more stiffness and weakness than those patients with osteoarthritis. In the wet form, there are exuberant granulations and marginal erosions that cause severe destruction of the proximal humerus. In addition, there is progressive erosion of the humeral head into the glenoid. In the resorptive type, destruction and resorption of the bone is the outstanding feature. These various clinical types have significant implications on performing shoulder arthroplasty. In the dry type, there is usually adequate bone stock for reconstruction, but in the others the bone is often deficient, usually soft and easily fractured.

Although many believe that a high-riding humerus in a patient with rheumatoid arthritis and glenohumeral joint destruction is a definitive sign of a massive rotator cuff tear, the rotator cuff is intact in most shoulder arthroplasties performed on patients with rheumatoid arthritis. In fact, the reported incidence of full-thickness rotator cuff tears has varied from only 10% to 40% in patients undergoing shoulder arthroplasty for rheumatoid arthritis. The initial cause of the humeral ascent is thought to be loss of the superomedial aspect of the articular surface. The glenohumeral fulcrum is lost, which causes an imbalance of the force couple between a strong deltoid and a weak, poorly rehabilitated rotator cuff. Thus, the rotator cuff is no longer able to function as an efficient humeral head depressor. Once the articular surface becomes more involved, the disease process progresses. Although rotator cuff tears in the shoulder with inflammatory arthritis are usually caused by tendon invasion by the inflammatory process, superior translocation of the humerus in the later stages of the disease also causes impingement erosion of the cuff. End-stage rheumatoid arthritis, therefore, is characterized by severe central and medial erosion of the upper glenoid toward the coracoid base associated with a large or massive rotator cuff defect resulting in an extremely painful shoulder with very limited function (Fig. 2). This is similar to arthrokatadysis in the hip.

This cascade of events has led authors to recommend early shoulder arthroplasty prior to irreparable bone damage and cuff degeneration. Early replacement arthroplasty of a rheumatoid shoulder can result in excellent function, whereas surgery on an end-stage rheumatoid shoulder with a massive rotator cuff tear and bone loss may achieve acceptable pain relief but disappointing function. As stated by Neer, "the answer to an easier and more successful arthroplasty on a rheumatoid shoulder has become clear. The operation should be performed prior to the development of severe bone loss and rotator cuff damage." Thus, shoulder arthroplasty is

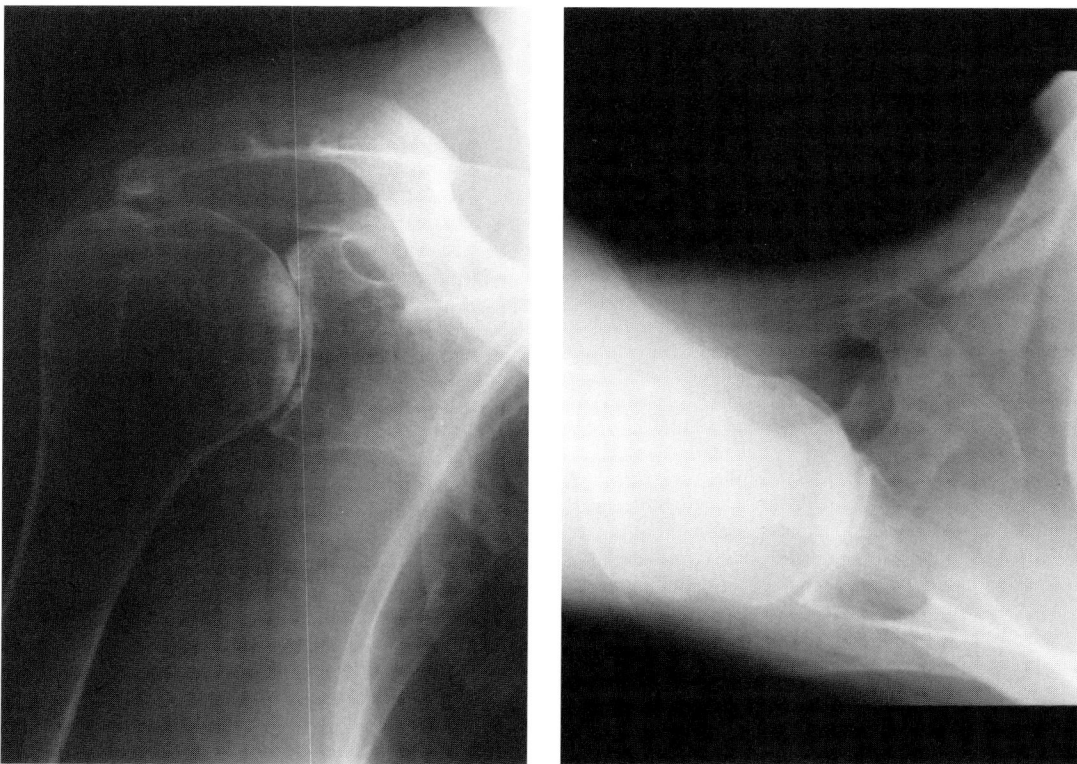

Fig. 1 Radiographs of a rheumatoid shoulder with moderate arthritic involvement. **Left,** Anteroposterior view shows characteristic osteopenia and loss of glenohumeral joint space but maintenance of humeral head sphericity and minimal marginal osteophyte formation. **Right,** Axillary view demonstrates central glenoid wear pattern seen with rheumatoid arthritis as opposed to posterior humeral head subluxation and posterior glenoid wear usually seen in osteoarthritis.

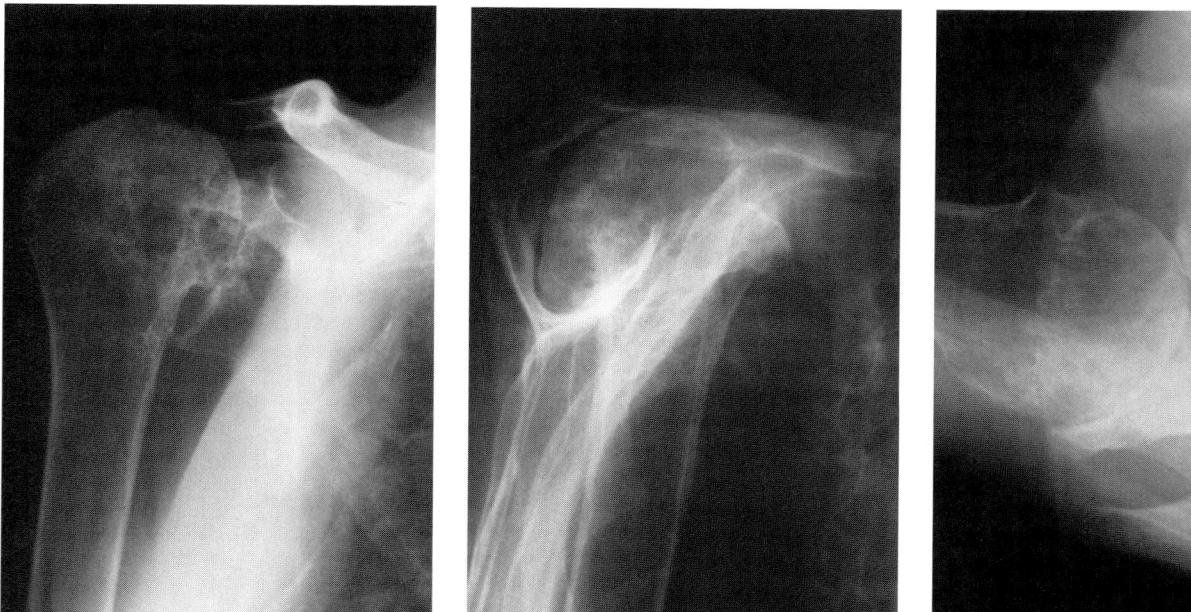

Fig. 2 Radiographs of end-stage rheumatoid arthritis. **Left,** Anteroposterior view shows complete loss of glenohumeral joint space with erosion of the superior glenoid and subchondral cystic changes in the humeral head. **Center,** Outlet view shows superior and anterior subluxation of the humeral head with loss of the acromial humeral distance consistent with massive rotator cuff tear. **Right,** Axillary view shows severe central erosion of the glenoid and insufficient glenoid bone stock to securely fix a glenoid component.

recommended early in this clinical spectrum, thereby minimizing the need for potentially harmful medications and avoiding further bone and soft-tissue destruction.

Clinical Presentation

It is rare for a patient with rheumatoid arthritis to initially present with monarticular shoulder involvement; however, it may occur. If a rheumatoid patient presents with an acutely painful, swollen shoulder and no history of trauma, the physician should always consider the possibility of septic subacromial bursitis and/or septic glenohumeral arthritis. In addition to a detailed history, physical examination, plain radiographs, and screening laboratory tests (complete blood count with differential, erythrocyte sedimentation rate, and C-reactive protein), aspiration of the bursa and/or glenohumeral joint should be performed. A cell count suggestive of rheumatoid or other inflammatory arthritis ranges from 10,000 to 50,000/mm^3; a cell count over 75,000/mm^3 is strongly suggestive of a septic process.

The cause of shoulder pain in patients with rheumatoid arthritis is often difficult to determine. These patients usually have associated cervical spine disease with possible radiculopathy or myelopathy. They may also have pain derived from the acromioclavicular joint, subacromial bursa, rotator cuff, or glenohumeral joint. In addition, referred discomfort and limitation of function of the elbow and hand when performing manual muscle testing of the shoulder can make assessment difficult. For example, a patient with glenohumeral degeneration from rheumatoid arthritis may also have pain from coexisting acromioclavicular (AC) arthritis. If the surgeon neglects to address the concomitant AC arthritis at the time of shoulder arthroplasty, the outcome will be disappointing. A thorough preoperative clinical evaluation must be done because of the potential for polyarticular involvement of the shoulder joint complex.

Despite the clinician's best efforts, the presenting symptoms and radiographic appearance of the rheumatoid shoulder may often fail to indicate the precise etiology of pain. Differential anesthetic injections of the AC joint, subacromial space, and/or glenohumeral joint are beneficial in evaluating these patients with shoulder girdle pain. In a recent study of 75 rheumatoid shoulders, local anesthetic injections of 1% xylocaine, followed by corticosteroid injections if indicated, were found to be beneficial for determining the most appropriate nonsurgical or surgical treatment. A subsequent study of patients with rheumatoid arthritis revealed that extraglenohumeral joint surgery (eg, bursectomy, acromioplasty, and distal clavicle excision) that was based on the response to preoperative injection testing resulted in no or minimal postoperative pain in 19 of 22 shoulders at an average 30-month follow-up, even in the presence of mild radiographic glenohumeral joint involvement. Thus, by combining a detailed history and physical examination with differential xylocaine injections, the etiology of shoulder pain in patients with early rheumatoid involvement of the shoulder can generally be isolated. It should be noted, however, that by the time most patients with rheumatoid arthritis are considered for surgery, the glenohumeral joint is often obviously symptomatic and arthritic. For this reason, repeated deep injections are not recommended because of the risk of contributing to soft-tissue deterioration and the possibility of introducing infection.

The radiographic appearance of the rheumatoid shoulder parallels that of other joints subjected to the rheumatoid process. Osteopenia, juxta-articular erosions, and cystic changes are common findings. Symmetric loss of joint space, subchondral sclerosis, and osteophytes are seen either later in the disease process or in the "dry" or "mixed" forms of inflammatory arthritis as described by Neer. Humeral head ascent is often seen on the anteroposterior radiograph, and central glenoid erosion can be seen on the axillary lateral view. Computed tomography can be used to determine the presence and size of subchondral cysts and delineate the amount of bone available for glenoid resurfacing. Ultrasound may be used to assess the status of the rotator cuff, but is technically difficult and highly operator-dependent. Magnetic resonance imaging (MRI) is useful for the preoperative diagnosis of rotator cuff tears and is currently favored over arthrography because it is noninvasive, more accurate, and is useful for quantifying the size of a rotator cuff defect. MRI may also demonstrate intra-articular pathology in rheumatoid arthritis better than plain films, but whether this is of clinical benefit has yet to be determined.

Nonsurgical Management

Conservative treatment of the rheumatoid shoulder should incorporate a team approach with a rheumatologist, orthopaedic surgeon, and physical therapist. The contribution from each specialty is important, and a close working relationship with open communication is essential to derive the most benefit from nonsurgical management.

The medical treatment of the patient with a symptomatic shoulder and inflammatory arthritis is coordinated by the rheumatologist. Many different medications are available to decrease both symptoms and disease progression, including salicylates, analgesics, nonsteroidal anti-inflammatory drugs, gold salts, corticosteroids, chloroquine, sulfasalazine, D-penicillamine, and methotrexate. In the last decade, the major change in the therapeutic approach to the medical treatment of rheumatoid and other inflammatory arthritides has been the universal acceptance and widespread use of methotrexate. However, there are medications that should and should not be used with methotrexate, and potential side effects should be monitored.

The rheumatoid shoulder is prone to stiffness. Early attempts at detection and treatment of loss of motion are beneficial. Physical therapy with low heat, analgesia, and assistive exercises may be done several times a day, usually at home. Emphasis is placed on regaining and maintaining forward elevation and internal and external rotation. It is important to avoid excessive stretching and/or strengthening exercises in the acutely inflamed shoulder because these actions may exacerbate irritation and inflammation. Isometric exercises and gentle pendulum exercises should be performed during this period. An injection of a mixture of corticosteroid and xylocaine is helpful in the acutely inflamed glenohumeral joint or subacromial space. Numerous corticosteroid injections should be avoided. Once the acute inflammation subsides, active-assisted exercises are begun to improve strength and function.

The role of the orthopaedic surgeon in the conservative management of the rheumatoid shoulder is to monitor the status of the soft tissues (including capsule and rotator cuff) by physical examination and bone and articular surfaces by radiographs. If stiffness occurs, gentle manipulation after an injection may be beneficial. However, manipulation under general anesthesia is discouraged in the management of the stiff, rheumatoid shoulder because of the risk of fracture of osteogenic bone and of rotator cuff avulsion. If adequate conservative measures fail, arthroscopic or open release(s) are preferable but more often are performed in conjunction with the procedures discussed in the next section.

Once destruction of the articular surfaces and/or rotator cuff has occurred, nonsurgical management has failed and prompt reconstructive surgery should be considered. Severe bony erosion and soft-tissue damage, particularly of the rotator cuff, will significantly compromise the outcome of surgery.

Surgical Management

Synovectomy/Bursectomy

Synovectomy for isolated glenohumeral synovitis may be indicated within a narrow time frame during the disease process of the rheumatoid shoulder. This procedure is useful in those few patients with inflammatory arthritis who present with signs of intra-articular inflammation and synovitis but still have a congruent joint and no evidence of cyst formation or joint degeneration. In most medical communities, the rheumatologist is the gatekeeper for the care of the rheumatoid patient. Consequently, the orthopaedic surgeon rarely encounters patients who meet these criteria, thus emphasizing the need for improved communication among those physicians caring for rheumatoid patients. Petersson reported the results of 15 patients with rheumatoid arthritis who underwent open glenohumeral synovectomy. The indications were severe, protracted shoulder disability in which a regimen of oral medications as well as intra-articular injections was unsuccessful and in which articular surfaces were normal or near-normal. At an average follow-up of 2 years, two patients had undergone subsequent shoulder arthroplasty and two others had painful, arthritic shoulders; however, pain relief, improved function, and slowing of the progression of the disease occurred in the other 11 patients. Pahle and Kvarnes have also reported encouraging results from open synovectomy while noting that the best results are obtained in those rheumatoid shoulders with normal or near-normal preoperative radiographs.

The arthroscopic approach enables better glenohumeral joint visualization than the open technique and thus provides a theoretically better ability to perform a synovectomy. Arthroscopic findings include synovial hyperemia, hypertrophic villi, and rice bodies (Fig. 3). Arthroscopic synovectomy can be performed in combination with removal of loose bodies, debridement of bursal and joint-sided rotator cuff fraying, and debridement of labral lesions. Early results using the arthroscopic approach have been encouraging. As noted above, the majority of patients referred to the orthopaedist with rheumatoid inflammation of the shoulder have significant cartilage and/or bone destruction at the time of presentation and are not candidates for synovectomy alone.

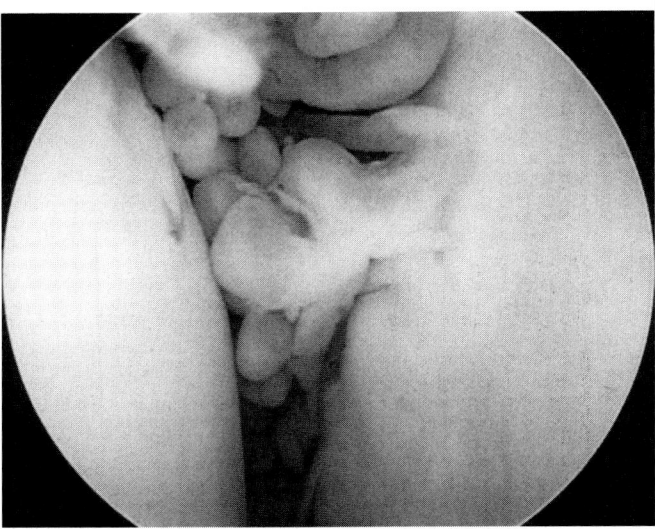

Fig. 3 Arthroscopic photograph from posterior portal showing intact humeral (**left**) and glenoid (**right**) articular cartilage. Exuberant hyperemic synovitis with hypertrophic villi is evident.

Occasionally the subacromial bursa may be the primary site of involvement in patients with inflammatory arthritis characterized by villous hypertrophy and marked lymphocytic infiltration of the thickened bursal tissue. Huge enlargements of the subacromial and subdeltoid bursa have been reported, at times mimicking a chest wall neoplasm. The bursa is filled with rice bodies and with less fluid than would be expected, simulating a solid mass. In patients with rheumatoid arthritis, subacromial bursectomy and acromioplasty are performed for the same indications as in those patients with subacromial impingement syndrome without rheumatoid arthritis—namely failure of nonsurgical management consisting of medications, subacromial anesthetic injection(s), and physical therapy. There is no predetermined amount of time before surgery should be recommended in a patient in whom nonsurgical treatment has been unsuccessful. However, several months to a year of a supervised nonsurgical regimen is usually necessary for the physician to ascertain the degree and pattern of shoulder involvement for an individual patient before specific surgical recommendations are made. Intuitively, patients with rheumatoid arthritis may be better served by relatively earlier subacromial bursectomy and decompression prior to the development of rotator cuff damage by degradative lymphocytic enzymes. Simpson and Kelly recently reported promising early results after bursectomy, acromioplasty, and distal clavicle excision in patients with rheumatoid arthritis. Preoperative local anesthetic injections were used to localize the sites of pain and serve as a basis for the surgical procedure performed. These authors have shown that extraglenohumeral joint procedures planned according to the results of preoperative injection testing can play a useful role in the management of the shoulder in rheumatoid arthritis, even if mild glenohumeral joint involvement has been documented radiographically (Fig. 4). The long-term results of this approach, however, are not yet available.

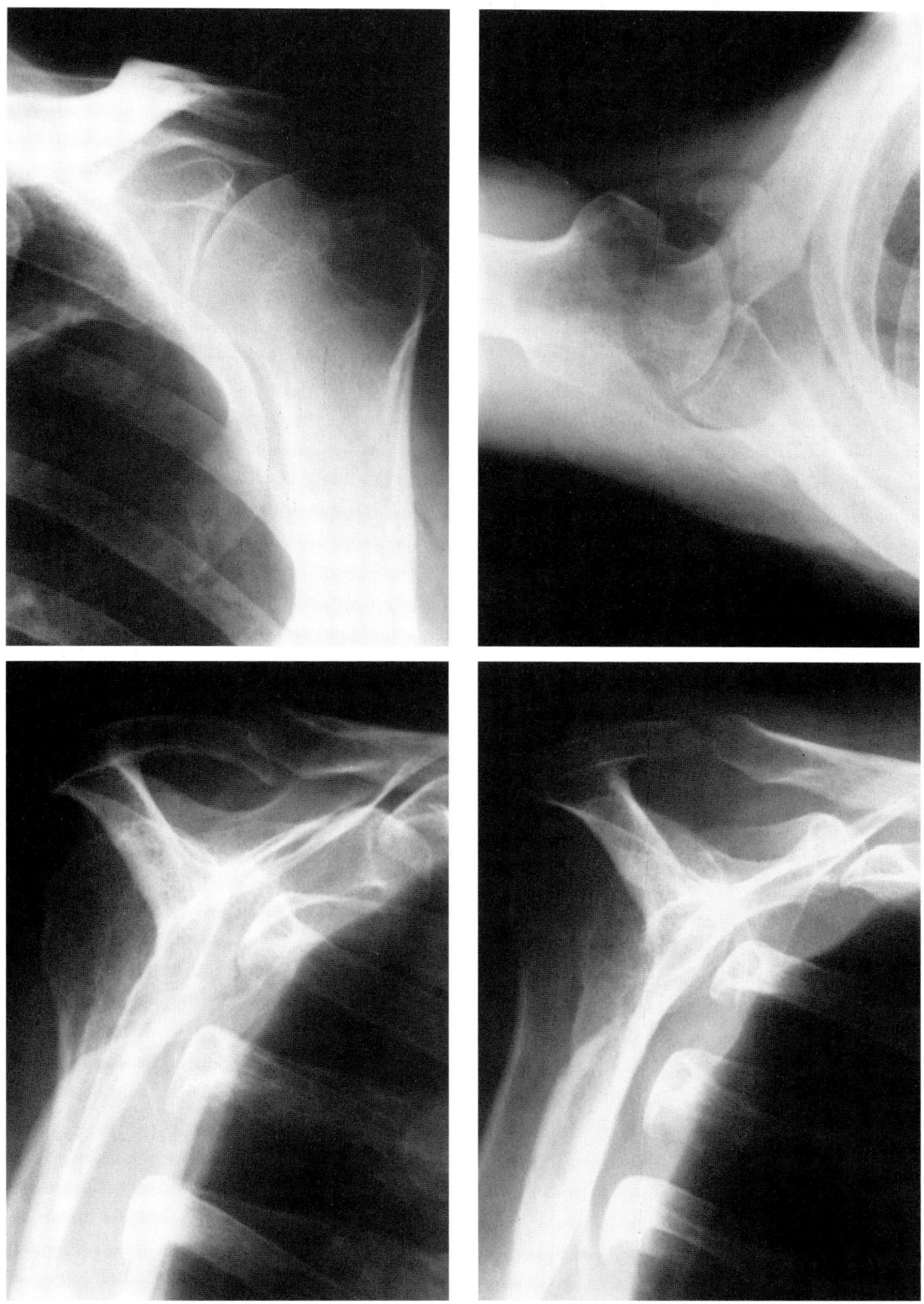

Fig. 4 Radiographs of a patient with early rheumatoid arthritis of the shoulder. **Top left,** Glenohumeral joint space is maintained. **Top right,** The axillary view reveals classic peripheral subchondral erosion. **Bottom left,** This patient presented with subacromial symptomatology and an associated type III acromial morphology. **Bottom right,** Arthroscopic synovectomy and acromioplasty were performed, which significantly ameliorated the patient's complaints.

As mentioned previously, the AC or sternoclavicular (SC) joints may also be symptomatic in patients with rheumatoid arthritis. If the physical examination and differential injection(s) verify AC or SC arthritis, resection of the distal or medial clavicle, respectively, can be performed. If the costoclavicular ligaments have been rendered incompetent with SC arthritis, reconstruction of these ligaments and medial clavicle excision should be performed simultaneously.

Rotator Cuff Repair

Numerous studies have reported that satisfactory results in both pain relief and functional improvement can be expected in approximately 85% of patients in whom surgical repair of a rotator cuff tear is performed. These results, however, are based on all diagnoses. The subset of patients with inflammatory arthritis have not been specifically evaluated. Patients with rheumatoid arthritis rarely have an isolated rotator cuff tear. The more common scenario is one in which the patient presents with shoulder pain, weakness, and radiographic findings of proximal humeral migration and a narrowed joint space.

Rotator cuff repair may be indicated in the unusual patient with rheumatoid arthritis who presents with signs and symptoms of primary subacromial pain without evidence of glenohumeral joint destruction. After glenohumeral synovectomy and subacromial bursectomy are performed, repair of a small full-thickness rotator cuff tear may yield a favorable outcome. However, the long-term results may not be as predictable or satisfactory as in those patients without inflammatory arthritis.

Shoulder Arthroplasty

Because resection arthroplasty and arthrodesis fail to consistently provide pain relief and maintenance of function, glenohumeral arthroplasty remains the most commonly performed procedure for the arthritic shoulder with inflammatory arthritis. Shoulder arthroplasty is recommended for painful glenohumeral incongruity that has not responded to nonsurgical management. Before proceeding to the operating room, the patient must be carefully evaluated for active or potential sites of infection. In rheumatoid patients on long-term regimens of steroid medication, the skin is atrophic and prone to breakdown. Rheumatoid foot deformities commonly create pressure sores and ulcerations. In addition, the patient should be instructed about and motivated to perform postoperative physical therapy.

In the rheumatoid patient with upper extremity involvement in multiple joints, the issue regarding the appropriate sequence of surgery is controversial. Although some have suggested that shoulder arthroplasty should take precedence over elbow arthroplasty and hand surgery, other authors believe that elbow replacement, if performed prior to shoulder arthroplasty, provides the upper limb with more improved function. Most agree, however, that the first surgical priority should be the joint(s) that cause(s) the patient the most pain and disability. If one joint is not any more or less disabling than the others in a single extremity, surgical priority must be determined. Because the function of the shoulder and elbow are to position the hand in space, hand and wrist function should be maximized prior to shoulder or elbow surgery. Neer has stated that shoulder arthroplasty should take precedence over elbow arthroplasty for a number of reasons. Improved shoulder range of motion after shoulder arthroplasty may decrease the functional stresses on the arthritic elbow. In addition, with the absence of referred pain from the shoulder to the elbow, the need for total elbow arthroplasty may be delayed or obviated. Most importantly, maximizing rotator cuff function in the rheumatoid upper extremity is essential. Delay in addressing the pathomechanics of the rheumatoid shoulder will compromise the integrity of the rotator cuff and adversely affect overall function of the upper extremity. Conversely, the severity of elbow involvement prior to total elbow arthroplasty in rheumatoid arthritis has not been shown to alter outcome. In addition, if total elbow arthroplasty is performed first, there is concern that the total elbow replacement is at risk for periprosthetic fracture as rotational forces are placed on the humerus when the shoulder is dislocated for the shoulder arthroplasty procedure. When there is severe involvement of both shoulders, bilateral arthroplasties are performed, usually with a 3- to 6-month interval between procedures.

A few technical considerations bear mentioning. If a full-thickness cuff tear is present, it is usually small and easily repaired using standard techniques. The coracoacromial (CA) ligament, however, is maintained to provide a buttress to anterosuperior humeral ascent. The tendon of the long head of the biceps is commonly torn, but if not, all efforts should be made to preserve it. There is commonly an impressive synovitis extending from the joint down the bicipital tendon sheath; this synovitis is decompressed and debrided during the exposure. If an AC arthroplasty is to be performed, the superior AC ligaments should be preserved to maintain stability of the distal clavicle.

In a recent review of total shoulder replacement in rheumatoid arthritis, it was found that nearly half of the press-fit humeral components demonstrated progressive radiographic loosening as opposed to no signs of loosening in the cemented humeral components, supporting the fact that the humeral component should be cemented. A bone or synthetic cement plug is recommended because subsequent elbow reconstruction may be necessary later. Furthermore, the humeral diaphyseal bone is usually extremely osteoporotic and predisposed to fracture during the procedure. Long-stem humeral prosthesis components should be available to bypass an intraoperative humeral shaft fracture should it occur.

One of the most controversial issues in shoulder arthroplasty in general, and shoulder arthroplasty for inflammatory arthritis in particular, is whether to perform a total shoulder arthroplasty or hemiarthroplasty. The decision of whether to use a glenoid component is based primarily on three factors: whether the rotator cuff is intact or repairable such that it can center the humeral head on the resurfaced glenoid, whether there is sufficient bone stock to support a glenoid component, and whether there is sufficient joint volume available for a glenoid component (determined by the status of the soft-tissue envelope).

If there is a massive rotator cuff tear or a thin, atrophic cuff that no longer functions as an efficient humeral head depressor, superior glenoid rim loading ("rocking horse glenoid") occurs, thereby increasing the chance for mechanical loosening. As described above, in shoulders with advanced inflammatory arthritis, the humeral head is often translated superiorly, articulating with the CA arch. Attempts to constrain the glenoid superiorly (with an overhang) have been generally abandoned because of increased rates of loosening and lack of functional improvement. The use of hemiarthroplasty in these shoulders maintains this new fulcrum with the superior glenoid and CA arch, often resulting in surprisingly good postoperative function. The lack of glenoid resurfacing has not been shown to adversely affect pain relief in patients with severe rheumatoid arthritis, perhaps because joint compressive forces in these patients are reduced. Although a bipolar prosthesis has been offered as a compromise between hemiarthroplasty and total shoulder replacement, the large amount of bone resection required for implantation, difficulties with rotator cuff reapproximation with the large bipolar implant, and the lack of follow-up data preclude its general acceptance.

The bone stock available for implantation is the second important factor in deciding whether to use a glenoid component. The glenoid bone in rheumatoid shoulders is commonly deficient with a superior and central "protrusion" pattern of destruction; this often leaves the inferior glenoid pole intact, giving the face of the glenoid a cephalic tilt. A reamer or burr is used to contour the inferior glenoid bone and readjust the orientation of the glenoid face prior to placement of the glenoid component. A smaller-sized glenoid component is often used with either pegged fixation or fixation with a keel cut shorter than normal. If the bone cannot be sculpted to support the component, or if the bone stock is so deficient that anchorage of a glenoid component is thought to be compromised, a hemiarthroplasty alone is preferred. The use of glenoid bone grafting is not recommended in patients with inflammatory arthritis as fixation and incorporation of the bone graft is generally poor because of the osteogenic bone.

Circumferential contraction of the joint volume in patients with long-standing rheumatoid arthritis may also preclude the placement of a prosthetic glenoid despite extensive surgical releases. Forcing a glenoid component into an overly tight joint space will limit postoperative range of motion and function. In severe cases, the tissues are inordinately tight, making it impossible to accommodate both the prosthetic humeral head and glenoid components while allowing a functional amount of soft-tissue laxity.

Although glenoid resurfacing is often avoided in patients who are young and active, young patients with rheumatoid arthritis may perhaps be the best suited for total shoulder arthroplasty. These patients usually live relatively sedentary lifestyles, have disease involvement of the elbow, wrist, and hand, and consequently are unlikely to place high physical demands on their shoulder arthroplasty. With competent rotator cuff musculature, they are at less risk of eccentric glenoid component loading and early mechanical failure. Thus, patients with cartilage loss, painful glenoid incongruity, relatively normally functioning rotator cuff muscles, adequate bone stock, and functional soft-tissue laxity are excellent candidates for glenoid resurfacing. Hopefully, patients with rheumatoid arthritis who have these characteristics will consult with the orthopaedic surgeon before severe bone loss, superior humeral migration, and rotator cuff pathology preclude an optimal result from shoulder arthroplasty.

If humeral hemiarthroplasty is chosen for the rheumatoid patient with a massive rotator cuff tear, some modifications of the surgical technique are advisable. Care is taken to maintain the CA ligamentous arch to superiorly contain the humeral head. The subscapularis tendon is usually inferiorly retracted, and the head protrudes superiorly, creating a boutonnière-type deformity. The subscapularis can usually be mobilized so that there is sufficient tendon for superior transposition. It is important to examine the posterior undersurface of the acromion because the leading edge of the rotator cuff may be adherent to this undersurface. The remaining posterior rotator cuff tissue is carefully mobilized to cover as much of the posterior-superior humerus as possible. However, to avoid weakness of external rotation, the remaining intact insertion of the posterior cuff is never detached. Several #2 nonabsorbable sutures are placed through the greater tuberosity for reattachment of the posterior and superior cuff, and through the lesser tuberosity for reattachment of the subscapularis prior to implantation of the prosthesis.

Modular humeral components are extremely helpful in this setting. Once the humeral stem has been cemented in place, various humeral head sizes allow the surgeon to pull the rotator cuff tissues into proposed alignment to assess the stability of the construct and the ability to repair the rotator cuff over the humeral head. The aim is to adequately fill the joint space while permitting rotator cuff repair under minimal tension and to avoid overstuffing this space in order to provide functional laxity. Complete superior coverage may be obtained by transposing the subscapularis superiorly and by repairing the remnants of the posterior cuff and supraspinatus. When tissue is too deficient or is unable to hold sutures, attention is focused on achieving stable anterior and posterior buttresses to maximize postoperative stability.

Results/Outcome

The results of shoulder arthroplasty for inflammatory arthritis have been favorable. Pain relief is reliably achieved, with most studies reporting over 90% satisfactory relief of pain. Functional improvement, however, has been less reliable in this subset of patients than in those patients with osteoarthritis or osteonecrosis. Improvements in range of motion, strength, and performance in activities of daily living are dependent on the preoperative status of the rotator cuff, surrounding soft tissues (eg, capsule), and glenoid bone.

Barrett and associates, in a review of 114 patients with polyarticular rheumatoid arthritis who had 140 total shoulder replacements, showed that 93% of patients had excellent pain relief. However, more modest improvements in active elevation (average of 34°) were dependent on the severity of the disease. As a result of their inferior findings associated with severe rheumatoid involvement, the authors advocated prompt total shoulder arthroplasty once the significant clinical and radiologic findings can no longer be controlled by conservative means. An inordinate delay in treatment allows further soft tissue and bone destruction by the inflammatory process and compromises results. Neer reported on 50 rheumatoid shoulders with greater than 2-year follow-up in his classic 1982 article. Forty-seven of 50 had satisfactory results after total shoulder replacement, and unsatisfactory ratings in three were caused by functional limitations rather than continued pain. Figgie and associates had similar findings in their evaluation of 50 total shoulder replacements in 36 patients with inflammatory arthritis; pain relief was nearly universal and functional results were related to the status of the rotator cuff and motivation of the patient.

Boyd and associates, in a retrospective review of 95 patients who had either humeral head or total shoulder replacements for rheumatoid arthritis, found that total shoulder replacement achieved complete pain relief more reliably than humeral head replacement (total shoulder replacement, 48%; humeral head replacement, 29%) and that functional improvements in range of motion occurred more often in those patients with total shoulder replacement than with humeral head replacement (total shoulder replacement, 37° improvement in elevation; humeral head replacement, 14° improvement in elevation). These more favorable results with total shoulder replacement were believed to be because these patients had diffuse cartilage abnormalities caused by their inflammatory arthropathy, a factor that humeral head replacement alone did not address. Shon and associates recently reviewed 46 shoulders in 36 patients who underwent arthroplasty for inflammatory arthritis. Glenoid resurfacing was performed in the absence of significant glenoid bone loss, massive rotator cuff tears, or severe soft-tissue contractures. Outcomes were comparable in the 20 total shoulder replacements and 26 humeral head replacements in regard to pain relief; (total shoulder replacement, 90% satisfactory pain relief, humeral head replacement, 92%), but range of motion and functional improvements were greater in the total shoulder replacement group. Results were more favorable in those patients with less severe disease.

Complications

Although the incidence of complications after shoulder arthroplasty has been less than for other major joint reconstructions, they are more common in patients with rheumatoid arthritis than in those with arthroplasties for other diagnoses. Although many complications are potentially avoided by proper indications, technique, and rehabilitation, some are unavoidable. It is important for the reconstructive shoulder surgeon to be aware of these potential complications, educate the patient about the relative risks, and be prepared to address these complications as indicated.

Infection
The shoulder is preferentially protected from infection, with its abundant blood supply and excellent soft-tissue coverage. Fortunately, the occurrence of infection after shoulder arthroplasty in general is rare. However, patients with rheumatoid or other inflammatory arthritides who have shoulder arthroplasty may be more likely to develop a postoperative infection because of such factors as their systemic disease process, immunosuppression, concomitant steroid dependence, and poor tissue healing. Great care must be taken preoperatively to decrease the likelihood of infection, including maximizing preoperative nutrition status and the patient's general medical condition, adhering to standard strict sterile techniques, and close monitoring of the wound postoperatively. Whether antibiotic-impregnated cement is an effective prophylaxis against infection in shoulder arthroplasty is unknown.

When infection occurs after arthroplasty, an aggressive surgical approach is indicated. If an early infection with a sensitive organism is present, aggressive irrigation and debridement of the shoulder and maintenance of the arthroplasty may be possible. However, if a resistant organism is present or if the infection is subacute or chronic, a two-stage reimplantation is recommended. If removal of the humeral cemented stem can be achieved without complete destruction of the humeral bone stock, an antibiotic-impregnated spacer in the shape of a hemiarthroplasty is used to maintain a soft-tissue spacer for the ensuing reimplantation while also delivering local antibiotics. If there is no radiographic evidence of loosening at the cemented humeral stem, a cement spacer can be fashioned in the shape of a modular head to serve the same purpose, while avoiding the complications associated with trying to remove a well-cemented humeral stem component from severely osteogenic bone. Intravenous and oral antibiotics during the treatment period should be supervised by an infectious disease physician. Long-term suppressive antibiotic therapy is often indicated.

Fracture
The risk of incurring an intraoperative humeral shaft fracture is significant. Rheumatoid bone is extremely soft and the cortices are thin. Fractures can occur with dislocation of the humeral head, canal reaming, or reduction of the prosthesis. Great care must be taken during extension and external rotation of the shoulder when dislocating the humeral head in an effort to avoid fracture of the tuberosity or humeral shaft. If during the procedure a humeral shaft fracture occurs near the tip of the prosthesis, a long-stemmed prosthesis may be required to bypass the fracture. In this situation, a barrier should be used on the outside surface of the humeral shaft to avoid extravasation of cement into the soft tissues and potential radial nerve injury. Oblique fractures of the humeral shaft are treated similarly. In this instance, the rehabilitation should be modified in the postoperative period to avoid excessive rotation exercises for an 8- to 12-week period to allow sufficient fracture healing. Periprosthetic fractures treated with long-stem humeral components and cables have been demonstrated to be stable without the need to alter the rehabilitation.

Tuberosity fractures should be managed in the same fashion as four-part fractures. Fixation via nonabsorbable nylon sutures through the junction of the rotator cuff and tuberosities is used. These sutures should be attached to both the fin of the prosthesis and the proximal shaft. Postoperatively, active motion should be avoided until tuberosity healing has occurred.

Postoperative fractures can be treated conservatively if the fracture is stable. However, if the fracture is unstable, further surgery is required. Internal fixation may be difficult, requiring special plates that incorporate cerclage wires as well as screws. In addition, autologous bone graft, allograft cortical struts, methylmethacrylate, and/or long-stemmed prostheses may be necessary. Bonutti and Hawkins have suggested that periprosthetic fractures of the proximal humerus have a high incidence of nonunion, and surgical treatment should be considered.

Instability

Direct anterior or posterior instability after shoulder arthroplasty for rheumatoid arthritis is uncommon. However, a specific type of postoperative instability deserves mention when discussing the rheumatoid population. Anterosuperior instability, caused by a large or massive rotator cuff tear and lack of anterosuperior glenohumeral restraints, is a very difficult complication to manage. Patients often lose the ability to raise and rotate their arm as the glenohumeral fulcrum is lost. With attempts at elevation, the prosthetic humeral head subluxates superiorly and anterior to the distal clavicle and acromion.

Because no ideal treatment for this complication currently exists, prevention must be emphasized. Care must be taken to preserve the CA ligament, anterior acromion, and biceps tendon. Mobilization and repair of concomitant rotator cuff tears should be done at the time of arthroplasty, achieving as much anterior and superior humeral head coverage as possible. If an anterior acromioplasty is performed, a minimal amount of bone should be resected with an emphasis on maintaining the anterior length of the acromion. The CA ligament should be repaired with the deltoid using nonabsorbable suture passed through the acromial bone. In addition, the size and orientation of the humeral component may also help prevent this complication. In patients whose humeral head is articulating with the superior glenoid and CA arch and who are found to have a massive rotator cuff tear at the time of surgery, the use of too small a modular humeral head component, along with excessive anteversion of the component, may predispose the patient to anterosuperior instability. Thus, in this setting an adequate-sized humeral head component that articulates with the contours of the superior glenoid, distal clavicle, and acromial undersurface should be used. Also, by placing the component in relatively more retroversion (~40°), stability will be enhanced.

If symptomatic postoperative anterosuperior instability occurs, the salvage procedures currently available are technically difficult, provide marginal results at best, and are associated with high complication rates. Arthrodesis is an option, but the associated bone loss from the previous arthroplasty may require allograft interposition to achieve a successful fusion. Resection arthroplasty may alleviate the superior instability, but pain relief is unreliable and function is significantly limited. Revision shoulder arthroplasty with CA arch reconstruction has been attempted in this situation, but results are preliminary.

Glenoid Loosening

Fortunately, the incidence of glenoid component failure requiring revision surgery from all diagnoses is low, averaging 3%. Most identifiable causes of aseptic glenoid loosening relate to either improper indications or to the technical aspects of glenoid resurfacing. As mentioned, a glenoid component should not be placed in shoulders where superior eccentric loading of the glenoid component caused by rotator cuff deficiency is present. In addition, with small rheumatoid bony glenoids that cannot reliably anchor a glenoid component, humeral head replacement alone should be performed.

The most common technical cause of aseptic glenoid loosening is inadequate initial stability of the glenoid component. The new glenoid reamers available for contouring the glenoid bone have improved the ability to match the back of the glenoid component to the prepared glenoid surface. Although the incidence of radiolucent lines at the glenoid bone cement interface has generally not correlated with clinical loosening, their common presence has caused concern and is often implicated as rationale for avoiding glenoid resurfacing. There is no standard system for description of these radiographic findings, and reproducible projections permitting serial evaluations of the bone cement interface are nearly impossible. A precise mechanism for comparison views using fluoroscopy has only recently been introduced.

The presence of radiolucent lines about the glenoid component is said to increase the chance of glenoid revision surgery by only approximately 5%. Many of these lines are noted to be present immediately postoperatively and do not progress. In a report on glenoid lucent lines, 69% were found before the patients' hospital discharge, and a statistical correlation was found between the incidence of lucent lines and the surgeon(s) involved. Whether the incidence of initial or progressive radiolucent lines about glenoid prostheses is increased in patients with inflammatory arthritis has not been shown.

Symptomatic glenoid loosening or failure requiring glenoid component revision is rare. This is not to say, however, that glenoid radiolucencies have no clinical merit. The high percentage of glenoid lucent lines is of concern and requires continued investigation.

Other Complications

Complications such as nerve injuries, heterotopic bone, thromboembolism, and postoperative rotator cuff tears have not been shown to be significantly more prevalent in patients with rheumatoid or other inflammatory arthritis versus other diagnostic categories.

Summary

The patient with inflammatory arthritis of the shoulder presents a number of difficult diagnostic and therapeutic challenges to the orthopaedist. Our goal is to obtain optimal pain relief and to preserve maximal shoulder function as the various stages of the rheumatoid process are encountered. There are multiple potential sources of shoulder pain in the rheumatoid patient, including AC and SC arthritis, subacromial and rotator cuff pathology, and glenohumeral synovitis and arthritis. Referred pain from the cervical spine must also be considered. In addition to the requisite careful history and physical examination, differential xylocaine injections can be helpful to delineate the primary cause of pain.

Nonsurgical measures including medications, physical therapy, and judicious use of corticosteroid injections are indicated for the early symptoms of the rheumatoid shoulder. Frequent communication between the rheumatologist, orthopaedist, and physical therapist is essential to provide the best care for these patients.

Preoperative evaluation must consider the patient's overall medical condition, the systemic involvement of the inflammatory disease, and the concomitant involvement of the ipsilateral neck and upper extremity before proceeding with surgery on the shoulder. When indicated, arthroscopic synovectomy, subacromial bursectomy, and rotator cuff repair when necessary can be very beneficial. Ultimately, shoulder arthroplasty performed prior to the development of severe osteoporosis and bone loss, and before superior humeral head migration compromises the integrity of the rotator cuff, will yield gratifying results with regard to pain relief and function.

Selected Bibliography

General

Ennevaara K: Painful shoulder joint in rheumatoid arthritis: A clinical and radiological study of 200 cases, with special reference to arthrography of the glenohumeral joint. *Acta Rheumatol Scand* 1967;11(suppl):1-116.

A classic description is presented of the clinical and radiographic findings in shoulders with rheumatoid arthritis, ranging from early to end-stage disease.

Petersson CJ: Painful shoulders in patients with rheumatoid arthritis: Prevalence, clinical and radiological features. *Scand J Rheumatol* 1986;15:275-279.

One hundred five shoulder joints with rheumatoid arthritis were examined; the mean patient age was 62 years and mean duration of disease 17 years. Ninety-six patients (91%) reported shoulder problems, with 33 having severe painful shoulder disability. With increasing duration of rheumatoid arthritis, there was progression of destructive changes and a decrease in functional motion.

Pathophysiology

Cosgarea AJ, Weng MS, McIntyre JM, et al: Giant synovial cyst of the shoulder presenting as a chest wall mass. *Am J Orthop* 1995;24:432-434.

Huston KA, Nelson AM, Hunder GG: Shoulder swelling in rheumatoid arthritis secondary to subacromial bursitis. *Arthritis Rheum* 1978;21:145-147.

This article describes how marked swelling of the shoulders secondary to rheumatoid arthritis is evaluated and managed; a histologic description of the bursal tissue is also provided.

Neer CS II (ed): *Shoulder Reconstruction.* Philadelphia, PA, WB Saunders, 1990, pp 143-271.

This chapter presents Neer's experience with shoulder arthroplasty in general, with a section devoted specifically to rheumatoid arthritis. He discusses the pathophysiology of the rheumatoid shoulder, and the unique technical considerations of glenohumeral arthroplasty in this setting.

Nonsurgical Management

Kelly IG: The source of shoulder pain in rheumatoid arthritis: Usefulness of local anesthetic injections. *J Shoulder Elbow Surg* 1994;3:62-65.

The technique and efficacy of local differential anesthetic injections to assist in the determination of the most appropriate form of surgical or nonsurgical management of the rheumatoid shoulder are described.

Kremer JM: The changing face of therapy for rheumatoid arthritis. *Rheum Dis Clin North Am* 1995;21:845-852.

Past and present prescribing patterns are reviewed for patients with rheumatoid arthritis and how methotrexate has become the centerpiece around which other therapies are built is discussed. Recent advances on the medical management of rheumatoid arthritis are also discussed.

Surgical Management

Barrett WP, Thornhill TS, Thomas WH, et al: Nonconstrained total shoulder arthroplasty in patients with polyarticular rheumatoid arthritis. *J Arthroplasty* 1989;4: 91-96.

A retrospective review is presented of 114 patients with polyarticular rheumatoid arthritis who had 140 total shoulder arthroplasties. Ninety-three percent had excellent pain relief; however, functional improvements were less dramatic. The authors advocate shoulder arthroplasty before inordinate delay allows further soft-tissue and bony destruction by the inflammatory process, which may compromise the ultimate result.

Bennett WF, Gerber C: Operative treatment of the rheumatoid shoulder. *Curr Opin Rheumatol* 1994;6:177-182.

An excellent review of the diagnosis and treatment options of the rheumatoid shoulder is presented, along with an annotated reference list.

Bonutti PM, Hawkins RJ: Fracture of the humeral shaft associated with total replacement arthroplasty of the shoulder: A case report. *J Bone Joint Surg* 1992;74A: 617-618.

Boyd AD Jr, Thomas WH, Scott RD, et al: Total shoulder arthroplasty versus hemiarthroplasty: Indications for glenoid resurfacing. *J Arthroplasty* 1990;5:329-336.

In a review of 64 Neer hemiarthroplasties compared to 146 Neer total shoulder arthroplasties in patients with all diagnoses, 95 patients had rheumatoid arthritis. Preoperative proximal migration of the humerus did not directly correlate with major cuff disruption, but did relate to an atrophic cuff in 71% of cases. Their results support the recommendation of total shoulder arthroplasty with glenoid resurfacing in patients with rheumatoid arthritis except in patients with inadequate bone stock to support a glenoid component.

Shon FG, Connor PM, Levine WN, et al: Abstract: Shoulder arthroplasty for rheumatoid arthritis. Proceedings of the American Academy of Orthopaedic Surgeons 64th Annual

Meeting, San Francisco, CA. Rosemont, IL, American Academy of Orthopaedic Surgeons, 1997, p 52.

A review is presented of 46 shoulder arthroplasties in 37 patients with rheumatoid arthritis at an average follow-up of 56 months. Glenoid resurfacing was performed in the absence of significant glenoid bone loss, massive rotator cuff tears, or severe soft-tissue contractures. Twenty-six (57%) hemiarthroplasties and 20 (43%) total shoulder replacements were performed. Both groups had over 90% pain relief, but range of motion and functional improvements were greater in the total shoulder replacement group.

Results/Outcome

Brems JJ, Wilde AH, Borden LS et al: Glenoid lucent lines. *Orthop Trans* 1986;10:231.

Campbell JT, Moore RS, Iannotti JP, et al: Periprosthetic humeral fractures: Mechanisms of fracture and treatment options. *Orthop Trans* 1996;20:59.

Figgie HE III, Inglis AE, Goldberg VM, et al: An analysis of factors affecting the long-term results of total shoulder arthroplasty in inflammatory arthritis. *J Arthroplasty* 1988;3:123-130.

This article presents a review of 36 patients with 50 total shoulder arthroplasties for inflammatory arthritis. There were 40 excellent/good results and ten fair/poor results; satisfactory pain relief was achieved in 48 shoulders. Functional results were related to the biologic condition and motivation of the patient, status of the rotator cuff, and the prosthetic alignment.

Franklin JL, Barrett WP, Jackins SE, et al: Glenoid loosening in total shoulder arthroplasty: Association with rotator cuff deficiency. *J Arthroplasty* 1988;3:39-46.

Friedman RJ, Ewald FC: Arthroplasty of the ipsilateral shoulder and elbow in patients who have rheumatoid arthritis. *J Bone Joint Surg* 1987;69A:661-666.

Friedman RJ, Thornhill TS, Thomas WH, et al: Non-constrained total shoulder replacement in patients who have rheumatoid arthritis and class-IV function. *J Bone Joint Surg* 1989;71A:494-498.

Kelly IG: Unconstrained shoulder arthroplasty in rheumatoid arthritis. *Clin Orthop* 1994;307:94-102.

An excellent review on the current surgical concepts for the rheumatoid shoulder is presented.

Kelly IG, Foster RS, Fisher WD: Neer total shoulder replacement in rheumatoid arthritis. *J Bone Joint Surg* 1987;69B:723-726.

Forty-two total shoulder arthroplasties were performed in 37 patients with rheumatoid arthritis. At a minimum 12-month follow-up, pain relief was present in 88% of shoulders; functional improvements were documented with activities of daily living, but patients with a large preoperative rotator cuff tear achieved less dramatic functional improvements.

Lee DH, Niemann KM: Bipolar shoulder arthroplasty. *Clin Orthop* 1994;304:97-107.

Matthews LS, LaBudde JK: Arthroscopic treatment of synovial diseases of the shoulder. *Orthop Clin North Am* 1993;24:101-109.

McCoy SR, Warren RF, Bade HA III, et al: Total shoulder arthroplasty in rheumatoid arthritis. *J Arthroplasty* 1989;4:105-113.

Twenty-nine total shoulder arthroplasties were performed in 26 patients with rheumatoid arthritis. At an average follow-up of 37 months, 93% experienced satisfactory pain relief. However, functional limitations persisted in those patients with preoperative rotator cuff tears.

Neer CS II, Watson KC, Stanton FJ: Recent experience in total shoulder replacement. *J Bone Joint Surg* 1982;64A:319-337.

This classic article reviews the results of total shoulder arthroplasty for all diagnostic categories, 50 of which were rheumatoid shoulders with greater than 2-year follow-up. Forty-seven of 50 achieved satisfactory pain relief; the three unsatisfactory results were caused by functional limitations rather than continued pain.

Pahle JA, Kvarnes L: Shoulder synovectomy. *Ann Chir Gynaecol Suppl* 1985;198:37-39.

The technique and results of open synovectomy of the rheumatoid shoulder with a mean follow-up of 5.3 years are described. In only six of 54 shoulders was a total replacement arthroplasty necessary, indicating the potential benefit of this procedure. The best results were obtained in early cases with minimal radiographic changes.

Petersson CJ: Shoulder surgery in rheumatoid arthritis. *Acta Orthop Scand* 1986;57:222-226.

Simpson NS, Kelly IG: Extra-glenohumeral joint shoulder surgery in rheumatoid arthritis: The role of bursectomy, acromioplasty, and distal clavicle excision. *J Shoulder Elbow Surg* 1994;3:66-69.

In 22 painful rheumatoid shoulders, bursectomy, acromioplasty, and distal clavicle excision were performed based on findings from preoperative differential anesthetic injections. At an average follow-up of 30 months, 19 of 22 shoulders had minimal pain and external rotation and elevation had improved in most.

Sneppen O, Fruensgaard S, Johannsen HV, et al: Total shoulder replacement in rheumatoid arthritis: Proximal migration and loosening. *J Shoulder Elbow Surg* 1996;5:47-52.

This is a prospective long-term follow-up study (average 92 months) of 62 Neer II arthroplasties for rheumatoid arthritis. Results revealed proximal humeral migration in 55% of patients, 40% incidence of progressive glenoid loosening, and loosening in five of 12 uncemented press-fit humeral components. Despite these findings, 89% achieved satisfactory pain relief and functional improvement.

Thomas BJ, Amstutz HC, Cracchiolo A: Shoulder arthroplasty for rheumatoid arthritis. *Clin Orthop* 1991;265:125-128.

This is a review of 30 shoulders in 24 patients followed for a minimum of 2 years; pain relief was good and functional recovery coincided with disease severity. The authors also showed that 15 of 30 shoulders showed superior subluxation postoperatively, despite attempts at rotator cuff repair at the time of surgery. Two standard glenoid components (7.7%) required revision for loosening.

Complications

Bigliani LU (ed): *Complications of Shoulder Surgery.* Baltimore, MD, Williams & Wilkins, 1993.

This text includes several chapters on the complications associated with shoulder arthroplasty in general. Specific information is presented on the issues of humeral and glenoid component loosening, glenoid bone deficiency, periprosthetic humeral fractures, and sepsis in the context of shoulder arthroplasty for rheumatoid arthritis.

25

Management of Osteoarthritis of the Shoulder

Gary W. Misamore, MD

Etiology

The etiology of osteoarthritis of the glenohumeral joint is either primary or secondary. The pattern of pathologic changes to the joint are similar in both circumstances, but in some situations, the treatment may vary.

In primary osteoarthritis, no specific cause for the arthritis can be identified. It is not clear if some of these cases are caused by a degenerative metabolic breakdown of articular cartilage or by an abnormality of the biomechanical properties of the subchondral bone causing excess stresses and shear on the articular cartilage, resulting in eventual breakdown of the cartilage.

Secondary osteoarthritis exists when an obvious cause for the development of arthropathy is identified. The most common etiology associated with secondary osteoarthritis of the shoulder is trauma. Fracture, instability, and surgery are the most common traumatic insults to the shoulder that may lead to secondary osteoarthritis.

Capsulorrhaphy arthropathy is arthritis associated with instability. It develops following a surgical procedure, which results in significant restriction of shoulder motion. The most common scenario for arthritis of instability is when anterior instability is treated by surgery, which overtly tightens the anterior soft tissue, resulting in significant contractures that restrict external rotation. The excessive anterior soft-tissue tightness increases the joint compressive force and pushes the humeral head posteriorly, causing increased wear on the posterior glenoid. Radiographically, this condition is identical to primary osteoarthritis.

Intraoperative fracture of the glenoid during a glenoid osteotomy for posterior instability can also result in shoulder arthritis. The arthritis occurs when attempts are made to lever the glenoid surface into anteversion before the osteotomy approaches the anterior cortex. Fracture extending from the anterior extent of the osteotomy to the articular surface, rather than to the anterior scapular neck, causes chondral damage and deforms the contour of the glenoid surface. This damage can precipitate development of arthritis with destruction of the glenoid, and then the humeral head.

Development of osteoarthritis as a result of untreated shoulder instability requiring shoulder arthroplasty occurs in approximately 21% of shoulders by 10 years. There are reports of osteoarthritis occurring many years subsequent to a single event of dislocation. Arthritis may occur following a successful surgery in which stability is achieved and good motion is maintained; however, this scenario is relatively uncommon. Traumatic glenohumeral arthritis is common following unreduced posterior dislocation of the shoulder. If the humeral head remains locked behind the glenoid, there is a posterior lateral head impression fracture. The posterior glenoid rim causes significant additional wear on the humeral head, resulting in destruction of both the cartilage and bone.

Although arthritis associated with surgery is most common following instability repairs, any surgery during which metallic implants are placed about the joint can result in joint injury if any part of the implant impinges on the articular surface. Placement of staples or screws in the glenoid during surgery for instability is the most frequent cause of arthritis related to metallic implants. Additionally, any surgery that results in significant soft-tissue contractures can cause abnormal joint compressive forces that may result in secondary osteoarthritis.

Fractures of the proximal humerus and the glenoid can be complicated by subsequent arthritis. Although displaced intra-articular fractures of the glenoid are not common, significant joint incongruity can result from these injuries such that the risk of arthritis is significant. Fractures of the proximal humerus most commonly associated with subsequent osteoarthritis include head-splitting fractures and three- or four-part fractures that result in malunion or nonunion or posttraumatic osteonecrosis.

Nontraumatic osteonecrosis of the proximal humerus can result in secondary osteoarthritis if collapse of the humeral head causes significant deformity resulting in joint surface incongruity. Factors associated with nontraumatic osteonecrosis may include use of corticosteroids, alcoholism, Caisson disease (decompression sickness), Gaucher's disease, renal transplantation, systemic lupus erythematosus, pancreatitis, hyperuricemia, and familial hyperlipidemia.

Infrequent causes of shoulder osteoarthritis include radiation necrosis, congenital developmental skeletal abnormalities such as epiphyseal dysplasia, and metabolic disorders. Metabolic abnormalities associated with osteoarthritis include Paget's disease, ochronosis, gout, and chondrocalcinosis (pseudogout).

Evaluation

Clinical evaluation of arthritis of the shoulder follows standard orthopaedic assessment of the musculoskeletal system. The diagnosis of osteoarthritis is easily made with history, physical examination, and radiographs. Laboratory studies are sometimes useful in elucidating the etiology of the arthritis. Rarely, electromyography may be indicated to evaluate for possible neuropathy affecting the extremity.

Patient history is relatively consistent. Pain is nearly always the chief complaint. Pain often occurs at rest but is exacerbated with use of the extremity, and is frequently present at night. The pain is typically vague and diffuse about the shoulder, and is common in the axilla and upper arm. Restricted motion and crepitus are also common complaints.

Examination reveals painful, restricted motion and crepitus. Subtle loss of the rounded contour of the superior lateral shoulder and prominence of the coracoid may be noted if a fixed posterior subluxation of the humeral head occurs because of significant glenoid erosion.

The radiographic features of osteoarthritis of the shoulder include joint space narrowing, sclerosis and cystic changes in the subchondral bone, and osteophyte formation. When glenoid erosion is present, most bone loss occurs in the posterior portion of the glenoid, which results in retroversion of the glenoid surface and posterior displacement of the humeral head relative to the plane of the scapular body. The magnitude of glenoid bone loss can be difficult to evaluate on plain radiographs. A limited axial computed tomography scan can be useful in assessing the glenoid version and bone loss. The amount of glenoid bone and resultant distortion of glenoid version should be determined preoperatively with imaging studies because intraoperative assessment is more difficult.

Treatment

Nonsurgical treatment of glenohumeral osteoarthritis includes gentle range-of-motion exercises, rest or avoidance of provocative activities, and use of nonsteroidal anti-inflammatory drugs. Judicious use of interarticular injection of corticosteroids can provide temporary relief of the arthritis.

When nonsurgical management is not effective, and the patient's symptoms are severe enough to justify more definitive treatment, surgical intervention is considered. Surgical options include joint debridement with synovectomy and release of contractures, osteotomies of the humerus and glenoid, resection arthroplasty, arthrodesis, and prosthetic replacement arthroplasty.

Although debridement, synovectomy, and release of contractures have been used in some cases of inflammatory arthritis, few series of patients with osteoarthritis treated in this way have been reported. Neer described four cases of osteoarthritis treated with open cheilectomy (spur removal) as dismal failures. Green and Norris reviewed the results of arthroscopic debridement in glenohumeral osteoarthritis; in 75% of patients studied, symptoms were worsened. Removal of the spurs for advanced arthritis did not address the cartilage loss; however, it provided more stiffness. Only a few reports of very small numbers of patients, typically with arthritis associated with significant loss of external rotation following surgery for anterior instability, have been published. Subscapularis recession or lengthening may be beneficial before more severe glenohumeral arthritis develops.

Periarticular osteotomy of the glenoid neck and proximal humerus has had limited acceptance. Its effectiveness in the treatment of osteoarthritis is unknown. Very limited reports on this technique have been published, but primarily have focused on patients with rheumatoid arthritis.

Resection arthroplasty has been used infrequently in the past, primarily for treatment of infection. It has been reported to have minimal success in the management of rheumatoid arthritis. The Jones procedure to resect the humeral head for fractures had poor results. These results inspired Neer to develop the humeral head replacement in 1951. There are no published series dealing with this treatment for osteoarthritis. Because prosthetic arthroplasty is a better choice in nearly all circumstances, there likely is no place for resection arthroplasty in the treatment of routine osteoarthritis.

Arthrodesis may be an option for treatment of osteoarthritis in cases complicated by loss of both the deltoid and rotator cuff or by infection, or as a salvage operation after prior failed reconstructive procedures. In uncomplicated cases of osteoarthritis, prosthetic replacement provides far superior results.

Prosthetic arthroplasty has become the most popular option for surgical treatment of osteoarthritis. Proximal humeral replacement for trauma, first reported in 1953, was quickly adapted to the treatment of arthritis. Many implant materials and designs have been used over the last 30 years. Total shoulder arthroplasty using a nonconstrained design consisting of polyethylene glenoid and metallic humeral implants has been the most successful type of prosthetic arthroplasty. Constrained implants, designed to compensate for instability of the joint or insufficiency of the rotator cuff or deltoid muscles, have been associated with an unacceptable rate of loosening. These implants have not typically been successful in restoring satisfactory function.

Posterior glenoid bone loss commonly occurs in advanced glenohumeral osteoarthritis and must be addressed during arthroplasty surgery. Mild to moderate glenoid deformity can be corrected by surgically lowering the prominent anterior glenoid with restoration of normal glenoid version. Alternatively, and less desirable, the glenoid implant can be placed on the uncorrected, retroverted glenoid. Appropriate adjustments of the humeral component version are made to compensate for the glenoid retroversion in order to make the system balanced and stable. If severe glenoid bone loss is present, bone grafting can be performed or, in rare circumstances, a custom implant can be used.

Hemiarthroplasty with a proximal humeral head implant can be a reasonable alternative to total joint replacement in some situations. When glenoid bone loss is so severe that satisfactory fixation or orientation of a glenoid component cannot be assured, hemiarthroplasty should be considered. Although tears of the rotator cuff are uncommon in association with glenohumeral arthritis, rotator cuff insufficiency can result in abnormal mechanics, causing excessive load on the edge of the glenoid, and possibly leading to a high rate of glenoid loosening. Hemiarthroplasty may be advisable when a rotator cuff tear is irreparable in order to avoid the increased risk of glenoid implant failure.

Bipolar arthroplasty has been suggested as a salvage procedure to consider when a massive rotator cuff tear is present in the arthritic shoulder. Results of that procedure have been poor because of unpredictable pain relief and minimal functional improvement.

Prosthetic glenoid fixation with methylmethacrylate has been highly successful in most reports and is still necessary to fulfill Food and Drug Administration requirements. Good results have been reported with bone ingrowth fixation of the glenoid implant. However, long-term results of that technique are not available and its possible advantages are not yet clear. Press-fit fixation of the humeral implant without cement has been successful and can be considered when there is good humeral bone stock. Loosening of the humeral component has been rare when cemented; Cofield has reported that greater than 50% of the uncemented humeral components shift or subside after 10 to 15 years.

Attention to detail in performance of shoulder arthroplasty is critical to success. Precise fitting of the prosthesis, release of soft-tissue contractures with balancing of the soft-tissue tension, and balancing of the version of the implants with correction of deformity resulting from bone loss or fracture are important points in the surgical technique. No amount of postoperative rehabilitation can compensate for intraoperative errors that can leave the shoulder unstable, stiff, or with improper tensioning of the muscle units about the joint.

Postoperative rehabilitation after replacement arthroplasty must be individually determined in each case based on the surgeon's assessment of the stability of the joint and the quality of the bone and soft-tissue repairs. Early motion after surgery is preferred whenever possible, with progression to muscle strengthening and active use of the arm dictated by the security of healing of the soft tissues and bone.

Complications

Approximately 10% of shoulder arthroplasties are associated with some type of complication. When complications do occur, they usually are significant and adversely affect the outcome.

The most common intraoperative or perioperative complications are instability and fracture. Instability is most often a result of technical error in which appropriate balancing of glenoid and humeral version and soft-tissue tension is not achieved during surgery. Periprosthetic humeral shaft fractures occur intraoperatively with inadequate soft-tissue releases and overreaming. By extending the incision, cerclage cables around a long stem humeral component permit secure fixation without alteration of the rehabilitation. Postoperative impingement, the next most common complication, may occur when the humeral head is positioned too low relative to the height of the greater tuberosity. Infection and nerve injury are uncommon. Each of these complications occurs in less than 1% of cases. Postoperative heterotopic ossification is rare.

Late complications after arthroplasty, occurring months or years following surgery, are more common than perioperative complications. Postoperative prosthetic loosening, rotator cuff tearing, and prosthetic instability are the most frequently reported late complications. Humeral fracture about the prosthetic stem and late infection caused by hematogenous seeding of the prosthetic joint are seen infrequently.

Results/Outcomes

There are very few reports of nonprosthetic surgical treatment for osteoarthritis. There are few reported series of patients with osteoarthritis treated by synovectomy and debridement or by resection arthroplasty. Bigliani reported favorable results in arthroscopic synovectomy in early glenohumeral osteoarthritis. With advanced osteoarthritis, debridement and spur removal offer some relief, but stiffness and nerve injury are possible. Only two author groups have reported results of periarticular osteotomy. Reasonable improvement in pain and motion are reported, but the numbers of patients with osteoarthritis in those reports are limited, and thus, results are not conclusive. Arthrodesis can be effective for relief of glenohumeral pain, but postoperative motion is severely restricted and scapular aching is common. There are no recent reports of arthrodesis for treatment of osteoarthritis. That procedure has been rarely performed in recent years because of the success of prosthetic arthroplasty.

Results of prosthetic replacement arthroplasty are superior to other forms of treatment of glenohumeral osteoarthritis. Pain relief is reasonably predictable and some improvement of motion is usually obtained. Relief of pain seems to be slightly better in total joint arthroplasty than in hemiarthroplasty. Although results have varied more widely after hemiarthroplasty, most series report 80% to 100% of patients obtaining good pain relief if glenoid erosion has not occurred. Once posterior glenoid erosion occurs, the success rate falls to 33%. Following total shoulder replacement arthroplasty, most studies report similar good results ranging from 85% to 100%. However, the results have been more predictable with total shoulder arthroplasty because few reports of total shoulder arthroplasty show results below that range, whereas more studies of hemiarthroplasty have a higher incidence of poor results. In Zuckerman and Cofield's review, less than 50% of those who received humeral head replacements for osteoarthritis had satisfactory pain relief at 10-year follow-up. Twenty-six percent were revised to total shoulder replacements for untreated glenoid arthritis.

Nonconstrained total joint arthroplasty has demonstrated better results than more constrained prosthetic types. Use of constrained implants has been reported to result in an increased incidence of radiographic lucent lines and clinical loosening of the prosthesis.

Reported results following prosthetic arthroplasty must be viewed cautiously because long-term survival rates and results are not clearly documented. Late prosthetic loosening may result in deterioration of results with time. Radiographic lucent lines around the glenoid prosthesis have been reported to occur frequently in most series. One report documented glenoid lucent lines to be present in 93% of patients. Although the presence of lucent lines on radiographs has not been related to clinical loosening of the glenoid prosthesis in short-term follow-up, there remains concern that the rate of prosthetic loosening will increase over time. The crux of the issue is better pain relief and stability in the face of more advanced glenoid wear with total shoulder replacement, versus the difficulty of performing glenoid replacement and the long-term propensity for particulate disease and glenoid loosening.

Selected Bibliography

Arntz CT, Jackins S, Matsen FA III: Prosthetic replacement of the shoulder for the treatment of defects in the rotator cuff and the surface of the glenohumeral joint. *J Bone Joint Surg* 1993;75A:485-491.

The authors performed hemiarthroplasty on 21 shoulders over a 9-year period for treatment of pain due to massive tear of the rotator cuff combined with glenohumeral arthritis. Eighteen shoulders were evaluated with follow-up ranging from 25 to 122 months. Postoperatively, active elevation was improved in all shoulders, and significant improvement of pain was noted in 15 shoulders. Three patients had continued significant pain postoperatively that resulted in the need for revision surgery. Technical points that the authors emphasized were preservation of the coracoacromial arch, debridement of subacromial scar and nonfunctional cuff tissue, and insertion of an appropriate size humeral component to avoid excessive tightness.

Ballmer FT, Lippitt SB, Romeo AA, et al: Total shoulder arthroplasty: Some considerations related to glenoid surface contact. *J Shoulder Elbow Surg* 1994;3:299-306.

Two commonly used shoulder arthroplasty systems were studied to evaluate joint surface contact. Wide variations were found in ranges of motion providing full surface contact. Undesirable bone and soft-tissue contact occurred and unwanted translations of the humeral head on the glenoid were observed when full surface contact was not present.

Bonutti PM, Hawkins RJ: Fracture of the humeral shaft associated with total replacement arthroplasty of the shoulder: A case report. *J Bone Joint Surg* 1992;74A: 617-618.

Boyd AD Jr, Thomas WH, Scott RD, et al: Total shoulder arthroplasty versus hemiarthroplasty: Indications for glenoid resurfacing. *J Arthroplasty* 1990;5:329-336.

Campbell JT, Moore RS, Iannotti JP, et al: Periprosthetic humeral fractures: Mechanisms of fracture and treatment options. *J Bone Joint Surg* 1996;20:58.

Cofield RH: Total shoulder arthroplasty with the Neer prosthesis. *J Bone Joint Surg* 1984;66A:899-906.

Cofield RH, Daly PJ: Total shoulder arthroplasty with a tissue-ingrowth glenoid component. *J Shoulder Elbow Surg* 1992;1:77-85.

A tissue-ingrowth glenoid component was implanted during 32 total shoulder arthroplasties in 29 patients. Seventeen of these patients suffered from osteoarthritis and seven from traumatic arthritis. Follow-up ranged from 29 to 80 months. Good relief of pain was achieved in 27 (84%) of the 32 shoulders. Reoperation was necessary in four patients because of complications or poor results. In three of these four patients, the glenoid tray remained securely fixed. The fourth reoperation was necessitated by joint sepsis and the glenoid was found to be loose. Dissociation of the polyethylene insert from the glenoid tray occurred in two patients. Complete lucent lines around the glenoid implant were present on radiographs in seven (22%) of the 31 noninfected shoulders, and three (10%) glenoid trays had shifted, suggesting gross loosening.

Collins D, Tencer A, Sidles J, et al: Edge displacement and deformation of glenoid components in response to eccentric loading: The effect of preparation of the glenoid bone. *J Bone Joint Surg* 1992;74A:501-507.

The effect of eccentric loading of glenoid components was studied in cadaveric scapulae. The study evaluated three methods of glenoid preparation. Simple removal of cartilage using a curet resulted in the greatest displacement and deformation of the implant. Contouring of the glenoid to approximate the shape of the implant using a hand-held power burr improved the results. The least displacement and deformation occurred after contouring with a power reamer sized to match the radius of the back of the glenoid component. Creation of posterior glenoid bone loss by osteotomy of the posterior 25% or 33% of the glenoid did not affect the results.

Edelson JG: Patterns of degenerative change in the glenohumeral joint. *J Bone Joint Surg* 1995;77B:288-292.

Examination of 486 skeletons of subjects over the age of 60 years was performed. Three patterns of degeneration were noted. Type I (29.6% of skeletons) revealed changes consistent with rotator cuff disease. The head was sclerotic, there was rounding and dissolution of the greater tuberosity, and only minor osteophyte formation. There were minor osteophytes about the glenoid. The acromion was eroded and thinned. Type II (3.5% of skeletons) revealed a pattern consistent with primary osteoarthritis. Osteophytes were more prominent and the greater tuberosity was preserved. Type III (4.7% of skeletons) showed more advanced distortion of the glenoid and significant flattening of the humeral head. In types I and II, the changes were bilateral whereas in type III the changes were unilateral.

Fenlin JM Jr, Ramsey ML, Allardyce TJ, et al: Modular total shoulder replacement: Design rationale, indications, and results. *Clin Orthop* 1994;307:37-46.

This report reviews the results of total shoulder arthroplasty performed in 47 shoulders in 40 patients using a modular implant system. Osteoarthritis was the diagnosis in 22 cases. Eighteen of the 22 shoulders (82%) with osteoarthritis and 15 of 17 (88%) with rheumatoid arthritis had satisfactory pain relief. In osteoarthritis cases, range of motion improved from an average of 107° elevation preoperatively to 145° postoperatively and external rotation improved from 23° to 31°. In rheumatoid arthritis, elevation improved from 90° to 125° and external rotation improved from 33° to 44°. Revision surgery was necessary in three cases during the period of follow-up, which ranged from 24 to 93 months.

Friedman RJ, Hawthorne KB, Genez BM: The use of computerized tomography in the measurement of glenoid version. *J Bone Joint Surg* 1992;74A:1032-1037.

Computed tomography (CT) was performed on 20 shoulders with arthritis (ten with osteoarthritis) and compared to 63 controls. Control measurements were obtained from chest CT scans of patients with no radiographic evidence of shoulder disease. Arthritic shoulders had significantly more retroversion of the glenoid caused by bone erosion from the disease process. Glenoid orientation averaged 11° of retroversion in arthritic shoulders and 2° of anteversion in the control group.

Iannotti JP, Gabriel JP, Schneck SL, et al: The normal glenohumeral relationships: An anatomical study of one hundred and forty shoulders. *J Bone Joint Surg* 1992;74A:491-500.

The dimensions of the humeral and glenoid articular surfaces of 140 cadaveric shoulders were measured. Wide variability in the size of humeral heads was noted. The radius of curvature of the glenoid averaged 2.3 mm greater than the radius of the humeral head. There was direct correlation between lateral offset and the size of the humeral head. The most superior aspect of the humeral head was above the tip of the greater tuberosity at an average of 8 mm. The authors conclude that restoration of the lateral humeral offset is important during prosthetic reconstruction to optimize the mechanics of the shoulder.

Lee DH, Niemann KMW: Bipolar shoulder arthroplasty. *Clin Orthop* 1994;304:97-107.

Fourteen patients were treated with bipolar arthroplasty as a salvage procedure for arthritis combined with a massive tear of the rotator cuff. Only one patient had osteoarthritis; the rest had inflammatory arthritis or failed total shoulder arthroplasty. Follow-up ranged from 2 to 4.8 years. Although pain relief was good for patients with rheumatoid arthritis, other patients had less satisfactory results. Bipolar cup dislocations occurred in two patients and subluxations occurred in one patient.

Moeckel BH, Altchek DW, Warren RF, et al: Instability of the shoulder after arthroplasty. *J Bone Joint Surg* 1993;75A:792-797.

Ten patients who suffered shoulder instability after replacement arthroplasty were reviewed. Seven had anterior instability and three had posterior instability. Disruption of the subscapularis and capsule occurred in all cases of anterior instability. Following secondary repair of the subscapularis and capsule, instability was resolved in four patients but recurred in three patients. In those three cases, Achilles tendon allograft was used to reconstruct the anterior soft tissues, after which all three shoulders were stable. External rotation was very limited in all shoulders following reconstruction for anterior instability. Causes of posterior instability included excessive glenoid retroversion, excessive humeral retroversion, and soft-tissue laxity. In patients with implant malposition, stability was achieved following revision of the components. In the patient with soft-tissue laxity, instability recurred after posterior capsular plication and the patient was finally treated with resection arthroplasty.

Mullaji AB, Beddow FH, Lamb GH: CT measurement of glenoid erosion in arthritis. *J Bone Joint Surg* 1994;76B:384-388.

Computed tomography was performed on 45 arthritic shoulders (34 rheumatoid and 11 osteoarthritic) and compared with scans in 19 normal shoulders. In rheumatoid disease, there typically was superior erosion that altered the vertical inclination of the glenoid. Associated with the superior erosion, there also were abnormalities of version. The glenoid was anteverted in some cases and retroverted in others. In osteoarthritis, posterior erosion resulting in retroversion of the glenoid was routinely found. The authors point out the implications of these abnormalities as related to performance of glenoid replacement.

Neer CS II: Replacement arthroplasty for glenohumeral osteoarthritis. *J Bone Joint Surg* 1974;56A:1-13.

Norris BL, Lachiewicz PF: Modern cement technique and the survivorship of total shoulder arthroplasty. *Clin Orthop* 1996;328:76-85.

Thirty-eight total shoulder arthroplasties were reviewed with follow-up from 2 to 9.5 years. Neer II components were implanted with cement fixation for all glenoids and cement fixation for 32 humeral components. At follow-up, there was little or no pain in 36 shoulders. No revisions were performed, although in one patient there was significant radiographic lucency about both implants with shift in position. Radiolucent lines around more than 50% of the bone-cement interface occurred about three humeral implants and two glenoid replants. Survivorship of the arthroplasty was 97% at 5 years and 93% at 8 years.

Norris TR, Iannotti JP: Prospective evaluation of fractures affcting the outcome of shoulder arthroplasty for osteoarthritis, in Vastamaki M, Jalovaara P (eds): *Surgery of the Shoulder.* Amsterdam, The Netherlands, Elsevier Science, 1995, pp 323-333.

Post M, Jablon M: Constrained total shoulder arthroplasty: Long-term follow-up observations. *Clin Orthop* 1983;173:109-116.

26

Osteonecrosis and Other Noninflammatory Degenerative Diseases of the Glenohumeral Joint Including Gaucher's Disease, Sickle Cell Disease, Hemochromatosis, and Synovial Osteochondromatosis

C. Craig Satterlee, MD

Osteonecrosis, also known as avascular necrosis or ischemic necrosis, is a condition in which compromised circulation to an area of bone results in death of that bone. Involvement of the humeral head is second in frequency only to the femoral head. Following is a discussion of the etiology, evaluation, types of treatment, and results of treatment of posttraumatic and nontraumatic osteonecrosis, along with a discussion of Gaucher's disease, sickle cell disease, hemochromatosis, and synovial osteochondromatosis.

Posttraumatic Osteonecrosis

Posttraumatic osteonecrosis of the shoulder most commonly occurs after a fracture disrupts the blood supply of the humeral head. The blood supply of the proximal humerus is via an anastomotic network supplied primarily by the anterolateral branch of the anterior circumflex artery (Fig. 1). This branch runs parallel to the lateral aspect of the long head of the biceps and enters the head proximally where the intertubercular groove meets the greater tuberosity. If this vessel is disrupted, only an anastomosis distal to the injury can compensate for the loss of its blood supply. The posterior humeral circumflex supplies only the posterior greater tuberosity and posterior-inferior head. The vessels entering the epiphysis via the rotator cuff have not been shown to provide much vascularization of the humeral head. Disruption of the blood supply either by trauma or surgical intervention may result in osteonecrosis. In fractures with minimal displacement the incidence of osteonecrosis is rare; however, it ranges from 3% to 25% in three-part fractures and up to 90% in four-part fractures.

Evaluation

Persistent pain after treatment and healing of a fracture may lead to the clinical suspicion of osteonecrosis (Fig. 2). Anteroposterior and axillary radiographs are useful in identifying resorption or collapse of the humeral head. Although magnetic resonance imaging (MRI) is the most sensitive study to detect or confirm osteonecrosis, the condition cannot be distinguished from bone contusion until 6 to 8 weeks postinjury. Single photon emission computed tomography (CT) bone scanning may be helpful if MRI is impractical or contraindicated.

Treatment

Treatment of posttraumatic osteonecrosis initially includes stretching exercises (for stiffness) and analgesic medication. Bone resorption or collapse may lead to pain and stiffness. Humeral head replacement or, if the glenoid is damaged, total shoulder replacement is indicated to relieve the pain and improve function. The procedure can be demanding. Extensive scar and capsular contracture may require release. Malunion or nonunion of the tuberosities may necessitate osteotomy and fixation (risking redisplacement). Soft-tissue disruption of the rotator cuff, deltoid, biceps, or capsule may require repair. Other complicating factors such as neurologic damage may be present.

Results of Surgical Treatment

The results of surgical treatment correlate directly with the degree of associated pathology. The results of arthroplasty for osteonecrosis are better after a previous surgery or minimally displaced fracture in which the rotator cuff and deltoid are functional. Most series combine posttraumatic osteonecrosis with other diagnoses such as posttraumatic arthritis, nonunion, and humeral shortening because the posttraumatic problems are often complex. The results infer improved range of motion and pain relief but outcomes are inferior when compared to those with acute arthroplasty.

Nontraumatic Osteonecrosis

Rather than being the direct result of an anatomic vascular disruption, nontraumatic osteonecrosis is a local pathologic event resulting in impaired blood flow and bone death. Outline 1 lists conditions associated with osteonecrosis. The etiology may be straightforward, complex, or idiopathic, and can be a source of controversy in particular cases. Osteonecrosis may be caused by external compression, as in Gaucher's disease, with marrow infiltration and increased interosseous pressure. Sickle cell disease causes osteonecrosis by embolization of red cell clumps to the involved area.

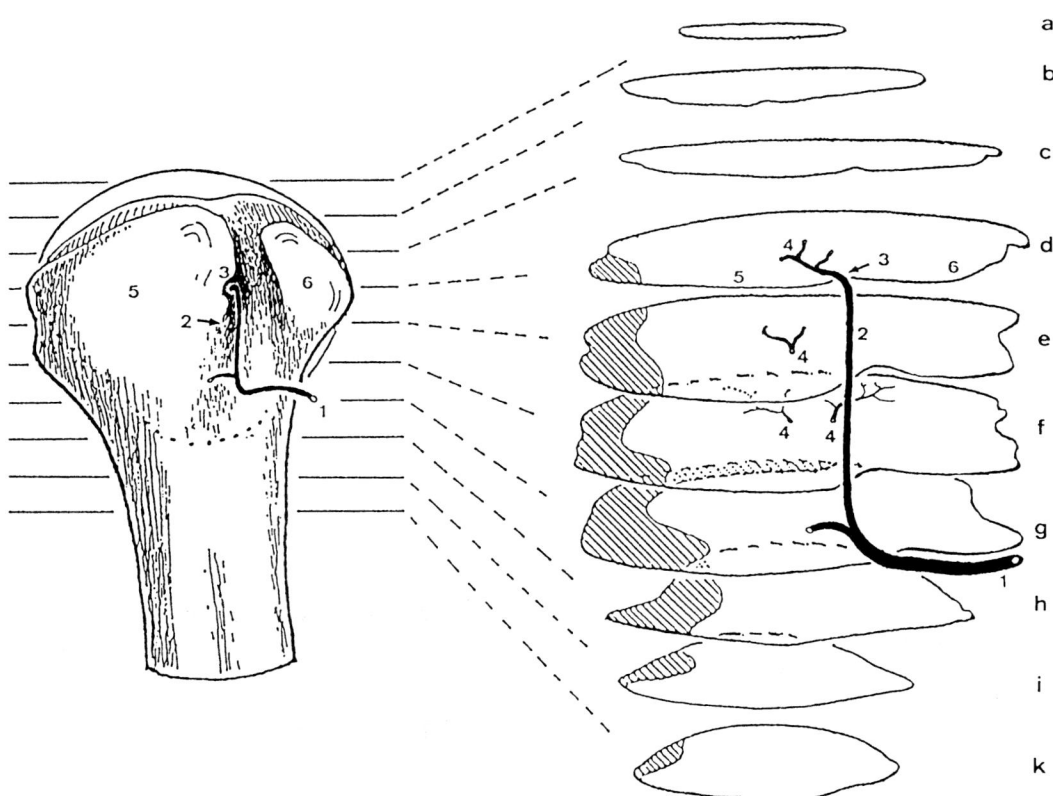

Fig. 1 Anterior aspect of a graphic representation of the right humeral head after selective injection of the anterior circumflex artery (1). The humeral head was cut into 4-mm-thick slices (a through k) and was analyzed microradiographically. Only the hatched area is not supplied by the anterior circumflex artery. 2 = anterolateral branch of the anterior circumflex artery, 3 = entry of the anterolateral branch into the humeral head, 4 = main stem of the arcuate artery, 5 = greater tuberosity, and 6 = lesser tuberosity. (Reproduced with permission from Gerber C, Schneeberger AG, Vinh T: The arterial vascularization of the humeral head. *J Bone Joint Surg* 1990;72A:1486-1494.)

Smoking increases the risk of osteonecrosis fourfold, presumably by local vascular spasm. Ethanol intake increases plasma fats and debris-potentiating embolization of bone. Steroid use causes osteonecrosis in a like manner. Osteonecrosis following electrical shock is reportedly due to bone "melting," although intravascular coagulation seems as plausible. Inflammatory vascular disease can increase the risk of osteonecrosis as can infiltrative diseases such as amyloidosis or sarcoidosis. In paraplegics, osteonecrosis of the shoulder develops as a result of increased bone load pressure under the weightbearing dome of the humeral head.

Evaluation

To assist in describing the indications and treatment of osteonecrosis, Neer adapted a classification system from Ficat and Enneking. In stage I, the head retains its normal shape. Radiographs may show slight mottling of the trabeculae or subchondral decalcification. MRI may detect the condition at this stage. Pain may or may not be present. In stage II, the articular surface is grossly round but may be indented with pressure and return to its normal shape. Radiographs show a meniscus sign that corresponds to minute subchondral fractures. Pain may be severe. Stage III is characterized by an area of loose articular cartilage that may form a flap. The glenoid surface remains intact. Stage IV involves arthritic changes of the glenoid from incongruity of the humeral head posteriorly, which can lead to posterior wear and subluxation.

Treatment and Results

In stages I and II, treatment is usually nonsurgical, especially if the patient has minimal or no pain. Stretching exercises to prevent stiffness and nonaddicting pain medications can be helpful.

The use of core decompression is controversial; some authors have said that the results are disappointing. Others report that clinical progression may not occur and recommend nonsurgical treatment. In one study including 14 patients in stage I or II undergoing core decompression, all had an excellent or satisfactory result. Eleven of the 14 had not deteriorated clinically at an average 5.6 years postoperatively. Because of the small number of patients studied, the influence of the natural course of the disease by core decompression remains uncertain.

In stage III, a humeral head replacement is usually performed for a painful shoulder (Fig. 3). Arthroplasty reportedly provides good pain relief in 91% to 100% of shoulders with

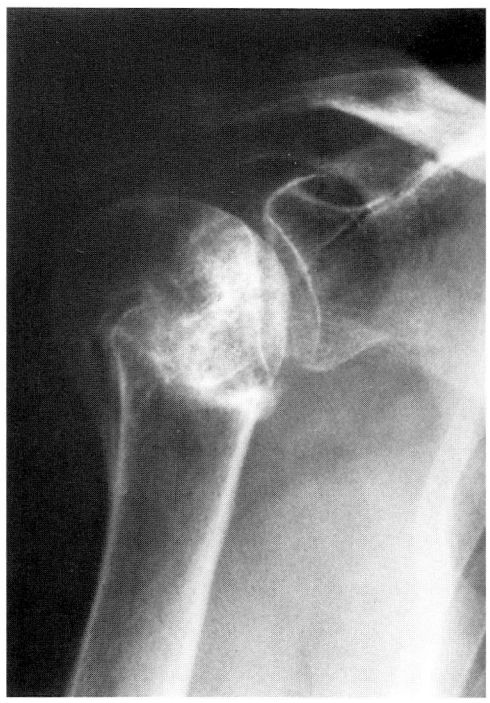 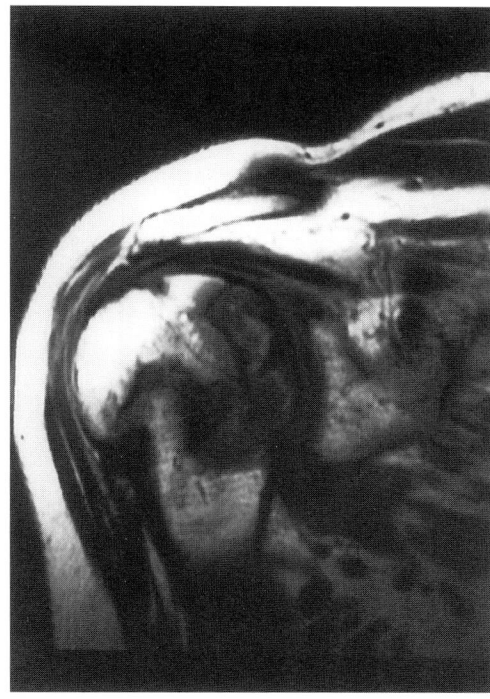

Fig. 2 **Left,** Radiograph of a one-part proximal humerus fracture that healed and became painful 1 year later. **Right,** MRI confirms osteonecrosis of the medial humeral head.

Outline 1. Conditions associated with osteonecrosis

Alcohol intake	Hyperlipidemia
Altitude exposure	Hypophosphatemia in renal
Antiphospholipid antibody	transplantation
syndrome	Intra-articular instillation of
Anabolic steroids	steroids
Arteriosclerosis	Liver disease
Brucellosis	Metabolic bone disease
Burns	Pancreatitis
Caisson disease	Paraplegia
Charcot joint	Pregnancy
Coagulopathy	Radiation
Collagen vascular disease	Sarcoidosis
Electrical shock	Sickle cell disease and variants
Fabry's disease	Smoking
Fracture	Systemic steroids
Gaucher's disease	Trauma
Gout	Tumors
Hemoglobinopathy	Vasculitis

osteonecrosis. Recent reports on modular implants indicate that this trend is continuing. The report on core decompression for stage III was good or excellent in seven of ten shoulders despite the fact that four showed radiologic progression. Two groups of patients tended to have less favorable arthroplasty results with stage III or IV osteonecrosis. These groups include patients with Gaucher's disease and sickle cell disease (discussed later in this chapter).

The preoperative diagnosis of glenoid involvement (stage IV) may be made radiographically or with CT. Sometimes the diagnosis is made at surgery in presumed stage III disease. Total shoulder arthroplasty (Fig. 4) is usually the procedure of choice unless contraindicated by the presence of a neuropathic joint, infection, paralysis, and/or loss of the cuff and deltoid muscles. Typically the cuff and deltoid are intact with good bone stock to support both components. However, there may be posterior subluxation requiring adjustment of the humeral component (less anteversion) to tense the posterior capsule or capsulorrhaphy. The results are similar to those for osteoarthritis (with the exceptions of Gaucher's and sickle cell disease).

Glenohumeral arthrodesis is recommended for the symptomatic shoulder with widespread muscle loss or high infection risk. Core decompression has not been shown to alter the progression of stage IV osteonecrosis. Nonsurgical treatment for osteonecrosis associated with a neuropathic joint is recommended because of persistent pain and instability after arthroplasty and difficulty obtaining union with arthrodesis.

Gaucher's Disease

Gaucher's disease is an autosomal recessive lysosomal storage disorder characterized by the accumulation of the glycolipid glucocerebroside. It has been classified into three major

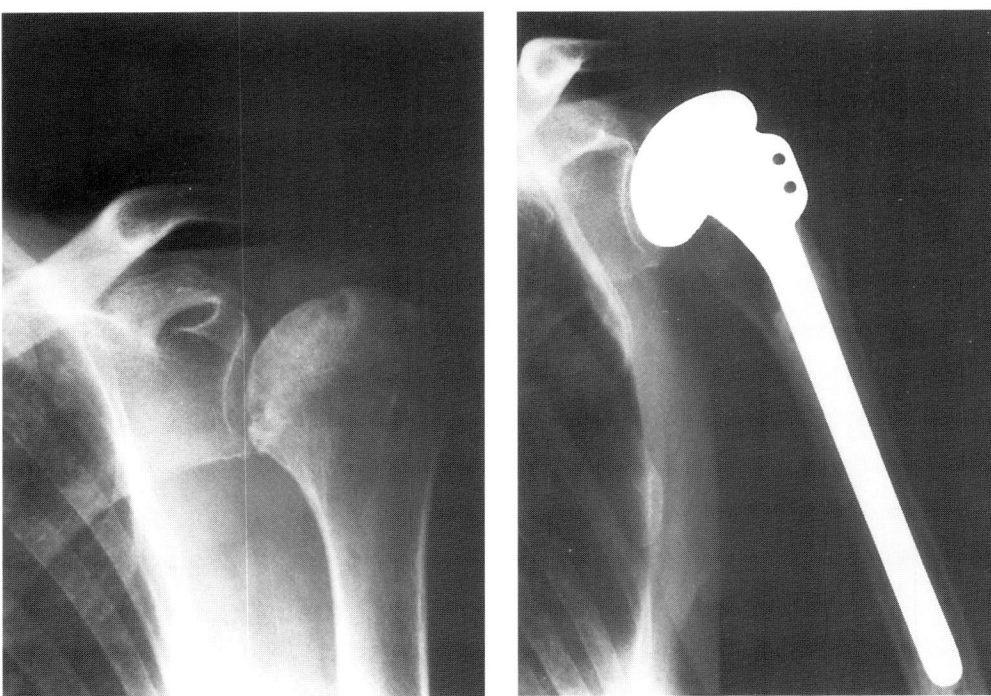

Fig. 3 **Left,** Radiograph of a shoulder with early grade III osteonecrosis. **Right,** Postoperative radiograph showing treatment with a humeral head replacement.

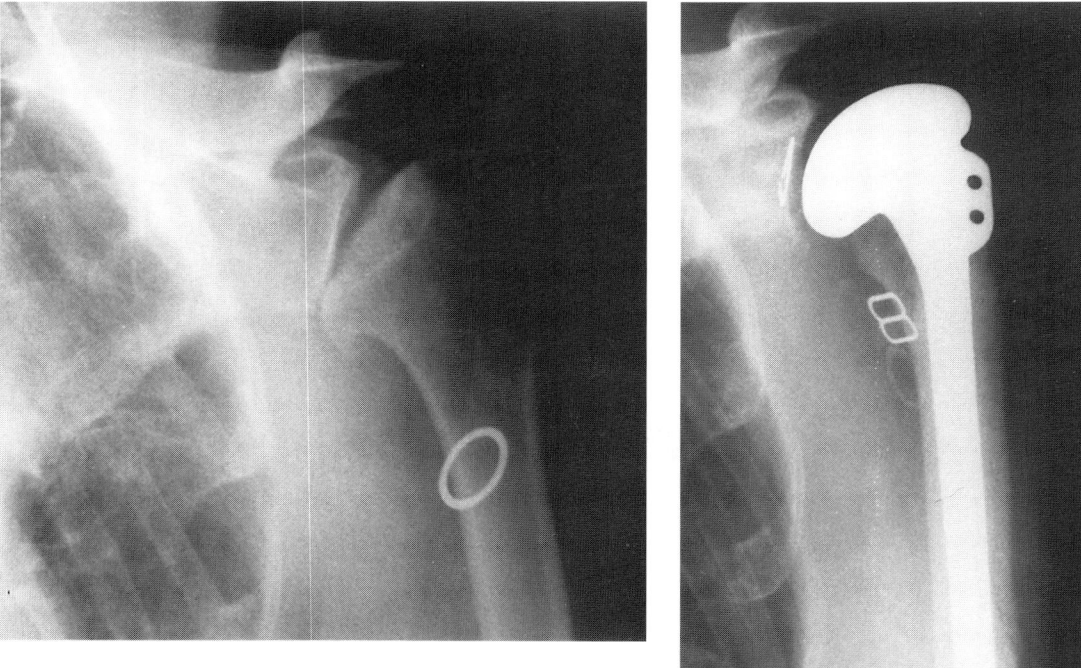

Fig. 4 **Left,** Radiograph showing humeral head collapse and glenoid erosion indicative of stage IV osteonecrosis. **Right,** Postoperative radiograph showing treatment with a total shoulder arthroplasty.

groups based on clinical manifestations. Type I disease is the least devastating form, has no neurologic involvement, and primarily involves Ashkenazi Jews. In contrast to those with type II and III disease, type I patients commonly present with orthopaedic problems. Bone involvement is often present, leading to bone marrow infiltration, infarcts, infection, and osteonecrosis. Surgery has most commonly been performed for symptoms secondary to osteonecrosis. Most of the reports are somewhat discouraging because the patients continue to have infarction pain and a higher risk of loosening and infection. It has been postulated that loosening in hip replacements was caused by continued Gaucher cell proliferation and erosion seen at revision surgery.

In the past there has been no useful medical treatment for underlying Gaucher's disease. The mannose-terminated enzyme alglucerase has recently been introduced with promising results. Concomitantly, reports of successful shoulder arthroplasty (> 2-year follow-up) have been made. At this time it would seem prudent to institute and/or continue medical treatment if arthroplasty is being considered for this condition. Future medical treatments, including gene therapy and bone marrow transplantation, are being investigated.

Sickle Cell Disease

Sickle cell disease and other hemoglobinopathies associated with hemolysis cause characteristic bone changes, including cortical thinning and intertrabecular and medullary widening. Patients with sickle cell disease have a higher incidence of gout, joint effusions, osteomyelitis, and bone infarctions. Septic arthritis is possible but not common. Osteonecrosis of the shoulder caused by end artery occlusion occurs with the associated bone changes previously described. There is radiographic evidence of shoulder osteonecrosis between 5.6% and 28% in patients with sickle cell disease.

Usually the patient does not present for orthopaedic evaluation until developing pain that coincides with humeral head collapse (Fig. 5). Infection is rare, but aspiration can confirm its presence. MRI may be helpful for diagnosis in rare cases presenting before collapse. Usually the diagnosis is made with plain radiograph changes combined with a history of the underlying sickle cell disease.

Treatment usually consists of arthroplasty as with other cases of osteonecrosis. There are a few reports of shoulder replacement surgery for osteonecrosis in sickle cell disease. The authors caution that patients are at a higher risk for postoperative infection, a condition that can be difficult to monitor because of fevers, elevated erythrocyte sedimentation rates, and bone infarction pain. Loosening has also been reported. However, patients can be extremely grateful for the relief of pain and recovery of use of their arms following arthroplasty. Patients with less severe disease forms such as thalassemia or sickle cell trait may have less severe systemic effects.

Hemochromatosis

Hemochromatosis, an autosomal recessive disorder, leads to an abnormally high intestinal absorption of iron, resulting in pathologic deposits of iron in the parenchymal cells of many organs. The exact mechanism of tissue injury is not known. Proposed mechanisms include lysosomal fragility, peroxidation of organelle membranes, or an effect on collagen biosynthesis leading to fibrosis. Clinical manifestations include liver disease, cardiomyopathy, arrhythmia, skin pigmentation, and endocrine dysfunction, especially diabetes mellitus. The gene is as prevalent in whites as is the sickle cell gene in blacks.

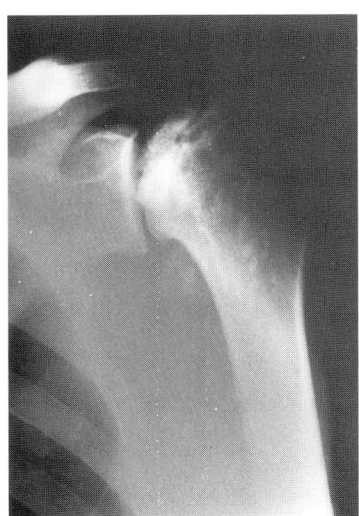
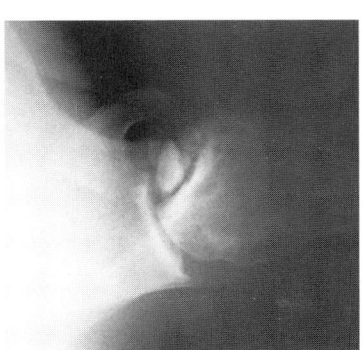
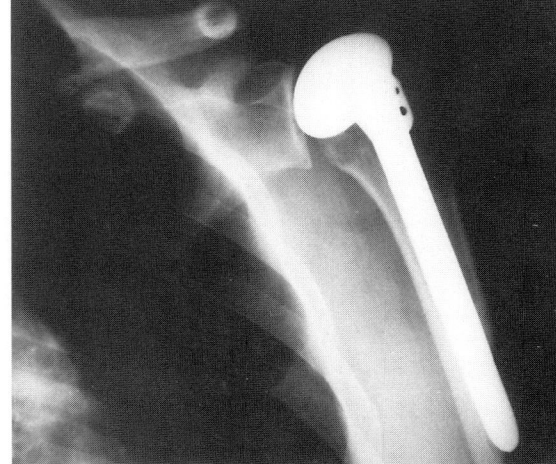

Fig. 5 Left, Sickle cell disease with osteonecrosis of the humeral head. **Center,** An axillary radiograph confirms collapse and fragmentation. **Right,** At surgery the glenoid was intact and a humeral head replacement was performed.

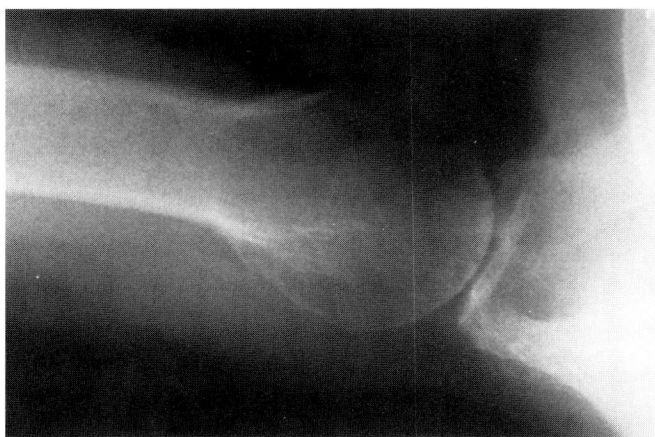 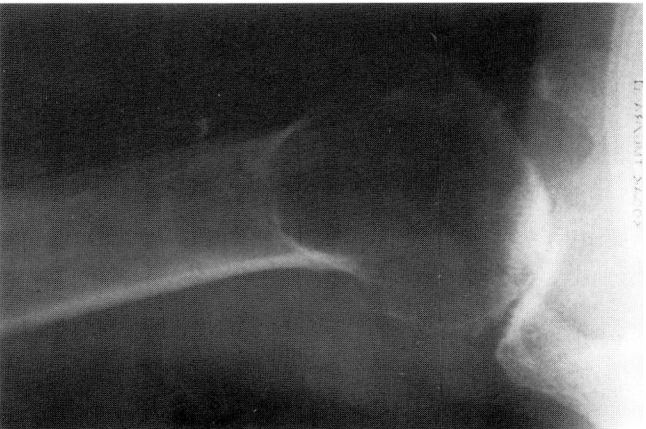

Fig. 6 A patient presented with shoulder pain and skin pigmentation. Laboratory testing revealed hemochromatosis. **Left,** An axillary radiograph at initial presentation shows mild joint space narrowing. **Right,** A radiograph 2 years later shows progressive arthropathy despite medical management.

Arthropathy is the presenting complaint in 44% to 64% of patients. Usually the hands and wrists are affected first, but the patient may present with shoulder pain and stiffness. Radiographs obtained early in the disease process may be unrevealing, but with time, joint space narrowing and progression to arthritis are apparent (Fig. 6). MRI is ineffective in detecting iron deposition in the cartilage before plain radiograph changes occur. Diagnostic screening is based on clinical manifestations combined with serum iron binding and total iron binding studies. Liver or duodenal biopsies are used by many clinicians to establish a probable diagnosis.

Medical treatment involves phlebotomy, which may take 2.5 years to unload excess body iron. Phlebotomy improves the visceral symptoms but not the arthropathy. The patients are more prone to infections with *Yersinia enterocolitica* as the organism requires an iron-rich environment. In one third of patients, death is a result of liver neoplasm.

Survival rates are improving as a result of earlier detection and treatment prior to the development of cirrhosis or diabetes. More patients are having normal lifespans. As this trend continues, arthroplasty may be indicated more frequently.

Synovial Osteochondromatosis

Synovial osteochondromatosis is a rare benign condition with metaplastic formation of hyaline cartilage nodules in the synovium that undergo enchondral ossification. The condition is most common in middle-aged men. Secondary osteoarthritis may develop.

Patients complain of progressive pain, swelling, crepitation, and decreased shoulder motion. Plain radiographs may show calcified cartilage nodes and associated changes of osteoarthritis. Arthrograms may show expanded capsule and filling defects from the cartilage nodules. MRI can reveal the condition because the nodules contain water and thus have a low signal intensity on T1-weighted images and a high signal intensity on T2-weighted images. CT scans can also show the nodules and the extent of defects.

Treatment usually involves synovectomy and, if arthritis is present, shoulder arthroplasty. Recurrence is rare and the results of arthroplasty are similar to those for osteoarthritis. Synovial osteochondromatosis rarely undergoes malignant transformation to chondrosarcoma.

Selected Bibliography

General

Cofield RH: Degenerative and arthritic problems of the glenohumeral joint, in Rockwood CA Jr, Matsen FA III (eds): *The Shoulder.* Philadelphia, PA, WB Saunders, 1990, pp 697-699.

Gerber C, Schneeberger AG, Vinh TS: The arterial vascularization of the humeral head: An anatomical study. *J Bone Joint Surg* 1990;72A:1486-1494.

Laing PG: The arterial supply of the adult humerus. *J Bone Joint Surg* 1956;38A:1105-1116.

Neer CS II: Glenohumeral arthroplasty, in Neer CS II (ed): *Shoulder Reconstruction.* Philadelphia, PA, WB Saunders, 1990, pp 194-202.

Osteonecrosis

Caldwell JR: Malpractice, steroids and avascular necrosis of bone. *J Fl Med Assoc* 1992;79:363-364.

In this editorial the author reviews the etiologies of avascular necrosis (AVN) and the legal ramifications. He states that "trial defeats in AVN-steroid cases might frequently result from a misunderstanding of AVN and failure to investigate the patients history enough to uncover more likely causes of AVN than steroid use."

Cruess RL: Osteonecrosis of bone: Current concepts as to etiology and pathogenesis. *Clin Orthop* 1986;208:30-39.

Dines DM, Warren RF, Altchek DW, et al: Posttraumatic changes of the proximal humerus: Malunion, nonunion, and osteonecrosis. Treatment with modular hemiarthroplasty or total shoulder arthroplasty. *J Shoulder Elbow Surg* 1993;2:11-21.

The authors performed 20 shoulder arthroplasties for chronic posttraumatic changes. Three patients had osteonecrosis. The postoperative scores of these patients were better than those of patients with nonunion or humeral head defects.

Gerber C, Lambert SM, Hoogewoud HM: Absence of avascular necrosis of the humeral head after post-traumatic rupture of the anterior and posterior humeral circumflex arteries. *J Bone Joint Surg* 1996;78A:1256-1259.

In a patient with angiographically documented rupture of the anterior and posterior humeral circumflex arteries, there was no evidence of avascular necrosis at 18 months by radiograph or MRI. These findings suggest intraosseous anastomosis from the deep brachial artery to the humeral head.

Govoni M, Orzincolo C, Bigoni M, et al: Humeral head osteonecrosis caused by electrical injury: A case report. *J Emerg Med* 1993;11:17-21.

A 52-year-old woman received a 220-volt electrical shock to the right hand and subsequently developed ipsilateral osteonecrosis of the humeral head.

Mont MA, Maar DC, Urquhart MW, et al: Avascular necrosis of the humeral head treated by core decompression: A retrospective review. *J Bone Joint Surg* 1993;75B:785-788.

In 20 patients, core decompression was performed on 30 shoulders. Twenty-two shoulders showed good or excellent results; the other eight required arthroplasty. All 14 shoulders with stage I or II radiologic changes at operation had good or excellent results.

Norris TR, Green A, McGuigan FX: Late prosthetic shoulder arthroplasty for displaced proximal humerus fractures. *J Shoulder Elbow Surg* 1995;4:271-280.

Twenty-three shoulders underwent arthroplasty for failed three- and four-part fractures. Nine shoulders had osteonecrosis; the condition was more common after open treatment than closed treatment.

Schlegel TF, Hawkins RJ: Displaced proximal humeral fractures: Evaluation and treatment. *J Am Acad Orthop Surg* 1994;2:54-66.

This article reviews the evaluation and treatment of proximal humerus fractures. Results and complications are discussed.

Steinberg ME, Steinberg DR: Osteonecrosis, in Kelley WW, Harris ED Jr, Ruddy S, et al (eds): *Textbook of Rheumatology,* ed 4. Philadelphia, PA, WB Saunders, 1993, vol 2, pp 1628-1650.

Gaucher's Disease

Balicki D, Beutler E: Gaucher disease. *Medicine* 1995;74:305-323.

This article reviews what has been learned about the fundamental nature of the disease and its diagnosis and treatment. A discussion of future directions is also presented.

Mankin HJ: Editorial: Gaucher's disease: A novel treatment and an important breakthrough. *J Bone Joint Surg* 1993;75B:2-3.

This editorial outlines past and present research and treatment of Gaucher's disease. Ceredase treatment appears promising in reducing the visceral and musculoskeletal manifestations such as fractures and bone infarctions.

Tauber C, Tauber T: Gaucher disease: The orthopaedic aspect. *Arch Orthop Trauma Surg* 1995;114:179-182.

In this series of seven case reports, there was one with bilateral osteonecrosis of the humeral heads. One shoulder was treated with a shoulder arthroplasty and had a good result at 2 years. The long-term effects on the skeleton of ceredase seem to be promising, but have yet to be determined.

Van Wellan PAJ, Haentjens P, Frecourt N, et al: Loosening of a noncemented porous-coated anatomic femoral component in Gaucher's disease: A case report and review of the literature. *Acta Orthop Beligica* 1994;60:119-123.

Typical lipid-laden Gaucher cells were found at the bone-prothesis interface of a total hip removed for loosening in a patient with Gaucher's disease. The authors hypothesize that loosening was caused by continued Gaucher cell proliferation and erosion of bone not specific to the type of prosthesis.

Sickle Cell Disease

David HG, Bridgman SA, Davies SC, et al: The shoulder in sickle cell disease. *J Bone Joint Surg* 1993;75B:538-545.

One hundred thirty-eight patients with sickle cell disease were reviewed for clinical and radiographic abnormalities of the shoulder. Twenty-eight percent had radiographic lesions that were frequently bilateral and only 53% had normal shoulder function. Two patients underwent arthroplasty and both loosened. Early diagnosis is important.

Milner PF, Kraus AP, Sebes JI, et al: Osteonecrosis of the humeral head in sickle cell disease. *Clin Orthop* 1993;289:136-143.

Two thousand twenty-four sickle cell patients were studied prospectively and followed for 5.6 years to determine the prevalence and incidence of osteonecrosis of the humeral head. At entry, 5.6% had radiographic evidence of osteonecrosis in one or both shoulders. Only 20.9% of patients reported pain or had limited range of motion at the time of diagnosis. Sickle cell disease is a frequent cause of osteonecrosis of the humeral head, especially in children and young adults.

Hemochromatosis

Conrad ME, Umbreit JN, Moore EG, et al: Hereditary hemochromatosis: A prevalent disorder of iron metabolism with an elusive etiology. *Am J Hematol* 1994;47:218-224.

This article reviews the etiology, prevalence, diagnosis, and treatment of hemochromatosis.

Eustace S, Buff B, McCarthy C, et al: Magnetic resonance imaging of hemochromatosis arthropathy. *Skeletal Radiol* 1994;23:547-549.

Ten patients with biopsy-proven hemochromatosis were studied prospectively. Plain radiographs and MRIs were taken of a symptomatic knee. MRI was not found to reliably detect intra-articular iron deposits in patients with hemochromatosis arthropathy and therefore is of limited value when clinical diagnostic uncertainty exists.

Faraawi R, Harth M, Kertesz A, et al: Arthritis in hemochromatosis. *J Rheumatol* 1993;20:448-452.

This study reviewed the clinical and radiograhic features of arthropathy in 25 patients with hemochromatosis. Arthropathy occurred in 16 (64%) and was the most common clinical feature at the time of diagnosis.

Synovial Osteochondromatosis

Porcellini G, Campi F, Brunetti E: Osteoarthritis caused by synovial chondromatosis of the shoulder. *J Shoulder Elbow Surg* 1994;3:404-406.

This case report describes metaplastic cartilage involvement of the rotator cuff leading to its destruction with arthropathy of the joint. Treatment consisted of synovectomy with loose body removal, humeral head replacement and subscaularis transfer. The result at 20 months' follow-up was satisfactory.

VI
Miscellaneous Shoulder Problems

Michael Watson, MA, MRCP, FRCS
Section Editor

27

Brachial Plexus Injuries

James D. Dalton, Jr, MD and Jon J.P. Warner, MD

Introduction

Patients with brachial plexus injuries exhibit a wide spectrum of involvement from annoying paresthesias to completely flail extremities with associated life-threatening injuries. Treatment of these patients is a challenge because of the anatomic variability of the plexus, difficulty of the neurologic examination, and the possibility of partial involvement of any part of the plexus. Furthermore, functional deficits in these patients may be multifactorial and not directly attributable to neurologic status. Advances in microsurgical and tissue transfer procedures have improved the functional outcome of severe plexus-injured patients; however, many of these patients still require a multidisciplinary approach to their care.

In order to systematically review the broad variety of lesions that affect the brachial plexus, an initial review of the clinically relevant anatomic features will be presented. This discussion will be followed by methods of evaluation, and then the following specific categories will be addressed: closed injuries (supraclavicular and infraclavicular), obstetric injuries, post-anesthetic injuries, open injuries, oncologic and radiation-induced injuries, and sports-related injuries to select peripheral nerves about the shoulder.

Anatomy

Disorders of the various components of the brachial plexus translate into predictable neurologic deficits. Knowledge of the brachial plexus anatomy along with a thorough neurologic examination of the upper extremity are the mainstays of an accurate anatomic diagnosis.

Many anatomic variations of the plexus exist, including those with contributions from the C4 and T2 nerve roots. These variations are not necessarily bilateral. In one study, 24 out of 63 bilateral cadaveric dissections were found to be asymmetrical. The most commonly encountered brachial plexus formation is shown in the schematic representation in Figure 1. Cervical roots from C5 and C6 and from C8 and T1 combine to form trunks (C7 does not combine, and thus is its own trunk), which divide and then combine again to form cords. The cords arborize to form peripheral nerves.

Because recovery is less likely in patients with preganglionic lesions than in those with postganglionic lesions, several additional anatomic points should be made about the roots and the dorsal root ganglia. First, anatomic studies have demonstrated that cervical roots C5, C6, and C7 are well attached to the neural foramen and transverse processes through the meninges and an envelope of fascia. Roots C8 and T1 lack these strong attachments, thus making them more susceptible to a preganglionic avulsion from the spinal cord. This factor has major prognostic implications because a root avulsion from the cord has an extremely poor prognosis for recovery. Second, the presence of a Horner's syndrome may be indicative of preganglionic lesions at the T1 level. Therefore, a Horner's syndrome is a negative prognostic factor for the T1 root.

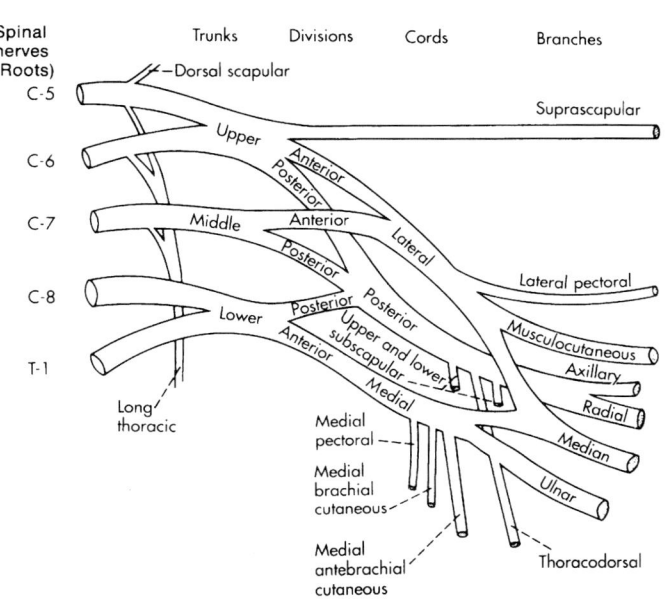

Fig. 1 Brachial plexus. (Reproduced with permission from Jenkins DB (ed): *Hollinshead's Functional Anatomy of the Limbs and Back*, ed 6. Philadelphia, PA, WB Saunders, 1991, pp 65-101.)

The dorsal scapular nerve, which innervates the rhomboids, and the long thoracic nerve arise from the C5 and C5-7 roots, respectively. If, on examination, the rhomboids and serratus anterior muscles are not paralyzed, then the lesion to the plexus can be considered to be at or distal to Erb's point (ie, postganglionic), which is where the fifth and sixth cervical roots join to form the upper trunk.

Finally, if electromyographic studies indicate that the posterior cervical musculature is denervated, then a preganglionic lesion exists. This denervation is present because the posterior primary ramus, which innervates the posterior cervical musculature, exits the root between the sympathetic ganglion and the spinal cord (Fig. 2).

Methods of Evaluation

When possible, a thorough history should be obtained for any patient with a suspected injury to the brachial plexus.

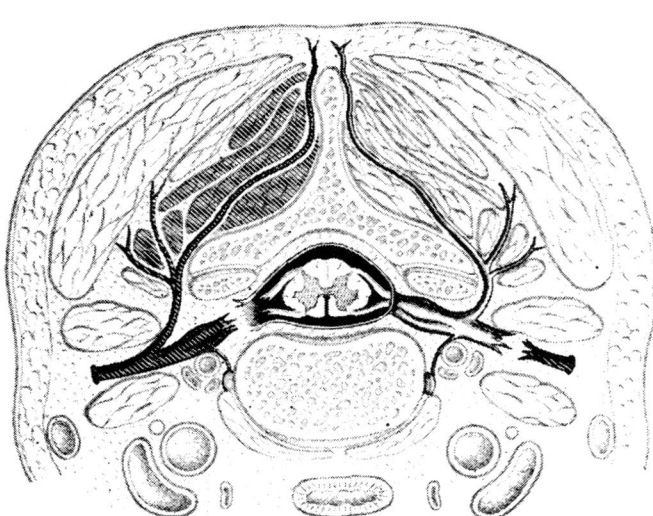

Fig. 2 The left side of the illustration shows a rupture distal to the dorsal root ganglion. The erector spinae musculature is not denervated. On the right, the root is avulsed (supraganglionic) and the erector spinae are denervated. (Reproduced with permission from Bufalini C, Pescatori G: Posterior cervical electromyography in the diagnosis and prognosis of brachial plexus injuries. *J Bone Joint Surg* 1969;51B:627-631.)

Occasionally, the patient may be unable to give a history because of associated injuries such as those to the head or airway. In these situations, witnesses or family members may provide key information that may help make management decisions easier. Hand dominance, occupation, mechanism of injury, preinjury function, and history of previous surgery to the neck or extremity are necessary items in the history about which to inquire. Also, factors such as preexisting neuropathy, psychiatric disease, substance abuse, and compliance may have a role in reconstructive surgical decision making as well.

An anatomy-based physical examination is extremely helpful in sorting out suspected lesions of the brachial plexus, and the examination should always be thoroughly documented and repeated on subsequent visits. Of major importance is the neurologic examination, which should include testing of dermatomal sensation, deep tendon reflexes, and motor strength. It is useful to begin the motor examination with an assessment of the muscles innervated by the C5 root, followed by those innervated by the C6 root, then the C7 root, and so on. Next, a sequential peripheral nerve examination of the musculoskeletal, axillary, radial, median, and ulnar nerves is conducted and the deficits noted. With the combined deficits of the roots and peripheral nerves noted, a general location of the lesion(s) can be determined. Next, an examination of the muscles innervated by those peripheral nerves that branch off of the roots, trunks, and cords of the plexus (ie, rhomboids, serratus anterior, pectoralis muscles, subscapularis, and latissimus dorsi) can usually provide the information necessary to focus in on the exact location of the deficit. The neurologic examination should also include the lower extremities. Spasticity of the ipsilateral lower extremity may indicate a concomitant cord injury at the site of root avulsion, and a preexisting neuropathy may also be detected.

For consistency, motor strength should be graded on a scale of zero to five based on the accepted notation system of the American Academy of Orthopaedic Surgeons and the British Medical Research Council. Grade 0 indicates complete paralysis. Grade 1 strength is a flicker of motion. Grade 2 strength is contraction with gravity eliminated. Grade 3 strength is contraction against gravity only. Grade 4 strength is contraction against some resistance, and grade 5 strength is normal contraction against powerful resistance.

The ipsilateral eye should be closely inspected for the presence of Horner's syndrome, which includes myosis (constriction of the pupil), ptosis (drooping of the lid), anhydrosis (lack of sweating on the affected side of the face), and enophthalmos (sinking in of the eyeball). The presence of Horner's syndrome implies that the preganglionic axons at the level of T1 have been disrupted. A positive percussion test (tingling distally in response to percussion over the plexus) implies that a postganglionic lesion exists. The finding of a positive Tinel's sign (distal migration of a positive percussion test on subsequent examinations) indicates that a postganglionic lesion is recovering. The function of the rhomboids (scapular retraction) and serratus anterior (scapular protraction) should be ascertained if possible. As previously mentioned, a functional serratus anterior muscle or rhomboid group in the setting of an upper root palsy implies a postganglionic lesion.

Cervical spine radiographs may demonstrate lateral tilt of the spine or transverse process fractures. Other disorders may be evident as well, such as fractures of the clavicle, humerus, first rib, or evidence of a scapulothoracic dissociation. A chest radiograph may demonstrate an elevated hemidiaphragm because of preganglionic contributions of C5 to the phrenic nerve. Electrodiagnostic studies may be of benefit as well. Electromyography will show evidence of denervation and involuntary motor action potentials 3 weeks after injury because of wallerian degeneration. Also, the segmentally innervated paraspinous musculature, the transverse spinous and the interspinosus intertransversalis, may show evidence of denervation at the associated level in preganglionic lesions (Fig. 2).

Nerve conduction velocity studies may be normal immediately after a root avulsion, but they should be abnormal across a discreet lesion more distal in the plexus. As wallerian degeneration begins in the motor axons, a discrepancy between motor and sensory nerve conduction occurs. Somatosensory-evoked potentials test the sensory conduction from the periphery to the cortex of the brain. In patients who have root avulsions, evoked potentials do not reach the cortex; however, they may still have normal peripheral sensory conduction.

Historically, myelography has been used to determine the presence of meningoceles, which were thought to be pathognomonic for nerve root avulsions. One study correlated myelographic findings with surgical findings and found that of 90 abnormal roots on myelogram, 70 were avulsions and 16 were distal lesions. False-positive results occurred in four. Combining myelography with computed tomography (CT) reduces false-positive results and raises the accuracy of diagnosis from around 84% to 94%. Magnetic resonance imaging

(MRI) of the plexus correlates well with CT myelograms and provides better visualization of injuries distal to the roots.

Axon reflex testing includes histamine sensitivity testing and the cold vasodilation test. The histamine sensitivity test is performed by injecting a small volume of 1% histamine phosphate into the skin. In a normally innervated area of skin, a triple response of local vasodilation, formation of a wheal, and a spreading vasodilatory response (flare) occurs. In an area of anesthetic skin that has been denervated by a preganglionic lesion, the triple response would be unaltered, indicating a poor prognosis for recovery. This condition occurs because the dendrites are still attached to their sensory bodies in the dorsal root ganglion. If the lesion is postganglionic, then the flare response will be absent because of the disruption of the axon from its body in the sympathetic ganglion. Therefore, the lack of a flare is a good prognostic indicator. One limitation of the histamine test is that it must be performed on an area with a flat skin surface. This surface can be found for every plexus root except C7, which innervates the long finger. The cold vasodilation test is useful when C7 injury is suspected. The test involves measuring the temperature of a cooled finger as it rewarms. In a normal digit, or one with a preganglionic lesion, a local vasodilatory effect is accompanied by a rise in temperature. This rise in temperature is not seen in a digit innervated by a nervous supply with postganglionic disruption.

Closed Injuries

In general terms, a peripheral nerve injury can be classified into one of three categories as described by Seddon. A neurapraxia results from a stretch injury. Neurapraxic lesions have intact nerve fibers, including axons, but have a functional conduction block. Neurapraxias usually resolve within 6 weeks. In mixed sensory and motor nerves, the motor component is usually affected to a greater extent than the sensory component. An axonotmesis is a disruption of the axons with intact Schwann sheaths, which are capable of guiding regenerating axons. The regeneration process occurs at a rate of approximately 1 mm/day. Because of wallerian degeneration, there is complete motor and sensory loss with fibrillations and no voluntary action potentials seen with electromyography at 3 weeks. The prognosis is good for a complete or nearly complete recovery from an axonotmesis. The most damaging form of nerve injury is a neurotmesis, complete disruption of the axons and the surrounding nerve sheaths. Neurotmeses are most commonly produced by lacerations, missiles, and extreme traction injuries. There is a complete motor and sensory loss, and electromyographic findings at 3 weeks are similar to those of an axonotmesis. There is poor potential for complete recovery, even if surgery is performed (Fig. 3).

Closed injuries to the brachial plexus can be considered to be supraclavicular or infraclavicular. This method of categorization is relevant because it separates injuries by their mechanisms, anatomic location, and prognosis for recovery. Supraclavicular injuries are usually the result of a traction mechanism caused by high-energy trauma affecting the roots, trunks, and divisions. Infraclavicular injuries are usually the

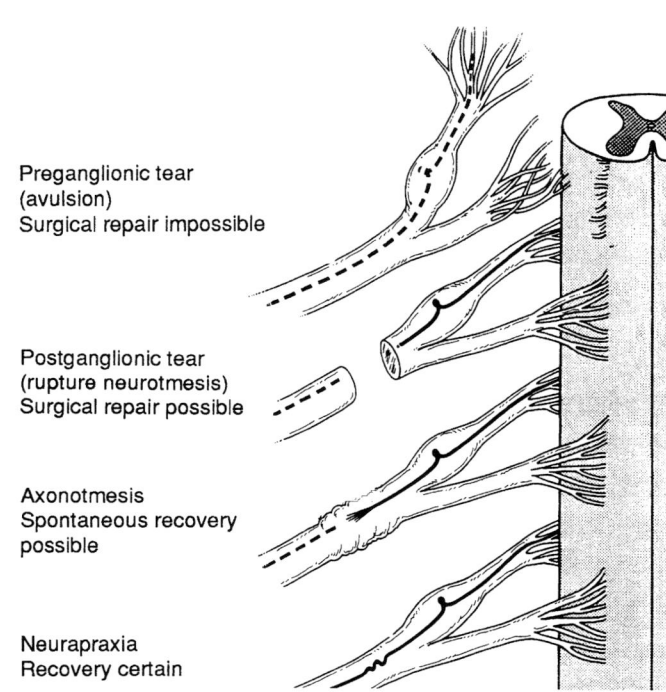

Fig. 3 A severe traction to the brachial plexus may cause nerve injuries of varying severity, including avulsion of the nerve root from the spinal cord (nonrepairable), extraforaminal rupture of the root or trunk (surgically repairable), or an intraneural rupture of fascicles (some spontaneous recovery possible). (Reproduced with permission from Green DP, Hotchkiss RN (eds): *Operative Hand Surgery*, ed 3. New York, NY, Churchill Livingstone, 1993, vol 2, p 1224.)

result of low-energy trauma resulting in a fracture or dislocation about the shoulder. The cords and peripheral nerves are the structures affected.

Supraclavicular traction injuries in adults usually fall into one of four neurologic patterns as described by Leffert (Table 1): (1) C5–6/Upper trunk lesion; (2) C5, C6, and C7 lesions; (3) C8 and T1 lesions; and (4) diffuse lesions of the plexus. Table 1 describes the characteristics and prognosis of each type of lesion pattern. Physical examination findings that are features of supraclavicular injuries include fracture of the clavicle or cervical transverse processes, Horner's syndrome, tenderness in the supraclavicular fossa, and injury to the dorsal scapular, suprascapular, and/or long thoracic nerves.

Infraclavicular injuries to the brachial plexus, as previously mentioned, are due to glenohumeral dislocations and humeral or scapular fractures. The axillary nerve is most predisposed to injury from an anterior dislocation. Anatomic studies have demonstrated that local traction occurs in the posterior cord, radial nerve, and axillary nerve when the humeral head is dislocated anteriorly and internally rotated. The lateral cord and musculocutaneous nerve become taut when the humeral head is dislocated anteriorly and externally rotated.

In general, recovery of infraclavicular brachial plexus injuries is better than that of supraclavicular injuries. The

Table 1. Closed supraclavicular brachial plexus injuries in adults

Pattern of Injury	Clinical Features	Muscles Affected*	Prognosis	Mechanism
C5, C6 upper trunk	Lack of shoulder control and elbow flexion; weak wrist extension; scapular winging if preganglionic; decreased sensation in C5 and C6 dermatomes; normal motor function in hand	Deltoid, Supraspinatus, Infraspinatus, Biceps, Brachialis, Brachioradialis, ECRB, ECRL, Rhomboids (if preganglionic), Serratus anterior (if preganglionic)	Good if postganglionic; if preganglionic, the extremity can be reconstructed to provide useful function	Traction with arm adducted
C5, C6, C7	Same as C5, C6 with loss of elbow, wrist, and finger extension	Same as C5, C6 plus triceps and finger extensors	Fair, but reconstruction to provide useful function is possible	Traction with arm adducted
C8, T1 (rare)	Horner's syndrome; intact shoulder function and elbow flexion; median and ulnar nerve palsies in hand	Intrinsics of hand, Finger flexors, Triceps (if C7 involved)	Fair, but useful hand function is possible with wrist arthrodesis and tendon transfer	Traction with arm abducted
Entire plexus	Horner's syndrome; flail, anesthetic arm; chronic pain	All plexus-innervated muscles to varying degrees	Poor	Major trauma, extreme traction

*ECRB = extensor carpi radialis brevis; ECRL = extensor carpi radialis longus

natural history of spontaneous recovery has been well documented by Leffert and Seddon and is based on cord involvement. In 13 patients in the posterior cord group, those with isolated axillary nerve injuries did poorer than those with posterior cord involvement, probably because of a selection bias in the study. In fact, most complete axillary palsies improve within 6 months. Watson-Jones reported on 15 patients with axillary nerve palsies, ten of whom recovered spontaneously within 6 months, and another three who recovered between 6 and 12 months. The two remaining patients had permanent paralysis of the deltoids.

In Leffert and Seddon's study, four of five patients with lateral cord or musculocutaneous nerve involvement regained biceps and brachialis function, and the fifth had powerful elbow flexion because of his brachioradialis. Medial cord recovery took the longest to occur. Thumb opposition and interossei function improved for up to 3 years in some patients with intrinsic paralysis. Overall, spontaneous recovery of infraclavicular injuries resulting in paralysis to the proximal muscles occurs in about 95% of patients, with slightly lower results for those with isolated deltoid palsies. Recovery of the hand intrinsics and median nerve sensibility occurs in over 80%, with ulnar sensibility occurring in approximately 60% of patients. In a group of 14 patients with diffuse infraclavicular palsies, all regained good or normal function proximal to the hand. The median and ulnar intrinsics lagged with 11 regaining median intrinsic function and 11 regaining ulnar intrinsic function up to 2 years after the injury. Unless there is evidence of a neurotmesis from a bone fragment or an accompanying vascular injury, closed infraclavicular lesions can be treated nonsurgically.

Treatment of Closed Injuries

When considering treatment options for an individual with a brachial plexus palsy, the patient's symptoms, including paralysis, sensory loss, joint contracture, and pain, must be clearly defined. Treatment should be tailored to each patient's specific complaints and needs. Treatment options include nonsurgical measures, surgical repair or reconstruction of the plexus, peripheral reconstruction, and palliation to alleviate pain.

Nonsurgical Treatment

The goals of nonsurgical treatment are to maintain preexisting passive motion, strengthen functional muscles and enhance overall extremity function, protect anesthetic areas of skin, prevent edema formation, and manage pain. Physical therapy is useful in maintaining passive motion; however, the patient should also be educated in a home program of range-of-motion exercises. Functional splinting may be helpful, but prolonged splinting in one position of any part of the extremity is ill-advised because joint contractures may develop. Hinged orthoses with cable or spring mechanisms may be useful as well. However, chronic edema may develop in response to dependent positioning, loss of vascular tone as a result of a sympathectomy effect, and coexisting soft-tissue trauma in the region of the plexus. If severe, this edema may lead to stiffness of the hand. Elevation of the area, use of a "statue of liberty" brace, elastic or air supports, and prompt treatment of any infection will keep edema to a minimum.

In patients with areas of anesthetic skin, education is the mainstay of treating sensory deficits. This education parallels the treatment program for diabetic patients with neuropathy. Patients should avoid exposing the area of injury to extreme temperatures. Daily inspections, with a mirror if necessary, of all areas of the insensate skin must be carried out. Management of chronic pain in patients with brachial plexus injuries can be difficult. The exact mechanism of the pain response in these patients is poorly understood, but patients with total plexus lesions tend to have more pain than those with partial injuries. Occasionally, a subluxated or dislocated joint, a fracture nonunion, or posttraumatic arthritis of the acromioclavicular and sternoclavicular joints will be found to be the source of pain. Often, social or psychological factors, including depression, contribute to pain. Referral to a pain clinic or consultation with an anesthesiologist who manages chronic pain is usually beneficial. Most pain control programs are multifaceted and may include physical therapy, psychological counseling, biofeedback, hypnosis, acupuncture, transcutaneous nerve stimulation, and pharmacologic agents. It is beyond the scope of this review to describe the different pharmacologic treatments and their side effects; however, a multifaceted pharmacologic approach using antidepressants, carbamazepine (Tegretol), and analgesics may be beneficial for the patient with chronic brachial plexus pain.

Surgical Treatment
Surgical treatment of closed supraclavicular injuries has received much attention since the early 1900s. Initial attempts at surgical repair or neurolysis of damaged nerves were unsuccessful. As techniques and equipment improved, so did the results of neurolysis and autografting plexus injuries. Modern advances have produced free muscle transfer and neurotization.

Currently, there is no universally accepted algorithm of treatment for patients with supraclavicular lesions. Several general statements can be made, however. First, the patients who have the most to gain by a neural procedure are those with complete loss of the C5, C6, and C7 root functions. Second, nerve grafting is often possible because rupture, not avulsion, of the upper roots usually occurs. Third, if avulsion of the upper roots does occur, or grafting is unsuccessful, then a neurotization procedure (or free muscle transfer) may be the only surgical option that will facilitate return of function. Fourth, avulsion of the C8 and T1 roots makes grafting impossible; however, if instead these roots rupture, grafting may provide protective sensation. Because of muscle atrophy, it is unlikely that grafting of a lower root or trunk will result in meaningful motor function in the hand because of the course over which the regenerating nerve has to travel to reinnervate the finger flexors and intrinsics. Fifth, in a child, any complete lesion regardless of the level should be repaired or grafted if possible. And sixth, the surgical results reported by most authors indicate that the best results are obtained if surgery is performed 3 to 6 months postinjury.

The results from nerve grafting using modern techniques are good. A nerve graft is indicated in a rupture or transection if the distance between the two stumps does not allow coaptation without tension. Free nerve grafts, vascularized pedicle nerve grafts, or free vascularized nerve grafts may be used. The viability of a free nerve graft is enhanced with grafts of small diameter; therefore, smaller nerves such as the sural or medial antebrachial cutaneous are optimal. The viability of the vascularized nerve grafts depends on their blood supply, and these grafts can be of larger diameter than nonvascularized grafts. Interestingly, neither vascularized nor nonvascularized nerve grafts have demonstrated superior results over the other. Using the criteria of shoulder joint stability and strong, active elbow flexion, good results can be achieved in 75% to 85% of the cases.

Neurotization or nerve transfer is the only neural-directed surgical alternative in root avulsion injuries. In neurotization, a healthy, less important nerve is mobilized from its bed and separated from its muscular insertion. It is then coupled directly, or via free grafts, to the distal stump of a nonfunctioning nerve. Overall, the best reported results of neurotization are those of reinnervating the lateral cord or musculocutaneous nerve with an intercostal nerve. Most studies indicate that this procedure yields strong elbow flexion in 50% to 60% of patients; however, a recent Japanese study reported 87% grade 3 or 4 strength in 112 patients. Three factors that contribute to good results are surgery within 5 months, patient age 50 years or younger, and use of adjuvant surgical procedures such as tendon transfers and arthrodeses. Patients who have undergone intercostal nerve transfer may exhibit a synkinesis between their elbow flexors and intercostal muscles that can be demonstrated with coughing or sneezing. Eventually, they learn to flex their elbow independent of respiration. Other nerves that are used for elbow flexion are the phrenic and spinal accessory. The spinal accessory nerve is used to neurotize the suprascapular and axillary nerves. Success rates for this procedure vary, but in the largest reported series of 22 patients, the success rate was 36% (Fig. 4).

Patients without a viable brachialis or biceps brachii muscle may be candidates for a free muscle transfer, such as a free vascularized gracilis muscle. Several cases of successful free gracilis transfers have been reported using intercostal nerves as donors. Free muscle transfers may be combined with other procedures to restore elbow and hand function. In one series of ten patients with complete avulsion of the entire brachial plexus, flexion and extension of both the elbow and fingers were restored using a double free muscle transfer coupled with neurotization procedures to improve sensibility. Shoulder arthrodeses were also performed. Five of the ten patients reportedly use their hands in activities of daily living.

Reconstructive Procedures
Peripheral reconstructive procedures should be considered when, after all methods of evaluation have been exhausted, there is indisputable evidence that neurologic recovery is highly unlikely, or that enough time has passed without progression of functional recovery. Arthrodeses and tendon transfers are the primary reconstructive procedures available; however, palliative procedures including amputations and the dorsal root entry zone (DREZ) ablation procedures will be discussed in this section as well.

Shoulder arthrodesis should be considered in the treatment of a painful, subluxated, or dislocated joint in which functional control is absent. The scapulothoracic musculature should be nearly normal in its function. Rowe recommends fusing the glenohumeral joint in 15° to 20° of abduction, 25° to 30° of flexion, and 40° to 50° of internal rotation in order to allow for personal hygiene, feeding, and to prevent excessive strain on the scapulothoracic musculature. For upper trunk lesions, arthrodesis of the shoulder can be combined

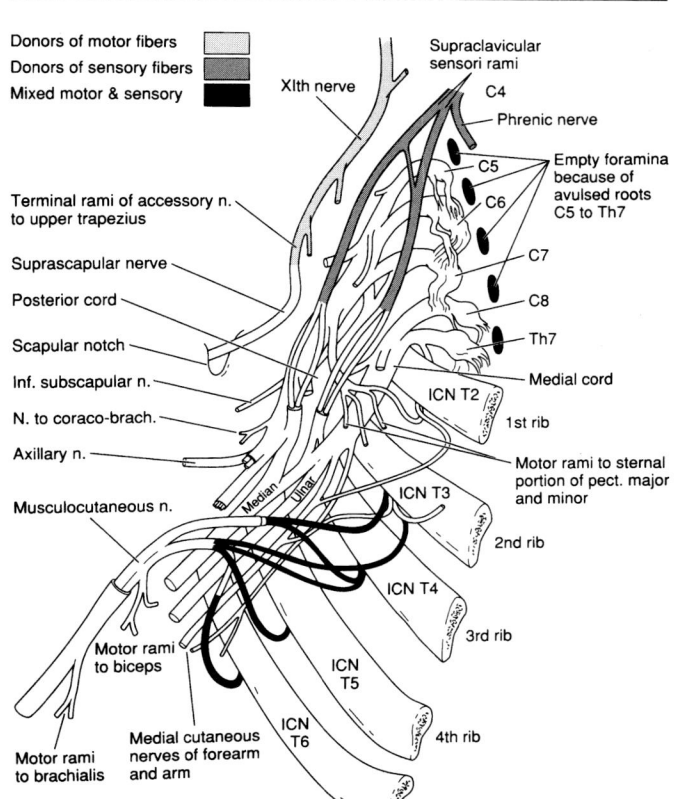

Fig. 4 The donor nerves and their destinations in a case of avulsion of all five roots is illustrated. (Reproduced with permission from Narakas AO, Hentz VR: Neurotization in brachial plexus injuries: Indication and results. *Clin Orthop* 1988;237:43-56.)

with other reconstructive procedures, such as one to improve elbow flexion, to produce a very functional upper extremity. It should be kept in mind that a glenohumeral arthrodesis limits the surgeon's ability to position the patient on the operating table to some degree, and that distal procedures may be more easily accomplished prior to arthrodesis of the shoulder. Some patients with long-standing contractures and bony changes may benefit from a derotational humeral osteotomy.

Most adult patients with paralysis of the shoulder benefit from arthrodeses; however, the occasional patient with partial paralysis may benefit from a soft-tissue procedure to enhance function, including capsular releases and tendon transfers such as the L'Episcopo procedure, which involves transferring the latissimus dorsi and the teres major to the posterolateral humerus or cuff to improve external rotation. Anterior advancement of the posterior portion of the deltoid to replace a nonfunctional anterior segment has also been described.

The restoration of elbow function plays a vital role in converting a nonfunctional extremity into a functional one. Because flexion is the single most important function of the elbow, most tendon transfers about the elbow have focused on this issue. The sternocleidomastoid (Bunnell), the pectoralis major (Clarke), the pronator-flexor group (Steindler), the triceps (Bunnell, Carroll), and the latissimus dorsi (Hovnanian) have been used to achieve active elbow flexion. When considering a transfer to establish elbow flexion, the excursion of the muscle, alignment of the transfer, cosmetic appearance, and preoperative range of motion are factors that must be considered. The goal of surgery is to have good strength throughout a functional range of motion (30° to 130°) without excessive pronation, which would render the upper extremity less useful. The sternocleidomastoid transfer is rarely used because of the odd web that appears in the neck when it contracts and the fact that some patients must preposition their head to gain forceful elbow contraction. The Steindler flexorplasty has historically been the most popular transfer, but its disadvantages include weakness, possibility of flexion contracture, and its tendency to cause pronation. Disadvantages of the pectoralis transfers are that they require stable or arthrodesed shoulders and that establishing the correct tension in the transfer is often difficult. However, these transfers do restore supination, power, and cosmesis. The power and excursion of the latissimus dorsi is equivalent to that of the pectoralis transfer. Unfortunately, the latissimus dorsi is often denervated along with the elbow flexors and is frequently unavailable. The triceps transfer results in good excursion, strength, and cosmesis. Its major drawback is the lack of active elbow extension.

Tendon transfers for the paralyzed hand in patients with brachial plexus palsies are the same as those for more distal nerve injuries and will not be covered in this chapter. One point on hand and wrist management that should be mentioned is the consideration of a wrist arthrodesis. A common strategy for augmenting hand function in a brachial plexus injured patient with a flail hand and wrist is arthrodesis of the wrist and use of whatever functioning muscle-tendon units are available to maximize finger control.

Occasionally, patients with flail, anesthetic arms may wish to have ablation surgery. Attempts at reconstructive surgery may have failed, or these patients may not be reconstructive candidates at all. They may simply feel encumbered by the weight of the arm, or are unable to properly care for their anesthetic skin. For these select patients, amputation can truly be a viable option. The amputation can be at virtually any level, depending on the specific needs of the patient. The amputation can also be combined with a shoulder arthrodesis or a functional prosthesis to enhance the overall usefulness of the extremity. Patients who request amputation for pain of neurologic origin should not be considered as candidates because they do not benefit from an amputation or disarticulation.

Palliative Treatment

Patients with intractable pain of neurologic origin that does not respond to nonsurgical measures should be considered for DREZ ablation as described by Nashold. Bruxelle reported on 20 of 24 patients with neurologic pain of "unbearable intensity" who had good results (defined as 75% or more pain relief) following the DREZ procedure. Reported complications of the procedure include cerebrospinal fistulas, sensory and motor deficits in the ipsilateral lower extremity, sensory changes in the thoracic region, persistent tingling sensations in the involved upper extremity, and postsurgical depression.

Obstetric Injuries

In the past, brachial plexus injuries occurring at birth have been attributed to compression injuries caused by conditions such as intrauterine pressure on the arm and axillary pressure during delivery. It is now nearly universally accepted that the etiology of obstetric injuries to the brachial plexus is traction on the supraclavicular components of the plexus. Because of the advent of better obstetric care, the severity of such birth-related injuries has decreased over the past several decades, but the incidence has not significantly changed. The reported incidences during the past several decades have ranged from 0.3 to 2.5 palsies per 1,000 live births. Risk factors that are associated with these injuries include prolonged labor, breech presentation, high birth weight, forceps delivery, and shoulder dystocia.

A brachial plexopathy should be suspected in any neonate with a normal passive range of motion and asymmetric active motion. The differential diagnosis may include pseudo-paralysis from a periarticular fracture, dislocation, or epiphyseal injury. Radiographs may be helpful in the identification of a fracture, but initial radiographs may be normal in a neonate with an epiphyseal separation. Radiographic findings consistent with a brachial plexus palsy include an elevated and rotated scapula, increased metaphyseal-glenoid distance, and delayed development of the humeral epiphysis.

Three major patterns of brachial plexus injuries are seen in neonates. Type I is the most common, involving the C5, C6/upper trunk complex. This form of obstetric palsy, described by Duchenne and Erb, comprises approximately 60% to 80% of all cases seen. The type II, or Erb-Duchenne-Klumpke palsy, involves the entire plexus and carries the worst prognosis for spontaneous recovery. This form of injury occurs in less than 25% of the cases. The type III palsy's pattern of injury is to the lower roots including C7, C8, and T1. This pattern is the least common, comprising approximately 10% of the lesions and is termed Klumpke's palsy.

Erb-Duchenne's palsy, or type I, involves those muscles innervated by C5 and C6. These include the supraspinatus, infraspinatus, teres minor, deltoid, biceps, brachialis, coracobrachialis, brachioradialis, extensor carpi radialis brevis, extensor carpi radialis longus, and extensor carpi ulnaris. Patients with this particular type of palsy characteristically exhibit some degree of loss of shoulder abduction, humeral external rotation, elbow flexion, wrist extension, and supination. The resultant position of the upper extremity is referred to as the "waiter's tip" position. It is important to note that passive motion in the newborn is normal.

Without proper treatment, secondary contractures and deformities occur in the older child and the adult. Loss of passive motion may be caused by loss of the antagonistic action of the internal rotators and adductors of the shoulder. The anterior and inferior shoulder capsule becomes contracted. Muscle paralysis and weakness coupled with these contractures result in an abnormal scapular rhythm during shoulder elevation, abduction, and forward flexion. Bony changes occur as well. The scapula may be undersized compared to the normal side, and the glenoid may take on a flattened appearance. Eventually, the articular incongruity may lead to degenerative arthritis.

Associated changes seen in the elbows of patients with Erb-Duchenne's palsy include flexion and pronation contractures. Bony deformities about the elbow are seen in about 30% of patients with Erb-Duchenne's palsy, and 16% to 25% of the elbows have posterior dislocations of the radial heads. The earliest abnormal radiographic finding in the elbow is clubbing of the radial head.

There is great variability in the amount of spontaneous recovery reported with Erb-Duchenne's palsy. This variability is likely caused by the different levels of injury severity and the extent of involvement of the plexus. A complete recovery is more likely if a neurapraxia or axonotmesis exists as opposed to a neurotmesis. In general, recovery is faster and more complete in palsies involving the upper roots because the upper roots usually stretch or rupture and only rarely do they avulse off of the spinal cord. In contrast, a recent report demonstrates an 81% rate of upper root avulsion in breech babies with brachial plexus palsies.

Initial management involves maintaining passive motion, judicious use of orthoses only to avoid contractures, and encouraging the child to use the involved arm or hand to the greatest extent possible. Limiting the use of the normal arm in an attempt to make the child use the affected arm is not recommended. With nonsurgical treatment, complete spontaneous recovery of C5 and C6 lesions is seen approximately 80% to 90% of the time. Recovery will occur in most infants within 3 months of birth; however, significant recovery can still be seen up to 12 months after birth.

Surgical treatment for an Erb-Duchenne's palsy should be considered when no evidence of recovery is apparent at 3 months of age. In one study of obstetric palsies, a baseline electromyogram was performed shortly after the diagnosis was made, and then repeated at 3 months if the infant had not regained biceps or deltoid function. The electromyogram and clinical findings were discussed with the parents, and microsurgical reconstruction of the neural elements was performed in those cases with no clinical improvement at 3 months. At 2 years postoperatively, there was improved ability for the biceps, deltoid, and external rotators of the shoulder to contract.

Two comments should be made about managing possible surgical candidates. If neurologic reconstruction is to be considered, a thorough and completely documented neurologic examination should be performed shortly after birth by an experienced examiner. Ideally, this person should be the physician who will be involved with the surgical decision making. Also, it cannot be stressed enough that passive motion must be maintained until motor function is restored. If contractures develop in the shoulder or elbow, the ultimate functional result may still be poor.

In those cases in which there is residual impairment in the older child, a number of reconstructive procedures exist. As previously mentioned, management of these cases is considerably less complicated if passive motion has been maintained through physical therapy. If a fixed contracture of the shoulder is present, however, an open anterior release as described by Fairbanks and Sever may be performed. The release can be combined with a transfer of the teres major and latissimus dorsi tendons to the posterolateral aspect of the proximal humerus or rotator cuff in order to convert them into external rotators (L'Episcopo procedure). In cases of excessive humeral head retroversion, subluxation, dislocation, or flattening, a soft-tissue procedure alone may be inadequate to treat the internal rotation deformity, and a rotational humeral osteotomy may be required. Leffert prefers the osteotomy in the midteen or young adult as opposed to the infant.

Loss of elbow flexion can be treated by one of several different procedures. The most common tendon transfers to obtain elbow flexion are the Clarke pectoralis major transfer, the Steindler flexorplasty, transfer of the triceps, and transfer of the latissimus dorsi. The pectoralis major tendon may be transferred, in part or in its entirety, to the ulna with a fascial graft extension, or by using the long head portion of the biceps muscle (Clarke, Brooks, and Seddon). The Steindler flexorplasty is accomplished by transferring the common origin of the flexor-pronator mass to a more proximal and anterolateral location on the humerus, a complication of which is the development of a pronation deformity in the forearm. The triceps tendon transfer (Bunnell, Carroll) is performed by dividing the triceps tendon at its insertion, routing it laterally around the elbow, and inserting it via a fascial graft into the tuberosity of the radius. Active elbow extension is lost with a triceps tendon transfer. The latissimus dorsi transfer (Hovnanian) involves mobilizing the origin of the latissimus off of the ribs and scapula and transferring it to the distal biceps tendon insertion.

Involvement of the entire brachial plexus is characteristic of the type II, or Erb-Duchenne-Klumpke palsy. This type of palsy carries the worst prognosis for spontaneous recovery. Patients with this type of palsy have variable presentations, depending on the severity of upper root involvement. The lower roots, C8 and T1, are almost always avulsed off the cord with scant hope for recovery. This is true for the type III, or Klumpke's palsy, as well. Little is written about the management of newborns with complete or lower root palsies. It seems reasonable to manage the complete palsies as one would manage Erb-Duchenne palsies and attempt a neural reconstruction of everything possible if there is no evidence of deltoid or biceps function at 3 months. The hand, in the meantime, should be kept supple until recovery of the more proximal muscles has plateaued. At that point, a decision regarding which type of reconstruction is most appropriate should be made. Free tissue transplant for elbow flexion or prehension, tendon transfers, amputation with prosthetic fitting, an orthosis, or simple observation are the treatment options. Orthoses or amputations with prosthetic fitting may be the most functional reconstructive options if hand sensibility is poor.

Postanesthetic Brachial Plexus Palsy

The etiology of postanesthetic brachial plexus palsies is excessive traction on the plexus in an unconscious patient. Compression of the plexus by the clavicle was thought to play a role as well, but this has not been shown to be the case. The clavicle may, however, function as a fulcrum that prevents further elongation of the plexus when the arm is abducted and the neck extended and tilted toward the contralateral side. Postanesthetic palsies may also be seen in cardiac patients following median sternotomies. These palsies are a result of excessive plexus tension caused by posterior displacement of the clavicles as the sternum is spread with sternal retractors.

In general, upper trunk lesions are more common, and muscle paresis is more common than true paralysis. The natural history of postanesthetic brachial plexus palsies is usually complete, spontaneous recovery within 8 weeks. Very mild neurapraxias may last only a couple of hours, and severe palsies may continue to improve for up to 1 year. Treatment should focus on splinting coupled with range-of-motion exercises to prevent contractures until motor function improves.

Certain steps should be taken to prevent the occurrence of position-related palsies. Patients with preexisting neuropathies or a history of postanesthesia palsy should be given extra attention during the positioning process. The arms should not be abducted past 90°, or extended to any degree. Arm boards should be padded well enough to allow for slight shoulder flexion (elbows anterior to the plane of the chest). The head and neck should be in neutral alignment with the torso, and medially-placed shoulder braces should not be used with the patient in the Trendelenburg position. When the patient is in the lateral decubitus position, a roll or pad should be placed beneath the downside hemithorax to elevate it and prevent compression of the axillary contents. No roll or pad should be placed directly beneath the axilla.

Paresthesias, pain, and occasionally weakness have been described following regional block anesthesia to the brachial plexus. These symptoms may be a result of local needle damage, toxicity or irritation from a component in the anesthetic, a mass effect from the anesthetic or local hematoma, or edema. Symptomatic treatment is indicated until symptoms resolve, usually within several weeks.

Open Wounds

Open wounds to the brachial plexus are uncommon occurrences, accounting for only 5% or 6% of all brachial plexus injuries. A number of factors must be considered when evaluating a patient with an open brachial plexus injury. The first consideration is whether or not there is an associated injury. Many open wounds to the brachial plexus may also cause injuries to nearby structures including vessels and intrathoracic contents, resulting in life-threatening hemorrhaging, breathing, or circulatory problems. Routine trauma life-support procedures should be employed with any penetrating wound that involves the brachial plexus.

Another important consideration in open brachial plexus injuries is the mechanism of the injury. The mechanism of injury has important prognostic and management implications. A sharp, lacerating type of mechanism usually produces a neurotmesis. Lacerating injuries are usually caused by stab wounds with a sharp object such as a knife or an edge of broken glass. These injuries usually produce clean edges, making them amenable to primary repair. Advantages of primary repair include less surrounding scar tissue, making identification easier and iatrogenic injury less likely. Also, prompt repair makes retraction of the cut ends less of an issue, alleviating the need for a nerve graft, or at least reducing the length of a needed graft. There is no study to suggest that the end results of a primary repair are better than those of delayed primary or secondary repair. Thus, if special equipment or adequate operating room personnel are not available at the time of presentation, or if the surgeon is exhausted, surgery can be delayed.

Gunshot wounds cause varying degrees of injury to the brachial plexus, depending on the amount of energy that is transferred from the missile to the tissue. Low-energy involvement may cause neurapraxias and axonotmeses; however, high-energy transfers may result in neurotmeses and segmental nervous tissue loss. Blasts from small caliber handguns usually cause neurapraxias or axonotmeses and do not require emergent exploration unless there is an accompanying injury to a more vital structure. Close-range shotgun and large-caliber rifle injuries may cause a great amount of tissue damage as a result of secondary missiles and the effect of temporary cavitation. Initial management of high-energy wounds should consist of irrigation and debridement. Primary repair is usually not possible because of coexisting life- or limb-threatening injuries that must be dealt with first. In these cases, identifying and tagging the ends of the plexus with nonabsorbable sutures of different colors make identification easier at a later date. Ideally, the stumps are identified and the sutures are placed in a loop stitch fashion to connect the matching ends and thus prevent retraction of the stumps. As a result, primary repair is possible and shorter grafts may be used.

A third consideration in managing these injuries is the physical, mental, and social well-being of the patient. Extensive microsurgical reconstruction efforts may be thwarted by the patient with substance abuse problems who cannot control his/her environment or loses consciousness with the reconstructed plexus under tension. Patients who have attempted suicide and damaged their plexus in the process may not be good candidates until they have been stabilized with appropriate psychiatric treatment. Patients with medical problems that are believed to interfere with wound healing and nerve regeneration (smoking, radiation/chemotherapy, and steroids) may have poorer results compared to healthy individuals.

The fourth consideration is the location and extent of injury to the plexus. Less extensive or partial injuries must be weighed against the risk of surgery and the chance that an open exploration may cause additional damage. Lesions affecting the C5 and C6 roots or upper trunk leave fewer residual deficits after healing than do lesions affecting the lower cervical and T1 roots. Recovery of primary repairs performed on the lower plexus may take longer than 1 year. Nonfunctioning intrinsic muscles of the hand may suffer irreversible atrophy by the time they become reinnervated by regeneration.

Oncologic and Radiation-Induced Injuries

Brachial plexus-related pain and dysfunction are known complications of cancer and are usually caused by metastatic disease or radiation injury. It is important to distinguish between the two causes for prognostic and treatment reasons. However, the differentiation between them is not always easy to make. Factors associated with metastatic brachial plexopathy are: (1) pain as the presenting symptom; (2) presence of a Horner's syndrome; (3) predominant involvement of the lower trunk and its branches; (4) a well-defined mass on MRI scan; and (5) a rapid deterioration of symptoms over a period of days to weeks. Factors associated with radiation-induced brachial plexopathy include: (1) the absence of pain; (2) the presence of paresthesias or numbness; (3) predominant involvement of the upper trunk and its branches; (4) a diffuse or ill-defined mass, or loss of tissue planes on MRI scan; and (5) myokymic discharges and/or fasciculations on electromyographic examination.

The prognosis of metastatic brachial plexopathy is poor. Radiation therapy can provide relief in approximately 50% of the patients. Nonsurgical measures including physical therapy, modalities, antidepressants, steroids, nonsteroidal anti-inflammatory drugs, carbamazepine, and narcotics may be helpful. Paravertebral nerve blocks may be useful in patients with involvement of one or two roots. In cases of unbearable pain unresponsive to nonsurgical measures, dorsal rhizotomies or dorsal root entry zone ablation procedures may be indicated. Amputation is not helpful as a pain-relieving procedure.

The prognosis of radiation-induced brachial plexopathy is variable. Approximately 80% of the cases improve spontaneously and 20% progressively deteriorate. Early physical therapy to prevent adhesive capsulitis is indicated. Pharmacologic therapy similar to that described for metastatic brachial plexopathy may be helpful as well. Surgical procedures including neurolysis, decompression, and neurolysis in conjunction with an omentoplasty have failed to give lasting pain relief.

Sports-Related Injuries

Sports-related injuries to the brachial plexus are well-known occurrences and can be quite problematic to an otherwise healthy athlete who is eager to compete. Fortunately, sports-related brachial plexus injuries are usually not severe (with the exception of motorcycle riding) and most respond to nonoperative therapy. Selective brachial plexus-related sports injuries are presented below.

Burners/Stingers

This form of brachial plexus injury occurs frequently in football players and is believed to be caused by either: (1) traction on the upper roots and/or trunk with the ipsilateral shoulder depressed and the head tilted toward the opposite side; or (2) compression of the upper plexus between the shoulder pad and the superomedial pole of the scapula. Burners or stingers usually last a few seconds or minutes; however, prolonged burners lasting several weeks have been described. Players typically remove themselves from the game and as they leave the field, the affected upper extremity hangs passively or may be cradled by the opposite extremity. Sideline evaluation should include an examination of the cervical spine and a neurologic examination of the extremities. Complete resolution of symptoms is required before returning to play. Recurrent episodes of burners or prolonged symptoms should be a reason to investigate with radiographic studies (including flexion and extension cervical spine views). Players with a Torg ratio of less than 0.8 have three times the risk of incurring burners, and an MRI scan may help rule out cervical stenosis in these patients. Symptomatic treatment and generalized strengthening of the trapezius and cervical musculature are indicated as well.

Long Thoracic Nerve Palsy
An injury to the long thoracic nerve causes serratus anterior dysfunction, resulting in scapular winging, and has been reported in swimmers, tennis players, wrestlers, weight lifters, and ballet dancers. Athletes may complain of shoulder pain after an acute injury or repetitive activity, and may eventually complain of weakness as well. Electromyographic studies of the serratus anterior muscle may reveal positive sharp waves, fibrillation potentials, polyphasic motor units, or decreased recruitment. There is no consensus on treatment regimens for this disorder. Most authors agree with abstaining from the activity that caused the injury. Some authors have advocated the use of a modified thoracolumbar orthosis with a scapular pad to decrease tension on the nerve and to prevent excessive stretching of the serratus anterior muscle. The prognosis for substantial recovery is good, but complete recovery and return to sport may not be possible in many cases, and athletes should be counseled regarding this. Patients with chronic long thoracic palsies that do not recover and are symptomatic may get relief with a pectoralis major transfer.

Suprascapular Nerve Palsy
Palsy of the suprascapular nerve can be caused by direct trauma, or compression from a ganglion, fracture callus, the transverse suprascapular ligament, or within the spinoglenoid notch. This condition has been well-described in volleyball players and baseball pitchers and may result in paralysis of the infraspinatus and, to a lesser extent, the supraspinatus muscles. Patients may present with weakness and atrophy in the infraspinatus and supraspinatus fossae. Pain may be a component; however, in one series of 96 volleyball players, 12 were found to have a suprascapular neuropathy and all were asymptomatic. Electrodiagnostic studies can confirm the diagnosis. In symptomatic patients with pain or weakness, exploration and decompression may be beneficial.

Summary

Despite the vast and growing number of surgical procedures, management of the severely involved brachial plexus-injured patient remains challenging. Balancing the many factors that contribute to a good result is often more difficult than the technical aspects of the most complicated operation. Motion, strength, sensibility, excursion, pain, cosmesis, and social and psychological problems are all factors that must be properly addressed by the treating physician.

Selected Bibliography

General Considerations
Leffert RD (ed): *Brachial Plexus Injuries.* New York, NY, Churchill Livingstone, 1985.

This is the most comprehensive and authoritative text on brachial plexus injuries available.

Anatomy
Kerr AT: The brachial plexus of nerves in man, the variations in its formation and branches. *Am J Anat* 1918;23:285-395.

This is a classic anatomic study of the variations seen in the brachial plexus. Bilateral dissections in 63 cadavers were used. Asymmetrical findings were present in 24 cadavers.

Methods of Evaluation
Frot B: Opaque cervical myelography in traumatic paralysis of the brachial plexus. *Rev Chir Orthop Reparatrice Appar Mot* 1977;63:67-72.

This article describes a large series of patients with brachial plexus injuries who underwent cervical myelogram and had their results correlated with surgical findings. Of 90 abnormal roots on myelogram, only 70 were avulsions.

Penfield W: Late spinal paralysis after avulsion of the brachial plexus. *J Bone Joint Surg* 1949;31B:40-41.

Lower extremity spasticity is reported after a root avulsion, indicating damage to the spinal cord.

Roger B, Travers V, Laval-Jeantet M: Imaging of posttraumatic brachial plexus injury. *Clin Orthop* 1988;237:57-61.

The authors correlated surgical findings of brachial plexus injuries with preoperative studies including myelogram, CT-myelogram, and MRI. The accuracy of the myelogram was 84% and the CT-myelogram was 94%. MRI correlated well with the CT-myelogram and offered better visualization of distal lesions.

Closed Injuries
Leffert RD: Brachial-plexus injuries. *N Engl J Med* 1974;291:1059-1067.

This review article is most valuble for its anatomic considerations, classification schemes, and section on evaluation of patients with plexus injuries.

Leffert RD, Seddon H: Infraclavicular brachial plexus injuries. *J Bone Joint Surg* 1965;47B:9-22.

This article documents the generally favorable prognosis for spontaneous recovery seen with infraclavicular brachial plexus injuries.

Treatment of Closed Injuries
Bruxelle J, Travers V, Thiebaut JB: Occurrence and treatment of pain after brachial plexus injury. *Clin Orthop* 1988;237:87-95.

Twenty-four patients with severe, intractable neural pain from brachial plexus injuries underwent a dorsal root entry zone ablation

(Nashold procedure) for pain relief. Twenty patients had good pain relief at a minimum of 2 years follow-up.

Doi K, Sakai K, Kuwata N, et al: Double free-muscle transfer to restore prehension following complete brachial plexus avulsion. *J Hand Surg* 1995;20A:408-414.

This is a report of ten patients evaluated after a minimum of 12 months after the second stage of a double free vascularized muscle transfer. Several of the patients also underwent arthrodeses of their shoulders and wrists. Five of the ten patients reported use of the hand for activities of daily living.

Friedman AH, Nunley JA II, Goldner RD, et al: Nerve transposition for the restoration of elbow flexion following brachial plexus avulsion injuries. *J Neurosurg* 1990;72:59-64.

Of 16 patients who underwent intercostal to musculocutaneous nerve neurotization, seven obtained good elbow flexion. Of four who underwent free vascularized gracilis graft with neurotization, two obtained good elbow flexion.

Obstetric Injuries

Geutjens G, Gilbert A, Helsen K: Obstetric brachial plexus palsy associated with breech delivery: A different pattern of injury. *J Bone Joint Surg* 1996;78B:303-306.

Of 36 babies who had an obstetric palsy of the upper roots, 81% had avulsions.

Jackson ST, Hoffer MM, Parrish N: Brachial-plexus palsy in the newborn. *J Bone Joint Surg* 1988;70A:1217-1220.

Twenty-one obstetric brachial plexus palsies were followed without surgery; full recovery at an average of 3 months (2 weeks to 2 months) was noted in 17. The incidence of this group of injuries was 2.5 per 1,000 live births.

Oncologic and Radiation-Induced Injuries

Kori SH: Diagnosis and management of brachial plexus lesions in cancer patients. *Oncology* 1995;9:756-760,765.

This article is a review of the literature that addresses those factors associated with metastatic brachial plexopathy and radiation-induced brachial plexopathy.

White SM, Witten CM: Long thoracic nerve palsy in a professional ballet dancer. *Am J Sports Med* 1993;21:626-628.

This case report and review of the literature addresses sports-induced scapular winging and its treatment.

Sports-Related Injuries

Black KP, Lombardo JA: Suprascapular nerve injuries with isolated paralysis of the infraspinatus. *Am J Sports Med* 1990;18:225-228.

Four patients with shoulder pain and weakness are found to have isolated infraspinatus paralysis caused by suprascapular neuropathy distal to the supraspinatus innervation.

Ferretti A, Cerullo G, Russo G: Suprascapular neuropathy in volleyball players. *J Bone Joint Surg* 1987;69A:260-263.

This report describes isolated paralysis of the infraspinatus muscle in 12 of 96 elite volleyball players. All 12 players were asymptomatic.

Markey KL, Di Benedetto M, Curl WW: Upper trunk brachial plexopathy: The stinger syndrome. *Am J Sports Med* 1993;21:650-655.

This article is a four-phase study that involves interviewing, examining, and performing electrodiagnostic testing on football players with symptoms of "stingers." Compression of the lateral cord caused by the ipsilateral shoulder pad was believed to be the mechanism of injury, and an orthosis designed to pad the area above Erb's point may reduce the occurrence and severity of the injury.

Meyer SA, Schulte KR, Callaghan JJ, et al: Cervical spinal stenosis and stingers in collegiate football players. *Am J Sports Med* 1994;22:158-166.

The relationship between the occurrence of "stingers" and cervical spinal stenosis was studied. Football players with a Torg ratio of less than 0.8 had three times the risk of incurring stingers.

Ringel SP, Treihaft M, Carry M, et al: Suprascapular neuropathy in pitchers. *Am J Sports Med* 1990;18:80-86.

Slowing of nerve conduction velocity was discovered in baseball pitchers as the season progressed, providing evidence that entrapment is not always the cause of suprascapular neuropathy. A cadaveric study demonstrates five possible sites of trauma to the nerve.

28
Frozen Shoulder
Timothy D. Bunker, FRCS

Frozen shoulder is the most enigmatic of all the conditions that occur around the shoulder in that the condition can be difficult to define and to treat. Recent research has revealed that the pathology of frozen shoulder is that of fibromatosis of the capsule, and in particular, the coracohumeral ligament and rotator interval tissues. Frozen shoulder is similar to Dupuytren's disease in that it affects the shoulder and leads to contracture of the capsule, causing a global restriction of passive joint movement. This knowledge allows rational decisions to be made about treatment options.

Definition

The term "frozen shoulder" is misused, and coming to a consensus on a definition for frozen shoulder has proven elusive. The term was coined in 1934 by Codman, who stated that frozen shoulder was characterized by slow onset, pain near the insertion of the deltoid, inability to sleep on the affected side, painful and restricted elevation and external rotation, and a normal radiologic appearance. This description cannot be improved on six decades later.

The problem is that this definition is still too general, because it could be applied to a patient with a cuff tear, although the likelihood of an entirely normal radiograph is slim. A great deal of confusion exists because any shoulder that is stiff and painful is described as frozen by general practitioners, and all too often even by orthopaedic surgeons. In Wiley's study, arthroscopy was performed on 150 patients referred with a given diagnosis of frozen shoulder, and the diagnosis could be confirmed in only 37. In Bayley's study of a large series of patients with a presumed diagnosis of frozen shoulder, arthroscopy revealed that one half had some other pathology and the other half had frozen shoulder.

As a result of these studies, the stiff painful shoulder can be classified into two groups. Patients with primary frozen shoulders are those who fit Codman's criteria and in whom all other pathology is excluded. Patients with secondary frozen shoulders are those who fit Codman's criteria but in whom the condition is secondary to soft-tissue injury, fracture, arthritis, hemiplegia, or any other known cause. This chapter will focus on primary frozen shoulder.

Zuckerman attempted to obtain a consensus definition of frozen shoulder from the American Shoulder and Elbow Surgeons. Ninety-eight percent agreed that frozen shoulder exists. Ninety-two percent said that it was a condition with a global loss of both active and passive shoulder movement. Fifty-eight percent said that they would like a better or tighter definition.

Terminology

Frozen shoulder has been plagued not only by a lack of a standard definition but also by the plethora of terms ascribed to it. Many of these terms attribute a false pathology to the condition. Periarthritis was the term used by Duplay in 1872. Many physicians and rheumatologists use the term "capsulitis", implying that inflammation is present; however, this is not an accurate description. Neviaser called it "adhesive capsulitis", which not only implies that it is inflammatory, but leads to the belief that there are adhesions within the joint (although Neviaser never said there were adhesions, he did say that the capsule stuck to the head as if an adhesive had been applied). There are no adhesions in this condition. The term "checkrein shoulder" has also been used. However, frozen shoulder remains the most popular term for this condition and has the merit of implying no false pathology.

Incidence

Frozen shoulder is actually quite rare. Of 1,324 consecutive new patients attending my shoulder clinic, 70 fit the criteria of having primary frozen shoulder, an incidence of just 5%. The diagnosis was confirmed by shoulder arthroscopy unless specifically contraindicated.

Previous studies have probably overreported the incidence because other shoulder disease was not so rigorously excluded. One study suggested an incidence of 2% of the population, and another, 2.3%.

Clinical Presentation

The patient, who is in late middle age (average 56 years), presents with an insidious onset of true shoulder pain. Men are affected as often as women, the left shoulder as often as the right. The patient has difficulty sleeping on the affected side.

The patient will usually have tried all conservative modalities of treatment without success before attending the shoulder clinic. Most have had at least one steroid injection and prolonged physiotherapy.

On examination, the patient may suffer from depression because of the relentless night pain. Examination of the shoulder is unremarkable. There is usually no wasting, in particular of the infraspinatus. The deltoid may be slightly wasted as a result of disuse. There may be tenderness lateral to the coracoid process, but this is unpredictable. The acromioclavicular joint is normal.

Active and, more importantly, passive movement is markedly restricted. Most authors suggest that combined elevation is less than 100°. In my series, combined elevation was 83.2°.

Most authors agree that passive external rotation should be less than 50% of the unaffected side. A reduction of passive external rotation is the pathognomonic sign of frozen shoulder. Patients with rotator cuff disease will often have restriction of elevation, although the passive range is greater than the active range. However, most patients with cuff disorders maintain a good range of passive external rotation. In massive rotator cuff tears there can be secondary shortening of the coracohumeral ligament that acts as a checkrein to external rotation, but usually the other signs of cuff tear (sulcus, eminence, wasting of cuff, subacromial crepitus, upward subluxation of head, weakness of cuff) are quite obvious by this stage. Gross limitation of passive external rotation is present only in three other conditions—arthritis, locked posterior dislocation, and frozen shoulder. In our series, the average external rotation was 9.4°.

Internal rotation is similarly restricted both actively and passively. Usually the patient can just reach to buttock level.

The shoulder, being stiff, is clearly stable. Neurologic examination is normal.

Associated Conditions

The relationship between diabetes and frozen shoulder is well documented. Patients with diabetes have a 10% to 20% incidence of frozen shoulder; this incidence rises to 36% in patients with insulin-dependent diabetes. Forty-two percent of patients with bilateral frozen shoulder are also diabetic. Although some researchers have stated that patients with diabetes often fail to benefit from manipulation, recent studies have disputed this theory.

Meulengracht and Schwarz found evidence of Dupuytren's contracture in 18% of their patients with frozen shoulder. In my study, I personally examined the hands of all 50 patients. Twenty-nine of 50 patients had a pit, nodule, or band of Dupuytren's contracture; Peyronie's disease is also common in this group. Dupuytren's contracture is also associated with diabetes.

Frozen shoulder has been associated with cardiac disease. Many patients with cardiac disease have elevated serum lipids. In one study, fasting serum lipid levels were tested and a significant elevation of cholesterol and triglyceride was found in patients with frozen shoulder. Elevated serum lipid levels are also found in patients with Dupuytren's contracture, and in patients with diabetes.

Frozen shoulder was believed to be related to abnormal emotional responses in patients. On the other hand, Quigley stated that the abnormal emotional responses of patients with frozen shoulder could be "as often the result of the painful shoulder as the cause." No psychologic evidence of personality disorders has been found in patients with frozen shoulder.

There may be an association between minor degrees of trauma and the onset of frozen shoulder. Frozen shoulder may, for instance, present following a Colles' fracture. Dupuytren's disease may also be initiated by minor trauma to the hand or, for instance, a Colles' fracture.

Frozen shoulder has been recorded in patients recovering from neurosurgery. It is highly likely that these patients were on antiepileptic treatment, the most common combination at the time being phenytoin and phenobarbitone. Phenytoin is associated with Dupuytren's disease and phenobarbitone with frozen shoulder, and phenobarbitone is also associated with elevated serum lipid levels.

Diagnostic Tests

Complete blood count, erythrocyte sedimentation rate, and HLA-B27 are all normal in frozen shoulder. Plain radiographs, by definition, must be normal, although some disuse osteopenia is allowed.

Neviaser in 1962, using arthrography, showed that there was a characteristic reduction in joint volume in frozen shoulder, with a lack of filling of the axillary fold and the subscapular recess (the rotator interval) (Fig. 1).

Emig and associates examined nine patients with frozen shoulder using magnetic resonance imaging (MRI) and found that the capsule was thickened, averaging 5.2 mm thick in the frozen shoulder group against 2.9 mm thick in the control group ($p < 0.01$). They could find no significant difference between coracohumeral thickness or the rotator interval on coronal oblique scans, but this is a difficult plane for examining such structures.

In another study, coronal oblique scans of the rotator interval were obtained in 14 patients with frozen shoulder. Although clear thickening of the coracohumeral ligament was present on some of the scans, this finding was not significant.

The arthroscopic findings in frozen shoulder are consistent. Joint volume is reduced, the subscapularis recess is obliterated, and the rotator interval is often obliterated with scar

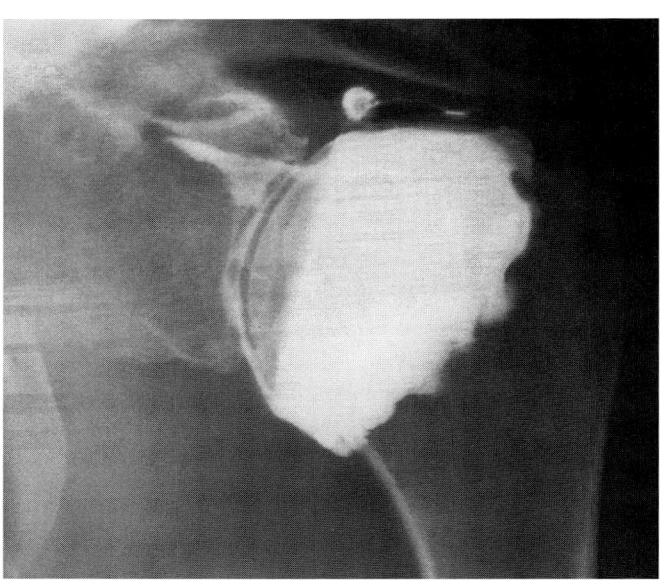

Fig. 1 Arthrogram of frozen shoulder, showing contracted, small-volume joint.

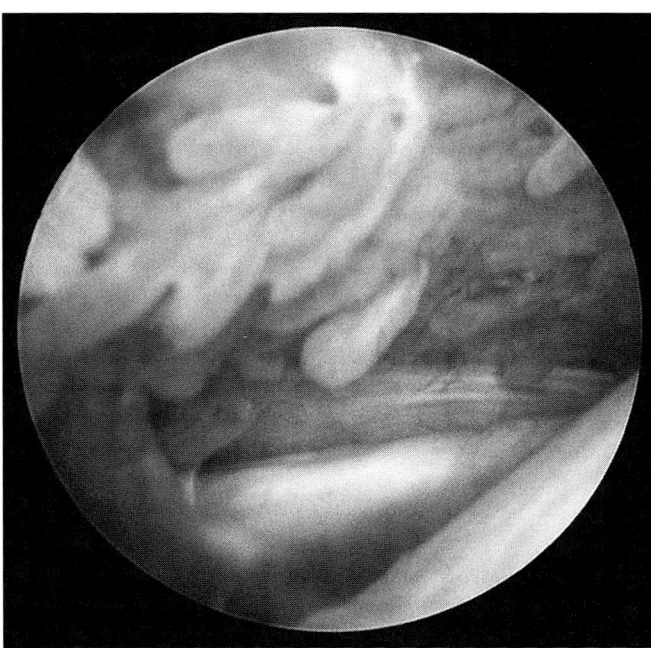

Fig. 2 Arthroscopic appearance of rotator interval in frozen shoulder showing villous synovitis.

tissue covered in a highly vasculitic synovium with papillary infolding. The axillary recess is tight and of reduced volume. There are no adhesions (Fig. 2).

In Wiley's 1991 study, a uniform arthroscopic appearance (a patchy vascular reaction around the biceps and the opening into the subscapularis recess, ie, the rotator interval) was found in 37 patients. Joint capacity was reduced. In no patient was the infraglenoid recess obliterated, and there were no adhesions.

Ogilvie-Harris and Wiley reported a reduced joint capacity and a mild synovitis. There appeared to be an extrasynovial contracture of the soft tissues in the anterior part of the joint.

Uitvligt's study showed a thickened capsule and small joint capacity in 20 patients. Nineteen patients had a synovitis of the rotator interval that was present to a marked degree in the subscapular recess in 12. Five patients had a synovitis of the posterior capsule, and four in the axillary recess. After manipulation, the infraglenoid recess was seen to be torn.

Esch stated that arthroscopy showed a thickened, scarred rotator interval, synovitis with adhesions around subscapularis, and chronic subacromial synovitis.

My colleagues and I have performed shoulder arthroscopies in 26 consecutive patients. The consistent findings were scarring in the rotator interval area with obliteration of the subscapularis recess. In two patients the scarring was so thick in this area that the long head of the biceps tendon was buried within the scar.

Findings of Surgical Exploration

The early macroscopic descriptions of frozen shoulder are still accurate. The thickening and contraction of capsule that peeled from the humeral head, similar to adhesive plaster from the skin, was termed "adhesive capsulitis". This term is often misused in describing adhesions within the joint. No adhesions have been reported in numerous recent arthroscopic studies.

In 1949, Simonds described the rotator cuff in frozen shoulder as looking like a vascular leathery hood with no obvious demarcation between the tendons. The demarcation between the tendons is now called the rotator interval, and it is this rotator interval that is obliterated on arthrograms and at arthroscopy.

The coracohumeral ligament has been described as a tough, inelastic band of fibrous tissue between the coracoid process and the tuberosities of the humerus, where it acts as a powerful checkrein. Division of this ligament allows early restoration of scapulohumeral movement.

The major cause of restricted glenohumeral movement was found to be a contracture of the coracohumeral ligament and rotator interval. The coracohumeral ligament was contracted and converted into a thick, fibrous cord. Release of this contracted ligament relieved pain and restored motion.

Over the past 5 years, my colleagues and I have studied 20 patients with frozen shoulder. The findings are consistent. The coracoacromial ligament is always normal. When the coracoacromial ligament is excised, an abnormal thickening can be seen in the rotator interval area. It is my belief that the rotator interval area is distorted by the scarring and contracture of the coracohumeral ligament, which obliterates the normal sulcus of the rotator interval. It is difficult to determine the exact location of the superior edge of the subscapularis tendon, which is highly abnormal. It is also difficult to define where the anterior edge of the supraspinatus tendon is. If the arm is now externally rotated, this scarred area tightens and then can be seen to be acting as a checkrein to external rotation. Division of this scarred area allows immediate and complete external rotation in the majority of patients. The scarred area is highly vascular and, when divided, it bleeds forcefully. In two or three patients, the contracture extended into the anterior and superior capsule and external rotation was regained with a manipulation at this point.

With the rotator interval now opened, the entire rotator interval area is excised to reveal a normal long head of biceps tendon, a normal humeral head, a normal glenoid, and no adhesions.

Pathology

The cause of frozen shoulder has been uncertain since it was first described. Possible causes included an autoimmune connective tissue disorder, recurrent hemarthrosis, reactive arthropathy, infection, trauma, algodystrophy, suprascapular nerve entrapment, and rotator cuff degeneration. All of these factors have been examined and disproven. The following paragraphs will discuss the macroscopic and histologic evidence collected by those surgeons who have performed open surgical release of frozen shoulders.

The few studies of tissue from patients with frozen shoulder have suggested either an inflammatory process or a fibromatosis. Neviaser's 1945 study of ten cases is often cited.

Thickening and contracture of the capsule with considerable or extensive fibrosis were found in six cases, but the increased cellularity was interpreted as a result of inflammatory changes. In another study, dense collagen fibers, increased vascularity, and the presence of "histiocytes" (which we now term fibroblasts) were found in four shoulders; however, it was concluded that frozen shoulder was an inflammatory condition.

In yet another study, 32 patients with frozen shoulder were examined. Histologic findings were described in some, but not all, patients. Degeneration of collagen fibers, round cell infiltration, increased vascularity, thickening of the synovial membrane, and evidence of increased fibrosis were noted. It was concluded that the cause of these findings was a low grade inflammation. It should be noted that these studies were performed between 1945 and 1952, when small round cell infiltration was nearly always inflammatory. Although it was recognized that some of these cells were fibroblasts, such techniques as immunocytochemistry that are now available to differentiate small round cells into fibroblasts and inflammatory cells were not available at the time these studies were carried out.

In a 1969 study, it was noted that the capsule was dense or compact with an increased cell population, most of which were fibroblasts; it was suggested that histologically this tissue was identical to Dupuytren's tissue. In 1981, the histology of the capsule in a diabetic patient with frozen shoulder was described as similar to Dupuytren's contracture. In 1989, in 17 patients with frozen shoulder, the capsule showed fibrosis, but cell type was not examined. In a 1994 study, arthroscopic biopsy specimens obtained from 15 patients showed diffuse capsular fibroplasia, thickening, and contracture.

My colleagues and I resected the thickened rotator interval tissues in 12 consecutive patients. The tissue showed nodules and laminae of collagen with a high cell population of fibroblasts and myofibroblasts as identified by immunocytochemistry (Fig. 3). Leukocytes and macrophages were scanty and were never seen in the nodules or laminae, only on the periphery and around small blood vessels. These findings were identical both histologically and by immunocytochemistry with six control cases of palmar Dupuytren's tissue.

It appears, therefore, that frozen shoulder is a disease characterized by fibrosis of the shoulder joint capsule, histologically similar to Dupuytren's contracture, leading to a contracture of the coracohumeral ligament that acts as a checkrein to passive glenohumeral movement and external rotation in particular.

If frozen shoulder is similar in pathology to Dupuytren's contracture, then it would fall into the group of diseases termed the fibromatoses. The fibromatoses are tumorous proliferations intermediate in their biologic behavior between benign fibrous lesions such as nodular fasciitis and malignant lesions such as malignant fibrous histiocytoma. The superficial fibromatoses are Dupuytren's contracture of the palm, Garrod's knuckle pads, plantar fibromatosis of Ledderhose, and Peyronie's penile fibromatosis. Clonal chromosomal abnormalities have been found in many of these conditions, clonality being defined as the observation of two or more cells with the same structural aberrations or supernumerary chromosomes.

In Dupuytren's contracture, clones of cells trisomic for chromosome 8 have been noted, and trisomy 8 has also been

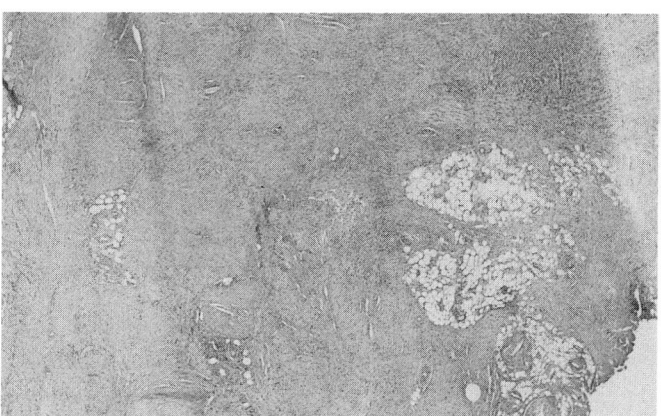

Fig. 3 Histology of coracohumeral ligament in frozen shoulder showing transformation to dense collagen.

found in Peyronie's disease. In tissue cultured from the capsule of the shoulder in seven patients with frozen shoulder and examined for chromosomal abnormalities, trisomy 7 and trisomy 8 were found. This gives further weight to the hypothesis that frozen shoulder is a fibrosing disease.

Functional Anatomy of the Rotator Interval

The rotator interval is the gap in the capsule between the subscapularis and supraspinatus. This area is roofed by the coracohumeral ligament, which spans the area from the coracoid to the intertubercular groove of the humerus similar to the ridge of a tent. The inside of the tent leads into the subscapular recess, which passes under the coracoid ensheathing the superior edge of the subscapularis. The long head of the biceps passes obliquely across this area, as if it were within the tent, before entering into the pulley system of the intertubercular sulcus.

Recent studies showed that the coracohumeral ligament was a consistent and well-developed structure that originated from the coracoid and inserted variably into the rotator interval, supraspinatus, or subscapularis. Conversely, Cooper and associates in 1993 stated that the coracohumeral ligament is not a real ligament but merely a folded part of the capsule of the joint that becomes prominent when the shoulder is externally rotated.

In yet another study, it was suggested that in order to understand the coracohumeral ligament, its counterpart in the hip should be studied. The analogous structure is the iliofemoral ligament. Although it is not a true ligament, but rather a thickening of the joint capsule of the hip, this structure is still regarded by some as the strongest ligament in the body. The iliofemoral ligament arises from the inferior iliac spine, which is the analog of the coracoid process, and runs down to insert between the greater and lesser trochanters. The reflected head of the biceps femoris is the analog of the long head of the biceps. It runs over the iliofemoral ligament, in contrast to the course of the long head of biceps in the shoulder, which runs under the coracohumeral ligament. However, in evolutionary terms, the long head of the biceps was also extra-articular; indeed, if a shoulder of lamb is dissected, it will be extra-articular. The long head of the biceps seems to have dropped down through the coracohumeral ligament as the coracoid enlarged.

Because the coracohumeral ligament is hidden from view by the coracoacromial ligament, it has been neglected, but attention has recently been drawn to it both in instability and contracture of the shoulder joint.

In 1992, a cadaver test was performed on the shoulder, with the rotator interval being divided first, and then imbricated. Imbricating the interval limited shoulder joint movement globally, but mostly restricted external rotation. Conversely, dividing the rotator interval allowed an increase in global shoulder movement and particularly external rotation.

Natural History of Frozen Shoulder

The classic understanding that frozen shoulder is a disease with three phases of pain, stiffening, and thawing leading to resolution in 2 years may be optimistic.

Frozen shoulder is defined as a disease of insidious onset leading to true shoulder pain, felt in the deltoid and radiating down toward the elbow. The pain is very severe at night. It is difficult to reconcile this pain with recent knowledge about the pathology of the condition. After all, it is very rare for Dupuytren's contracture to be painful in origin. In its formative phase Dupuytren's contracture can be painful, but patients rarely present at this stage but at the final stage of contracture. The pain of frozen shoulder, however, is severe and it is unlikely that this pain is caused by the forming contracture itself.

The same is true of plantar fibromatosis; it is rarely painful except when the nodule is large enough to feel like a pebble. However, if the pain of frozen shoulder was caused by the nodule pressing on the coracoacromial ligament, this pain should remain consistent, and not ease after approximately 6 months. Arthroscopically, a vascular synovitis is noted and it is possible that the synovitis is responsible for the pain.

In frozen shoulder, perhaps the pain can be explained not by the fibrosing pathology but by the environment in which this pathology occurs. Harryman and associates have shown how imbrication or contracture of the rotator interval causes obligatory anterosuperior translation of the humeral head and leads to impingement. This causes pain of an impingement type, pain on movement, and night pain. The pain of frozen shoulder is very similar to this description.

Once again, if the histology is fibrosis, similar to Dupuytren's contracture, why should the stiffness subside? The answer is that the shoulder, being capable of global movement, probably can compensate for a contracture in one area of the capsule by stretching out in another area. The movement is abnormal and the center of rotation is shifted, but the range increases sufficiently for the shoulder to be able to compensate. In this manner the obligatory anterosuperior translation caused by the contracture is circumnavigated, the impingement eases, and the pain diminishes.

As to whether all patients improve by 2 years, Shaffer (1992) showed that they did not. In the most detailed long-term study of the natural history of frozen shoulder, 50% of the patients studied had either mild pain or stiffness or both at an average of 7 years after the onset of the disease. None of the patients reported the pain as more than mild and the stiffness was mainly in external rotation. Functional restriction was small.

There may be several reasons why the literature is optimistic in terms of the natural history of this condition. Many of the original studies came to no consensus on diagnostic criteria, had poor methodology with no controls, and poor follow-up. However, the best reason as to why the condition has been reported optimistically is that ultimately the residual functional disability is neither frequent nor substantial, and most people adapt to their functional restrictions.

According to Neer, elevation of 150°, external rotation to 50°, and internal rotation to T8 is sufficient for normal function. Older patients with fewer functional demands can tolerate even more restriction in one plane. Finally, because restriction is mainly in external rotation and most functional demands of the shoulder depend on elevation, it may be easier for the patient to compensate for this loss.

Treatment

Conservative

Treatment options consist of physiotherapy, manipulation, steroid injection, manipulation under anesthetic, and surgical release.

Physiotherapy and home stretching include passive stretching and range-of-motion exercises. Warming of the tissues should be followed by pendulum exercises, moving on to pulley exercises, wallbars, pushing external rotation with a stick, and forcing internal rotation by toweling the back.

During the early phase of the disease, these exercises may be painful, and theoretically could cause microtearing of the forming contracture and stimulate further fibrosis. However, these exercises are very helpful in the later stages of the disease, acting in one of two ways. If the fibrosing checkrein is small and thin, it may be stretched out at this stage. If the fibrosing checkrein is too thick to stretch, then the other areas of the capsule that are not affected to such a degree, such as the infraglenoid recess, can be stretched. This action leads to gains in elevation and therefore a vast improvement in function, although external rotation may remain restricted, much as in Shaffer's long-term study of the natural history of the disease.

Such physiotherapy stretching exercises are essential after manipulation under anesthesia or surgical excision to keep up the benefit attained during the manipulation.

Steroid Injection

Steroid injections have been given empirically in frozen shoulder. Some studies show a beneficial effect from the use of intra-articular steroids.

Steroid was injected subcutaneously around the nodules of patients with Dupuytren's contracture prior to excision. Those injected 24 hours prior to excision showed no changes within the tissue although the lumens of the vessels on the periphery of the nodules, which were normally occluded, were opening.

When the tissue that had been injected 4 to 6 days preoperatively was examined, there were striking changes histologically. There were numerous ghost cells among the fibroblasts. The absence of an inflammatory reaction in association with this cell death suggests that a process of planned cell death, or apoptosis, was occurring rather than necrosis. The normally present proinflammatory cytokines were all absent. These changes only affected nodules that were active and did not cause changes in the collagen of mature cords. Because the histology of frozen shoulder and Dupuytren's contracture is similar, these findings certainly make a case for considering steroid injection in the treatment of frozen shoulder.

Manipulation Under Anesthesia

Studies by Codman and others precipitated concern that manipulation could cause tearing of the rotator cuff, dislocation, or humeral fractures. As a result, manipulation under anesthesia went out of vogue through the middle part of this century. Rest seemed to be more desirable to the patient than any form of treatment.

Professor Sir John Charnley was intrigued by frozen shoulder as well as by joint replacement. In 1959, he published a paper on his personal results of manipulation in this condition. Prior to this investigation, he set out to find out what was the prevailing orthodox attitude to manipulation. He sent a questionnaire to Fellows of the British Orthopaedic Association. Of the respondents, 70% stated that they would never manipulate a frozen shoulder, because all shoulders would eventually get better and some could be harmed by manipulation. Charnley manipulated the frozen shoulders of 35 patients and showed that in none did it do any harm, that early manipulation did not prolong treatment, that pain relief was the most important result of manipulation, and that the duration of symptoms after manipulation was fairly constant, averaging 10 weeks, no matter how long the symptoms had been present before the manipulation. Charnley insisted on one matter of technique: that external rotation should be released before abduction was attempted or dislocation could occur.

Manipulation has attained the status of the most predictable form of treatment for frozen shoulder in the last half of this century. In a very carefully controlled study, it was shown that 75% of patients obtained a near-normal range of motion, and 79% were relieved of their pain. Seventy-five percent returned to work within 9 weeks of manipulation.

There is one group, however, who have a poor response to manipulation, and that is the patients with diabetes. Janda and Hawkins showed that any improvement in movement and diminution in pain disappeared by 4 weeks after manipulation and suggested that manipulation should not be attempted in these patients.

Surgical Release

Surgical release for frozen shoulder has been undertaken in very limited numbers and with limited evaluation in the past. In 1989, Ozaki and associates described their method of open surgical release for frozen shoulder in 17 patients and recommended this method for patients in whom nonsurgical treatment has failed. However, open surgical release remains a poorly recognized and little performed procedure.

My colleagues and I have performed an open surgical release in 20 patients who failed to respond to conservative methods and manipulation. The release is performed through a deltoid muscle-splitting incision centered over the medial third of the coracoacromial ligament. The fibers of the deltoid lie in a plane perpendicular to Langers lines at this point; therefore, a gridiron incision has to be made, the skin being incised along Langers line, and undermined so that the gridiron split can be made in the deltoid.

The whole of the coracoacromial ligament is then cleaned with a pledget before being completely excised. The scarred nodular area of the coracohumeral ligament now comes into view, and is better appreciated with the arm in external rotation when the ligament can be seen and felt as a checkrein from the coracoid to the intertubercular sulcus. Because the rotator interval is obliterated by scar, it is difficult to judge where rotator interval ends and subscapularis or supraspinatus start. The checkrein is divided; care should be taken not to incise the long head of the biceps, which runs just underneath.

The edges of the rotator interval can be seen and felt more easily from inside the joint, and all the tissues that make up the rotator interval are now excised so that there is a gaping hole between the top edge of the subscapularis and the leading edge of the supraspinatus. Finally, an arthroscopic duckbill punch is taken and the scarred area is excised down to and below the coracoid process.

At the time that the checkrein is incised and divided, the shoulder contracture is felt to release and external rotation is regained. Occasionally a final manipulation is required to regain a full 80° of external rotation. The shoulder is then flexed to split the infraglenoid recess. Bupivacaine with adrenaline 1:200,000 is instilled. No attempt is made to close the rotator interval, the split in deltoid is allowed to close, and the skin is closed with a subcuticular suture.

Postoperatively, a roller towel support is used overnight. No sling is allowed and physiotherapy is instituted to maintain the gained range of motion.

Arthroscopic Surgical Release

If an open surgical release can be performed, then it is only a matter of time before an arthroscopic technique will supercede it. There have been several series of arthroscopic release for resistant frozen shoulder, but most of them have been seriously flawed.

In a recent study, arthroscopic debridement of the joint following manipulation was performed in 40 patients. In ten other patients, arthroscopic release of the rotator interval, subacromial bursectomy, and in some an arthroscopic acromioplasty, excision of the coracoacromial ligament, the coracoacromial ligament, and the coracohumeral ligament were performed.

In another study, arthroscopic release of the infraglenoid recess followed by a gentle manipulation was performed in 26 shoulders (Fig. 4).

In yet another study, the coracohumeral ligament was sectioned with electrocautery in 14 patients, and was followed by subacromial bursectomy and manipulation. Results were satisfactory in all 14 patients. This group of patients had failed to improve with manipulation.

Arthroscopic excision of the rotator interval and coracohumeral ligament shows promise both in theory and in practice in selected patients with primary frozen shoulder who have failed to respond to conservative measures or manipulation under anesthetic.

Summary

Primary frozen shoulder is a disease characterized by insidious onset of true shoulder pain with a global restriction of both active and passive shoulder movement, especially external rotation. Primary frozen shoulder is caused by a Dupuytren's-like contracture of the coracohumeral ligament, which acts as a checkrein to passive shoulder movement and external rotation in particular. The condition is best treated by manipulation under anesthesia, and in those cases that fail to improve by manipulation, surgical release, either by open or arthroscopic methods, should be performed.

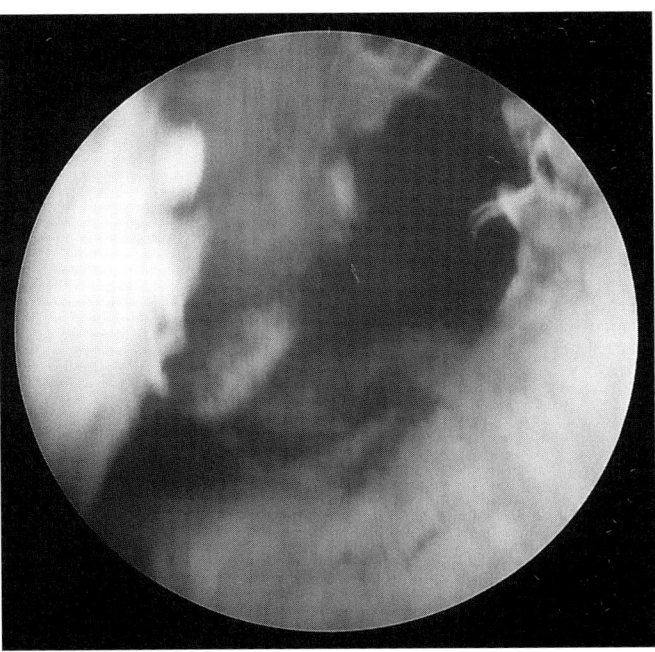

Fig. 4 Arthroscopic appearance of infraglenoid recess following manipulation showing tear between capsule and neck of humerus.

Selected Bibliography

Definition

Codman EA (ed): Tendinitis of the short rotators, in *The Shoulder: Rupture of the Supraspinatus Tendon and Other Lesions in or About the Subacromial Bursa.* Boston, MA, Thomas Todd and Co, 1934.

Wiley AM: Arthroscopic appearance of frozen shoulder. *Arthroscopy* 1991;7:138-143.

Zuckerman JD, Cuomo F, Rokito S: Definition and classification of frozen shoulder: A consensus approach. *J Shoulder Elbow Surg* 1994;3:S72.

This article, under the auspices of the American Shoulder and Elbow Surgeons, takes a consensus approach at defining frozen shoulder.

Terminology

Bunker TD: Time for a new name for frozen shoulder. *Br Med J* 1985;290:1233-1234.

Duplay ES: De la periarthrote scapulohumerale. *Arch Gen Med* 1872;20:513-542.

Neviaser JS: Adhesive capsulitis of the shoulder. *J Bone Joint Surg* 1945;27:211-222.

Quigley TB: Checkrein shoulder, a type of frozen shoulder. *Surg Clin North Am* 1969;43:1715-1720.

Incidence

Bridgman JF: Periarthritis of the shoulder and diabetes mellitus. *Ann Rheum Dis* 1972;31:69-71.

Lundberg BJ: The frozen shoulder: Clinical and radiographical observations. The effect of manipulation under general anesthesia: Structure and glycosaminoglycan content of the joint capsule. Local bone metabolism. *Acta Orthop Scand* 1969;119(suppl):1-59.

Associated Conditions

Bunker TD, Anthony PP: The pathology of frozen shoulder: A Dupuytren-like disease. *J Bone Joint Surg* 1995;77B: 677-683.

This article presents the histology and immunocytochemistry of the shoulder joint capsule in patients who have undergone open release for frozen shoulder.

Bunker TD, Esler CN: Frozen shoulder and lipids. *J Bone Joint Surg* 1995;77B:684-686.

Patients with frozen shoulder have elevated levels of serum lipids, a condition that is also found in patients with Dupuytren's disease in the hand.

Bunker TD, Lagas K, DeFerme A: Arthroscopy and manipulation in frozen shoulder. *J Bone Joint Surg* 1994;76B(suppl 1):53.

In patients with frozen shoulder, the rotator cuff interval area appears normal on arthroscopic evaluation.

Emig EW, Schweitzer ME, Karasick D, et al: Adhesive capsulitis of the shoulder: MR diagnosis. *Am J Roentgenol* 1995;164:1457-1459.

These authors showed that thickening of the shoulder capsule in patients with frozen shoulder can be seen on coronal MRI scans.

Esch JC: Arthroscopic treatment of resistant primary (idiopathic) frozen shoulder. *J Shoulder Elbow Surg* 1994;3:S71.

The response to arthroscopic debridement was investigated in patients with frozen shoulder. This treatment method proved to be a useful adjunct to manipulation.

Fisher L, Kurtz A, Shipley M: Association between cheiroarthropathy and frozen shoulder in patients with insulin-dependent diabetes mellitus. *Br J Rheumatol* 1986;25:141-146.

Havel RJ: Disorders of lipid metabolism, in Beeson PB, McDermott W, Wyngaarden JB (eds): *Textbook of Medicine*, ed 15. Philadelphia, PA, WB Saunders, 1979, vol 2, pp 2002-2011.

Janda DH, Hawkins RJ: Shoulder manipulation in patients with adhesive capsulitis and diabetes mellitus: A clinical note. *J Shoulder Elbow Surg* 1993;2:36-38.

Manipulation was not successful in patients with diabetes mellitus and adhesive capsulitis.

Lequesne M, Dang N, Bensasson M, et al: Increased association of diabetes mellitus with capsulitis of the shoulder and shoulder-hand syndrome. *Scand J Rheumatol* 1977;6:53-56.

Meulengracht E, Schwartz M: Course and prognosis of periarthrosis humeroscapularis with special regard to cases with general symptoms. *Acta Med Scand* 1952;143:350-360.

McLaughlin HL: On the frozen shoulder. *Bull Hosp Jt Dis* 1951;12:126-131.

Ogilvie-Harris DJ, Wiley AM: Arthroscopic surgery of the shoulder: A general appraisal. *J Bone Joint Surg* 1986;68:201-207.

Pal B, Anderson J, Dick WC, et al: Limitation of joint mobility and shoulder capsulitis in insulin- and non-insulin-dependent diabetes mellitus. *Br J Rheumatol* 1986;25: 147-151.

Sanderson PL, Morris MA, Stanley JK, et al: Lipids and Dupuytren's disease. *J Bone Joint Surg* 1992;74B:923-927.

This article points out that in patients with Dupuytren's disease, serum lipid levels are elevated.

Uitvligt G, Detrisac DA, Johnson LL, et al: Arthroscopic observations before and after manipulation of frozen shoulder. *Arthroscopy* 1993;9:181-185.

In this article, the authors note that there is an abnormality of the rotator interval tissues in patients with frozen shoulder, and that following manipulation, a tear or rent can be seen in the inferior, and sometimes, the anterior, capsule.

Wright V, Haq AM: Periarthritis of the shoulder: I. Aetiological considerations with particular reference to personality factors. *Ann Rheum Dis* 1976;35:213-219.

Wright V, Haq AM: Periarthritis of the shoulder: II. Radiological features. *Ann Rheum Dis* 1976;35:220-226.

Findings of Surgical Exploration

DePalma AF: Loss of scapulohumeral motion (frozen shoulder). *Ann Surg* 1952;135:193-204.

Neer CS II, Satterlee CC, Dalsey RM, et al: The anatomy and potential effects of contracture of the coracohumeral ligament. *Clin Orthop* 1992;280:182-185.

The coracohumeral ligament can be thickened and contracted in a number of conditions around the shoulder, including frozen shoulder.

Simonds FA: Shoulder pain: With particular reference to the "frozen" shoulder. *J Bone Joint Surg* 1949;31B:426-432.

Pathology

Bonnici AV, Birjandi F, Spencer JD, et al: Chromosomal abnormalities in Dupuytren's contracture and carpal tunnel syndrome. *J Hand Surg* 1992;17B:349-355.

These authors have demonstrated clonal chromosomal abnormalities in patients with Dupuytren's contracture.

Hannafin JA, DiCarlo EF, Wickiewicz TL: Adhesive capsulitis: Capsular fibroplasia of the glenohumeral joint. *J Shoulder Elbow Surg* 1994;3:S5.

Arthroscopic biopsies of the capsule were obtained in patients with frozen shoulder, and diffuse capsular fibroplasia was seen in these patients.

Kay NRM, Slater DN: Fibromatoses and diabetes mellitus. *Lancet* 1981;2:303.

Neviaser JS: *Arthrography of the Shoulder: The Diagnosis and Management of the Lesions Visualized.* Springfield, IL, Charles C Thomas, 1975, pp 60-66.

Sergovich FR, Botz JS, MacFarlane RM: Nonrandom cytogenic abnormalities in Dupuytren's disease. *N Engl J Med* 1983;308:162-163.

Wurster Hill DH, Brown F, Park JP, et al: Cytogenetic studies in Dupuytren's contracture. *Am J Hum Genet* 1988;43:285-292.

Functional Anatomy of the Rotator Interval

Cooper DE, O'Brien SJ, Arnoczky SP, et al: The structure and function of the coracohumeral ligament: An anatomic and microscopic study. *J Shoulder Elbow Surg* 1993;2: 70-77.

A number of shoulders were dissected to examine the rotator interval. It was shown that the rotator interval was not a true ligament but a thickening of the capsule in the rotator interval area.

Edelson JG, Taitz G, Grishkan A: The coracohumeral ligament: Anatomy of a substantial but neglected structure. *J Bone Joint Surg* 1991;73B:150-153.

Harryman DT II, Sidles JA, Harris SL, et al: The role of the rotator interval capsule in passive motion and stability of the shoulder. *J Bone Joint Surg* 1992;74A:53-65.

Locating the rotator interval reduced the range of shoulder movement, and external rotation in particular.

Treatment

Charnley JC: Periarthritis of the shoulder. *Postgrad Med J* 1959;384-388.

Fazzi UG: Dupuytren's disease: The use of corticosteroids. *J R Coll Surg Edinb* 1995;40:76.

   Steroids were injected into nodules of Dupuytren's disease and the effects examined when the nodules were excised. There was apoptosis or cell death of fibroblasts within the nodules.

Midorikawa K, Hara, Shibata, et al: Manipulation of frozen shoulder: Application of arthroscopic surgery. *J Shoulder Elbow Surg* 1994;3:S42.

   The coracohumeral ligament was sectioned arthroscopically, with release of the frozen shoulder.

Ozaki J, Nakagawa Y, Sakuri G, et al: Recalcitrant chronic adhesive capsulitis of the shoulder: Role of contracture of the coracohumeral ligament and rotator interval in pathogenesis and treatment. *J Bone Joint Surg* 1989;71A:1511-1515.

Segmuller HE, Taylor DE, Hogan CS, et al: Arthroscopic treatment of adhesive capsulitis. *J Shoulder Elbow Surg* 1995;4:403-408.

   The infraglenoid recess was sectioned arthroscopically in a patient with frozen shoulder, resulting in release of the frozen shoulder.

29

Suprascapular Nerve Entrapment

Martti Vastamäki, MD, PhD

The diagnosis and treatment of neurologic entrapment syndromes about the shoulder can be challenging. Suprascapular nerve entrapment is the most common of these entrapment syndromes, occurring in 1% to 2% of patients with shoulder pain or muscle weakness. Kopell and Thompson described suprascapular nerve entrapment at the suprascapular notch in 1959. In 1982, Aiello and associates described suprascapular nerve entrapment at the spinoglenoid notch.

Anatomy

The suprascapular nerve is derived from the upper trunk of the brachial plexus formed by the C5 and C6 nerve roots. It enters the supraspinatus fossa through the suprascapular notch, passing below the superior transverse scapular ligament. It is important to remember that the suprascapular artery and veins pass above this ligament. The notch may be low and narrow and the nerve can be adherent to the notch. After passing the notch, the suprascapular nerve supplies one or two branches to the supraspinatus muscle and provides articular twigs to the glenohumeral and coracoacromial joints and also to the coracoclavicular ligament. It then passes into the infraspinatus fossa around the lateral margin of the scapular spine or the spinoglenoid notch. In most cases, an osteofibrous orifice is enclosed by the spinoglenoid ligament, an aponeurotic band that separates the supraspinatus and infraspinatus muscles. Normally there is no sensory function arising from the suprascapular nerve to the skin. However, this nerve may at times provide sensory branches to innervate the skin of the posterior shoulder, medial to the deltoid.

Etiology

Patients with suprascapular nerve entrapment normally have a history of trauma or some kind of exertion. Trauma can be direct, such as a blow to the shoulder region or a fall onto the shoulder, or indirect, such as a fall onto an outstretched hand, causing twisting and stretching of the shoulder. When there has been no definitive injury, activities that require repeated wide excursions of the scapula, such as baseball, volleyball, tennis, weightlifting, hammering, throwing, or bearing heavy articles, can be factors related to injury.

In some cases, the suprascapular nerve lesion is not caused by entrapment or stretching. Tumors and stab wound lesions of this nerve are very rare. More common is the so-called mononeuritis of the suprascapular nerve, an involvement of a single nerve such as that seen in some patients with anterior interosseous syndrome, or in patients with an isolated serratus palsy with winging of the scapula. One rare cause of suprascapular nerve entrapment at the suprascapular notch is fracture of the superior lateral angle of the scapula.

Evaluation

A poorly localized, dull ache over the posterior and lateral area of the shoulder is a typical symptom of suprascapular nerve entrapment at the suprascapular notch. The pain may radiate medially and upward into the neck and laterally down the arm, but it is usually not more distally. Weakness of the shoulder, particularly in the movements of abduction and external rotation, is a common complaint. In advanced cases, wasting of the spinati muscles can be observed. In most cases, however, atrophy is not present. This adds to the difficulty in diagnosing this condition.

A sharp pain in the shoulder may be felt in connection with the trauma or exertion. Thereafter, the pain may be brought on by movement and exertion of the shoulder girdle. Over time, the pain becomes constant and is severe enough to disturb sleep. Without any atrophy of the spinati muscles, the patient may be unable to lift the arm above the horizontal level, and may be unable to lie on the affected side. In many cases, the onset of symptoms is insidious with a vague shoulder pain that has persisted for years as the only symptom.

In clinical examination of suprascapular nerve entrapment at the suprascapular notch, tenderness over the notch, in the triangle between the clavicle and the scapular spine, is almost invariably present (Fig. 1). Tenderness of the trapezoid area is a very common finding in a painful shoulder, but in suprascapular nerve entrapment the maximal tenderness is localized over the suprascapular notch. The power of active abduction and external rotation is usually reduced. The spinati muscles, particularly the infraspinatus, may be atrophied (Fig. 2). The acromioclavicular joint may be tender, mediated by the articular twigs of the suprascapular nerve.

The pain accompanying suprascapular nerve entrapment at the spinoglenoid notch is usually milder than that accompanying entrapment at the suprascapular notch. The pain is located at the infraspinatus area. Tenderness over the spinoglenoid notch may be marked. Except for atrophy of the infraspinatus muscle, which can be remarkable, local findings are not as prominent.

The diagnosis of suprascapular nerve entrapment is based on a careful, thorough history, physical examination, and electroneuromyography. Electromyographic findings such as delayed conduction velocity and fibrillation potentials are definitive. Unfortunately, an electromyogram can be entirely normal in some cases. A correct diagnosis can be missed in these patients if their only complaint is poorly localized shoulder pain.

In the absence of decisive findings, other conditions causing symptoms similar to those accompanying suprascapular nerve entrapment should be excluded, such as a rotator cuff tear, impingement syndrome, acromioclavicular joint disease, and cervical disk disease.

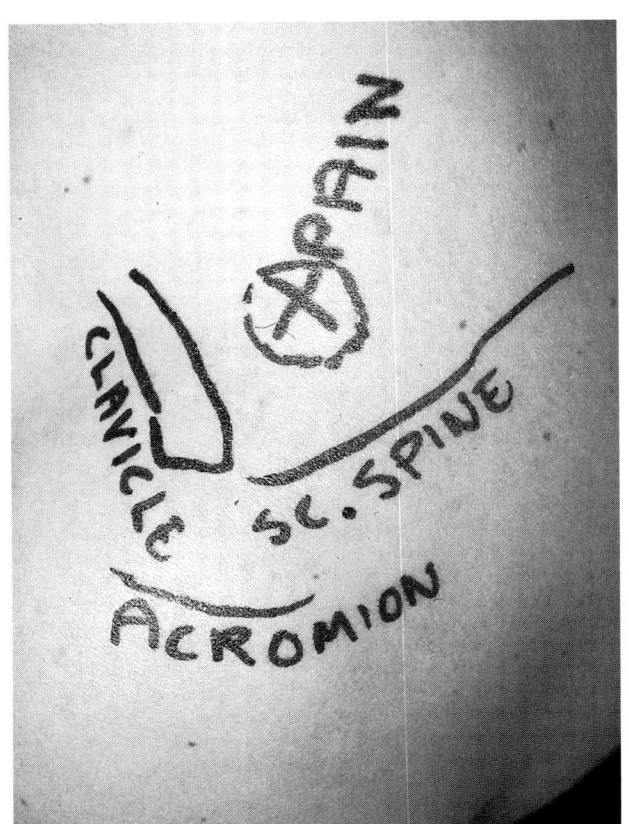

Fig. 1 Location of tenderness over the suprascapular notch.

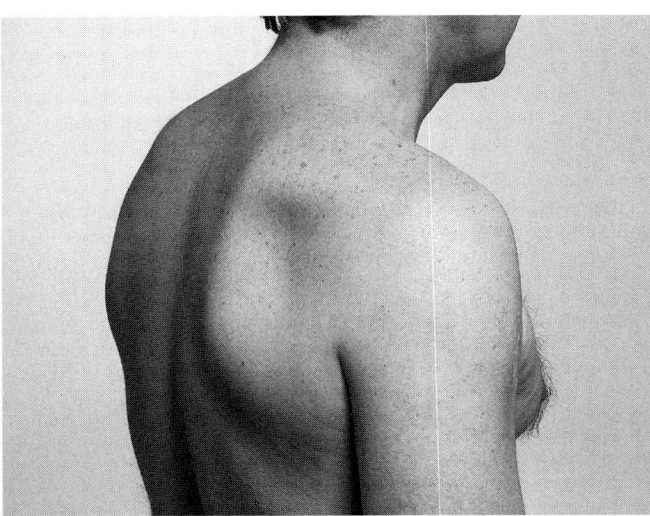

Fig. 2 Atrophy of the infraspinatus muscle on the right side.

Normally, the infraspinatus muscle is more affected, and the supraspinatus can be asymptomatic and normal for a long time as well in suprascapular nerve entrapment at the suprascapular notch. As in other entrapments, the first electrical finding is a prolonged conduction time. The normal conduction time from Erb's point to the supraspinatus muscle is about 2.7 ms, and to the infraspinatus, 3.3 ms.

Treatment

Rational management of severe peripheral nerve entrapment is decompression of the nerve. The management of suprascapular nerve entrapment does not differ from this generally accepted principle. Of course, conservative treatment such as rest, analgesics, physical therapy, and perhaps local corticoid injections should be offered. Nerve entrapment caused by acute trauma or exceptional single exertion without any marked anatomic compression may improve with conservative treatment.

If the pain does not subside with conservative treatment or if the nerve does not show any signs of recovery in 1 to 2 months in patients with atrophy, surgical treatment is a consideration. Surgical treatment is advisable in some patients during the first weeks after the onset of symptoms. More than half of the cases will recover without surgery.

There is no reason to postpone surgical release of the suprascapular nerve if the diagnosis is assured by prominent atrophy of a spinatus muscle and there are no signs of recovery in 1 to 2 months. Pain is not a factor in this instance. However, if the patient has severe pain, prompt surgical treatment should be undertaken, as in other nerve entrapments. But if the pain is diminishing and the strength of the shoulder is improving, follow-up is necessary. Recovery in these patients is usually spontaneous, particularly if the cause of the suprascapular nerve entrapment has been some type of injury. In this instance, the entrapment has been initially caused by stretching of the nerve, leading to compression at the notch. After conservative treatment, the nerve will do well as in other neurapraxias.

There are at least three approaches to explore the suprascapular notch—anterior, superior, and posterior. The anterior approach over the medial aspect of the coracoid process is less advisable because of the risk to the elements of the brachial plexus and vessels. The superior or cranial (distal trapezius-splitting) approach, which I advocate, is easiest to perform and has the shortest recovery time, but may be technically difficult in patients with a well-developed musculature. The posterior trapezius elevating approach advocated by Post provides the most accessibility to the suprascapular notch, but some immobilization after surgery is required.

The superior transverse scapular ligament, as well as the suprascapular nerve, are identified during surgery, most suitably by means of electrical stimulation if the nerve is still functioning. The ligament is sectioned, taking care not to injure the nerve, suprascapular artery, and veins. It may be advisable to perform notch resection if the suprascapular notch is very narrow and deep.

During surgery for spinoglenoid notch entrapment, the skin incision goes along the scapular spine, the deltoid muscle is released subperiosteally from its insertion to the scapular spine, and the infraspinatus muscle is gently retracted to expose the suprascapular nerve where it enters the infraspinatus fossa through the spinoglenoid notch. The inferior transverse spinoglenoid ligament compressing the infraspinatus branch of the suprascapular nerve should be excised. If this ligament does not exist, the nerve is only liberated from any scar tissue tethering the nerve to the periosteum. Mostly, the mechanism of suprascapular nerve entrapment at the spinoglenoid notch in such cases is some kind of repetitive strain to the infraspinate branch of the suprascapular nerve such as that seen in volleyball players. Nottage advises that glenohumeral arthroscopy precede all suprascapular nerve decompressions. Concomitant intra-articular pathology has been found in more than 50% of 36 cases.

Complications

Complications in the surgical treatment of suprascapular nerve entrapment are very rare. I have seen one postoperative minor hematoma in need of special treatment. When retracting the supraspinatus muscle, care should be taken to avoid lesion to the supraspinatus branches. One also should remember that some branches to the supraspinatus may go over the superior transverse scapular ligament. Thus, it is always important to use electric stimulation during surgery if the nerve still is functioning. A lesion of suprascapular vessels would be difficult to treat but is easy to avoid by careful dissection. Cadaver dissections are advised before surgery on patients is attempted.

Results

The most dramatic effect of the operation is prompt disappearance of the pain, as in all nerve entrapments after surgery. Of course, muscle atrophy and weakness improve more slowly according to severity of the nerve injury.

In the largest study on suprascapular nerve entrapment, published in 1993 by Vastamäki and Göransson (56 operations, mean follow-up 5.6 years), 81% of the patients were improved. The strength of flexion, abduction, and especially of external rotation improved markedly. However, some patients remained symptomatic. The poor results may be explained by misdiagnoses and operation in the wrong area. Some of the patients might have had "mononeuritis" at the suprascapular nerve, for which surgical treatment is not required. I cannot distinguish nerve entrapment from mononeuritis; therefore, I have had to explore the nerve. Some patients in the study were believed to have nerve entrapment at the suprascapular notch when in fact the correct diagnosis was nerve entrapment at the spinoglenoid notch. This misdiagnosis came about because I did not become acquainted with the spinoglenoid compression until 1986. Electrodiagnostic studies should be able to differentiate the two sites of compression. Both the supraspinatus and infraspinatus must be tested.

The results of smaller studies by many other authors have been beneficial. Of course, an atrophy that persists for many years very seldom disappears.

Selected Bibliography

Aiello I, Serra G, Traina GC, et al: Entrapment of the suprascapular nerve at the spinoglenoid notch. *Ann Neurol* 1982;12:314-316.

Berry H, Kong K, Hudson AR, et al: Isolated suprascapular nerve palsy: A review of nine cases. *Can Neurol Sci* 1995;22:301-304.

In nine patients, suprascapular nerve palsy occurred following serious accidents associated with fractures of the cervical vertebrae, clavicle, or scapula and after weightlifting, wrestling, and a fall on the elbow or shoulder. In contrast to published studies, none of the patients presented with spontaneous shoulder pain, nor with limited involvement of the infraspinatus muscle.

Eggert S, Holzgraefe M: Compression neuropathy of the suprascapular nerve in high performance volleyball players. *Sportverletz-Sportschaden* 1993;7:136-142.

In 36 high-performance volleyball players, ten had an atrophy of the infraspinatus muscle. On the basis of these findings, a prospective study was carried out. Thirty-two players were examined as to the extent to which a functional impairment of the suprascapular nerve occurred in the pursuit of the competitive sport of volleyball. The study revealed a functional impairment of the suprascapular nerve in 45% of the patients who were examined both clinically and neurophysiologically.

Fritz RC, Helms CA, Steinbach LS, et al: Suprascapular nerve entrapment: Evaluation with MR imaging. *Radiology* 1992;182:437-444.

Twenty-seven masses were identified adjacent to the suprascapular nerve on magnetic resonance (MR) images of the shoulder; there were 21 ganglion cysts, two synovial sarcomas, one Ewing sarcoma, one chondrosarcoma, one metastatic renal cell carcinoma, and one hematoma associated with a fracture. MR imaging may facilitate the diagnosis of suprascapular nerve entrapment in patients with shoulder pain of unclear origin when perineural masses and atrophy of the spinatus musculature are present.

Glennon TP: Isolated injury of the infraspinatus branch of the suprascapular nerve. *Arch Phys Med Rehabil* 1992;73:201-202.

Goldberg RS, Post M: Compression neuropathies about the shoulder. *Ann Chir Gyn* 1996;85:159-165.

Kopell HP, Thompson WA: Pain and the frozen shoulder. *Surg Gynecol Obstet* 1959;109:92-96.

Sjöström L, Mjöberg B: Suprascapular nerve entrapment in an arthrodesed shoulder. *J Bone Joint Surg* 1992;74B: 470-471.

Torres-Ramos FM, Biundo JJ Jr: Suprascapular neuropathy during progressive resistive exercises in a cardiac rehabilitation program. *Arch Phys Rehabil* 1992;73: 1107-1111.

A 56-year-old man developed left shoulder pain 3 weeks after starting a cardiac rehabilitation program that consisted of submaximal aerobic and progressive resistive exercises. Pain in the left shoulder intensified and weakness developed 1 week later. Suprascapular neuropathy was diagnosed and should be considered as a cause of shoulder pain and weakness in a person involved in a strengthening exercise program.

Vastamäki M, Göransson H: Suprascapular nerve entrapment. *Clin Orthop* 1993;297:135-143.

Fifty-four patients with suprascapular nerve entrapment were evaluated 5.6 years after surgical release. A supposed causative factor was exertion at work or vacation in 36 patients. A new cranial approach is advocated. The most dramatic effect of the operation was prompt disappearance of the pain in 24 patients and marked diminishing in 15.

30
Lesions of the Superior Aspect of the Shoulder

Felix H. Savoie, MD and Larry D. Field, MD

Introduction

The variations in the normal anatomy of the labrum and capsular ligaments of the superior aspect of the glenohumeral joint often make interpretation of pathologic lesions and diagnosis of injury in this area difficult. Arthroscopy, which has advanced the understanding of the function of all shoulder structures, seems especially relevant in the area of the superior aspect. The ability to directly visualize the intra-articular structures has allowed the discovery of many new lesions. Injuries may occur as an entire avulsion (superior labrum anterior and posterior (SLAP) lesion), an isolated biceps tendon avulsion, a biceps–superior glenohumeral ligament injury, or as an injury to the anterosuperior quadrant (superior and medial glenohumeral ligament avulsion). The superior labrum and its attached biceps tendon and superior and middle glenohumeral ligaments represent a functional stabilizer of the glenohumeral joint. Diagnosis and management of injuries will be discussed here.

History

Snyder, in 1990, was the first to use the term "SLAP" lesion to refer to the superior labrum, anterior to posterior avulsion. He noted these lesions occurred in only 27 of more than 700 arthroscopic shoulder cases, and classified them into four categories based on the physical characteristics of the lesions (Fig. 1). However, Andrews in 1985 observed lesions involving the biceps tendon and anterior superior labrum in throwing athletes. The injury described was remarkably similar to the type II SLAP lesion noted by Snyder. Grauer and associates described a continuum of injuries occurring to the superior labrum, biceps tendon, and rotator interval in these patients. They also noted the extreme anatomic variability in this region. Field and Savoie noted the presence of an anterosuperior instability in these patients, attributing this to the loss of function of the superior glenohumeral ligament-biceps tendon complex. They described the first clinical examination technique for this injury (SLAP test).

Snyder recommended repair of these injuries in his preliminary report but provided no follow-up data. Field and Savoie described a repair technique for the unstable type II and IV lesions using the Caspari suture punch with excellent results. Yoneda also described a similar repair technique for the unstable SLAP tears. Recent reports have described the use of absorbable tacks, as well as anchor-suture combinations, for these injuries. Since these early efforts, much has been written regarding the superior quadrant of the shoulder.

Diagnosis

Patient History

There are no unique signs for lesions of the superior labrum. The presenting history is variable, including falls directly onto the lateral aspect of the shoulder, somewhat sudden downward force applied to an outstretched supinated arm, or vague discomfort with overhead use. Patients with these injuries complain of pain, decreased endurance with use of the shoulder, popping, or sliding, especially with overhead use, as well as problems sleeping on the shoulder at night.

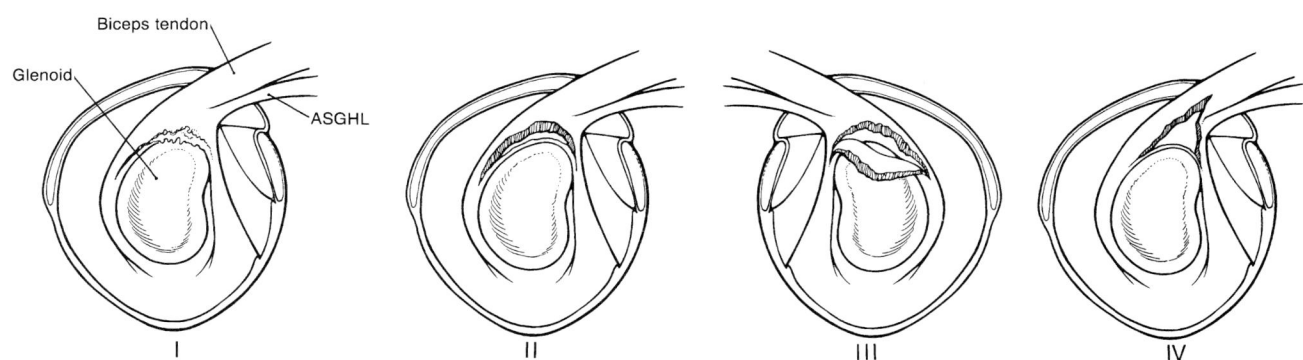

Fig. 1 The four types of superior labral lesions described by Snyder. Type I, degenerative fraying of the labrum. ASGHL = anterior superior glenohumeral ligament. Type II, avulsion of the superior labrum and biceps tendon from the superior glenoid. Type III, a bucket handle tear of the superior labrum, preserving the connection of the labrum to the glenoid. Type IV, a type II or III lesion with extension into the biceps tendon.

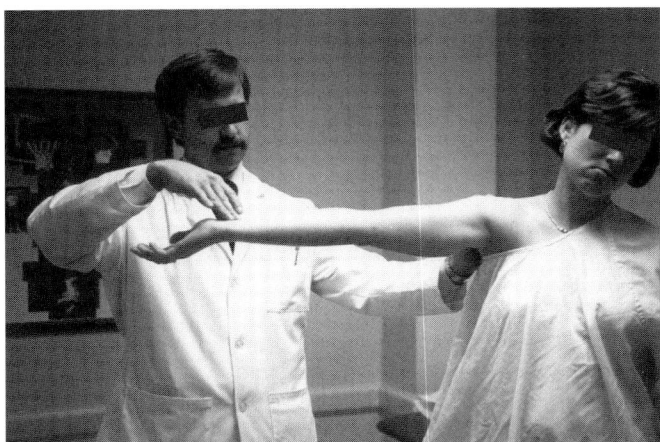

Fig. 2 The SLAP test. The thumb of the left hand of the examiner is pushing the humeral head in a superior direction as the patient resists the downward force on the abducted and supinated forearm.

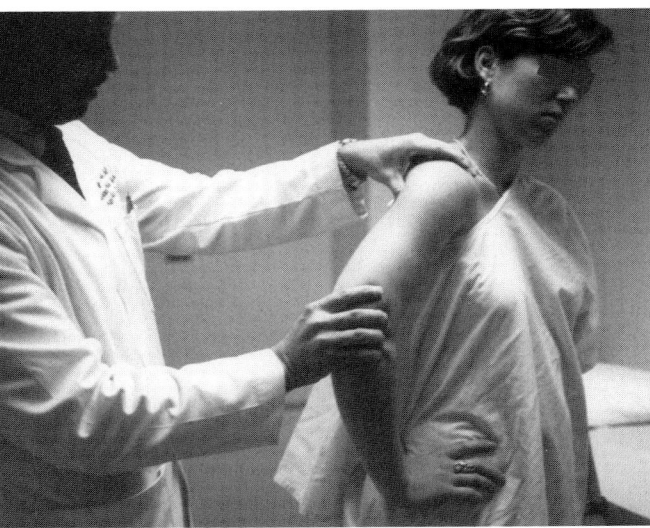

Fig. 3 Kibler test for anterior/superior labral lesions.

Physical Examination

Examination findings are more specific. Active and passive range of motion are usually normal. Standard impingement signs of pain on frontal flexion (Neer's sign), rotation from external rotation to internal rotation in 90° of abduction and forced cross chest flexion in internal rotation (Hawkin's sign) are often positive because of secondary rotator cuff irritation. Although the standard apprehension position may be mildly painful, Jobe's augmentation and relocation tests are usually negative.

There are four specific clinical examination tests described for lesions in this area. The SLAP test is used in the diagnosis of unstable type II and IV superior labral lesions (Fig. 2). The arm is held abducted to 90° with the hand fully supinated. The examiner places one hand on the shoulder with the thumb in the 6 o'clock position inferiorly (in the axilla). The opposite hand is used to exert downward force on the outstretched hand of the patient, creating a fulcrum of the thumb shifting the humeral head in a superior direction. Crepitation, buckling, and pain represent a positive finding.

In another maneuver, the patient places the injured extremity on the ipsilateral hip, finger anteriorly, and thumb posteriorly. The examiner then pushes upward and forward on the elbow. Pain and crepitation are produced when a tear is present (Fig. 3). This test will be positive for SLAP tears, anterosuperior labral tears, and middle glenohumeral ligament avulsions.

In the O'Brien test for SLAP lesions (Fig. 4), the examiner places the patient's arm in 90° of flexion, full internal rotation, and cross chest adduction. The patient is then asked to resist the downward force on the hand. This position winds the long head of the biceps around the humeral head, producing traction on the glenoid attachment of the biceps. Pain or buckling indicates a positive test. This maneuver differs from the standard acromioclavicular (AC) joint compression test by the rotated position of the arm (internally rotated in the O'Brien test, neutral in the AC compression test).

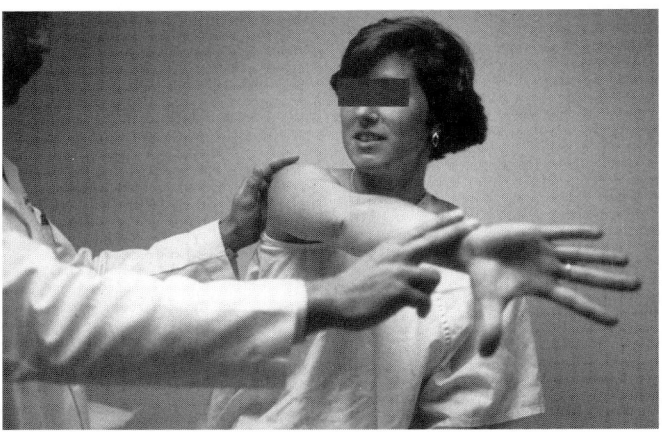

Fig. 4 The O'Brien test for SLAP tears.

The fourth specific examination technique involves a "load and shift" or fulcrum maneuver. This test can be used to examine any area of the shoulder, and with practice this would appear to be the most specific and sensitive of the examination techniques. In this test the hand of the examiner is positioned as in the SLAP test of Field. The thumb is used to exert a force in the direction of the area to be tested (ie, 12 o'clock for SLAP tears, 1 o'clock for superior glenohumeral ligament injuries, 3 o'clock for middle glenohumeral ligament tears, etc), while the opposite hand of the examiner pulls the flexed and neutrally rotated elbow in the opposite direction (Fig. 5).

Although each of these maneuvers may be helpful in the diagnosis, one additional test is often positive in these patients

ity with associated secondary rotator cuff tearing (superior labrum anterior cuff).

Diagnostic Studies

The extreme variability of the anatomy in this area makes diagnostic studies difficult to interpret, leading to considerable interobserver disagreement. Standard arthrograms and ultrasonography, while less expensive, are usually ineffective in the anterior superior corner. An arthrogram supplemented by computed tomography is more valuable, especially in true avulsions of the entire superior labrum. However, a significant false positive rate exists, which indicates the difficulty in differentiating normal anatomy from pathology.

Magnetic resonance imaging (MRI) has shown the most promise in evaluation of this area. Initial reports seem to show a high sensitivity and specificity in the detection of labral lesions, but interobserver and intraobserver correlations are poor. Dynamic imaging has been more accurate. Recent reports have also demonstrated improved accuracy through the use of magnetic resonance arthrography. Injection of the joint with saline or gadolinium prior to MRI allows detection of tears and avulsions often unseen on regular studies. Additionally, the smooth contour noted on normal anatomic variance can be visualized with these more refined tests, decreasing the incidence of false positives. Additional factors improving accuracy are the use of a dedicated shoulder coil and experience in orthopaedic imaging by the radiologist.

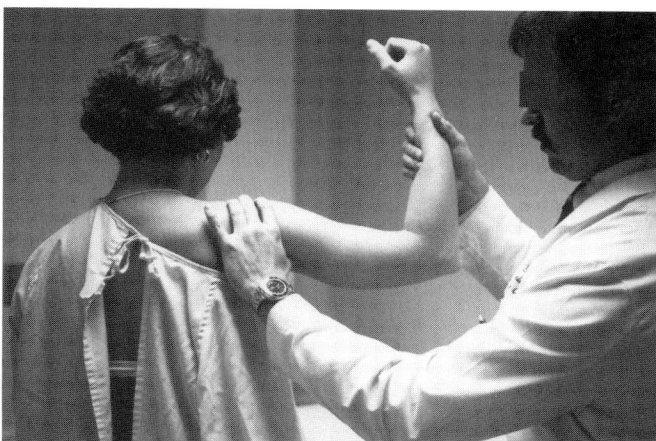

Fig. 5 The load and shift maneuver to evaluate the superior labrum.

Nonsurgical Management

Lesions of the superior labrum may go undetected for a number of years; studies show an average delay from onset to definitive treatment of 29 months. Many of these patients function reasonably well during this delay, although slow deterioration during this time is common. Selective use of nonsteroidal anti-inflammatory medications, isolated corticosteroid injections, and rotator cuff rehabilitation exercises may decrease symptoms to a manageable level in many patients, obviating the need for surgical intervention. Emphasis on rotator cuff and periscapular exercises that limit forward flexion to less than 90° is often beneficial.

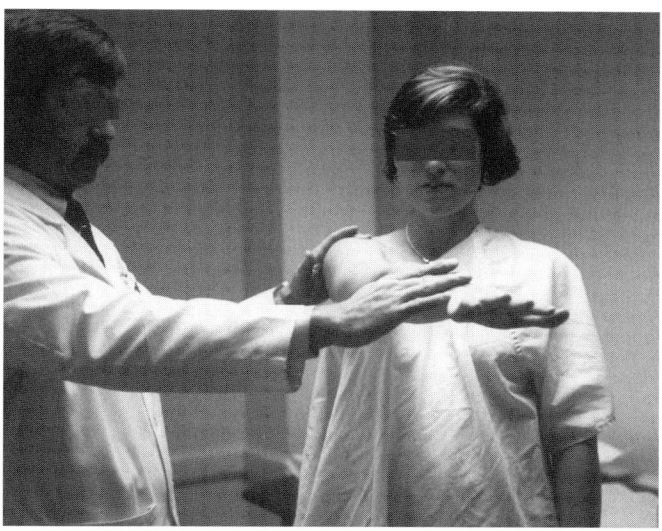

Fig. 6 The Whipple test for anterior supraspinatus tears.

Surgical Management

SLAP lesions are best managed using arthroscopic techniques. Extreme caution should be used in the evaluation of this area. Normal variants with age-related fraying greatly outnumber pathologic lesions.

There are many surgical options in repairing these lesions. Repairs fall into three basic categories: absorbable tack/rivet techniques, transglenoid (Caspari or Morgan) techniques with absorbable suture, and anchor techniques with absorbable or nonabsorbable suture. The initial step in all techniques is to define the lesion, debride the frayed/damaged tissue and, if repair is required, abrade the glenoid beneath the tear (Fig. 7).

In addition to being absorbable, tacks are advantageous because they are easy to use. The disadvantage to using these

and is particularly valuable in identifying rotator cuff pathology. The Whipple test is generally positive only in patients with a tear of the anterior part of the supraspinatus in addition to the instability. In this test, the arm is placed in 90° frontal flexion with the elbow straight and the palm facing toward the floor. The arm is adducted slightly so that the hand is in front of the opposite shoulder (Fig. 6). The patient is then asked to resist a downward force. Pain and buckling represent positive findings, indicating a partial or complete rotator cuff tear involving the anterior aspect of the supraspinatus tendon. A positive Whipple test in combination with one or more of the above provocative maneuvers indicates a variant of the subluxation impingement syndrome or anterior superior instabil-

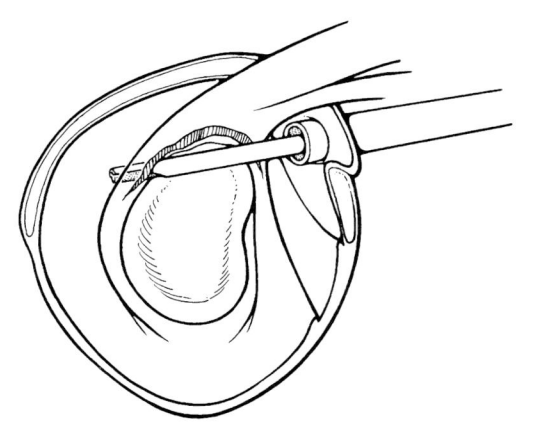

Fig. 7 The initial step in repair of the superior labrum is to adequately debride and abrade the superior labrum and superior glenoid.

devices is their sometimes tenuous hold on the tissues, difficulty obtaining a proper angle of insertion without violating the rotator cuff, and rapidity of absorption.

Suretac Technique

A standard diagnostic arthroscopy is performed with the arthroscope in the posterior portal. Once the superior labral lesion has been noted, fixation using a Suretac fixation device can be initiated. The initial step in all techniques is a debridement of the lesion to stable tissue followed by abrasion of the superior glenoid neck.

Standard Technique In this technique, the drill and wire are inserted through the labrum into the glenoid neck. The optimal portal for Suretac placement in the anterior superior corner is an anterior superior portal through the rotator interval. The guide is used to hold the superior labrum in anatomic position and the drill is inserted through the labrum into the glenoid neck. Once drilled into position, the hexhead nut on the drill bit is loosened and the guide wire advanced by tapping it until it engages the posterior cortical rim of the glenoid neck. The drill is then removed and the Suretac device inserted over the wire and tapped into position, securing the anterior superior corner of the labrum. The advantage of this standard technique is its simplicity. The disadvantage involves passage of the drill bit through the soft tissues, possibly diminishing the hold of the Suretac on the superior labrum. These steps can be repeated using a posterior superior portal with placement of a posterior Suretac when necessary (Fig. 8).

Revised Technique In this technique the drill is inserted directly on the bone, creating a pilot hole to the appropriate depth. The Kirschner wire is then used to "spear" the unstable superior labrum. The wire is then guided into the previously drilled hole and the Suretac is inserted over the wire, fixing the labrum to the underlying bone of the glenoid neck. This technique allows improved soft-tissue fixation because there is no drilling through the labrum.

Caspari Technique

The Caspari suture technique was the first described for the treatment of superior labral detachment lesions of the shoulder. The reported success rate is quite high, and it is the only technique for which long-term results are available. Advantages of this technique include the establishment of multiple fixation points and the use of a superior stitch to maintain downward pressure on the entire avulsed labrum as well as the use of absorbable suture material. The disadvantage is the transglenoid drill hole and the associated risks of neurovascular damage.

In this technique, the standard diagnostic arthroscopy, debridement, and superior glenoid abrasion are performed. The suture punch cannula is then inserted through a standard anterior portal. The initial stitch is made with a curved suture punch placed over the biceps tendon and into the posterior superior corner of the tear. This stitch is then retrieved out the anterior portal. A second stitch can be placed again over the biceps tendon adjacent to the first one and slightly more anterior in position. The next stitch is placed inferior to the biceps at approximately the 12 o'clock position on the glenoid. Additional stitches are then placed into the base of the biceps,

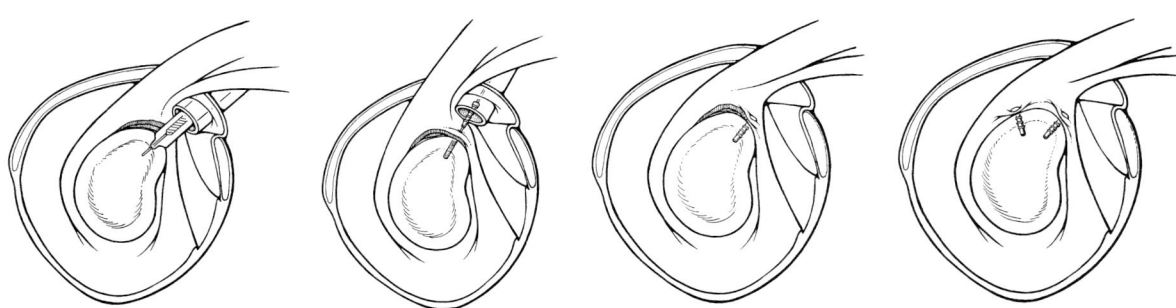

Fig. 8 Suretac technique. **Far left,** Once the debridement and abrasion are completed, a pilot hole is drilled into the superior glenoid just anterior to the biceps tendon. **Center left,** The labrum is then "spread" with the guide wire and the wire inserted into the drill hole. **Center right,** The Suretac fixation device is then inserted over the wire, stabilizing the superior labrum to the superior glenoid. **Far right,** The steps are then repeated using an additional posterior portal to place a posterior Suretac and complete the procedure.

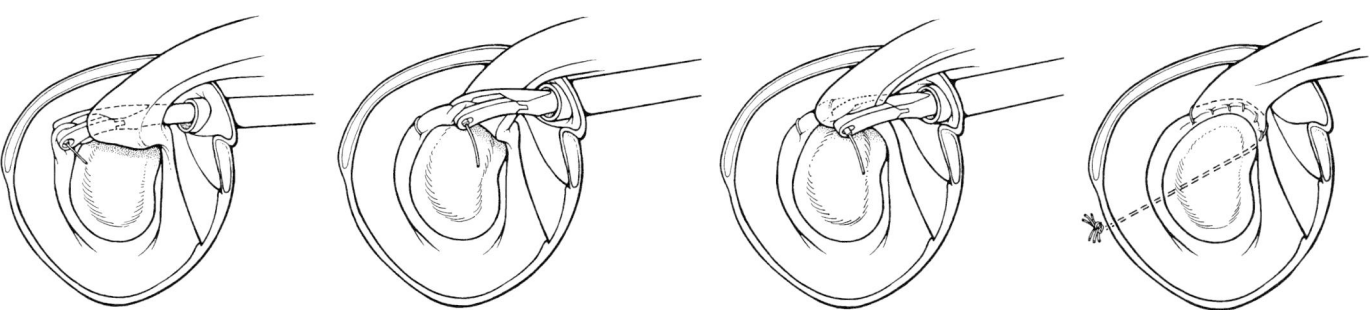

Fig. 9 Caspari technique. **Far left,** Once the debridement and abrasion are completed, the suture punch device is placed into the anterior portal, over (superior to) the biceps and into the labrum at the posterior superior corner of the avulsion. **Center left,** The next suture is placed into the labrum at the straight superior (12 o'clock) position. **Center right,** The third stitch is placed at the base of the biceps and the fourth is placed into the tendon of the biceps to relieve tension on the repair. Additional sutures are placed into the superior glenohumeral ligament and superior labrum as needed. A Beath pin is then drilled transglenoid and the sutures are pulled posteriorly and tied over the infraspinatus fascia **(far right).**

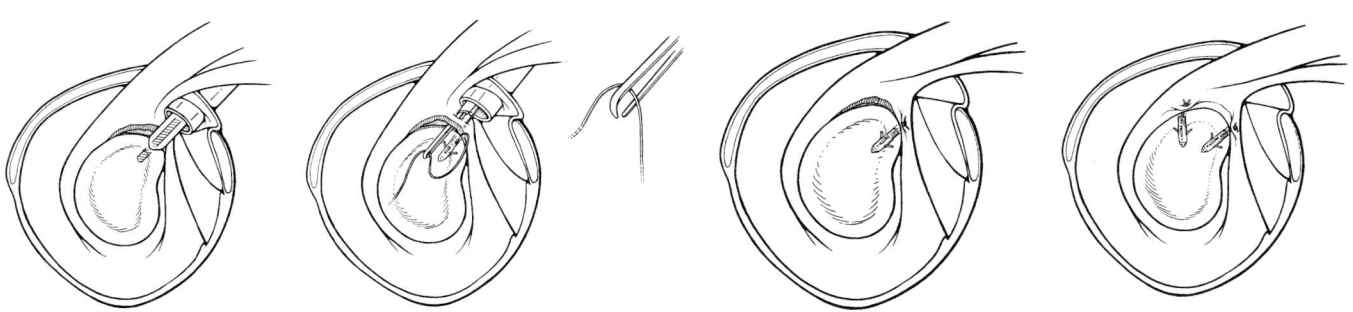

Fig. 10 Anchor technique. **Far left,** Once the debridement and abrasion are completed, the pilot hole for the suture anchor is drilled into the superior glenoid just anterior to the biceps tendon insertion. **Center left,** The anchor is inserted into the drill hole and the sutures attached to the anchor retrieved through the labrum. **Center right,** These sutures are tied, repairing the anterior aspect of the avulsion. **Far right,** These steps are then repeated for the placement of the posterior anchor.

the biceps tendon, and superior glenohumeral ligament. The Beath pin is then drilled through the glenoid neck with care being taken to orient it to exit inferiorly and medially on the scapula, penetrating the skin posteriorly in the region of the medial border of the scapula. The sutures are then pulled through to the posterior aspect of the shoulder and tied down to the thick fascia along the medial border of the scapular (Fig. 9).

Anchor Technique

Recent use of anchors with attached absorbable or nonabsorbable sutures has gained popularity. An advantage of these devices is the ability to attach the labrum directly to the glenoid while avoiding transglenoid drilling. The disadvantages include the presence of permanent implants and the need for arthroscopic knot tying.

In this technique, the arthroscope is placed posteriorly and a standard diagnostic arthroscopy, debridement, and abrasion is accomplished. Through an anterior superior portal established in the rotator interval, a suture anchor is placed into the superior glenoid neck by drilling a pilot hole and placing the anchor into position. The sutures attached to the anchor are then passed through the superior labrum using a suture retriever, a double 2-0 Prolene, or a suture shuttle. These sutures are then tied together using an arthroscopic knot pusher with either a mattress or simple stitch. In this area, a mattress suture is preferred to avoid placing the suture knots near the articular cartilage. Additional anchors are placed posterosuperiorly using a posterior superior portal through the interval between the infraspinatus and supraspinatus (Fig. 10).

Open Technique

Many surgeons may not have the equipment or technical skills to perform an arthroscopic repair. In these cases, an open repair through an anterior superior approach may be used because it involves visualization of the detached complex and the ability to directly repair the injury without arthroscopic techniques. However, a drawback to open repair is the need to partially detach the deltoid muscle origin, split the coracoacromial ligament, and separate the rotator interval to gain access to the superior labrum.

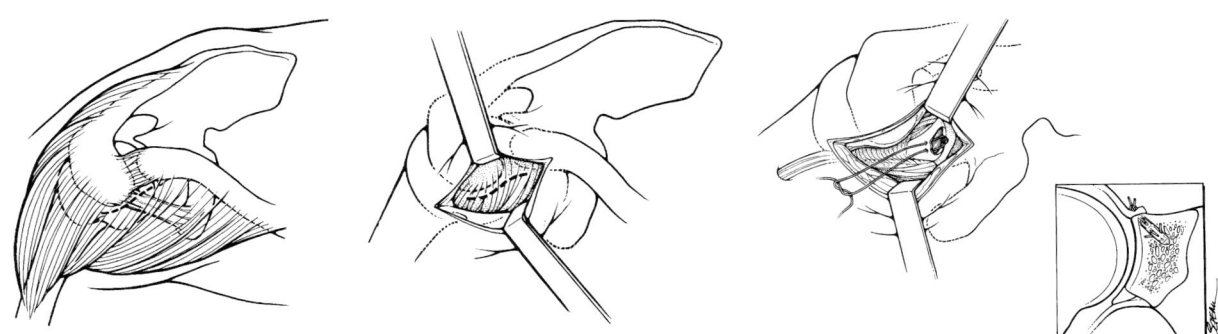

Fig. 11 Open technique. **Left,** A limited superior approach may be used to repair these lesions. The initial incision is just anterior to the acromion. **Center,** The fibers of the anterior head of the deltoid are separated and the rotator interval identified. **Right,** The interval is incised, allowing access to the superior labrum and biceps tendon **(inset).** Any of the previous repair techniques may be used under direct vision to complete the repair.

A standard superior approach to the rotator cuff may be used, which involves an incision along the anterior margin of the acromion. The deltoid is then detached from the anterior acromion and the coracoacromial ligament visualized. The coracoacromial ligament is then incised to obtain access to the subacromial area. Using the biceps tendon as a guide, the rotator interval is identified and a longitudinal incision made anterior to the tendon of the supraspinatus, allowing direct visualization of the superior aspect of the labrum and the biceps tendon. The superior labrum can then be repaired using an open version of one of the previously described techniques (Fig. 11).

Postoperative Course

The patient is placed in an immobilization device with the elbow flexed at 90° and the arm slightly abducted and internally rotated. The device is removed for showers and gentle passive exercises within a pain-free range of motion beginning on postoperative day one. After approximately 3 weeks, the immobilization device is discontinued and an active shoulder exercise program is initiated. After 6 weeks, sport- or work-specific conditioning programs are introduced so that normal function is achieved by 10 to 16 weeks.

Results

Success rates of better than 90% have been reported with the use of arthroscopic techniques. The key to appropriate management of superior labral detachments centers around proper diagnosis. Once the diagnosis has been made through appropriate history, physical examination, and diagnostic studies, arthroscopic or open repair can be performed with high probability of success.

Selected Bibliography

Andrews JR, Carson WG Jr, McLeod WD: Glenoid labrum tears related to the long head of the biceps. *Am J Sports Med* 1985;13:337-341.

This is the first report of anterosuperior instability with biceps–labral injuries in throwing athletes. A description of pathology and mechanism of injury is included.

Field LD, Savoie FH III: Arthroscopic suture repair of superior labral detachment lesions of the shoulder. *Am J Sports Med* 1993;21:783-790.

Field and Savoie described a repair technique for unstable type II and IV lesions in 20 patients using the Caspari suture punch. The concept of anterosuperior instability and diagrams of the repair technique are included.

Grauer JD, Paulos LE, Smutz WP: Biceps tendon and superior labral injuries. *Arthroscopy* 1992;8:488-497.

This is a combined anatomic and clinical paper describing the spectrum of injuries occurring in the anterosuperior quadrant. Variations in normal anatomy are also discussed.

Kibler WB: Specificity and sensitivity of the anterior slide test in throwing athletes with superior glenoid labral tears. *Arthroscopy* 1995;11:296-300.

Kibler describes his maneuver for diagnosing anterosuperior labral injuries. The patient places the hand of the injured extremity on the ipsilateral hip, finger anteriorly and thumb posteriorly, while the examiner pushes the elbow superiorly.

Maffet MW, Gartsman GM, Moseley B: Superior labrum-biceps tendon complex lesions of the shoulder. *Am J Sports Med* 1995;23:93-98.

Diagnostic tests, provocative maneuvers, incidence, and management of superior labral injuries in 84 patients are presented.

O'Brien SJ, Pagnani MJ, McGlynn SR, et al: A new and effective test for diagnosing labral tears and AC joint pathology. Proceedings of the American Academy of Orthopaedic Surgeons 63rd Annual Meeting, Atlanta, GA. Rosemont, IL, American Academy of Orthopaedic Surgeons, 1996, p 106.

The O'Brien test for SLAP lesions is performed by placing the patient's arm in 90° of flexion, full internal rotation, and cross chest adduction. The patient is then asked to resist the downward force on the hand. This position winds the long head of the biceps around the humeral head, producing traction on the glenoid attachment of the biceps.

Pagnani MJ, Deng XH, Warren RF, et al: Effect of lesions of the superior portion of the glenoid labrum on glenohumeral translation. *J Bone Joint Surg* 1995;77A:1003-1010.

This anatomic study describes the instability resulting from superior labral detachment.

Rodosky MW, Harner CD, Fu FH: The role of the long head of the biceps muscle and superior glenoid labrum in anterior stability of the shoulder. *Am J Sports Med* 1994;22:121-130.

A dynamic cadaveric model is used to evaluate the role of the superior labrum-biceps tendon in instability.

Savoie FH III, Caspari RB: Instability of the shoulder: Superior, posterior, and multidirectional, in McGinty JB, Caspari RB, Jackson RW, et al (eds): *Operative Arthroscopy*, ed 2. Philadelphia, PA, Lippincott-Raven, 1966, pp 709-723.

This article illustrates the concept of anterosuperior instability and describes examination and repair techniques.

Snyder SJ, Karzel RP, Del Pizzo W, et al: SLAP lesions of the shoulder. *Arthroscopy* 1990;6:274-279.

This report presents the classification system for superior labral detachment injuries. The mechanism of injury, delay in diagnosis, and early thoughts on repair are noted.

31

Calcifying Tendinitis, Chondrocalcinosis, Heterotopic Ossification, and Pigmented Villonodular Synovitis

Hans K. Uhthoff, MD, FRCSC, Hirotaka Sano, MD, and Joachim F. Loehr, MD, FRCSC

Calcifying Tendinitis

Calcific tendinopathy of the rotator cuff, also known as calcifying tendinitis, is a common disorder of unknown etiology in which multifocal, cell-mediated calcification of a living tendon is usually followed over time by spontaneous phagocytic resorption. After resorption or surgical removal of the deposit, the tendon reconstitutes itself. During the deposition of calcium, the patient may be either free of pain or suffer only a mild to moderate degree of discomfort, but the disease becomes acutely painful during resorption of calcium.

Calcifying tendinitis must be distinguished from degenerative or dystrophic calcifications that occur at the insertion into bone but not in the midsubstance of the tendon. Moreover, radiologic signs of degenerative processes are extremely rare in calcific tendinopathies.

Pathogenesis

The etiology of calcifying tendinitis is still a matter of controversy. Circumscribed tissue hypoxia and localized pressure are believed to be causative factors.

Two fundamentally different processes leading to formation of calcium deposits in the cuff, degenerative calcification and reactive calcification, have been proposed.

Degenerative Calcification Codman proposed that degeneration of the tendon fibers precedes calcification. Necrosis of the fibers is followed by dystrophic calcification. Degeneration of fibers of the rotator cuff tendons is usually attributed to the wear-and-tear effects of normal usage as well as to aging. Obviously, these two causes are interrelated. It is reasonable to assume that degeneration attributed to normal usage is because the glenohumeral joint is not only a universal joint, but probably the most used joint of the body.

Aging is considered to be the foremost cause of degeneration in cuff tendons. Brewer believes that with aging there is a general diminution in the vascularity of the supraspinatus tendon along with fiber changes. The well-delineated bundles of collagen or the fascicles that constitute the distinctive architecture of the tendon show the most conspicuous age-related changes that begin at the end of the fourth or during the fifth decade. The majority of the fascicles undergo thinning and fibrillation, both of which are defined as part of a degenerative process. Mohr and Bilger believe that the process of calcification starts with necrosis of tenocytes with concomitant intracellular accumulation of calcium, often in the form of microspheroliths, also known as psammomas. Contrary to Mohr and Bilger, psammomas were not observed during the early phases of formation in our studies, but were seen regularly during resorption. In addition, our electron microscopic examinations confirm that the electron-dense material is situated intracellularly. It is unfortunate, however, that these authors failed to distinguish between calcifications at the insertion and intratendinous calcifications, ie, the site of calcifying tendinitis, nor did they describe morphologic features characteristic of formation on one hand and of resorption on the other.

In general, supporters of the theory of degenerative calcification fail to take into consideration the typical age distribution and the course of the disease, as well as the morphologic aspects of calcific tendinopathy.

Reactive Calcification The process of calcification is actively mediated by cells in a viable environment. Moreover, there cannot be the slightest doubt that formation of the calcium deposit must precede its resorption. Consequently, we propose the following concept for the evolution of the disease, which can be divided into three distinct stages: precalcific, calcific, and postcalcific (Fig. 1).

In the precalcific stage, the site of predilection for calcification undergoes fibrocartilaginous transformation. This metaplasia of tenocytes into chondrocytes is accompanied by metachromasia, indicative of the elaboration of proteoglycan.

The calcific stage is subdivided into the formative, resting, and resorptive phases. During the formative phase, calcium crystals are deposited primarily into matrix vesicles that coalesce to form large areas of deposits. For the convenience of description, the term "formative phase" is used to denote this initial period of the calcific stage. If the patient undergoes surgery at this stage, the deposit appears chalk-like and has to be scooped out for removal. The fibrocartilaginous septae between the foci of calcification are generally devoid of vascular channels. They do not consistently stain positive for collagen type II, which is known to be a component of fibrocartilage. These fibrocartilaginous septae are gradually eroded by the enlarging deposits. Whereas during the phase of formation the foci of calcification are surrounded by fibrocartilage, during the resting phase fibrocollagenous tissue borders these foci. The presence of this tissue around the calcification indicates that the formation of deposit of a given focus is

---

This chapter is adapted from Uhthoff HK, Loehr JW: Calcific tendinopathy of the rotator cuff: Pathogenesis, diagnosis, and management. *J Am Acad Orthop Surg* 1997;5:183-191.

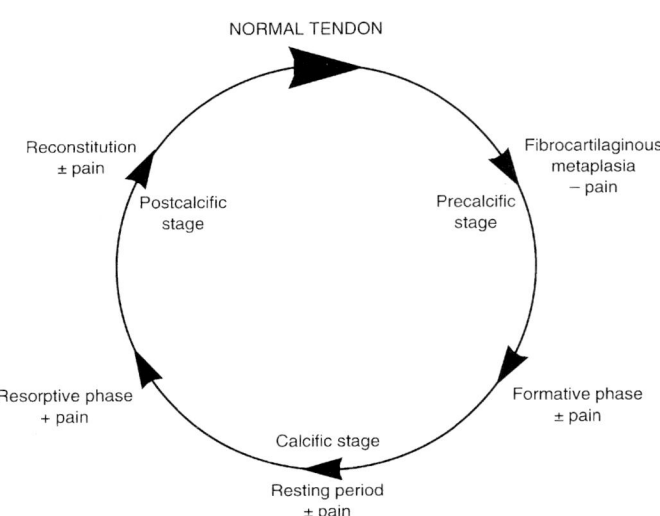

Fig. 1 Schematic representation of the progressive stages of calcific tendinitis. (Reproduced with permission from Uhthoff HK, Loehr JW: Calcific tendinopathy of the rotator cuff: Pathogenesis, diagnosis, and management. *J Am Acad Orthop Surg* 1997;5: 183-191.)

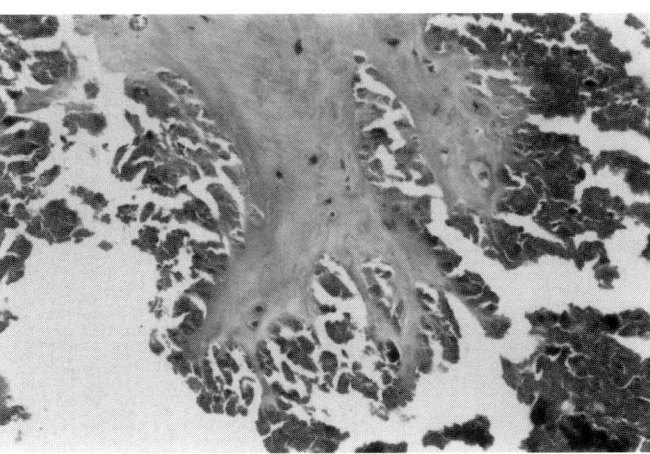

Fig. 2 This microphotograph illustrates the formative phase. Septae of fibrocartilaginous tissue are seen between calcium deposits. Masson's trichrome, magnification × 50. (Reproduced with permission from Uhthoff HK, Loehr JW: Calcific tendinopathy of the rotator cuff: Pathogenesis, diagnosis, and management. *J Am Acad Orthop Surg* 1997;5:183-191.)

terminated. Following a variable period of inactivity of the disease process, the spontaneous resorption of calcium is heralded by the appearance of thin-walled vascular channels at the periphery of the deposit. Soon after, the deposit is surrounded by macrophages and multinucleated giant cells that phagocytose and remove the calcium. At this stage psammoma bodies can be seen. If an operation is performed at this stage, the calcific deposit contains a thick, cream- or toothpaste-like material and often is under pressure.

Simultaneously with the resorption of calcium, granulation tissue containing young fibroblasts and new vascular channels begins to remodel the space occupied by calcium. These sites stain positive for collagen type III. As the scar matures, fibroblasts and collagen eventually align along the longitudinal axis of the tendon. During this remodeling process, collagen type III is replaced by collagen type I.

Although the pathogenesis of the calcifying process can be reasonably constructed from morphologic studies, it is difficult to resolve what triggers the fibrocartilaginous transformation in the first place. Codman's suggestion that tissue hypoxia is a primary etiologic factor is an attractive hypothesis because of the peculiarity of the tendon's blood supply and shoulder mechanics. We have found an increased frequency of HLA-Al in patients with calcifying tendinitis, indicating that these individuals may be genetically susceptible to the condition. Factors that trigger the onset of resorption also remain unknown.

Pathoanatomy

The calcium deposits are usually not in contact with the bony insertion but are at least 1.5 to 2 cm away from it. The presence of calcific deposits in subchondral bone has been described in only isolated reports. It is important to note that not all foci of calcification in a given patient are in the same phase of evolution; in general, one or another phase predominates. The morphologic aspect of an individual focus can vary from fibrocollagenous to foreign body-like granulomatous tissue. Because we believe that the disease starts with fibrocartilaginous metaplasia of tendinous tissue and ends with a tendon reconstitution, the histologic aspects of the consecutive stages will be described in sequence.

Under the light microscope, the calcific deposits appear multifocal, separated by fibrocollagenous tissue or fibrocartilage (Fig. 2). The latter consists of easily distinguishable chondrocytes, described by Archer and associates as chondrocyte-like cells, within a matrix showing varying degrees of metachromasia. The appearance of chondrocytes within the tendon substance near calcification has been documented by many authors since 1912. The ultrastructure of these chondrocytes shows that the cells often have a fair amount of cytoplasm containing a well-developed endoplasmic reticulum, a moderate number of mitochondria, one or more vacuoles, and numerous cell processes. The margin of the nucleus is indented. The cells are surrounded by a distinct band of pericellular matrix with or without an intervening lacuna. The above-described changes are compatible with the precalcific stage.

The fibrocartilaginous areas are generally avascular. The intercellular substance is metachromatic, and glycosaminoglycan-rich pericellular halos around rounded cells are prominent. Surprisingly, monoclonal collagen staining performed by Archer and associates did not reveal the presence of collagen type II; its presence was occasionally documented during our studies using collagen type II monoclonal antibodies (Fig. 3). The different outcome may be because of differences in tissue preparation, source of monoclonal antibodies, and staining technique.

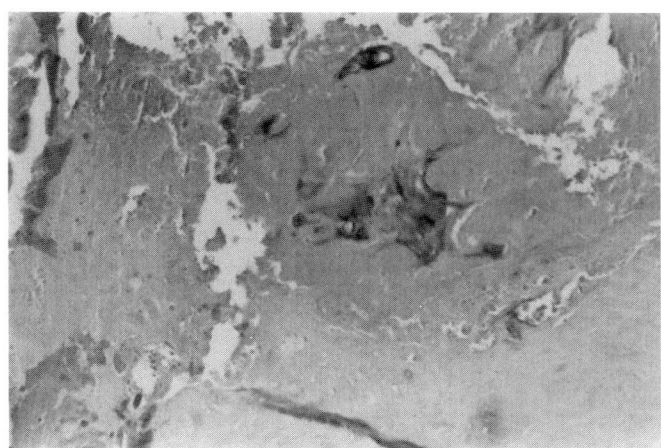

Fig. 3 During the formative phase some of the septae contain type II collagen. Immunohistochemical monoclonal staining for type II collagen, magnification × 50. (Reproduced with permission from Uhthoff HK, Loehr JW: Calcific tendinopathy of the rotator cuff: Pathogenesis, diagnosis, and management. *J Am Acad Orthop Surg* 1997;5:183-191.)

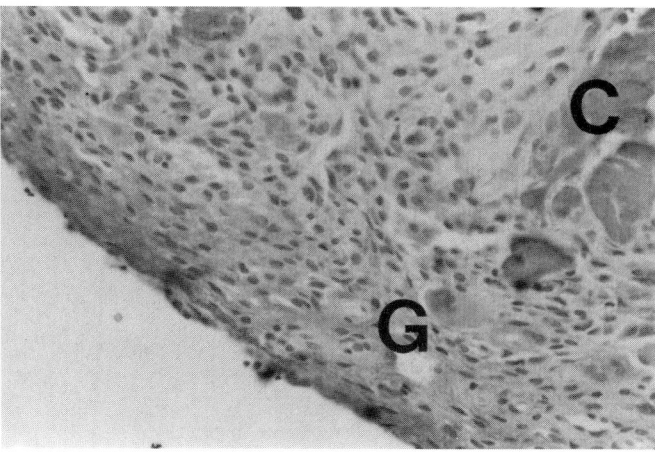

Fig. 5 Resorptive phase. Note the presence of giant cells (G) around calcium deposits (C). Masson's trichrome, magnification × 100. (Reproduced with permission from Uhthoff HK, Loehr JW: Calcific tendinopathy of the rotator cuff: Pathogenesis, diagnosis, and management. *J Am Acad Orthop Surg* 1997;5:183-191.)

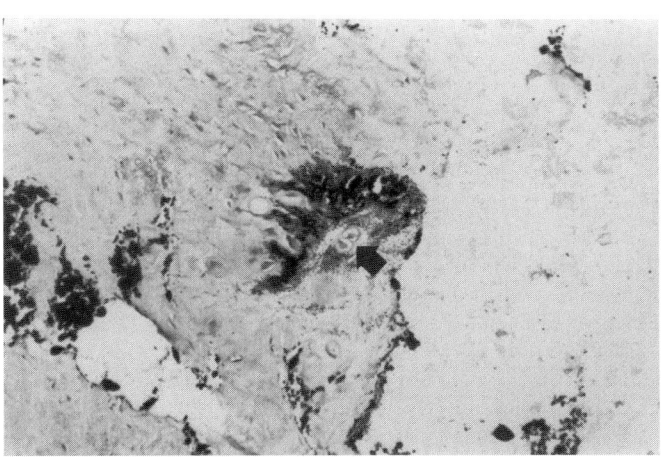

Fig. 4 Formative phase. Note the early calcifications around living chondrocytes (*arrow*). von Kossa × 50. (Reproduced with permission from Uhthoff HK, Loehr JW: Calcific tendinopathy of the rotator cuff: Pathogenesis, diagnosis, and management. *J Am Acad Orthop Surg* 1997;5:183-191.)

The first evidence of calcium deposition is the presence of loosely granular material that stains positive with the von Kossa method (Fig. 4). This material coalesces to form clumps. With the transmission electron microscope, aggregates of rounded structures containing crystalline material are found in a matrix of amorphous debris or irregularly fragmented collagen fibers. Irregularly rectangular crystals are sometimes found within membrane-bound structures resembling matrix vesicles, also called calcifying globules. Infrequently, crystalline densities seem to be embedded between collagen fibers. High-resolution transmission electron microscopy revealed that the crystals are much larger than the classic apatite crystals and have a different configuration.

During this formative phase, inflammation or vessels were notably absent. Other foci were surrounded by tendinous tissue, again without evidence of inflammation. These areas seem to correspond to the resting phase.

Still other foci showed the presence of young mesenchymal cells, epithelioid cells, leukocytes, a certain number of lymphocytes, and occasionally, giant cells. Presence of these cells is indicative of resorption. Indeed, the marked cellular reaction around calcific deposits, often called a calcium granuloma, is considered to constitute a characteristic lesion of calcifying tendinitis. The granulomatous appearance is caused by the presence of multinucleated giant cells (Fig. 5) and macrophages. Archer and associates interpreted the presence of the latter two cell types as a resorption phenomenon. The cellular reaction is often accompanied by capillary or thin-walled vascular channels around the deposits (Fig. 6). Phagocytosed material within macrophages or multinucleated giant cells can be easily discerned. The ultrastructure of these cells shows electron-dense crystalline particles in cytoplasmic vacuoles, but the crystals are somewhat different in appearance from those in the extracellular deposits. Some of the intracellular accumulations have a rounded aspect and are known as microspheroliths or psammomas (Fig. 7).

Small areas representing the process of repair can be found in the general vicinity of calcification, showing considerable variation in appearance. Granulation tissue with young fibroblasts and newly formed capillaries (Fig. 8) contrasts with well-formed scars with vascular channels and maturing fibroblasts that are in the process of alignment along the long axis of the tendon fibers. Using monoclonal antibodies against collagen type III, we were able to confirm collagen neoformation, most pronounced around vascular channels.

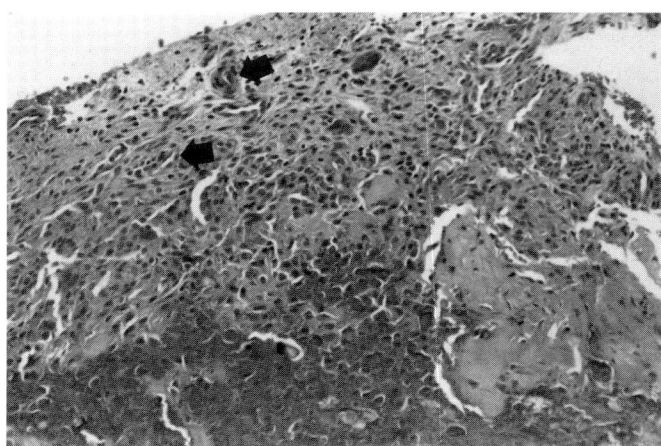

Fig. 6 Resorptive phase. Many thin-walled vascular channels (*arrows*) are seen in the vicinity of calcium deposits undergoing phagocytic resorption. Hematoxylin-eosin, magnification × 50. (Reproduced with permission from Uhthoff HK, Loehr JW: Calcific tendinopathy of the rotator cuff: Pathogenesis, diagnosis, and management. *J Am Acad Orthop Surg* 1997;5:183-191.)

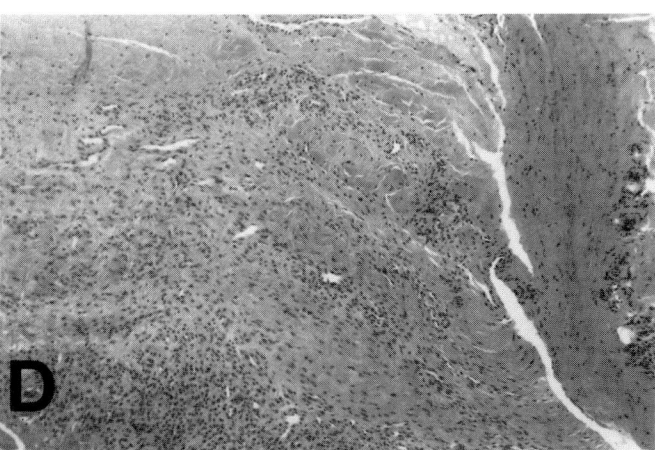

Fig. 8 Postcalcific stage. The calcific deposit is seen in the left lower corner (D). In its immediate vicinity there is still evidence of phagocytic resorption whereas further away fibroblasts elaborate new collagen. Hematoxylin-eosin, × 25. (Reproduced with permission from Uhthoff HK, Loehr JW: Calcific tendinopathy of the rotator cuff: Pathogenesis, diagnosis, and management. *J Am Acad Orthop Surg* 1997;5:183-191.)

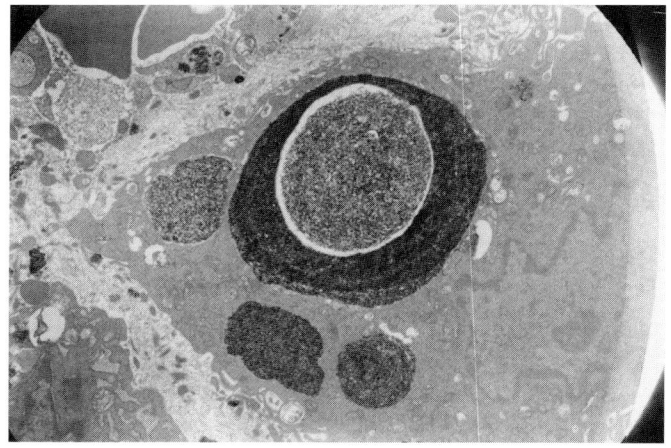

Fig. 7 This electron microphotograph shows a psammoma inside a macrophage beside three smaller accumulations of electron dense material. The multilayered structure of the psammoma is quite evident. Uranyl acetate and lead citrate, × 14,500. (Reproduced with permission from Uhthoff HK, Sarkar K: Calcifying tendinitis, in Rockwood CA Jr, Matsen FA III (eds): *The Shoulder*. Philadelphia, PA, WB Saunders, 1990, vol 2, pp 774-790.)

These changes correspond to the postcalcific stage of our schema (Fig. 1).

Diagnostic Techniques

Calcium deposits in calcifying tendinitis are most often localized in the supraspinatus tendon. In all instances of suspected calcification of the cuff, a radiograph must be obtained. The follow-up radiologic assessment identifies changes in density and in extent of calcification.

Initial radiographs should include an anteroposterior film in neutral rotation and in internal and external rotation. Deposits in the supraspinatus are readily visible on films in neutral rotation, whereas deposits in the infraspinatus and teres minor are best seen in internal rotation. Calcifications in the subscapularis occur only in rare instances, and a radiograph in external rotation will show them well. Axillary views are rarely indicated. Scapular views, however, will help to determine whether a calcification causes an impingement.

In the acute or resorptive phase, calcium deposits are often barely visible on radiographs; they may be visible on computed tomographic images. Magnetic resonance imaging could be indicated under rare circumstances. In T1-weighted images, calcifications appear as areas of decreased signal intensity, whereas T2-weighted images frequently show a perifocal band of increased signal intensity compatible with edema.

Radiographs not only confirm the absence or presence of calcium deposits, they also permit assessment of their extent, delineation, and density.

During the formative phase when pain is chronic or even absent, the deposit is dense, well-defined, and of homogeneous density (Fig. 9). During the resorptive phase, which is characterized by acute pain, the deposit is fluffy, cloud-like, and ill-defined, and its density is irregular (Fig. 10). Rupture of the calcific deposit into the bursa can only occur during the latter phase, given the toothpaste- or cream-like consistency during this phase. Radiographs then show a crescent-shaped radiodensity overlying the deposit (Fig. 11). In longitudinal studies, a change from a dense, well-delineated deposit to a fluffy, ill-defined one can be observed, but the opposite is never seen.

Most authors agree that radiologic evidence of degenerative joint disease is usually lacking in patients with calcific tendinopathies. This scenario holds true for patients in the

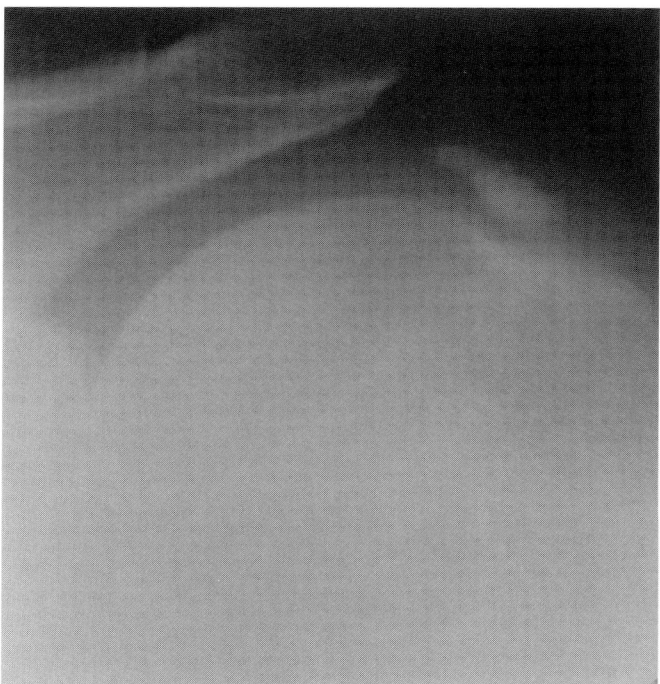

Fig. 9 Calcifying tendinitis in the formative phase. The deposit is dense, well-circumscribed, and homogenous. (Reproduced with permission from Uhthoff HK, Loehr JW: Calcific tendinopathy of the rotator cuff: Pathogenesis, diagnosis, and management. *J Am Acad Orthop Surg* 1997;5:183-191.)

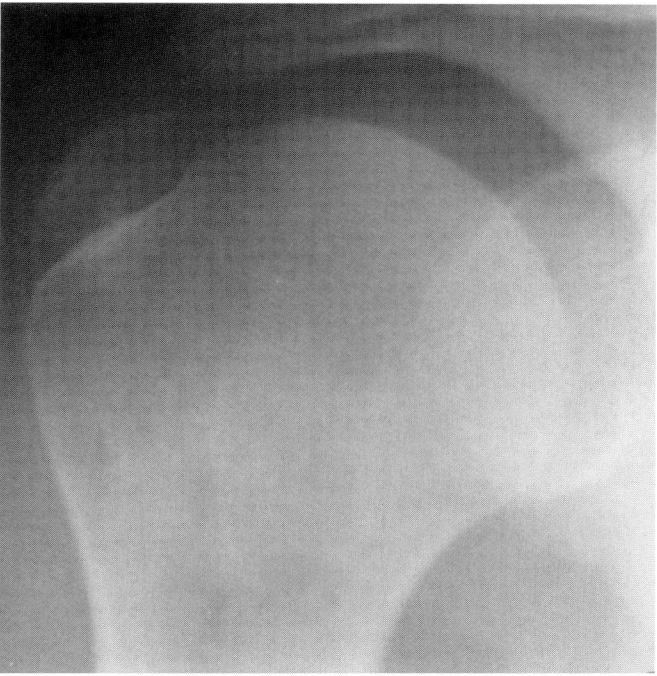

Fig. 10 Calcifying tendinitis in the resorptive phase. The deposit is fluffy and ill-defined. (Reproduced with permission from Uhthoff HK, Loehr JW: Calcific tendinopathy of the rotator cuff: Pathogenesis, diagnosis, and management. *J Am Acad Orthop Surg* 1997;5:183-191.)

fourth and fifth decades of life, when the disease peaks. It is therefore not surprising that in three of our patients in the seventh decade of life, acromioclavicular osteophytes were observed.

Calcifications seen in arthropathies have a quite different appearance; they are stippled and overlie the bony insertion and are always accompanied by degenerative bony or articular changes. These calcium deposits must be clearly distinguished from the reactive intratendinous calcifications.

According to Hartig and Huth, sonography is more sensitive than radiography in detecting calcium deposits. In 90% of 217 patients studied, the deposit could be visualized radiologically and 100% sonographically (as well as histologically). Sonography permits a more exact localization of the deposit without submitting the patient to radiation. Farin and Jaroma found radiography more reliable. Radiographs showed calcifications in 93 patients but sonography in only 87. Only radiography made the distinction between formative and resorptive phase possible.

Management

A distinction between formative and resorptive phase is important for proper management. During the formative phase, the pain is chronic in nature or even absent. On radiographs the deposit appears well-delineated, dense, and homogenous with a chalk-like consistency, and histologic observations show calcification around living chondrocytes. During resorption, on the other hand, the pain is acute, the deposit has a fluffy, ill-defined radiologic appearance, the consistency is cream- or toothpaste-like, and the histologic features are compatible with phagocytic resorption.

Conservative Management In order to avoid loss of mobility of the glenohumeral joint, the patient is instructed to participate in a daily exercise program and to keep the arm in abduction as often as possible. Abduction can be achieved by placing the arm on the backrest of a chair or, when lying down, by putting a pillow under the axilla. Application of moist heat is suggested when the symptoms are subacute. Although ultrasound is occasionally used in our physiotherapy department and has been beneficial to some patients, there is no evidence that ultrasound accelerates the disappearance of calcium.

During the formative phase when symptoms are chronic, intrabursal injections of corticosteroids are only done in the presence of an impingement syndrome. Needling of dense, homogenous deposits has never been attempted nor has lavage ever been successful, possibly because of the chalk-like consistency of the deposit.

During the resorptive phase, when the symptoms are acute or subacute and when radiographs indicate ongoing resorption, a lavage of the deposit is attempted using two large bore needles and 2% xylocaine. The site of lavage is determined radiologically and clinically. In the outflow liquid, calcium particles can be easily recognized. Even when lavage is not successful, the multiple perforations of the site of calcium

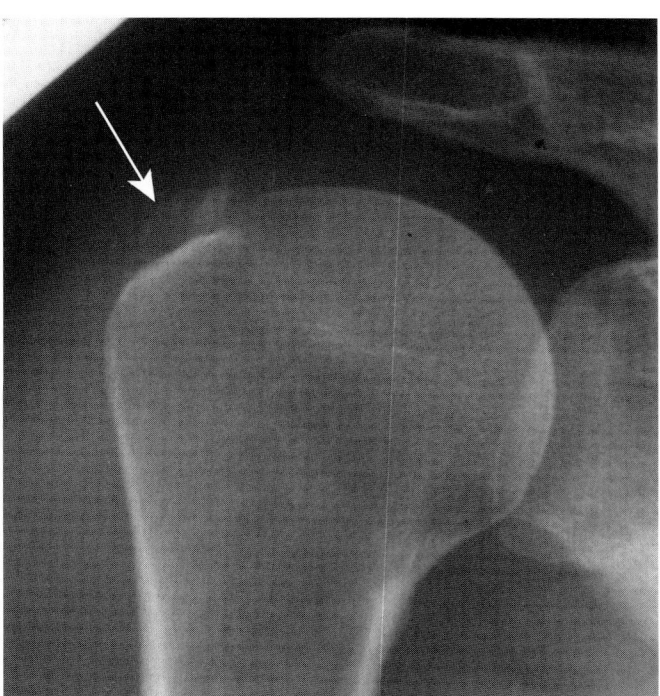

Fig. 11 Calcifying tendinitis in the resorptive phase. The calcium that has ruptured into the subacromial bursa is seen as a crescent-like shadow (*arrow*) overlying the intratendinous deposit. (Reproduced with permission from Uhthoff HK, Loehr JW: Calcific tendinopathy of the rotator cuff: Pathogenesis, diagnosis, and management. *J Am Acad Orthop Surg* 1997;5:183-191.)

deposition will decrease the intratendinous pressure and thus the pain. In a few instances lavage has been repeated. However, the surgeon should take caution not to exceed the toxic dosage of lidocaine in order to avoid the potential complication of a seizure.

Although we prescribe a 1-week regimen of nonsteroidal anti-inflammatory drugs, we have no proof of their beneficial action nor could we find a relevant publication to substantiate this regimen. The symptoms usually decrease after 1 week, at which time the patient is referred for physiotherapy. Clinical and radiologic assessment is performed every 4 weeks.

We never used ultrasound during this phase nor do we recommend radiotherapy. Extracorporeal shock wave therapy, a well-established technique known as lithotripsy in urology, has recently been used for treating calcific deposits. Rompe and associates reported on a series of 40 patients who received 1,500 impulses to the shoulder area under regional anesthesia during a single therapy session. Fifteen of these patients had no improvement, but in 25 a partial or complete disappearance of the calcific deposit was observed. A similar experience was reported by Loew and associates. Fourteen of 20 patients with "chronic, symptomatic calcifying tendinitis" experienced symptomatic improvement at the time of follow-up (limited to 12 weeks). These 14 patients developed local hematomas after this therapy. Thirty percent of the patients had an improvement of the Constant score and in seven the deposit disappeared completely. Extracorporeal shock wave therapy is still under investigation, and longer follow-up studies, a larger patient population, and reports from other centers are necessary before this technique can be recommended.

Surgical Management
Should conservative therapy fail during the formative phase, surgery may become necessary. Surgery is very rarely indicated during the resorptive phase when nature attempts, and usually succeeds with, the removal of the deposit.

Gschwend and associates formulated the three indications for surgery: progression of symptoms; constant pain interfering with activities of daily living; and absence of improvement of symptoms after conservative therapy. Surgery, be it arthroscopically or through an open approach, is performed on an outpatient basis.

Ark and associates believed that the advantages of arthroscopic surgery for calcifying tendinitis are a shorter rehabilitation time, possibly a better functional result, and a better cosmetic appearance than after open surgery. Postoperative management consists of range-of-motion exercises, starting with pendulum exercises, then going on to active-assisted exercises after the third day, and progressing to active exercises as tolerated. Usually no arm sling is necessary except for patient comfort at night.

It should be stressed once more that surgical removal is the exception and that it is indicated only when adequate conservative measures have failed and when symptoms interfere with work or activities of daily living. A sling is applied after surgery. We stress that this sling must be removed at least four times a day for pendulum and gentle, passive range-of-motion exercises. The sling is permanently removed after 3 days and active exercises are started. We encourage patients to keep the arm in abduction as often as possible. We have never resorted to postoperative corticosteroid injections.

Most authors see no or only a limited indication for an associated acromioplasty, and few seem to agree with Goutallier and associates that an isolated acromioplasty is sufficient.

In conclusion, the stage of disease must be determined for optimal treatment results. There are not two forms of calcifying tendinitis, a chronic and an acute one, but only two phases of the same disease. Should conservative care fail, surgery may become necessary, foremost in the formative phase of the disease.

Chondrocalcinosis

Chondrocalcinosis (CC) is a general term denoting deposition of calcium salts in hyaline and fibrocartilage of joints. Calcium salts can consist of calcium pyrophosphate dihydrate (CPPD), calcium hydroxyapatite, dicalcium phosphate dihydrate crystals, or a combination of these three. CC does not imply any symptomatology.

Intra-articular deposition of CPPD may lead to structural changes of cartilage and bone, a condition known as pyrophosphate arthropathy. This condition, which usually starts in the knee, is seen most often in the elderly and is rare in persons under 50 years of age. Twenty percent of all persons over 80 years of age are affected.

The clinical syndrome of acute synovitis associated with intra-articular CPPD deposits is termed pseudogout. This discussion will focus on pertinent features of CC and features special to the shoulder.

Familial CC was first described by Zitnan and associates, who later described radiologic signs of progression of this disease. The mode of transmission is believed to be autosomal dominant. In support of this mode of transmission is a recent study by Hughes and associates, who described a gene that causes CC and showed linkage with several polymorphic markers on chromosome 5p. Similar analysis was reported by Baldwin and associates. They found a genetic link between the disease and chromosome 8q in another family.

It is doubtful whether increased calcium concentration as present in hyperparathyroidism is responsible for the deposition of CPPD. Moreover, the articular symptoms persist after removal of the parathyroid adenoma. It has been speculated that the presence of inhibitory ions such as calcium, iron, and/or copper causes a reduced breakdown of inorganic pyrophosphate by alkaline phosphatase.

Reduced levels of hypophosphatase may also lead to CC. Repeated joint insults may also lead to CC, as does surgical trauma. It could well be that the resulting hemarthrosis favors the deposition of CPPD crystals. The precise relationship between osteoarthritis and CPPD deposition remains unknown. Despite the fact that both may coexist, both conditions can occur independently of the other.

The presence of microspheroids of hydroxyapatite in the joint fluid of the shoulder has been noted by McCarty and associates. This condition led to the term Milwaukee shoulder, which is also characterized by the presence of a massive cuff tear and degenerative osteoarticular changes. It is of interest to note that in an apparently identical condition described as cuff arthropathy, Neer and associates did not describe the presence of crystals. The incidence of CC of the shoulder in pseudogout can reach 50%. The clinical signs and symptoms of CC of the shoulder may mimic aseptic arthritis, as Hughes and associates have shown.

Pathology

Deposition of CPPD crystals is confined to the connective tissues of the locomotor system. Primary deposition occurs in the cartilage with secondary release into the joint fluid and uptake by synovial tissues. In the degenerating articular cartilage, microcrystalline CPPD deposits are seen early on, around hypertrophic chondrocytes. This early precipitation is followed in time by tophi-like accumulations. The surrounding cartilage may show loss of metachromasia and cloning of chondrocytes. In instances of severe cartilage changes, the trabeculae of the subchondral bone appear thickened and multiple cysts develop. Bone fragmentation and collapse will follow in time.

Diagnosis

The presence of chondrocalcinosis is confirmed by radiography. Whereas the articular cartilage shows fine to sometimes coarse and linear calcifications parallel to but separate from the subchondral bone (Fig. 12), deposits in other structures such as the labra of the glenohumeral joint and the menisci of knees have an irregular, mottled outline. In advanced cases of

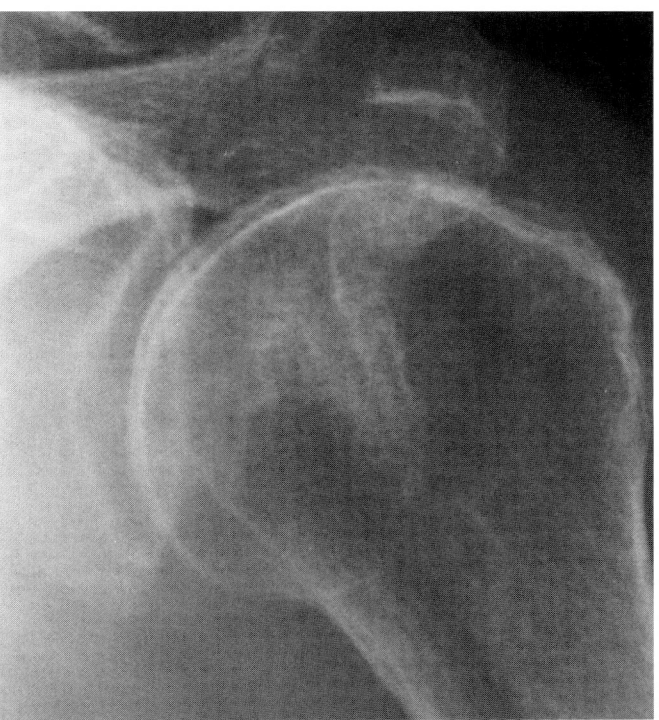

Fig. 12 Typical chondrocalcinosis of the left humeral head in a 75-year-old woman. Linear calcifications parallel to but separate from the subchondral bone are clearly seen. (Courtesy of Dr. Martin Lecompte, Quebec, Canada.)

CC, osteophyte formation and collapse of the subchondral bone are regularly observed. Bilateral and symmetrical involvement of joints is common in CC.

Because aspiration of joint fluid is not indicated in CC, no results have been reported. In pseudogout, however, the fluid is often turbid and blood-stained. Whereas CPPD crystals are usually not visualized by light microscopy, polarization reveals the presence of weakly birefringent crystals.

Therapy

Because there is no etiotropic treatment known for CC, the aim of therapy is nosotropic, ie, directed at the symptoms. Consequently, the mere presence of CC is not an indication for therapy. In the presence of effusion, joint aspiration followed by a corticosteroid injection should be considered. It must be noted, however, that the Gram stain has been negative, as well as results of culture.

Additional benefit can be gained from the prescription of simple analgesics and nonsteroidal anti-inflammatory drugs. Although colchicine has been recommended for treatment during an acute attack of pseudogout, its effect seems uncertain. Other supportive measures such as reduction of adverse mechanical stresses must form part of the overall treatment regimen. Underlying metabolic diseases should be identified and treated properly to decrease symptoms and to improve function.

Heterotopic Ossification

Heterotopic ossification (HO) has been reported in the past as a complication of acromial surgery. It has also been observed after traumatic acromioclavicular dislocations accompanied by disruption of the coronoid and trapezoid ligaments; it often follows the course of the coracoacromial ligament. Although rarely occurring after elective shoulder surgery, HO is a well-documented complication of proximal humeral fractures either managed by closed or open reduction or after prosthetic hemiarthroplasty.

An incidence ranging from 15% to 45% has been reported in patients in whom HO was believed to be responsible for an impaired function. In a retrospective study reviewing 333 patients who had an acromioplasty, or distal clavicle resection either by open or arthroscopic methods, a 3.2% incidence of HO was found. On radiographs, HO appeared as monolocular or as multilocular bone formations (Fig. 13). In 28 patients they were localized close to the acromion, but in 6 of them they encroached on the so-called "supraspinatus outlet," causing a recurrent impingement syndrome. Of 20 patients who underwent revision surgery, four developed a recurrence of heterotopic bone formation.

HO should not be confused with calcifications occurring in rotator cuff tendons nor with reactive ossifications of the shoulder because they might occur as a sequence of a posterior subluxation. These ossifications are also known as Bennett lesions.

Preventive measures either by radiotherapy or nonsteroidal anti-inflammatory medications, such as indomethacin, should be considered in patients with a risk for developing ectopic ossifications, particularly those who exhibit signs of hypertrophic pulmonary osteoarthropathy or ankylosing spondylitis.

Pigmented Villonodular Synovitis

Pigmented villonodular synovitis (PVNS) is a proliferative lesion affecting synovial tissues of joints and tendon sheaths, and presents as a monoarticular multifocal condition. The annual incidence in the United States has been reported as 1.8 patients per million, with the knee joint being affected most often (80%). PVNS of the shoulder is a rare disease and might occur as a single or multifocal process more likely to occur in the younger adult. The clinical presentation includes a slow, insidious onset of limitation of motion, swelling, and later on, pain.

Radiographically, subchondral and intraosseous cyst formations begin, more often in the humeral head than in the glenoid; secondary osteoarthrosis is common. The diagnosis is refined with imaging techniques such as computed tomography, which demonstrates a mass within the joint, and magnetic resonance imaging with different gradient echo sequences. While reports of larger series of PVNS have included various joints, studies of shoulder involvement are still limited to case reports.

The diagnosis is based on histologic examination. Any differential diagnosis has to include other synovial lesions. Hemosiderotic arthropathy or hemosynovitis resulting from multiple recurrent bleedings has a characteristic histologic appearance. The disease has been found in children and is known for its asymmetric presentation. Extra-articular synovial sarcoma or synovial hemangioma should also be considered, as should rheumatoid and tuberculous arthritis and hemophilic arthropathy.

The treatment concept based on experience gained in more commonly involved joints has been simple synovectomy for cases in which the villonodular synovitis has been circumscribed, whereas for those with diffuse destruction a shoulder replacement has been suggested in conjunction with a synovectomy. Incomplete synovectomy is likely to lead to the development of a local recurrence, whereas complete synovectomy seems to give the best results.

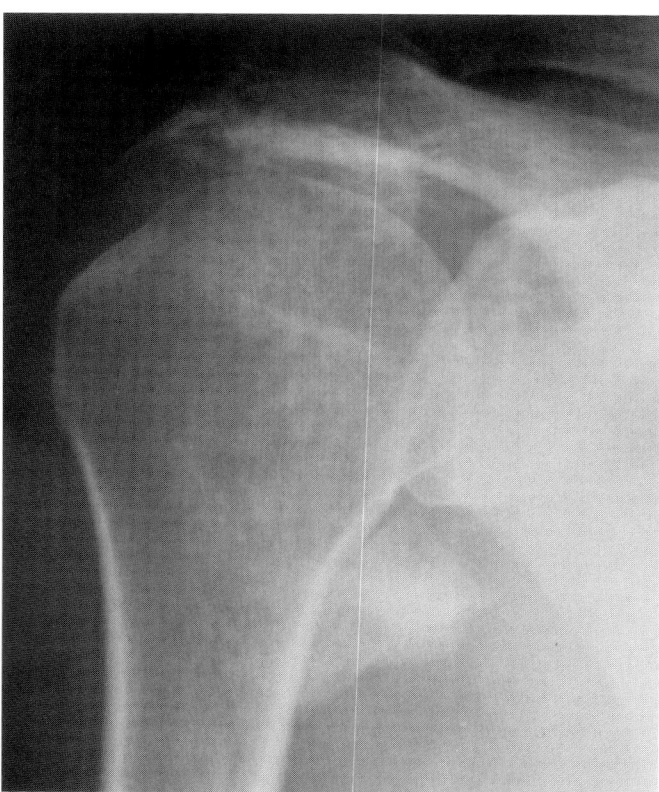

Fig. 13 Heterotopic ossification of the shoulder in a 46-year-old man.

Selected Bibliography

Calcifying Tendinitis

Archer RS, Bayley JI, Archer CW, et al: Cell and matrix changes associated with pathological calcification of the human rotator cuff tendons. *J Anat* 1993;182:1-11.

In this thorough study, the authors document the widespread labeling for chondroitin-4-sulphate/dermatan sulphate and the intense pericellular chondroitin-6-sulphate accumulation. They were unable to obtain a positive stain for type II collagen.

Ark JW, Flock TJ, Flatow EL, et al: Arthroscopic treatment of calcific tendinitis of the shoulder. *Arthroscopy* 1992;8:183-188.

In 23 patients who had shoulder pain for more than 1 year, the authors obtained good results in 11, satisfactory results in nine, and unsatisfactory ones in two. They conclude that arthroscopy is a reasonable alternative to open procedures.

Brooks CH, Revell WJ, Heatley FW: A quantitative histological study of the vascularity of the rotator cuff tendon. *J Bone Joint Surg* 1992;74B:151-153.

In this quantitative histologic analysis, the authors found that a zone of hypovascularity 15 mm in width exists close to the insertion into bone of supraspinatus and infraspinatus. They conclude that factors other than vascularity are important in tendinopathies.

Farin PU, Jaroma H: Sonographic findings of rotator cuff calcifications. *J Ultrasound Med* 1995;14:7-14.

From this study the authors conclude that plain radiographs should always be obtained before sonograms. Only radiographs allow a distinction between formative and resorptive phases, whereas sonograms proved to be superior in the detection of large and slurry calcifications and intrabursal accumulation of calcium.

Gärtner J: Tendinosis calcarea: Results of treatment with needling. *Z Orthop Ihre Grenzgeb* 1993;131:461-469.

Thirty-three patients treated with needling and lavage were followed for more than 1 year. In 23 patients, the deposit had disappeared at follow-up.

Hartig A, Huth F: Neue aspekte zur morphologie und therapie der tendinosis calcarea der Schultergelenke. *Arthroskopie* 1995;8:117-122.

In this report of 217 patients who underwent arthroscopy and removal of calcium deposit, preoperative sonographic examination and histologic assessment revealed the presence of calcium salts in 100%; radiographs showed the presence of calcium in only 90%. The authors warn that spontaneous resorption does not always occur.

Hsu HC, Wu JJ, Jim YF, et al: Calcific tendinitis and rotator cuff tearing: A clinical and radiographic study. *J Shoulder Elbow Surg* 1994;3:159-164.

In this study from Taiwan, the age of the 82 patients with calcifying tendinitis was much higher than in reported series. The incidence of arthrographic evidence of rotator cuff tearing was 28%. This incidence was predominant in men (77.9%).

Kempf JF, Bonnomet F, Nerrison D, et al: Arthroscopic isolated excision of rotator cuff calcium deposits, in Gazielly DF, Gleyze P, Thomas T (eds): *The Cuff*. Amsterdam, The Netherlands, Elsevier Science, 1997, pp 164-167.

The authors report on three different studies, all of which confirmed that no advantage could be gained by adding an acromioplasty. Furthermore, best results were noted when the deposit has been excised completely.

Loew M, Jurgowski W, Mau HC, et al: Treatment of calcifying tendinitis of rotator cuff by extracorporeal shock waves: A preliminary report. *J Shoulder Elbow Surg* 1995;4:101-106.

In 20 patients observed over a 12-week period, all underwent two sessions of shock with 2,000 pulses each (18 to 22 kV); 15 patients experienced a marked reduction in symptoms and a 30% improvement of their Constant score. More accurate details would have been helpful.

Lohr JF, Uhthoff HK: The microvascular pattern of the supraspinatus tendon. *Clin Orthop* 1990;254:35-38.

In this cadaver study, the microvascular pattern of the supraspinatus tendon was examined in 18 specimens. A hypovascular zone was seen close to the insertion. The frontal section, however, showed a sparse vascularity at the articular side of the tendon whereas the bursal side was abundantly supplied by vessels.

Mohr W, Bilger S: Basic morphologic structures of calcified tendopathy and their significance for pathogenesis. *Z Rheumatol* 1990;49:346-355.

These authors place the formation of psammoma bodies containing hydroxyapatite crystals at the beginning of the process of calcium deposition. They hypothesize that injury to cells leads to an intracellular accumulation of calcium that is subsequently extruded into the extracellular space. This paper does not seem to distinguish between calcifications inside the tendon and those at the insertion.

Molé D, Kempf JF, Gleyze P, et al: Results of endoscopic treatment on non-broken tendinopathies of the rotator cuff: 2. Calcifications of the rotator cuff. *Rev Chir Orthop Reparatrice Appar Mot* 1993;79:532-541.

This is essentially a review article. The authors conclude that arthroscopic treatment has reduced the morbidity when compared to open surgery. Moreover, the results are said to be superior.

Ollagnier E, Bruyère G, Gazielly DF, et al: Medical treatment of calcifying tendinopathies of the rotator cuff, in Gazielly DF, Gleyze P, Thomas T (eds): *The Cuff*. Amsterdam, The Netherlands, Elsevier Science, 1997, pp 147-151.

The authors report on their experience with anti-inflammatory radiotherapy (dosage not stated) in 47 patients. They obtained "good subjective results" in 68%. The time span from therapy to relief of pain was 43 days. It "appears to promote the radiographic disappearance of calcifications."

Re LP Jr, Karzel RP: Management of rotator cuff calcifications. *Orthop Clin North Am* 1993;24:125-132.

This article is a report on 112 patients with chronic calcifying tendinitis who underwent arthroscopic surgery. The approach led to an objective success in 89% and to a subjective success in 82%. After a follow-up of an average of 20.9 months, a disappearance of symptoms was noted in 88 patients. Total removal led to better results. An associated acromioplasty did not improve results.

Resch H, Povacz P, Seykora P: Excision of calcium deposit and acromioplasty, in Gazielly DF, Gleyze P, Thomas T (eds): *The Cuff.* Amsterdam, The Netherlands, Elsevier Science, 1997, pp 169-171.

The authors propose strict criteria for an additional acromioplasty such as a type III acromion in patients with diffusely spread calcium deposits and small deposits. Inflammation around the deposit and large deposits causing an impingement are not an indication for acromioplasty.

Rompe JD, Rumler F, Hopf C, et al: Extracorporeal shock wave therapy for calcifying tendinitis of the shoulder. *Clin Orthop* 1995;321:196-201.

This report covers 40 patients who underwent one shock treatment with 1,500 pulses. Follow-up time was 24 weeks. There was no improvement in 15 patients, and partial or complete disappearance of the deposit in 25.

Tillmann B: Rotatorenmanschettenrupturen. *Operative Orthopädie und Traumatologie* 1992;4:181-184.

This article is a study of the vascularity of the rotator cuff in an unstated number of specimens using India ink-gelatin. The author found an avascular area in the supraspinatus close to the bony insertion but not in the subscapularis or the infraspinatus.

Toriyama K, Fukuda H, Hamada K, et al: Calcifying tendinitis of the infraspinatus tendon simulating a bone tumor. *J Shoulder Elbow Surg* 1994;3:165-168.

In this study, calcification of the infraspinatus invading the greater tuberosity gave the impression radiologically of a bone tumor. Biopsy confirmed the presence of calcifying tendinitis.

Uhthoff HK, Sarkar K: Calcifying tendinitis, in Rockwood CA Jr, Matsen FA III (eds): *The Shoulder.* Philadelphia, PA, WB Saunders, 1990, vol 2, pp 774-790.

This review article includes 108 references. An updated version will be found in the second edition scheduled for publication in 1997.

Chondrocalcinosis

Abramson SB: Treatment of gout and crystal arthropathies and uses and mechanisms of action of nonsteroidal anti-inflammatory drugs. *Curr Opin Rheumatol* 1992:4;295-300.

This review article discusses the recent literature of the actions of nonsteroidal anti-inflammatory drugs on gout and crystal arthropathies, with 39 references.

Baldwin CT, Farrer LA, Adair R, et al: Linkage of early-onset osteoarthritis and chondrocalcinosis to human chromosome 8q. *Am J Hum Genet* 1995:56;692-697.

This study of a large New England family with early-onset CPPD and severe degenerative osteoarthritis shows a genetic linkage between the disease of this family and chromosome 8q.

Doherty M: Calcium pyrophosphate dihydrate, in Klippel JH, Dieppe P (eds): *Rheumatology.* St. Louis, MO, Mosby-Year Book, 1994, pp 1-12.

This is a comprehensive review article with 40 references and 20 schemata.

Hughes AE, McGibbon D, Woodward E, et al: Localisation of a gene for chondrocalcinosis to chromosome 5p. *Hum Mol Genet* 1995;4:1225-1228.

This study revealed the location of the gene causing chondrocalcinosis in a large family by typing all available family members.

Ishikawa K, Masuda I, Ohira T, et al: A histological study of calcium pyrophosphate dihydrate crystal-deposition disease. *J Bone Joint Surg* 1989;71A:875-886.

This splendidly illustrated study shows the histologic, ultrastructural, and crystalline structures of CPPD deposition.

Masuda I, Ishikawa K, Usuku G: A histologic and immunohistochemical study of calcium pyrophosphate dihydrate crystal deposition disease. *Clin Orthop* 1991;263:272-287.

This study documents the presence of dermatan sulfate proteoglycan, type I collagen, and S-100 protein in and around hypertrophic chondrocytes.

Menkès CJ, Chouraki L: Chondrocalcinose articulaire. Éditions Techniques. *Encycl Med Chir Appareil locomoteur* 1993;14-271A-10:1-10.

This is an excellent review article in French, with 109 references.

Heterotopic Ossification

Berg EE, Ciullo JV: Heterotopic ossification after acromioplasty and distal clavicle resection. *J Shoulder Elbow Surg* 1995;4:188-193.

Of 333 patients undergoing an isolated acromioplasty, or a distal clavicle resection, 40 patients were found to develop postoperative ectopic bone formation. Bone formation occurred after open as well as after arthroscopic procedures. In 22 patients heterotopic bone formation was observed close to the acromion, encroaching on the so-called "supraspinatus outlet." In 28 patients periclavicular heterotopic bone formation was found. Ossifications of the coracoacromial ligament were found to be asymptomatic. It is suggested that prophylactic treatment should be considered in patients demonstrating signs of pulmonary osteoarthropathy or active spondyloarthropathy.

Berg EE, Ciullo JV, Oglesby JW: Failure of arthroscopic decompression by subacromial heterotopic ossification causing recurrent impingement. *Arthroscopy* 1994;10:158-161.

In a series of patients treated by arthroscopic subacromial decompression, ten were noted to have developed heterotopic ossifications postoperatively. In ten other patients, HO occurred after an arthroscopic decompression and distal clavicle resection. None of the patients were manual laborers. HO occurred at one site only in seven patients and at two sites in three patients. Bone formation developed between 2 and 5 months postoperatively. Eight of the patients had evidence of recurrent impingement, and five patients went on to a revision procedure. The authors conclude that male patients with hypertrophic pulmonary osteoarthropathy should be considered at risk for heterotopic ossifications, warranting prophylactic measures.

Ferrari JD, Ferrari DA, Coumas J, et al: Posterior ossification of the shoulder: The Bennett lesion. Etiology, diagnosis, and treatment. *Am J Sports Med* 1994;22:171-176.

The authors report on an ossific lesion of the posterior inferior glenoid rim, situated extra-articularly. This Bennett lesion was associated with a posterior inferior subluxation in persons involved in repetitive overhead shoulder movements; it should not be confused with heterotopic ossification or triceps tendon injury.

Moeckel BH, Dines DM, Warren RF, et al: Modular hemiarthroplasty for fractures of the proximal part of the humerus. *J Bone Joint Surg* 1992;74A:884-889.

The results of treatment in 22 displaced proximal humerus fractures treated with a reconstructive hemiarthroplasty were reviewed. HO was present in nine shoulders, classified after the Brooker grading system from one to four. Except for two patients the ossification did not lead to an impairment of the clinical outcome.

Pigmented Villonodular Synovitis

Cotten A, Flipo RM, Mestdagh H, et al: Diffuse pigmented villonodular synovitis of the shoulder. *Skeletal Radiol* 1995;24:311-313.

This report deals with one patient treated for pigmented villonodular synovitis with a subtotal synovectomy. The different types of imaging are discussed. In particular, magnetic resonance imaging in different gradient echoes allows differentiation between hemophilic arthropathies and villonodular synovitis, or other synovial pathologic conditions.

France MP, Gupta SK: Nonhemophilic hemosiderotic synovitis of the shoulder: A case report. *Clin Orthop* 1991;262:132-136.

This is a case report of a 72-year-old man who underwent synovectomy of therapy-resistant shoulder pain. Histologic results demonstrated a hemosiderotic synovitis (not a pigmented villonodular synovitis) associated with repetitive inbleeding in a progressively destructed joint. Early recognition and therapy may prevent destruction of the joint and the cuff.

Kay RM, Eckardt JJ, Mirra JM: Multifocal pigmented villonodular synovitis in a child: A case report. *Clin Orthop* 1996;322:194-197.

The authors report on an 11-year-old boy with asymmetric multifocal pigmented villonodular synovitis of the shoulder. The patient was treated in different stages by excisional biopsy with no recurrence after 3 years. It is believed that pigmented villonodular synovitis should be considered in the differential diagnosis of any polycentric lesion.

Mulier T, Victor J, Van Den Bergh J, et al: Diffuse pigmented villonodular synovitis of the shoulder: A case report and review of the literature. *Acta Orthop Belg* 1992;58:93-96.

A patient presented with a painful shoulder and slow onset of swelling. During surgery a rotator cuff tear associated with a diffuse pigmented villonodular synovitis was found. An open synovectomy, acromioplasty, and cuff repair led to a good result.

32

Rehabilitation of the Shoulder

W. Ben Kibler, MD

Introduction

The ultimate goal of rehabilitation of the injured shoulder is maximum restoration of shoulder function. Function may be best summarized as "where anatomy meets physiology and biomechanics." Understanding normal physiology and biomechanics and the pathophysiology of shoulder injury will allow a more complete framework for organization of the rehabilitation process. Knowledge of normal shoulder function is essential for implementing efficacious shoulder rehabilitation. Protocols and guidelines that emphasize restoration of normal motions, force couples, and biomechanics will allow quickest return to activity.

Basic Concepts

Physiologic and Biomechanical Basis for Shoulder Rehabilitation: Mobility Versus Stability

The shoulder functions most effectively in a relatively limited set of anatomic conditions that create a balance between the mobility necessary to achieve the wide ranges of joint motion and disparate joint and bone positions that are necessary for athletic activity (Table 1), and the stability necessary to allow a normal path of the instant center of joint motion in the face of large forces and translatory and distraction loads that occur in normal throwing or serving (Table 2).

Mobility is possible because of the "large ball/small socket" bony arrangement of the shoulder and the voluminous glenohumeral joint capsule that does not restrict motion except at its extremes. The scapula is also highly mobile because of the limited bony constraint of the clavicle. The scapula can therefore retract and protract on the thoracic wall to follow the moving humerus, and rotate and elevate to avoid humeral impingement.

Stability is achieved by the interaction of bony, ligamentous, and muscular constraint systems that control the move-

Table 1. Normal joint motions and bony positions around the shoulder joint

Scapula	
Rotation through arc of 65° with shoulder abduction	
Translation on thorax up to 15 cm	
Glenohumeral	
Abduction	140°
Internal/External Rotation	90°/90°
Translation	
Anterior/Posterior	5 to 10 mm
Inferior/Superior	4 to 5 mm
Total Rotations	
Baseball	185°
Tennis	165°

Table 2. Forces and loads on the shoulder in normal athletic activity

Activity	Forces and Loads
Rotational velocities	
Baseball	7,000°/sec
Tennis serve	1,500°/sec
Tennis forehand	245°/sec
Tennis backhand	870°/sec
Angular velocities	
Baseball	1,150°/sec
Acceleration forces	
Internal rotation	60 N·m
Horizontal adduction	70 N·m
Anterior shear	400 N·m
Deceleration forces	
Horizontal abduction	80 N·m
Posterior shear	500 N·m
Compression	70 N·m

ment of the instant center of motion of the glenohumeral joint. In the midranges of motion, very little translation of the humerus occurs on the glenoid, but at the extremes of motion in flexion, abduction, or rotation, translation occurs within certain limits. This means that despite the anatomic "large ball/small socket" discrepancy, the glenohumeral joint does function as a ball-and-socket joint in most positions during throwing or serving, being stabilized by the ligaments mainly at the extremes of motion, and muscles at rest and during the midrange of motion.

Constraint Systems Around the Shoulder

The bony constraints do contribute to stability. The geometry of the joint surfaces allows smooth conformity of the humerus and glenoid of the scapula. The glenoid is enlarged and deepened by the labrum, which will increase the conformity, thereby increasing the "concavity-compression" effect that helps to control translation. The conformity is maximized by proper positioning of the scapula with the glenoid, in relation to the moving arm. This positioning will depend on proper scapular muscle activity. The glenohumeral joint has been statically compared to a "golf ball on a tee" in terms of its size relationships. A more appropriate description of the dynamic situation would be Rowe's comparison to a "ball on the seal's nose." As the ball (humerus) moves, the seal (scapula and glenoid) moves to maintain the balanced relationship.

The ligamentous constraints are the primary stabilizers at extremes of motion in rotation, abduction, or flexion. They control both anterior/posterior and superior/inferior translation, and control "coupled translation," or translation that occurs at the limit of normal rotation. Different parts of the ligamentous structures are the main restraints at different

Table 3. Force couples around the shoulder

Force Couple	Examples

Coordinated coactivation
  Low net torque
  Increased joint control
  Joint stability
	Upper trapezius/levator scapulae: Lower trapezius/serratus anterior to control scapular rotation
	Deltoid: Subscapularis/ infraspinatus/teres minor to control glenohumeral rotation

Agonist/antagonist
  Increased joint torque and motion
  Larger number of muscles, distant and local to joint
  Coordinated sequencing
	Trapezius/rhomboids: Serratus to control scapular retraction and protraction
	Pectoralis/latissimus dorsi: Posterior deltoid/infraspinatus/teres minor to control upper arm internal rotation

glenohumeral positions. The ligaments work in a static fashion to limit translation and rotation, but their stiffness and torsional rigidity are increased with concomitant muscle activity. Both rotator cuff activity and biceps activity have been shown to stiffen the capsule and decrease glenohumeral translation.

The muscular constraints work in several ways to allow stability. First, as has already been mentioned, they contribute to the other constraint systems by dynamic positioning of the scapula and by increasing capsuloligamentous stiffness. Second, they can act as dynamic ligaments when their passive elements are used to limit joint excursion when the muscles are put on stretch. Third, and most importantly, they act as parts of force couples around the joint, either controlling the joint motion, controlling the position of the bones and joint, or by controlling and directing the force through the joint.

Force Couples Around the Shoulder
Two types of force couples work around the shoulder joint (Table 3). The first is coactivation, or coordinated simultaneous activation of agonist and antagonist muscles about a joint. This activation creates low net torque around the joint but creates increased control of motion. The net effect of these activations is to increase joint stability. Examples of this activation would be upper trapezius/levator scapulae working with lower trapezius/serratus anterior muscles to control scapular rotation, and deltoid working with rotator cuff to control glenohumeral rotation.

The second force couple is agonist/antagonist activity, with coordinated excitation of the agonist and inhibition of the antagonist muscles. This activation will increase joint torque and motion, thereby increasing and transferring forces through the joint. These local activations are usually part of a sequence of activations involving other muscles and joints to develop ultimate force and momentum. Examples of this type of activation would include trapezius/rhomboids working with the serratus anterior muscle to move the scapula in relation to the moving arm, and pectoralis/latissimus dorsi working with posterior deltoid/infraspinatus/teres minor muscles to create glenohumeral internal rotation.

The Kinematic Chain
Sequential coordinated muscle activation is necessary to produce the torques and accelerations around the shoulder that allow normal shoulder function. The intrinsic shoulder musculature does not have the capability to generate the recorded values. Mathematical analysis, based on measured velocities throughout the tennis serve in elite players, shows that the shoulder link contributes about 13% of the total kinetic energy during the tennis serve, and is contributing 10% of the total forward arm velocity at the moment of ball impact (Table 4).

The sequential activation that occurs to assist the shoulder in most throwing or serving activities is a proximal to distal activation of the links in a kinematic chain. This proximal to distal sequencing allows generation, summation, and transfer of velocities, energy, and accelerations from the proximal segments of the legs and back through the shoulder, to be added to the contributions of the distal segments of the arm. The primary pattern of muscle activation for this link sequencing is a force-dependent, agonist/antagonist pattern, with each link being activated in the specific sequence for each shoulder activity. The shoulder not only functions as a small energy generator in this sequence, but also as a funnel for the transfer and concentration of the forces generated from the proximal links. The efficiency with which this is accomplished depends on the stability of the joint.

It appears that the primary force couple activation pattern of local muscles around the shoulder joint to allow this stability is the length-dependent, coordinated coactivation, stabilization pattern. This pattern would regulate the transferred forces, allow humeral head compression, allow ball-and-socket motion in the midranges of motion, and help stiffen the capsule at the extremes of motion.

The muscles around the shoulder, both locally and regionally, have major input into normal shoulder function, both as part of the muscular constraint system, but also in complementing the other constraint systems. This has important implications for shoulder rehabilitation because muscles can be effectively rehabilitated and conditioned in many ways.

Pathophysiology Accompanying Shoulder Injury
Shoulder pathology results from acute macrotrauma or chronic repetitive microtrauma. Each type of mechanism has characteristic presentations and associated anatomic and clin-

Table 4. Contributions of each shoulder link

Link	Velocity (m/sec)	Mass (kg)	Kinetic Energy (Joules)	%	Accel (m/sec/sec)	Force (Mass × Accel)	%
Hip/trunk	2.7	54	197.1	51	13.5	729	54
Shoulder	3.3	9	49.1	13	33	297	21
Elbow	6.4	4	82	21	53	212	15
Wrist	7.8	2	61	15	65	130	10

ical implications. It is important to note that chronic microtrauma injuries may produce a group of tissues that are not overtly symptomatic, but are objectively not normal. Examples are scarred posterior capsular tissues, resulting in restricted glenohumeral internal rotation; weak infraspinatus muscles, resulting in force couple imbalance; and inhibited lower trapezius and serratus anterior muscles, resulting in loss of scapular control. These abnormal tissues impose a biomechanical inefficiency on shoulder function, and may contribute to pathology or complicate rehabilitation. Acute macrotrauma injuries include fracture of the clavicle, acute traumatic shoulder dislocation, and acromioclavicular joint sprain. Examples of chronic microtrauma are rotator cuff tendinitis, nontraumatic capsuloligamentous instability, and attritional labral tears.

In the presence of macrotrauma or microtrauma, the pathologic process alters the normal bony, ligamentous, or muscular constraint systems so that the normal path of the instant center of rotation is not constrained. Pathology may involve only one of the constraint systems, but because the constraint systems interact to allow mobility while conferring stability, there is usually some involvement of several constraints. The constraint systems may fail individually (one system only; eg, clavicle fracture or acute Bankart lesion), concurrently (two or three at the same time; eg, rotator cuff tear with anterior dislocation), or consecutively (failure of one followed by failure of others; eg, posterior cuff weakness and inflexibility followed by anterior humeral translation and labral tear). The initiating factor in the pathology is commonly local, but alterations in other parts of the kinematic chain may produce loads or stresses that have clinical expression at the shoulder because of the shoulder's role as a funnel for developed forces.

From a rehabilitation standpoint, alterations in the muscular constraint system are the most important because these alterations can be modified and improved by appropriate protocols, and because of the important role the muscular system plays in complementing and increasing the efficiency of the other constraint systems.

The largest alterations in the muscular constraint system are caused by changes in the neurologic control of the muscle rather than by direct muscle injury. Neurologic changes affect the muscular constraint system by altering local strength development and the organization of the motor firing patterns necessary for force-dependent kinematic chain activity. Most of the muscle weakness seen in the postoperative or postinjury period is caused by decreased neural drive, a central nervous system-controlled combination of activation and coordination of muscle firing patterns. Central nervous system control of motor function is based, in part, on stored specific patterns of sequential muscle activation that guide a complex motor task. This motor pattern is learned through repetition and practice. The stored motor pattern can be recalled easily with little thought. Many factors, including joint effusions, pain from any source, disuse, and various abnormalities such as altered proprioception, decrease the neural drive stimulus and alter the stored patterns.

The force-dependent motor patterns responsible for smooth generation and transfer of force through a coordinated succession of joint positions and movements are highly dependent on the neurologic integrity of each of the joints. If the length-dependent patterns that operate around individual joints are not functioning correctly because of weakness, inhibition, or other problems with neural drive, then the force-dependent patterns break down and are altered, thereby decreasing the efficiency and maximal force production from that pattern.

Both anatomic and neurologic alterations in muscle may be present at the same time during the pathologic process. Their clinical effect is to decrease the amount and effectiveness of muscle strength production. These alterations are widespread in a muscle-dependent joint such as the shoulder and should be checked for closely.

Scapular muscle failure, which is commonly seen in shoulder pathology, appears to be a nonspecific response to glenohumeral pain, injury, or pathology. Disruption of the force couples has deleterious effects on the function of the scapula during overhead activities. Lack of acromial elevation, because of upper trapezius weakness, increases impingement with shoulder abduction. Trapezius, rhomboid, and serratus anterior muscle weakness impairs the scapula's ability to position itself as a congruent socket for the moving humerus; to stabilize itself as an anchor for origins of the rotator cuff, deltoid, biceps, and triceps; and to move smoothly from retraction to protraction during the throwing motion. These abnormalities of motion and position are called scapular dyskinesis. Finally, this weakness, by interrupting the kinetic chain, disrupts funneling of velocity and force, and does not allow a stable base for the arm to work.

Rotator cuff injury, caused either by impingement or by partial- or full-thickness tears, results in failure of energy and force production, but its most deleterious effects are on the force couples that position and stabilize the glenohumeral joint. Supraspinatus weakness decreases capsular stiffness and concavity/compression. Infraspinatus/teres minor weakness alters the deltoid force couple for abduction, leading to excessive superior translation. Subscapularis weakness can lead to overstretching of the anterior capsular structures and cause excessive anterior translation. Internal/external rotation force couple imbalance, with relatively strong internal rotators and relatively weak external rotators, decreases concavity/compression and, in concert with restricted glenohumeral internal rotation, increases anterior translation.

Pathology in other links of the kinematic chain may affect the muscular constraints. Biomechanical flaws or anatomic injuries, such as ankle sprains, knee pathology, or inflexibility or weakness of the back create a catch-up situation if the distal kinematic links have to increase their energy or force production to maintain normal force production at the hand. The arm muscles, with their smaller cross-sectional area, cannot initiate or maintain this higher level of activity and are at risk of fatigue and injury. Our studies have shown that, in a mathematical model, a decrease of 10% of trunk/leg kinetic energy requires an 18.5% increase in shoulder velocity or a 40% increase in shoulder mass to achieve the same resultant energy at the hand.

Guidelines for Implementing Shoulder Rehabilitation

The basic concepts reviewed earlier can be used to set up guidelines for efficacious shoulder rehabilitation. These guidelines can then be used to construct specific protocols that will achieve the goal of restoration of shoulder function.

Establishment of a Complete Diagnosis

The specific tissues that are overtly symptomatic must be identified, but this evaluation may only partially define the extent of the physiologic or biomechanical alterations that may be associated with overt shoulder pathology.

For example, rotator cuff tendinitis is commonly associated with glenohumeral rotational inflexibility, strength imbalance with force couple imbalance, and scapular dyskinesis. Often, distant kinetic chain links may also be involved, with hip rotational inflexibility or trunk muscular weakness.

Similarly, "impingement" should be considered more a clinical sign or symptom, rather than a specific diagnosis, because so many other shoulder alterations are associated with the impingement sign or test. Among them are microtrauma instability, superior labral pathology, capsular tightness, and scapular dyskinesis.

All of the local constraint systems, as well as the regional and distant links in the kinematic chain, need to be evaluated before a complete diagnosis is made. Traditional methods of examining shoulder function, such as instability testing, muscle strength and range of motion measurement, and neurologic testing, should be supplemented by evaluation of scapular position and motion, trunk posture, strength, and flexibility, and hip rotation and flexion flexibility.

Organization of Rehabilitation Progression

The rehabilitation protocol should be organized into successive phases. Each phase would have specific anatomic and functional goals, certain activity progressions, and specific entrance and exit criteria for movement between phases. Within each phase, the specific activities will be classified by type, frequency, intensity, and duration. Because these protocols are function-based, the protocols for specific diagnoses tend to progress to some common end points in later phases regardless of the starting point. There are three phases, based on anatomic healing of injured tissues.

Acute Phase The acute phase begins with the onset of clinical symptoms or injury, or when the patient is seen for rehabilitation. Patient injuries will vary widely, from acute fracture or dislocation to postsurgical repair to tendinitis.

The rehabilitation protocol during this phase will be the most diverse because of the wide spectrum of pathology and the variety of early treatments. During this phase, the goal is to create stable healing tissues that will allow tensile loading and will allow coordinated muscle firing, and to improve joint health to allow more advanced rehabilitation.

Recovery Phase Entry into this phase assumes that the tissues have healed enough to be loaded in tension and compression so that normal flexibility and strength can be reached. This phase is often the longest and most complex because it must address the physiologic and biomechanical alterations that may be associated with the clinical symptoms. However, normalization of these problems creates the conditions for normal function.

Functional Phase The functional phase is final preparation for and initiation into return to play. This is the final common pathway for the various protocols for the different injuries. Functional progressions, a series of exercises that simulate sport-specific activities and progress in difficulty toward normal play, are used to ensure that the athlete can respond to the normal demands inherent in sports.

Integration of the Kinematic Chain

Because the more proximal links in the kinematic chain are important in the development of normal force and velocity around and through the shoulder, and because deficits in flexibility, strength, and strength balance in these links are not uncommon in shoulder pathology, these links should be rehabilitated early in the protocol. Often they can be exercised quite intensely during the healing process. Correction of hip and trunk inflexibility or muscular weakness may be done, and aerobic and anaerobic endurance and power may be maintained.

Specific patterns for integration of the legs and trunk with the shoulder and arm are important. Three specific patterns that should be emphasized include hip and trunk rotation; hip stabilization with contralateral shoulder elevation, creating a diagonal force pattern (Fig. 1); and hip and trunk rotation with

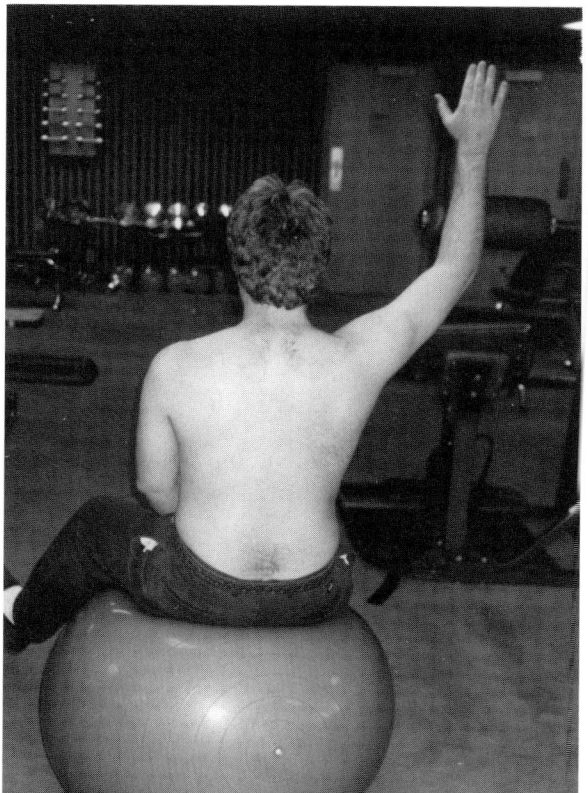

Fig. 1 Integrated kinematic chain—hip stabilization, shoulder elevation.

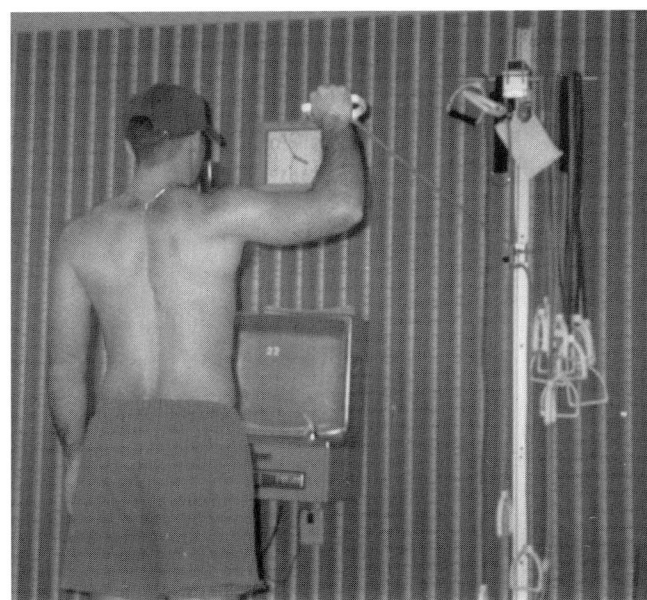

Fig. 2 Integrated kinematic chain—hip and trunk rotation, scapular retraction.

scapular retraction (Fig. 2). These three patterns create a stable base of muscular support to allow shoulder strengthening at the appropriate phase of healing.

Scapular Stabilization
The scapula is the base upon which the shoulder muscles contract, the humerus articulates, and the entire arm pivots. Scapular dyskinesis, or lack of coordination of normal scapular motion and position, negatively affects the scapula's ability to be an effective base. The scapular stabilizing muscles, especially the lower trapezius and serratus anterior, display disorganized firing patterns early in the pathologic process. This disorganization is usually caused by reflex-based inhibition rather than direct nerve or muscle injury, and can be corrected by specific exercises for the involved muscles. These exercises should be done early in rehabilitation, to stabilize the base for glenohumeral function. The most effective method for strengthening these muscles is through "closed chain" rehabilitation.

Closed Chain Rehabilitation
Closed chain exercises are those in which the distal end of the extremity meets a considerable resistance. This resistance creates a predictable pattern of joint positions and muscle contractions that is specific for the applied force. In the shoulder, the hand is placed on a wall or table, or a movable object on the wall or table, or is loaded with a heavy weight. Movement of the scapula and shoulder is then initiated so that the arm does not move. These exercises, by promoting co-contraction force couples, reproduce their stabilizing function and recall the length-dependent patterns. Also, because the joint does not move, there is minimal stress on the injured ligaments or capsular structures. Finally, they eliminate the deltoid portion of the abduction force couple, decreasing the chances of impingement.

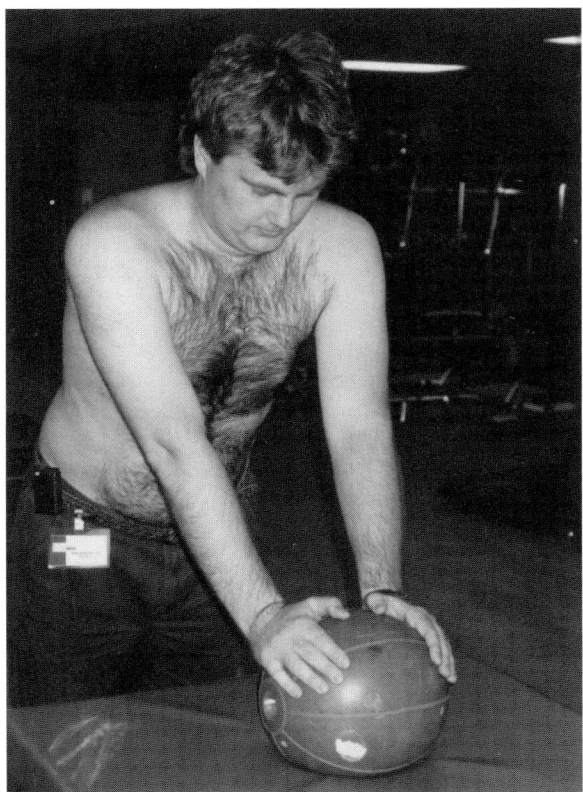

Fig. 3 Closed chain—early activity below 45° of abduction/60° of flexion.

Early in rehabilitation, these exercises may be done at arm positions of less than 45° abduction/60° flexion (Fig. 3). As soon as possible, the extremity should be progressed to 90° abduction, because this is the position of most shoulder functions. Exercises for scapular elevation/depression (Fig. 4) and retraction/protraction (Fig. 5) and glenohumeral compression and rotation (Fig. 6) can be done safely in this position.

Achievement of 90° of Abduction
The 90°-abducted position is the key to normal shoulder function. Almost every throwing or serving activity takes place close to this position. The normal force-dependent and length-dependent patterns operate only when the shoulder is in this position, and the normal ball and socket kinematics are present in this position. This position can be achieved within 3 to 4 weeks after labral or capsular surgery, and within 3 to 5 weeks after rotator cuff surgery. Just as in anterior cruciate ligament surgery, the desired position is checked and achieved at the time of surgery, so that early rehabilitation may be aggressive without imposing excessive shear. Early mobilization is done by active-assisted and passive techniques, but active mobilization should be instituted as well.

294 Miscellaneous Shoulder Problems

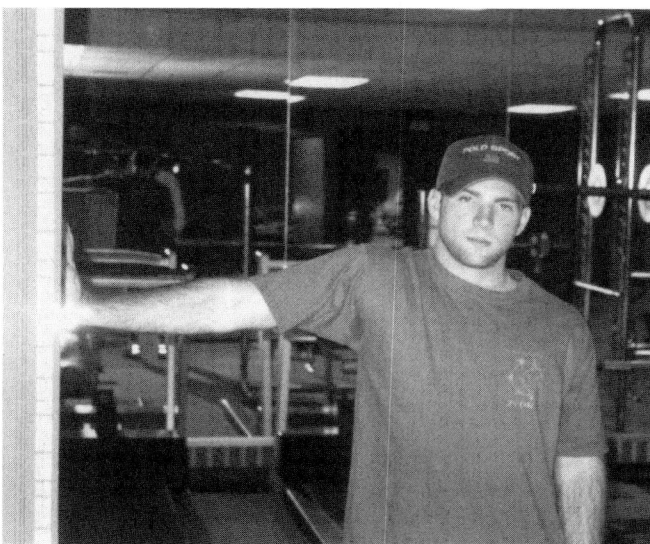 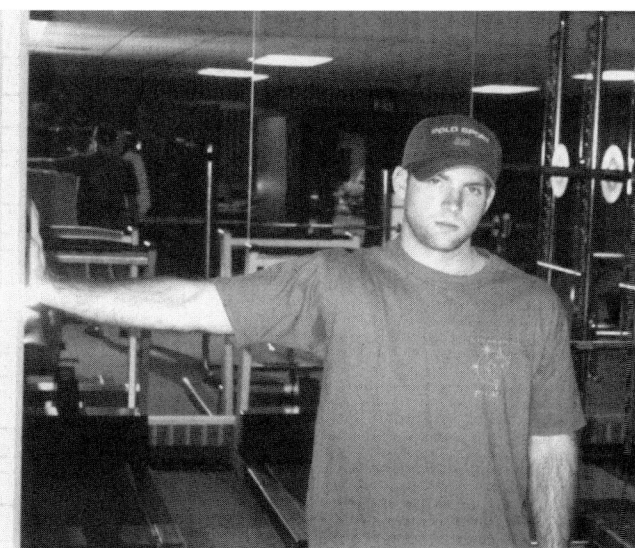

Fig. 4 Closed chain—scapular elevation/depression. **Left,** Scapular elevation; **right,** Scapular depression.

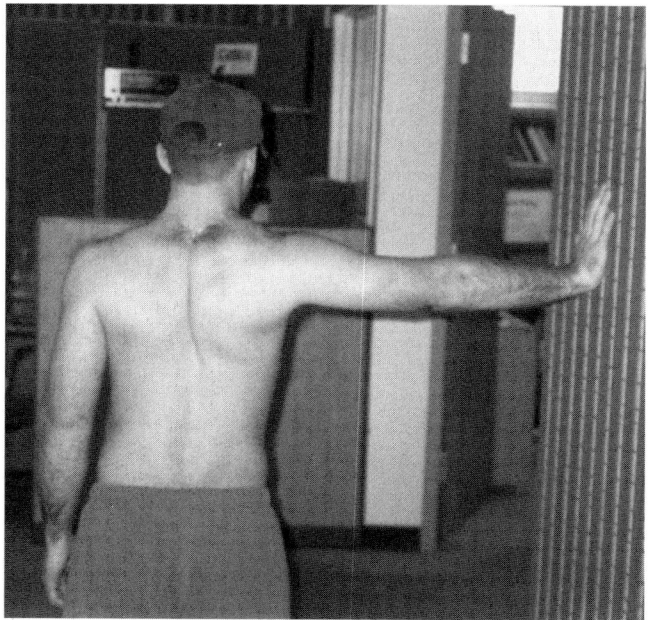 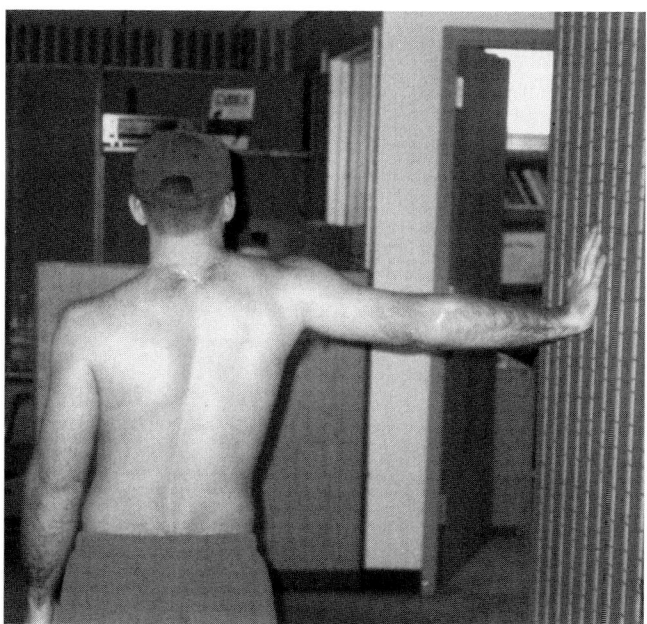

Fig. 5 Closed chain—scapular retraction/protraction. **Left,** Scapular retraction; **right,** Scapular protraction.

Rotator Cuff Exercises

Isolated rotator cuff exercises should be used later in rehabilitation, after the proper base has been established for their use. These exercises, because they are usually done in open chain fashion, require a stable scapula for muscle origin, and create shear stress across the glenohumeral joint early in initiation of joint motion. They should be used to strengthen isolated strength deficits in specific muscles. However, because shoulder function is determined by integrated, coordinated activation of the muscles, this method of isolated, individualized training plays a relatively small role in the total rehabilitation protocol.

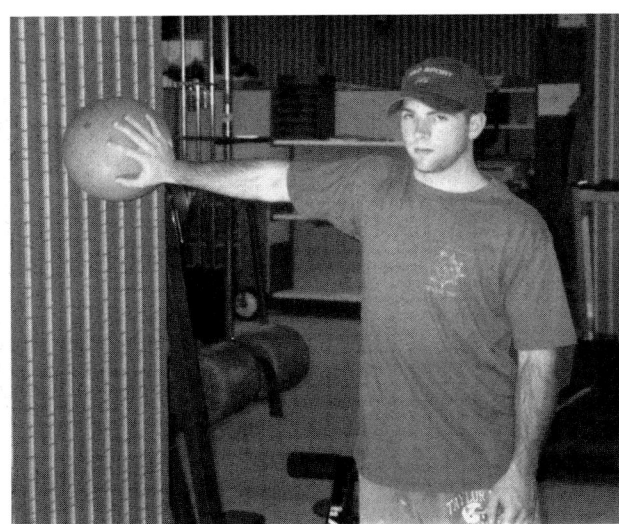

Fig. 6 Closed chain—glenohumeral rotation on a ball.

Plyometric Training

Open chain training involving agonist/antagonist force couples to develop power to move the shoulder, arm, and hand is important for total shoulder function and allows the fast ballistic movements that occur in throwing or swimming. Plyometric exercises, which involve a relatively slow prestretch that tensions the muscles and stores elastic energy, followed by a rapid explosive contraction, are the preferred method of training.

These exercises emphasize large ranges of motion, rapid joint motion, and forceful muscle contractions. They should, therefore, be used in later stages of rehabilitation, after tissue healing has occurred, closed chain exercises have stabilized the joint, and neurologic retraining has occurred.

These exercises should be done throughout the entire kinematic chain, because all parts are required to do plyometric type activity during the cocking, acceleration, and deceleration phases of throwing. At the shoulder, they should be done at 90° abduction (Fig. 7). Tubing, weights, and medicine balls may be used as resistance.

Specific Rehabilitation Program

There are no data to suggest that one specific shoulder rehabilitation protocol is the best. Most of the currently advocated protocols are based on the key concepts presented and adhere to the guidelines. A postoperative protocol that was developed in this manner will be presented to show implementation of the concepts and guidelines. Outcomes analysis has shown this to be efficacious; competitive athletes have resumed throwing at a mean of 2.5 months after arthroscopic labral surgery and 3.25 months after open instability reconstruction, while utilizing six to seven physical therapy visits.

Postoperative Rehabilitation Protocol

This general protocol will illustrate principles for rehabilitation of any postoperative problem. This protocol assumes sta-

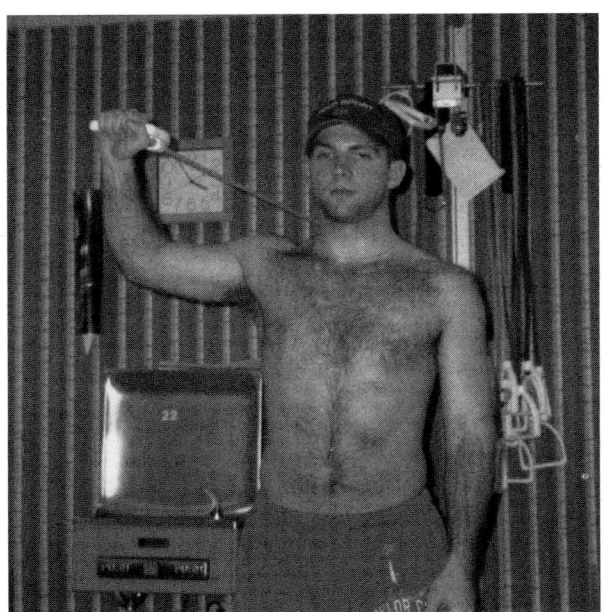

Fig. 7 Plyometrics—shoulder rotation at 90° of abduction.

ble repair of the labrum, capsule, or rotator cuff, and ability to achieve 90° abduction without impingement or excessive capsular stretch at the time of the operation. With postoperative labral repairs, shoulder reconstructions, and acromioplasties, the goal is 90° of passive or active-assisted abduction by 3 weeks, and with rotator cuff repairs, 90° passive or active-assisted abduction by 4 to 6 weeks.

Goals of the Acute Phase

The goals to be obtained during this phase are: (1) tissue healing; (2) reduce pain and inflammation; (3) reestablish nonpainful range of motion below 90° abduction; (4) retard muscle atrophy; (5) achieve scapular control; and (6) maintain fitness of other components of kinematic chain.

Criteria for movement out of the acute phase include progression of tissue healing (healed or sufficiently stabilized for active motion and tissue loading), passive range of motion 66% to 75% of opposite side, minimal pain, manual muscle strength in nonpathologic areas grades 4+/5, scapular control, with dominant side/nondominant side scapular asymmetry < 1.5 cm, and kinematic chain function and integration.

Tissue Healing Tissue healing is achieved with a combination of rest, short-term immobilization, physical therapy modalities, and surgery.

Pain and Inflammation There are several aggressive treatment options to control pain to decrease inhibition-based muscle atrophy and decrease scapular instability caused by serratus and/or trapezius inhibition. These include medications, either nonsteroidal or judicious use of steroids orally or by injection; modalities, usually ultrasound, twice per week for

2 weeks; cold compression devices; and joint protection, usually by sling or swathe, with gradual progression out of the sling.

Range of Motion Range of motion should be started in pain-free arcs, kept below 90° abduction, and may be passive or active-assisted. The degree of movement will be guided by the stability of the surgical repair. Types of range-of-motion exercises include Codman's or other pendulum exercises, manual capsular stretching and cross fiber massage, and use of a T-bar or ropes and pulleys.

Muscle Atrophy Early exercises to control muscle atrophy will include isometric exercises, with the arm below 90° abduction and 90° flexion. These exercises may be done by patients who have had labral or capsular repair, but not by those who have had rotator cuff repair.

Scapular Control Isometric scapular pinches and scapular elevation; closed chain weight shifts, with hands on table, shoulder flexed < 60°, abducted < 45°; and use of a tilt board or circular board weight shifts with the same range of motion limitations all help improve scapular control.

Fitness of Kinematic Chain Components Aerobic exercises, such as running, bicycling, or stepping; anaerobic agility drills; lower extremity strengthening, by machines, squat exercises, or open chain leg lifts; elbow and wrist strengthening by isometrics or rubber tubing; flexibility exercises, especially areas that are shown to be tight on the evaluation; and integration of the kinematic chain by leg and trunk stabilization on a ball, employing rotational and oblique patterns of contraction, all assist in maintaining fitness of the kinematic chain.

Goals of the Recovery Phase

The goals to be obtained during this phase are: (1) normal active and passive shoulder and glenohumeral motion; (2) improved scapular control; (3) normal upper extremity strength and strength balance; (4) normal shoulder arthrokinematics in single, then multiple planes of motion; and (5) normal kinematic chain and force generation patterns.

Criteria for moving out of the recovery phase include full nonpainful scapulothoracic motion, 90% normal glenohumeral motion, lateral slide asymmetry less than 0.75 cm, normal back motion, rotator cuff strength 4+/5 or higher, and normal kinematic chain function.

Range of Motion Range of motion exercises should start with active-assisted above 90° abduction with a wand and proceed to active-assisted, then active motion in internal and external with scapula stabilized. In this manner, glenohumeral rotation is normalized without substitution movements from the scapula.

Scapular Control Scapular proprioceptive neuromuscular facilitation patterns in diagonals, closed chain exercises at 90° flexion/90° abduction (scapular retraction/protraction and scapular elevation/depression), modified push-ups, regular push-ups, medicine ball catch and push, and dips can all be used to achieve scapular control.

Upper Extremity Strength and Strength Balance This goal can be achieved with glenohumeral proprioceptive neuromuscular facilitation patterns, closed chain exercises at 90° flexion then 90° abduction (glenohumeral depression and glenohumeral internal/external rotation), forearm curls, isolated rotator cuff exercises, and machines or weights for light bench press, military press, and pull downs. The resistance should initially be light, then progress as strength improves. Emphasis is placed on proper mechanics and technique, and joint stabilization.

Normal Shoulder Arthrokinematics Normal shoulder arthrokinematics includes the following factors: (1) Achieving smooth motion with the arm at 90° of abduction, which is the position where most throwing and serving activities occur. The periarticular soft tissues must be completely loose and balanced at this position. (2) Muscle activity at 90° abduction. Normal muscle firing patterns must be reestablished at this position, both in organization of force generation and force regulation patterns and in proprioceptive sensory feedback. Closed chain patterns are an excellent method to reestablish the normal neurologic patterns for joint stabilization. (3) Open chain exercises, including mild plyometric exercises, may be built upon the base of the closed chain stabilization to allow normal control of joint mobility.

Normal Kinematic Chain and Force Generation This goal may be achieved by normalization of all inflexibilities throughout chain; normal agonist/antagonist force couples in legs by squats, plyometric depth jumps, lunges, and hip extensions; trunk rotation exercises, with medicine ball or tubing; integrated exercises with leg and trunk stabilization (rotations, diagonal patterns from hip to shoulder, and medicine ball throws); and normal throwing or serving motion without resistance.

Goals of the Functional Phase

The goals of this phase are: (1) increase power and endurance in the upper extremity; (2) increase normal multiple-plane neuromuscular control locally, regionally, and in the entire kinematic chain; (3) instruction of the patient in rehabilitation activities; and (4) performance of sports-specific activity.

Criteria for return to play include normal clinical examination, normal shoulder arthrokinematics, normal kinematic chain integration, and completed progressions.

Power and Endurance in the Upper Extremity Power is the rate of doing work. Work may be done to move the joint and the extremity, or it may be done to absorb a load and stabilize the joint or extremity. Power has a time component, and for shoulder activity, quick movements and quick reactions are the dominant ways of doing work. Exercises to increase power and endurance should, therefore, be done with relatively rapid movements in planes that approximate normal shoulder function (ie, 90° of abduction in shoulder, trunk rotation, and diagonal arm motions, rapid external/internal rotation). Diagonal and multiplanar motions with tubing, light weights, small medicine balls, and isokinetic machines, along with plyometrics (wall push-ups, corner push-ups, weighted ball throws, and tubing) are good exercises. Tubing exercises may be used to mimic any of the needed motions in throwing or serving. Medicine balls are very effective plyometric devices. The weight of the ball creates prestretch and an eccentric load when it is caught, creates a resistance, and demands a powerful agonist contraction to propel it forward again.

Increase Multiple-Plane Neuromuscular Control In order to increase multiple-plane neuromuscular control, the force-dependent motor firing patterns should be reestablished. No subclinical adaptations, such as "opening up" (trunk rotation too far in front of shoulder rotation), three quarter arm positioning on throwing, or excessive wrist snap, should be allowed. Help in this area can be obtained by watching preinjury videos or by using a coach knowledgeable in the particular sport. Special care must be taken to integrate completely all of the components of the kinematic chain to generate and funnel the proper forces to and through the shoulder.

Rehabilitation The athlete who is injured while playing a sport will most likely be going back to the same sport and will be facing the same sports demands. The body should not only be healed from the symptomatic standpoint, but should be prepared for resuming the stresses inherent in playing the sport. A maintenance program is the best way to condition to prevent overload injuries and further problems in sport. General body flexibility, with emphasis on sport-specific problems (shoulder internal rotation and elbow extension in the arm, low back, hip rotation and hamstrings in the legs); strengthening (appropriate amount and locations of strength for sport-specific activities—quadriceps/hamstring strength for force generation, trunk rotation strength, strength balance for the shoulder); power (rapid movements in appropriate planes with light weights); and endurance (mainly anaerobic exercises, due to short duration, explosive, and ballistic activities seen in throwing and serving) are important exercises and should be based on the periodization principle of conditioning.

Sport-Specific Activity Sport- or activity-specific functional progressions of throwing or serving must be completed before full competition is allowed. These progressions will gradually test all of the mechanical parts of the throwing or serving motion. Very few deviations from normal parameters of arm motion, arm position, force generation, smoothness of all of the kinematic chain, and from preinjury form should be allowed because most of these adaptations will be biomechanically inefficient. The athlete may move through the progressions as rapidly as possible.

Selected Bibliography

Fleisig GS, Andrews JR, Dillman CJ, et al: Kinetics of baseball pitching, with implications about injury mechanisms. *Am J Sports Med* 1995;23:233-239.

This article presents a good review of biomechanics.

Howell SM, Galinat BJ, Renzi AJ, et al: Normal and abnormal mechanics of the glenohumeral joint in the horizontal plane. *J Bone Joint Surg* 1988;70A:227-232.

A very complete evaluation of glenohumeral motion and translation is presented.

Inman VT, Saunders JB Dec M, et al: Observations on the function of the shoulder joint. *J Bone Joint Surg* 1944;26:1-30.

This article is the classic study of joint motions and muscle activity of the shoulder joint.

Jobe FW, Kvitne RS, Giangarra CE: Shoulder pain in the overhand or throwing athlete: The relationship of anterior instability and rotator cuff impingement. *Orthop Rev* 1989;18:963-975.

An excellent review of concepts and classification of the instability/impingement spectrum is presented.

Kibler WB: Role of the scapula in the overhead throwing motion. *Contemp Orthop* 1991;22:525-532.

This article is an overview of scapular function and dysfunction.

Kibler WB, Livingston BK, Bruce RB: Current concepts in shoulder rehabilitation. *Adv Oper Orthop* 1995;3:249-300.

A detailed overview, with 150 references, of biomechanics, physiology, modalities, and methods of rehabilitation with specific protocols used at the Lexington Clinic Sports Medicine Center, is presented.

Kibler WB: Normal shoulder mechanics and function, in Springfield DS (ed): *Instructional Course Lectures 46.* Rosemont, IL, American Academy of Orthopaedic Surgeons, 1997, pp 39-42.

Kibler WB, Garrett WE Jr: Pathophysiologic alterations in shoulder injury, in Springfield DS (ed): *Instructional Course Lectures 46.* Rosemont, IL, American Academy of Orthopaedic Surgeons, 1997, pp 3-6.

Kibler WB, Livingston B, Chandler TJ: Shoulder rehabilitation: Clinical applications, evaluation, and rehabilitation, in Springfield DS (ed): *Instructional Course Lectures 46.* Rosemont, IL, American Academy of Orthopaedic Surgeons, 1997, pp 43-51.

The neurologic basis of shoulder function and dysfunction, concepts of pathophysiology, evaluation of the shoulder, and rehabilitation protocols are discussed.

Nichols TR: A biomechanical perspective on spinal mechanisms of coordinated muscular action: An architecture principle. *Acta Anat Basel* 1994;151:1-13.

An overview of force dependent and length dependent motor organization is presented.

Pink MM, Screnar PM, Tollefson KD, et al: Injury prevention and rehabilitation in the upper extremity, in Jobe FW, Pink MM, Glousman RE, et al (eds): *Operative Techniques in Upper Extremity Sports Injuries.* St. Louis, MO, Mosby-Year Book, 1996, pp 3-14.

This article presents review of principles and specific protocols used at the Kerlan-Jobe Clinic.

Speer KP, Garrett WE Jr: Muscular control of motion and stability about the pectoral girdle, in Matsen FA III, Fu FH, Hawkins RJ (eds): *The Shoulder: A Balance of Mobility and Stability.* Rosemont, IL, American Academy of Orthopaedic Surgeons, 1993, pp 159-172.

This chapter discusses how muscles function to control the many demands in athletic activities.

Steindler A (ed): *Kinesiology: The Human Body Under Normal and Pathological Conditions.* Springfield, IL, Charles C Thomas, 1970.

This article is the classic discussion of muscle activity, closed and open chain activities, and acquired muscle adaptations to use.

Wilk KE: Current concepts in the rehabilitation of the athlete's shoulder. *J South Orthop Assoc* 1994;3:216-231.

The shoulder rehabilitation program used at the American Sports Medicine Institute is discussed.

Wilk KE, Voight ML, Keirns MA, et al: Stretch-shortening drills for the upper extremities: Theory and clinical application. *J Orthop Sports Phys Ther* 1993;17:225-239.

This article gives a good description and application of plyometric exercises.

VII
Elbow Trauma/Fracture/Reconstruction

Shawn W. O'Driscoll, MD, PhD, FRCSC
Section Editor

33

Biomechanics and Functional Anatomy of the Elbow

Graham J.W. King, MD, MSc, FRCSC and Kai-Nan An, PhD

Introduction

An understanding of the functional anatomy and biomechanics of the elbow is an essential prerequisite to the effective treatment of elbow disorders. The elbow has a complex articulation, with three joints interacting during both normal function and in pathologic conditions. This chapter will discuss the functional anatomy and biomechanics of the elbow in order to improve understanding of the basic scientific rationale for the management of elbow disorders.

Functional Anatomy

Osteology

The articular surface of the distal humerus has two portions: a spool-shaped trochlea, which articulates with the greater sigmoid notch of the ulna, and a hemispherical capitellum, which articulates with the concave surface of the radial head (Fig. 1). The articular surface is situated anterior to the mid-axis of the humerus. This articular orientation must be reconstructed following a distal humeral fracture if a full arc of flexion-extension is to be realized. Plates can be applied low on the lateral column of the distal humerus because of the anterior orientation of the capitellum.

The proximal ulna has a unique osseous shape and articular surface that has important clinical implications (Fig. 2). The guiding ridge of the greater sigmoid notch runs longitudinally and articulates with the apex of the trochlear groove, whereas the medial and lateral portions articulate with the sloping surfaces of the trochlea. During flexion, the coronoid process of the ulna locks into the coronoid fossa of the distal humerus and the margin of the radial head is restrained by the radial fossa, further enhancing osseous stability. During extension, the tip of the olecranon is contained by the olecranon fossa, increasing the osseous stability of the joint in this position. The hyaline cartilage on the articular surface of the olecranon is usually discontinuous centrally, distributing the force on the articulation into two functional facets. Fractures often occur through this nonarticular portion because of weak subchondral bone at this location. To expose distal humeral fractures, olecranon osteotomies can be performed through the nonarticular portion without violating the hyaline cartilage. The irregular appearance of the articular cartilage can be confused with pathology in patients undergoing elbow arthroscopy.

The radial head consists of a concave dish that articulates with the capitellum and an articular margin that articulates with the lesser sigmoid (radial) notch of the ulna. Approximately 240° of the radial margin articulates with the ulna, while the remaining 120° is nonarticular and may be devoid of cartilage. Fixation of radial head fractures is possible by virtue of screws countersunk through the nonarticular margin of the radial head. Excision of wedge fragments comprising

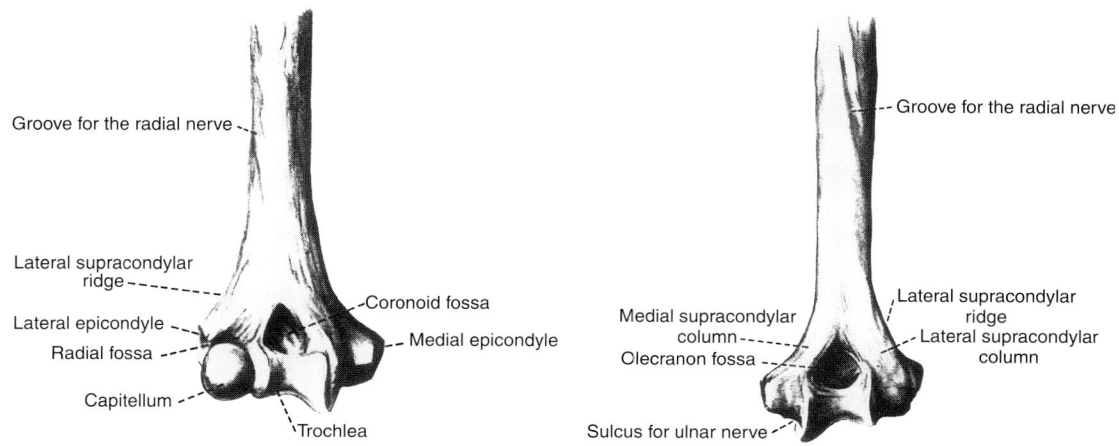

Fig. 1 Distal humerus. **Left,** Anterior aspect of the distal humerus. **Right,** Posterior aspect of the distal humerus. (Reproduced with permission from Morrey BF: Anatomy of the elbow joint, in Morrey BF (ed): *The Elbow and Its Disorders*, ed 2. Philadelphia, PA, WB Saunders, 1993, pp 16-52.)

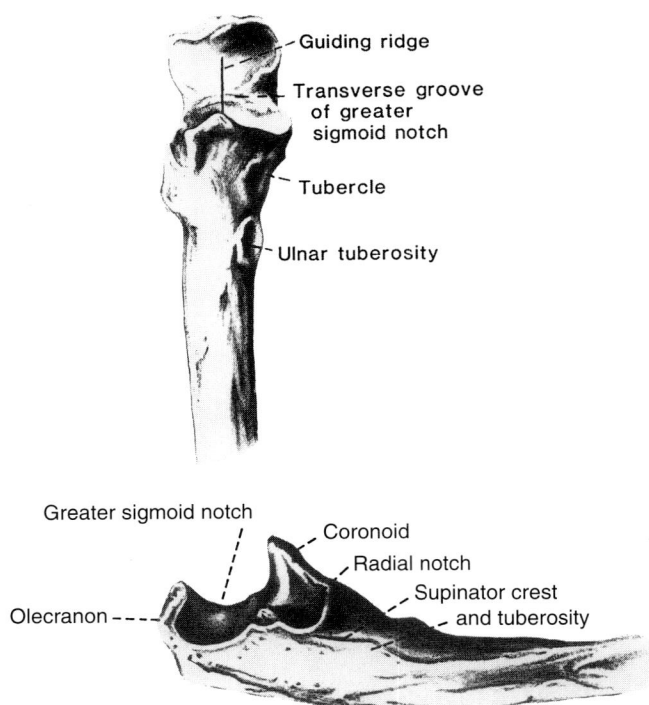

Fig. 2 Proximal ulna. **Top,** Anterior aspect of the proximal ulna, which articulates with the trochlea of the distal humerus. Note the nonarticular portion near the center of the greater sigmoid notch. **Bottom,** Lateral aspect of the proximal ulna. (Reproduced with permission from Morrey BF: Anatomy of the elbow joint, in Morrey BF (ed): *The Elbow and Its Disorders,* ed 2. Philadelphia, PA, WB Saunders, 1993, pp 16-52.)

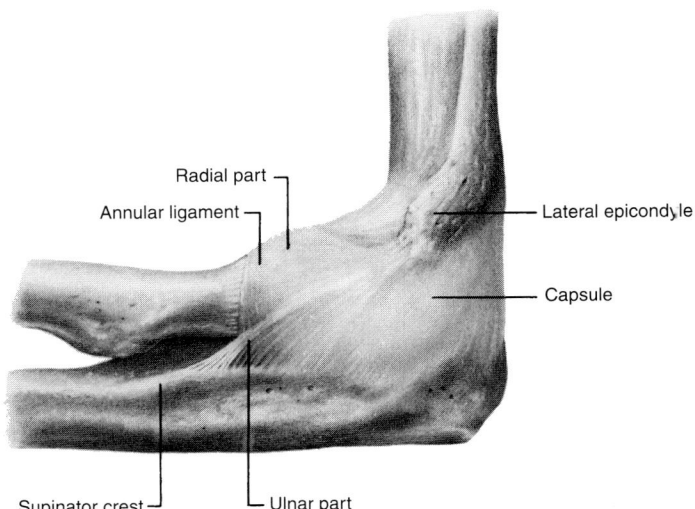

Fig. 3 Lateral collateral ligament complex. Representations of the three parts of the lateral ligamentous supports are shown. The ulnar part (lateral ulnar collateral ligament) passes from the lateral epicondyle to the supinator crest of the ulna. The radial part blends with the annular ligament. (Reproduced with permission from O'Driscoll SW, Horii E, Morrey BF, et al: Anatomy of the ulnar part of the lateral collateral ligament of the elbow. *Clin Anat* 1992;5: 296-303.)

less than 30% of the articular surface is possible if these fragments do not articulate with the proximal radioulnar joint. Recent data has demonstrated that the radial head is not a circular structure, but is elliptical in shape. The radiocapitellar dish is circular and offset from the neck of the radius. These anthropometric features may have important implications in the design of radial head hemiarthroplasties.

Capsuloligamentous Tissues

The capsule of the elbow attaches to the articular margins of the joint and blends with the fibers of the annular ligament. Anteriorly it includes both the coronoid and radial fossae; posteriorly it contains the olecranon fossa. The anterior capsule has transverse and obliquely directed bands that provide significant stability when taut in extension. The anterior capsule does not attach to the tip of the coronoid process, but is located an average of 6 mm distal to it. The attachment of the anterior capsule accounts for the excellent visualization of the coronoid that is possible during anterior elbow arthroscopy. It also explains how type I coronoid tip fractures cannot occur as a result of capsular avulsion; rather, they represent shearing injuries caused by joint subluxation. The lack of soft-tissue attachment also explains the significant incidence of nonunion and the development of intra-articular loose bodies.

Similarly, the posterior capsule becomes taut in flexion and may also have an important role as a static stabilizer in this position. The capsule of the elbow allows maximal distention with the elbow in 70° to 80° of flexion. Patients with hematomas or effusions who commonly hold their elbow in this position do so to minimize discomfort from capsular distention. The normal capsular volume is 25 ml; however, this volume is reduced in patients with elbow contractures. This reduction in capsular volume may lead to an increased risk for neural injury in patients undergoing elbow arthroscopy when capsular distention might not be sufficient for anterior displacement of the nerves.

The lateral collateral ligament (LCL) consists of three parts: the annular, radial, and ulnar parts (Fig. 3). The origin of the LCL on the lateral epicondyle is near the axis of rotation of the elbow; therefore, this ligament remains taut throughout the range of elbow flexion-extension with little change in the distance between the ligament origin and insertion (Fig. 4). As a consequence of its isometricity, division of the LCL is usually not required in patients undergoing surgery for long-standing elbow contractures. The annular ligament attaches to the anterior and posterior margins of the lesser sigmoid notch. The ligament's funnel shape helps stabilize the proximal radius throughout the range of prosupination. The radial part of the collateral ligament blends with the annular ligament and is an important stabilizer of the radial head. Indirectly, through the annular ligament, this structure also stabilizes the humeroulnar joint. The ulnar part (also known as the lateral ulnar collateral ligament) extends from the lateral epicondyle to the crista supinatoris of the ulna and has

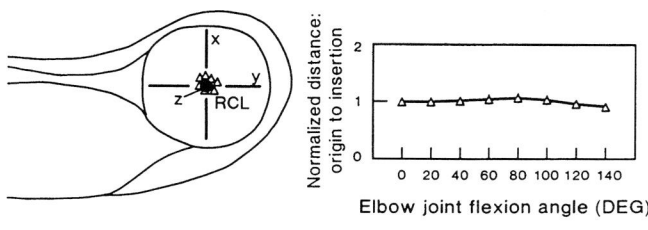

Fig. 4 Isometry of the radial collateral ligament. **Left,** Lateral view of the distal humerus demonstrating the close proximity of the radial collateral ligament (RCL) to the center of rotation of the elbow joint. **Right,** The distance between the origin and the insertion of the radial collateral ligament is essentially constant throughout the range of elbow motion. DEG = degrees. (Reproduced with permission from King GJW, Morrey BF, An KN: Stabilizers of the elbow. *J Shoulder Elbow Surg* 1993;2:165-174.)

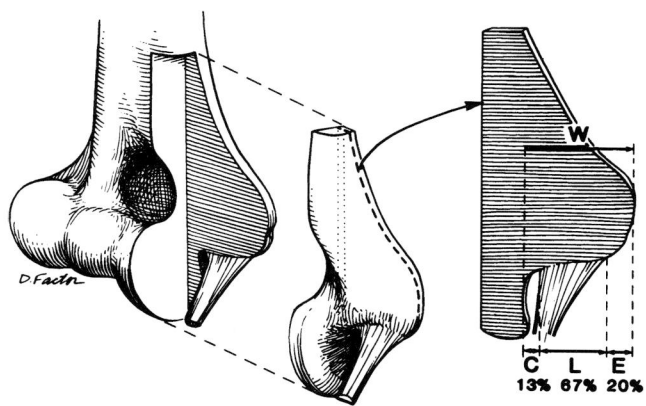

Fig. 6 Humeral origin of the medial collateral ligament. The humeral origin of the medial collateral ligament was investigated by performing orthogonal osteotomies in a series of cadaveric specimens. A 2-mm section through the widest part of the anterior band of the medial collateral ligament demonstrates the location of the humeral attachment **(right)**. W = width of medial epicondyle; C = distance from trochlea to attachment of medial collateral ligament; L = width of origin of the anterior band of the medial collateral ligament; E = distance from top of epicondyle to medial collateral ligament. (Reproduced with permission from O'Driscoll SW, Jaloszynski R, Morrey BF, et al: Origin of the medial ulnar collateral ligament. *J Hand Surg* 1992;17A:164-168.)

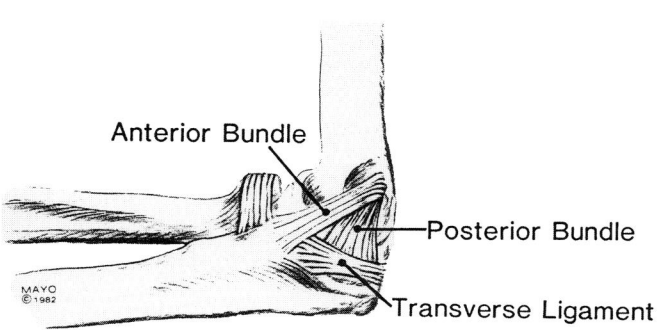

Fig. 5 Medial collateral ligament complex. Representation of the medial collateral ligament complex of the elbow. The anterior and posterior bundles are identified based on their site of attachment to the ulna. The transverse ligament has little functional importance. (Reproduced with permission from The Mayo Foundation, Rochester, MN.)

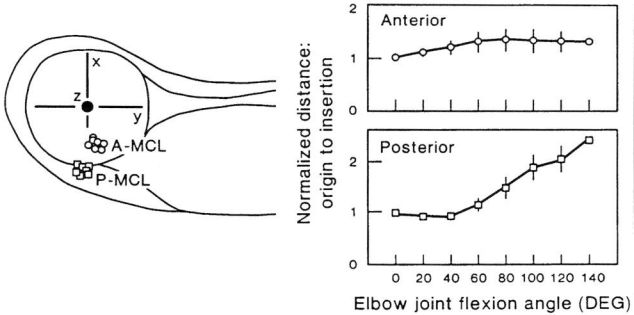

Fig. 7 Isometry of the medial collateral ligament complex. Medial view of the distal humerus **(left)**. Note that both the anterior and posterior bundles of the medial collateral ligament (A-MCL, P-MCL) are posterior to the axis of elbow motion. The distance between the origin and the insertion of the anterior and the posterior bundles increases with flexion, thereby increasing the stabilizing influence of the medial ligaments **(right)**. DEG=degrees. (Reproduced with permission from King GJW, Morrey BF, An KN: Stabilizers of the elbow. *J Shoulder Elbow Surg* 1993;2:165-174.)

been shown to be an essential stabilizer of the elbow. Disruption of the lateral ulnar collateral ligament has been demonstrated to be an important cause of both acute and recurrent dislocation of the elbow.

The medial collateral ligament (MCL) has three components: an anterior bundle, a posterior bundle, and a transverse portion (Fig. 5). The anterior bundle is stronger than the posterior bundle and its insertion into the anteromedial portion of the coronoid and greater sigmoid notch of the ulna gives it a significant mechanical advantage in controlling valgus-varus forces. The anterior bundle inserts an average of 18 mm posterior to the tip of the coronoid, and is therefore disrupted only in Regan type III fractures, which involve the majority of the coronoid. The posterior bundle is thin and fan-shaped, inserting into the posteromedial margin of the greater sigmoid notch. The transverse ligament is variable in its definition and appears to have a minimal role in stabilizing the elbow. The humeral attachment of the MCL arises from the anteroinferior surface of the medial epicondyle (Fig. 6). Excision of the medial epicondyle, a procedure frequently performed for the treatment of ulnar neuropathy, should be limited to 20% of the width of the medial epicondyle in the coronal plane to avoid violating this structure and potentially destabilizing the elbow. The humeral origins of both the anterior and posterior bundles are posterior to the axis of joint motion and are therefore more taut in flexion than in extension (Fig. 7). In a cadaveric study, Morrey and An measured an average 18% increase in the length of the anterior bundle from full extension to 120° of flexion. The posterior bundle of the MCL is even more posterior to the axis of motion than the anterior bundle, hence the length change in the posterior MCL was much greater, averaging 39% of the resting length. As a consequence, a cam effect occurs, which can necessitate partial division of the MCL to achieve complete elbow motion in some patients undergoing surgery for long-standing elbow contractures.

Muscles

The majority of the muscles crossing the elbow serve to rotate the forearm or flex and extend the wrist or fingers. Only a few muscles act primarily to move the elbow joint. By virtue of their joint reaction forces, all muscles that cross the elbow have the potential to provide increased joint stability by compressing the articular surfaces together. This stabilizing influence, however, is dependent on the position of the joint and the relative activity of the muscles acting across the articulation (resultant vector).

The primary elbow flexors are the biceps, brachialis, and the brachioradialis muscles. The biceps has a smaller cross sectional area than the brachialis; however, its mechanical advantage is greater because of its greater moment arm. The brachialis muscle has the largest cross sectional area; however, it also has the poorest mechanical advantage of the elbow flexors. Its insertion into the anterior aspect of the proximal ulna suggests that it may have a role as an anterior buttress, stabilizing the elbow against posterior subluxation. The brachioradialis is an important elbow flexor despite its relatively small cross sectional area. Arising along the lateral supracondylar ridge, the brachioradialis has the largest mechanical advantage of any of the muscles crossing the flexor surface of the elbow.

Elbow extension can be attributed almost exclusively to the triceps muscle, which consists of three parts: the long, lateral, and medial heads. The triceps attaches onto and around the tip of the olecranon. By virtue of its close relationship to the axis of joint motion, the moment arm of the triceps muscle is small, similar to that of the brachialis muscle anteriorly. With the elbow flexed, a considerable resultant vector of compressive force is applied across the elbow joint and may be an important dynamic stabilizing factor. The anconeus is a small muscle that is draped across the posterolateral aspect of the elbow covering the annular ligament and the radial head. Although its function remained unclear for some time, its origin near the lateral epicondyle and insertion broadly on the ulna suggest it is an important dynamic constraint to varus and posterolateral rotatory instability of the elbow.

Kinematics

The function of the elbow is to position and stabilize the hand in space for manual activities. The elbow allows primary motions in both flexion, extension, and prosupination. In view of the permitted motions in two degrees of freedom, the elbow has generally been described as a trochoginglymoid joint.

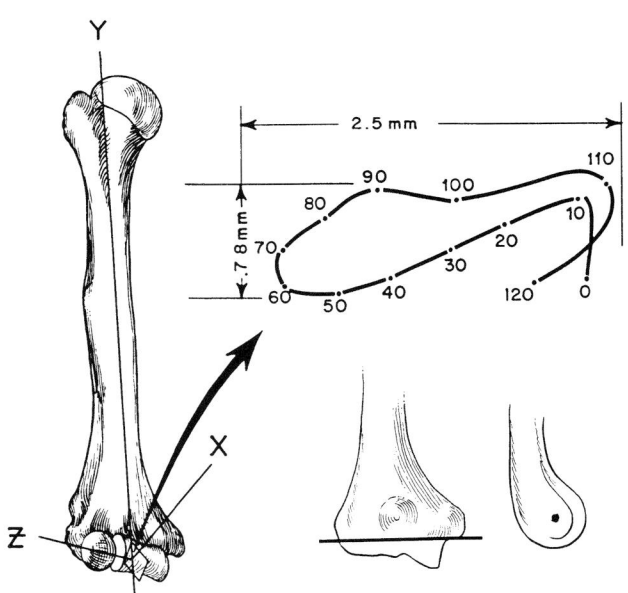

Fig. 8 Locus of instant centers of rotation of the elbow. The axis of rotation runs through the center of curvature of the capitellum and trochlea. (Reproduced with permission from An KN, Morrey BF: Biomechanics of the elbow, in Morrey BF (ed): *The Elbow and Its Disorders*, ed 2. Philadelphia, PA, WB Saunders, 1993, pp 53-72.)

Flexion-Extension

The range of elbow motion in the flexion and extension plane varies from approximately 0° to 145°. According to one study, approximately 30° to 130° of this total arc were necessary to perform most activities of daily living. The motion pathway of elbow flexion-extension has been shown to approximate that of a loose hinge joint. The flexion-extension axis follows a line that can be drawn between the center of the capitellum and the center of curvature of the trochlear groove (Fig. 8). External landmarks that are useful in defining this axis are the anteroinferior aspect of the medial epicondyle and the center of the arc of curvature of the capitellum. It has been demonstrated that the locus of instant centers of rotation is small, moving less than 4 mm throughout the arc of elbow flexion-extension. An understanding of the patterns of elbow motion has fostered the development of articulated external fixators and elbow distraction devices that are being increasingly used for reconstructive surgery and trauma, leading to the development and clinical application of loose hinge total elbow arthroplasty design.

It is important to understand that the axis of rotation does not correspond to the so-called carrying angle described for the elbow. The axis of rotation is approximately 3° to 5° internally rotated relative to the plane of the medial and lateral epicondyles and in 4° to 8° of valgus with respect to the long axis of the humerus. For clinical purposes, the carrying angle is defined as the angle between the long axis of the humerus and the long axis of the ulna measured in the frontal plane with the elbow in the extended position. Considerable variation in the carrying angle exists between patients. Carrying angles are generally higher in women than in men. The average carrying angle for men has been reported to vary between 10° to 15°, and is about 5° greater in women. The clinical implication is that in patients with elbow flexion contractures, the true carrying angle of the elbow cannot be measured and varus deformities may not be apparent until a flexion contracture is corrected.

Prosupination

Rotation of the radius occurs about the ulna at the proximal and distal radioulnar joints. The axis of forearm rotation has been demonstrated to pass through the center of the radial head and near the fovea of the distal ulna. Forearm rotation measured at the distal radioulnar joint is approximately 90° of supination and 80° of pronation. Several studies have shown that rotation of the ulna with respect to the humerus also occurs during forearm rotation. External rotation of the ulna occurs with supination of the forearm and internal rotation occurs with forearm pronation. In addition, the radius has been shown to migrate proximally with pronation and distally with supination.

Force Transmission

A number of approaches to the study of forces acting across the elbow have been performed. These have included two-dimensional and three-dimensional static and dynamic models with or without simulating activities at the level of the hand. To date, in vivo studies evaluating forces acting across the elbow joint, such as with the use of a telemetric prosthesis, have not been reported. Analytical models are based on knowledge of the muscles acting across the elbow, their lines of action and moment arms, muscle volumes, fiber lengths, and physiologic cross-sectional areas. In a three-dimensional model developed by Amis, maximal elbow joint forces were estimated to aid in the design of elbow implants. With triceps antagonism during isometric flexion, peak radiohumeral and ulnohumeral forces were calculated to be approximately 3200 N at 30° of flexion (greater than four times body weight). With biceps antagonism during isometric extension, peak ulnohumeral force was 30 to 100 N at 120° of flexion and peak radiohumeral force was 1400 N at 60° to 90° of flexion. An and associates showed that for strenuous weightlifting the resulting force on the ulnohumeral joint could range from one to three times the body weight, maximal at 30° of flexion. Push-up exercises exerted forces across the elbow joint averaging 45% of body weight.

The relative distribution of joint compression forces on the various facets of the elbow joint have been a focus of a number of investigators. Hall and Travell, using transducers in the radiocapitellar and ulnotrochlear joints, demonstrated that 57% of the force went through the radiocapitellar joint and 43% through the ulnohumeral joint. An and associates demonstrated a similar distribution of forces with the elbow in the extended position. Analytical models developed by Amis and associates have predicted similar distribution in forces that have been confirmed experimentally as outlined above. When the elbow is flexed, rotation of the forearm against resistance imposes a large torque across the articulation. Tension in the MCL was estimated to exceed double the body weight and triple the body weight at the radiohumeral joint. Because the strength of the MCL complex has been reported to average only 420 N in elderly cadaveric specimens, muscle forces are likely needed to protect the ligamentous structures from excessive loading. The frequent occurrence of MCL disruption and osteochondritis dissecans in throwing athletes may be explained by the high valgus torques placed across the elbow joint. In one study of baseball pitchers, the maximum compressive forces on the elbow joint were reported to be 780 N, approximately equal to body weight.

Geel and associates, using pressure-sensitive film in the intact elbow, have demonstrated that repair of the MCL complex reduced loading across the radiocapitellar joint in an unstable cadaveric model. Joint loading was demonstrated to increase in pronation and decrease in supination. The importance of the interosseous membrane has also been established based on these in vitro studies supporting in vivo clinical observations.

Stabilizers

Articular Surfaces

Proximal Ulna The greater sigmoid notch of the ulna articulates with the trochlea of the distal humerus. Progressive excision of the proximal ulna reportedly results in a stepwise decrease in the stability of the elbow. Eighty percent of valgus stress was resisted by the proximal portion of the greater sigmoid notch, whereas 65% of varus stress was primarily resisted by the distal portion of the joint surface. Excision of the proximal ulna for comminuted olecranon fractures has an important influence on the static constraint and stability of the elbow.

The coronoid process of the ulna is a key stabilizer of the elbow. Failure to reconstitute this structure after fractures has been correlated with elbow instability and a poor functional outcome. The coronoid process appears to be an essential osseous block to prevent posterior subluxation of the elbow joint, especially with the elbow in extension. The attachment of the anterior band of the MCL to the coronoid has important implications in the treatment of displaced type III coronoid fractures, in which there is significant elbow instability.

Proximal Radius The proximal radius articulates with the capitellum of the humerus and has been demonstrated to be an important stabilizer to valgus stress. A study by Morrey and An using a sequential sectioning protocol suggested that the radial head contributed about 30% of the valgus stability of the joint in both flexion and extension. A subsequent kinematic study with unconstrained loading, however, demonstrated that the radial head was a secondary restraint to valgus elbow stability and that the MCL was the primary stabilizer. Excision of the radial head with an intact MCL had a minimal effect on the valgus stability of the elbow. However, following division of the MCL, the radial head was observed to be essential in maintaining the valgus stability of the elbow.

Distal Humerus Although the contribution of the articular surface of the distal humerus to the stability of the elbow has not been quantified, the circular shape of the trochlea with its deep groove is important in stabilizing the ulnohumeral joint, just as the convex shape of the capitellum is important in stabilizing the concave radial head.

Capsuloligamentous Tissues

Medial Collateral Ligament Complex The anterior bundle of the MCL has been shown to be the primary stabilizer of the elbow against valgus. A number of kinematic studies have demonstrated moderate joint laxity after sectioning of the anterior bundle of the MCL, even in the presence of an intact radial head. Clinically, the functional importance of the anterior bundle of the MCL has been confirmed and ligament reconstructions have been developed and used to treat patients with a deficiency of this structure. The anterior bundle is greatly augmented by the surrounding tendons of the common flexor pronator origin, with which it is integrated.

The posterior bundle of the MCL has been shown to contribute little to the static stability of the elbow. In vitro mechanical testing has confirmed that the posterior bundle is approximately 61% as strong as the anterior bundle of the MCL, possibly also reflecting its relative significance.

Lateral Collateral Ligament Complex The LCL is the major stabilizing structure for both rotational and varus stability. Injury to the ulnar part of this ligament results in posterolateral rotatory instability of the elbow. Reconstruction of this ligament restores elbow stability and eliminates the lateral pivot shift for posterolateral rotatory instability both clinically and experimentally.

The LCL has recently been shown in an unconstrained testing system to have a major influence on both varus and rotational stability of the elbow. The humeral attachment of the LCL was divided, including both the radial collateral and lateral ulnar collateral ligament origins. After lateral ligament sectioning, a fivefold increase in varus and rotational laxity of the elbow was measured at higher angles of flexion, even in the presence of an intact articulation (Fig. 9). Preservation or repair of this ligament should be emphasized in patients undergoing surgical approaches to the lateral aspect of the elbow.

Capsule The anterior capsule of the elbow has been shown to be an important static valgus-varus stabilizer with the elbow in extension. In a study by Morrey and An, the capsule provided 30% to 40% of the resistance to valgus-varus loading and 85% of the resistance to distraction with the elbow in extension but only minor contributions in flexion.

Muscles

Limited data exist regarding the stabilizing influence of the muscles that cross the elbow. In one study, simulated muscle loading of the triceps, biceps, and brachialis in a cadaveric model resulted in a significant increase in elbow stability. Theoretical studies based on the cross-sectional area and the muscle moment arms suggest that the biceps, brachialis, and triceps apply a compressive force across the elbow and thereby should contribute to the stability of the elbow joint. Further studies using a rigid body spring model have demonstrated that the pattern and extent of muscle activation determines the direction and magnitude of the resultant joint force on the articulating surface. Provided that the flexor and extensor muscle forces are appropriately balanced, the muscles should stabilize the elbow as confirmed by simulated muscle loading in cadaveric studies and clinical observations. Motion analysis studies in baseball pitchers have demonstrated that the valgus forces acting on the MCL complex exceed its strength. Electromyographic studies in these pitchers suggest that muscle contraction may dynamically stabilize the elbow and protect the static ligamentous constraints. It is clear that more work is needed to improve our understanding of the function of muscles acting across the elbow.

Biomechanics of Total Elbow Arthroplasty

A number of prostheses have been designed and used for elbow joint replacement over the past 25 years. Although the success rate of these implants has generally been lower than that of other joints, recent publications have reported improved long-term survival rates that are approaching those of the hip and knee. Our understanding of the normal kinematics and stabilizers of the elbow has contributed to refinements in implant designs and their surgical application.

Whereas constrained total elbows have fallen into disfavor because of high rates of aseptic loosening, both semiconstrained and resurfacing implants have reported excellent results. Current implants can be considered either linked or unlinked. Semiconstrained implants are generally coupled together (eg, with an axis pin) to prevent separation. These implants allow a certain amount of varus-valgus and rotational toggle before reaching their laxity limit. While these "loose-hinged" implants have eliminated the problem of dislocation frequently seen with unlinked resurfacing implants, there has been concern about their potential to function as constrained implants in vivo. In one recent study that evaluated the in vitro kinematics of semiconstrained arthroplasty, the Mayo-modified Coonrad device was shown to have laxity values higher than the intact cadaveric elbow, but lower than the limits of the implant when balanced simulated muscle

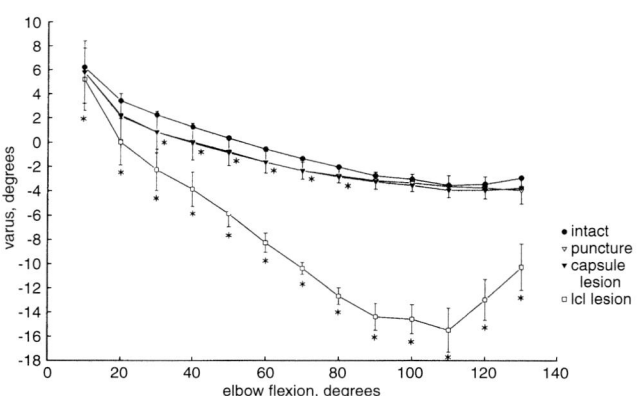

Fig. 9 Stabilizing influence of the lateral collateral ligament complex. Sectioning of the lateral collateral ligament complex caused a significant decrease in the varus-valgus stability of the elbow. (Reproduced with permission from Olsen BS, Vaesel MT, Søjbjerg JO, et al: Lateral collateral ligament of the elbow joint: Anatomy and kinematics. *J Shoulder Elbow Surg* 1996;4:103-112.)

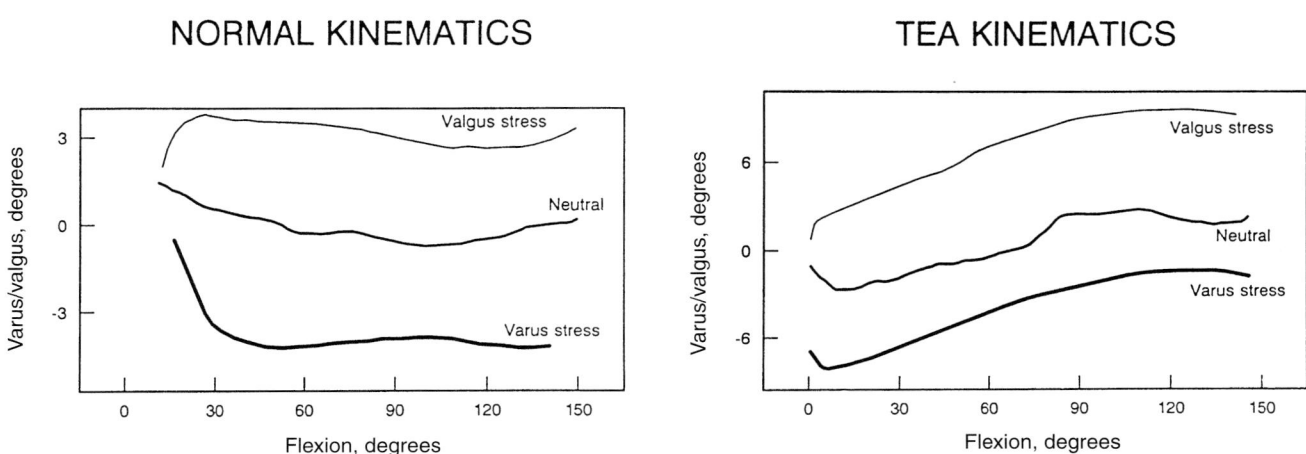

Fig. 10 Kinematics and laxity of a semiconstrained total elbow. Kinematics and laxity of a normal elbow in vitro subjected to balanced muscle loading **(left)**. Kinematics and laxity of an elbow following Mayo-modified Coonrad total elbow arthroplasty **(right)**. Note the increase in laxity relative to the intact joint; however, the laxity is lower than the toggle permitted by the implant. TEA = total elbow arthroplasty. (Reproduced with permission from O'Driscoll SW, An KN, Korinek S, et al: Kinematics of semiconstrained total elbow arthroplasty. *J Bone Joint Surg* 1992;74B:297-299.)

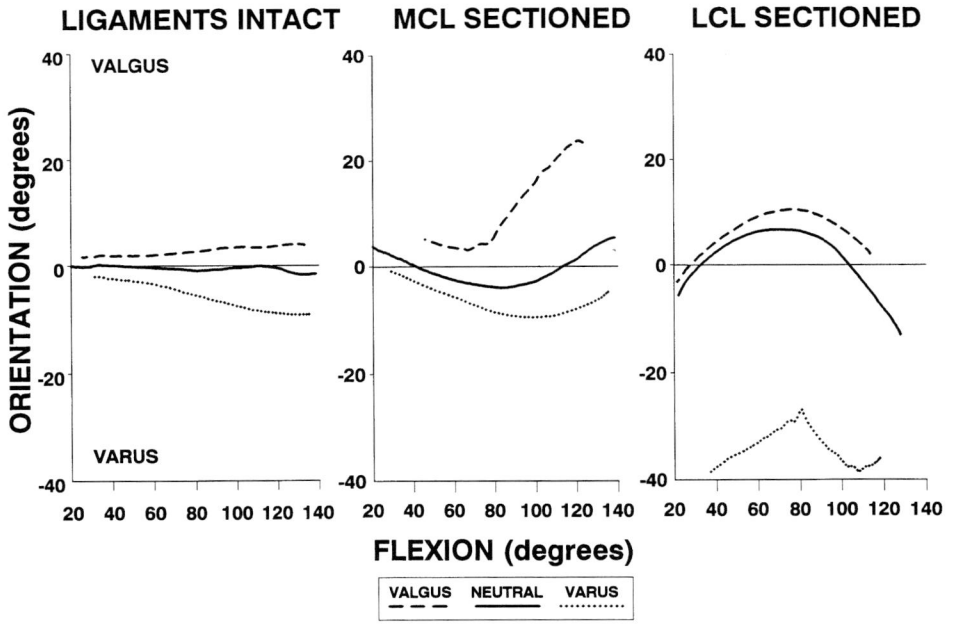

Fig. 11 Kinematics and laxity of a resurfacing total elbow: effect of collateral ligament sectioning. Kinematics and laxity of the elbow after arthroplasty with a capitellocondylar prosthesis subjected to balanced muscle loading in vitro **(left)**. After sectioning of the medial collateral ligament (MCL) with the lateral collateral ligament (LCL) intact, the elbow became markedly unstable with valgus loading **(center)**. Gross varus instability of the elbow occurred when the LCL complex was detached along with the lateral epicondyle (with the MCL intact) **(right)**. (Reproduced with permission from King GJW, Itoi E, Niebur G, et al: Motion and laxity of the capitellocondylar total elbow prosthesis. *J Bone Joint Surg* 1994;76A:1000-1008.)

loading was applied across the elbow (Fig. 10). This study suggests that the muscles absorb some of the forces and moments that act across the elbow and thereby minimize loading of the bone-cement interface as occurs with more constrained devices. This laboratory data may explain the low incidence of loosening that has been observed clinically with this and other semiconstrained devices.

Resurfacing elbow replacement arthroplasties have the theoretical advantage of load sharing with the capsuloligamentous stabilizers, potentially lowering the forces absorbed by the implant-bone interface. One of these implants, the capitellocondylar total elbow, has been widely used and is a subject of several clinical studies. Although one long-term study recently reported a low incidence of dislocation and loosening with this device, others have reported a much higher rate of implant instability and aseptic loosening. In a cadaveric study of 17 elbows, this prosthesis was able to restore acceptable patterns of motion and stability to the elbow given appropriate component positioning and soft-tissue balance. The collateral ligaments were demonstrated to be an essential stabilizer of this resurfacing implant. Gross instability was evident in the MCL or LCL deficient elbow (Fig. 11).

Based on the current laboratory data, resurfacing implants should be used only if there are adequate collateral ligaments and the components are accurately placed to restore normal kinematics and hence, soft-tissue balance. Linked implants should be considered the implant of choice in patients with either poor bone stock or ligament insufficiency.

Selected Bibliography

Amis AA, Dowson D, Wright V: Elbow joint force predictions for some strenuous isometric actions. *J Biomech* 1980;13:765-775.

Using a two-dimensional model of elbow loading, forces of up to 3 kN were predicted for some strenuous activities primarily because of the relatively long length of the forearm and the influence of muscle loading. The head of the radius was predicted to be important in force transmission across the elbow. Excision of the radial head was predicted to significantly increase loading across the ulnohumeral joint and the medial collateral ligament. The elbow was considered to be a "weightbearing joint."

An KN, Himenho S, Tsumura H, et al: Pressure distribution on articular surfaces: Application to joint stability evaluation. *J Biomech* 1990;23:1013-1020.

An KN, Hui FC, Morrey BF, et al: Muscles across the elbow joint: A biomechanical analysis. *J Biomech* 1981;14:659-669.

An KN, Kaufman KR, Chao EYS: Physiological considerations of muscle force through the elbow joint. *J Biomech* 1989;22:1249-1256.

An KN, Kwak BM, Chao EY, et al: Determination of muscle and joint forces: A new technique to solve the indeterminate problem. *J Biomech Eng* 1984;106:364-367.

An KN, Morrey BF: Biomechanics of the elbow, in Morrey BF (ed): *The Elbow and Its Disorders,* ed 2. Philadelphia, PA, WB Saunders, 1993, pp 53-72.

An KN, Morrey BF, Chao EYS: Carrying angle of the human elbow joint. *J Orthop Res* 1984;1:369-378.

An KN, Morrey BF, Chao EYS: The effect of partial removal of proximal ulna on elbow constraint. *Clin Orthop* 1986;209:270-279.

Cage DJN, Abrams RA, Callahan JJ, et al: Soft tissue attachments of the ulnar coronoid process: An anatomic study with radiographic correlation. *Clin Orthop* 1995;320:154-158.

The soft-tissue attachments on the coronoid were studied in 20 cadaveric elbows. The anterior bundle of the medial collateral ligament was attached an average of 18 mm dorsal to the tip of the coronoid. Only Regan type III fractures would include the ulnar insertion of this structure. The anterior capsule was attached an average of 6 mm distal to the coronoid tip and therefore type I fractures are unlikely to be caused by capsular avulsion. The brachialis has a broad attachment 26 mm in length averaging 11 mm distal to the coronoid tip.

Callaway GH, Field LD, O'Brien SJ, et al: The contribution of medial collateral ligaments to valgus stability of the elbow: A biomechanical study. *J Shoulder Elbow Surg* 1995;4:S58.

In a cadaveric study, the anterior bundle of the medial collateral ligament was found to consist of two functional bundles that tighten in reciprocal fashion during elbow flexion and extension. The anterior bundle of the medial collateral ligament was found to be the primary stabilizer to valgus loading. Complete division of this structure was found to result in only a small increase in valgus rotation that may be too small to be detectable by clinical examination.

Carret JP, Fischer LP, Gonon GP, et al: Cinematic study of prosupination at the level of the radiocubital (radioulnar) articulations. *Bull Assoc Anat* 1976;60:279-295.

Using photographic markers in cadaveric limbs, the instantaneous centers of forearm rotation were determined. The axis of rotation was found to vary throughout forearm prosupination demonstrating that the radial head not only rotates but also slides relative to the sigmoid notch of the ulna.

Chess DG, Leahey JL, Hyndman JC: Cubitus varus: Significant factors. *J Pediatr Orthop* 1994;14:190-192.

Using skeletal models of the upper limb, supracondylar osteotomies of the distal humerus were performed to create deformities of the distal humerus. Flexion contractures and posterior angulation of the distal humeral fragment were found to decrease the apparent cubitus varus deformity. Internal rotation of the distal humeral fragment worsened the deformity.

Conway JE, Jobe FW, Glousman RE, et al: Medial instability of the elbow in throwing athletes: Treatment by repair or reconstruction of the ulnar collateral ligament. *J Bone Joint Surg* 1992;74A:67-83.

Davidson PA, Pink M, Perry J, et al: Functional anatomy of the flexor pronator muscle group in relation to the medial collateral ligament of the elbow. *Am J Sports Med* 1995;23:245-250.

The flexor carpi ulnaris muscle was found to directly overlie the medial collateral ligament of the elbow in a series of anatomic dissections. The flexor digitorum superficialis was situated slightly anterior to the medial collateral ligament. Exercise and specific conditioning of these muscles may prevent injury or assist in rehabilitation of medial elbow instability, especially in overhand throwing athletes.

Donkers MJ, An KN, Chao EYS, et al: Hand position affects elbow joint load during push-up exercise. *J Biomech* 1993;26:625-632.

Forces exerted across the elbow were investigated in normal volunteers using a force plate and motion tracking device. Peak forces along the forearm axis averaged 45% of body weight. Torque values were reduced if the hands were positioned farther apart or more superiorly than normal. Valgus torque increased by 42% for one-handed push-ups.

Eckstein F, Lohe F, Hillebrand S, et al: Morphomechanics of the humero-ulnar joint: I. Joint space width and contact areas as a function of load and flexion angle. *Anat Rec* 1995;243:318-326.

Eckstein F, Lohe F, Muller-Gerbl M, et al: Stress distribution in the trochlear notch: A model of bicentric load transmission through joints. *J Bone Joint Surg* 1994;76B:647-653.

Eckstein F, Muller-Gerbl M, Steinlechner M, et al: Subchondral bone density in the human elbow assessed by computed tomography osteoabsorptiometry: A reflection of the loading history of the joint surfaces. *J Orthop Res* 1995;13:268-278.

The subchondral bone density of 36 cadaveric extremities was studied using computed tomography. The fovea of the radial head showed a central density maximum because of the flatter socket of the humeral radial joint leading to central load transmission. The trochlear notch usually presented a bicentric maximum density corresponding to the deeper socket of the humeroulnar joint yielding two functional facets.

Funk DA, An KA, Morrey BF, et al: Electromyographic analysis of muscles across the elbow joint. *J Orthop Res* 1987;5:529-538.

The electromyographic activity of eight elbow muscles was recorded during resisted motions. The muscle activity was found to be highly dependent on the angle of joint flexion and the direction of the motion. The activity in the major elbow muscles was found to be determined primarily by the size of the flexion and extension moments created about the elbow joint, but not by valgus and varus moments.

Fuss FK: The ulnar collateral ligament of the human elbow joint: Anatomy, function and biomechanics. *J Anat* 1991;175:203-212.

Gallay SH, Richards RR, O'Driscoll SW: Intraarticular capacity and compliance of stiff and normal elbows. *Arthroscopy* 1993;9:9-13.

The capsular capacity and compliance of stiff and normal elbows was measured in 11 patients. The capacity of the normal elbow was 14 × 2 ml and that of the stiff elbows was only 6 × 3 ml. The capsular compliance of the stiff elbow was 15% of normal. The position of minimal intra-articular pressure and maximal compliance was at 70° of flexion.

Hotchkiss RN, Weiland AJ: Valgus stability of the elbow. *J Orthop Res* 1987;3:372-377.

Josefsson PO, Gentz CF, Johnell O, et al: Surgical versus non-surgical treatment of ligamentous injuries following dislocation of the elbow joint: A prospective randomized study. *J Bone Joint Surg* 1987;69A:605-608.

Josefsson PO, Johnell O, Gentz CF: Long-term sequelae of simple dislocation of the elbow. *J Bone Joint Surg* 1984;66A:927-930.

King J, Brelsford HJ, Tullos HS: Analysis of the pitching arm of the professional baseball pitcher. *Clin Orthop* 1969;67:116-123.

King GJW, Itoi E, Niebur G, et al: Motion and laxity of the capitellocondylar total elbow prosthesis. *J Bone Joint Surg* 1994;76A:1000-1008.

The motion patterns and laxity of the capitellocondylar resurfacing total elbow arthroplasty were compared to those of the intact elbow in 17 cadaveric specimens. Whereas the laxity of the elbows was increased following joint replacement arthroplasty, there were no dislocations or malarticulations of the prostheses observed given appropriate implant positioning and soft-tissue tensioning. The ulnar collateral ligament was found to be vulnerable to injury during placement of the ulnar component. Sectioning of either the medial or lateral collateral ligament resulted in gross instability of the prosthetic joint, demonstrating the importance of soft tissue integrity when using unlinked resurfacing implant designs.

King GJW, Morrey BF, An KN: Stabilizers of the elbow. *J Shoulder Elbow Surg* 1993;2:165-174.

Lanz T, Wachsmuth W: *Praktische Anatomie,* ed 2. Berlin, Germany, Springer-Verlag, 1959, p 156.

Linscheid RL, Wheeler DK: Elbow dislocations. *JAMA* 1965;194:1171-1176.

Martin BF: The annular ligament of the superior radio-ulnar joint. *J Anat* 1958;92:473-482.

Mehlhoff TL, Noble PC, Bennett JB, et al: Simple dislocation of the elbow in the adult: Results after closed treatment. *J Bone Joint Surg* 1988;70A:244-249.

Morrey BF, An KN: Articular and ligamentous contributions to the stability of the elbow joint. *Am J Sports Med* 1983;11:315-319.

Morrey BF, An KN: Functional anatomy of the ligaments of the elbow. *Clin Orthop* 1985;201:84-90.

Morrey BF, An KN, Stormont TJ: Force transmission through the radial head. *J Bone Joint Surg* 1988;70A:250-256.

Morrey BF, Chao EYS: Passive motion of the elbow joint: A biomechanical analysis. *J Bone Joint Surg* 1976;58A:501-508.

Morrey BF, Tanaka S, An KN: Valgus stability of the elbow: A definition of primary and secondary constraints. *Clin Orthop* 1991;265:187-195.

Murray WM, Delp SL, Buchanan TS: Variation of muscle moment arms with elbow and forearm position. *J Biomech* 1995;28:513-525.

Using two cadaveric extremities to provide baseline data, a computer model was developed to investigate changes in muscle moment arms with elbow motion. The major muscles acting across the elbow were found to have varying moment arms (and thus varying strength) throughout both flexion-extension and prosupination.

O'Driscoll SW, An KN, Korinek S, et al: Kinematics of semiconstrained total elbow arthroplasty. *J Bone Joint Surg* 1992;74B:297-299.

The kinematics and laxity of the Mayo-modified Coonrad total elbow arthroplasty were compared to those of the intact elbow in 11 cadaveric upper limbs. Balanced muscle loading was applied across the joint by loading the biceps, brachialis, and triceps. The laxity of the elbows increased following joint replacement; however, the toggle in the implant exceeded this laxity. This suggests that muscles absorb some of the forces and thereby minimize loading of the prosthesis-bone interface of this loose-hinged implant.

O'Driscoll SW, Bell DF, Morrey BF: Posterolateral rotatory instability of the elbow. *J Bone Joint Surg* 1991;73A: 440-446.

O'Driscoll SW, Horii E, Morrey BF, et al: Anatomy of the ulnar part of the lateral collateral ligament (LUCL) of the elbow. *Clin Anat* 1992;5:296-303.

The three parts of the lateral collateral ligament complex of the elbow, radial part, ulnar part, and the annular ligament, are described. The ulnar part has also been termed the lateral ulnar collateral ligament, which has been demonstrated to be the primary constraint against posterolateral rotatory instability of the elbow.

O'Driscoll SW, Jaloszynski R, Morrey BF, et al: Origin of the medial ulnar collateral ligament. *J Hand Surg* 1992;17A:164-168.

The humeral origin of the anterior attachment of the medial collateral ligament was found to arise from the anteroinferior portion of the medial epicondyle. Excision of the entire medial epicondyle for the treatment of ulnar neuropathy may destabilize the elbow.

O'Driscoll SW, Morrey BF, An KN: Intraarticular pressure and capacity of the elbow. *J Arthrosc Rel Surg* 1990;6: 100-103.

O'Driscoll SW, Morrey BF, Bell DF: Posterolateral rotatory instability of the elbow: Clinical, pathoanatomic, and radiographic features. *J Bone Joint Surg* 1990;72B:543.

O'Driscoll SW, Morrey BF, Korinek S, et al: Elbow subluxation and dislocation: A spectrum of instability. *Clin Orthop* 1992;280:186-197.

Elbow subluxation and dislocation was investigated by sequential ligament release in a series of 13 cadaveric extremities. Dislocation was demonstrated to be the final of three stages of instability resulting from posterolateral rotation with soft-tissue disruption progressing from lateral to medial. Disruption of the lateral ulnar collateral ligament was considered to be an essential component of the pathoanatomy of elbow dislocation. Dislocation of the ulnohumeral joint was demonstrated to occur in the presence of an intact medial collateral ligament.

Olsen BS, Henriksen MG, Søjbjerg JO, et al: Elbow joint instability: A kinematic model. *J Shoulder Elbow Surg* 1994;3:143-150.

Olsen BS, Vaesel MT, Søjbjerg JO, et al: Lateral collateral ligament of the elbow joint: Anatomy and kinematics. *J Shoulder Elbow Surg* 1996;5:103-112.

In a cadaveric study, the lateral collateral ligament complex was found to be an important stabilizer of the humeroulnar joint in forced varus and external rotation. The contribution of the collateral ligament to elbow stability was minimal in extension; however, it increased at larger angles of flexion. Humeroulnar stability was observed to independent of forearm rotation during testing.

Osborne G, Cotterill P: Recurrent dislocation of the elbow. *J Bone Joint Surg* 1966;48B:340-346.

Regan W, Morrey B: Fractures of the coronoid process of the ulna. *J Bone Joint Surg* 1989;71A:1348-1354.

Regan WD, Korinek SL, Morrey BF, et al: Biomechanical study of ligaments around the elbow joint. *Clin Orthop* 1991;271:170-179.

Roetert EP, Brody H, Dillman CJ, et al: The biomechanics of tennis elbow: An integrated approach. *Clin Sports Med* 1995;14:47-57.

This is a review of important biomechanical factors in the pathogenesis of tennis elbow. The extensor carpi radialis longus and brevis muscles are highly active in all tennis strokes. Forces are highest on the backhand stroke. The use of a two-handed backhand decreases forces in the wrist extensors and reduces the clinical incidence of tennis elbow.

Schwab GH, Bennett JB, Woods GW, et al: Biomechanics of elbow instability: The role of the medial collateral ligament. *Clin Orthop* 1980;146:42-52.

Søjbjerg JO, Ovesen J, Gundorf CE: The stability of the elbow following excision of the radial head and transection of the annular ligament: An experimental study. *Arch Orthop Trauma Surg* 1987;106:248-250.

Søjbjerg JO, Ovesen J, Nielsen S: Experimental elbow instability after transection of the medial collateral ligament. *Clin Orthop* 1987;218:186-190.

Werner FW, An KN: Biomechanics of the elbow and forearm. *Hand Clin* 1994;10:357-373.

This is a good review article covering the biomechanics of both the elbow and forearm.

Werner SL, Fleisig GS, Dillman CJ, et al: Biomechanics of the elbow during baseball pitching. *J Orthop Sports Phys Ther* 1993;17:274-278.

Using a motion analysis system and electromyography, the kinematics and kinetics of baseball pitchers were measured. A varus torque of 120 Nm, acting to resist valgus stress, occurred near the time of maximal shoulder rotation. The medial collateral ligament may not be strong enough to resist this load without dynamic stabilizers. The triceps, flexor pronator muscles, and anconeus activity during peak valgus stress suggests that these muscles may be important dynamic stabilizers to prevent injury to the medial collateral ligament.

Zarzour ZDS, Cordy ME, Milne AD, et al: Abstract: An anthropometric study of the radial head and its relationship to implant design. *Trans Orthop Res Soc* 1995;20:690.

Anthropometric measurements of 28 cadaveric radial heads were performed using a coordinate measuring machine. The articular margin of the radial head was elliptical, with the difference between the maximum and minimum diameters averaging 1.7 ± 0.7 mm. The articulation between the radial head and capitellum was offset an average of 4.2 ± 2.5 mm from the radial neck. These anatomic features may have important implications in the design of a radial head hemiarthroplasty.

34

Athletic Injuries of the Elbow

James R. Andrews, MD and S. Wendell Holmes, Jr, MD

Introduction

Elbow injuries are becoming more common as participation in throwing and racquet sports increases. Although acute injuries occur, athletic injuries to the elbow are more commonly the result of chronic overuse. These injuries are usually the result of repetitive intrinsic or extrinsic overload resulting in repeated microrupture of tendons or ligaments. The most common problems include tendinitis (lateral, medial, and posterior), nerve dysfunction, and ligamentous injuries. Tendon ruptures about the elbow are rare but do occur.

Many elbow injuries result from valgus and extension overload caused by throwing or axial compression. A useful way of grouping these injuries is to classify them as medial tension injuries, lateral compression injuries, extension overload injuries, and tendinopathies. Nerve dysfunction usually falls into the medial tension category. Skeletally immature patients should be grouped separately because of their unique injury patterns involving the growth centers about the elbow.

Improved understanding of the biomechanics of the elbow has aided in the diagnosis and treatment of injuries to this joint. Elbow biomechanics has been especially well studied in the throwing athlete, specifically in baseball pitchers. The pitching motion is analogous to the overhead motions in other sports such as volleyball, the overhead serve in tennis, and swimming. Thus, some of the biomechanical principles of the pitching motion will also apply to the pathophysiology of elbow injuries in other sports.

Acute fractures and dislocations also occur in the athletic population. These injuries are discussed in detail in the chapters on elbow instability and fractures. Specific treatment options for athletes are related to rehabilitation plans, which should be modified in preparation for return to their particular sport.

A complete history, physical examination, and plain radiographs remain the cornerstones of diagnosis of elbow injuries. Magnetic resonance imaging (MRI) techniques continue to improve and this method is helpful in the diagnosis of elbow injuries, particularly soft-tissue injuries. Stress radiographs continue to play an important role in the diagnosis of elbow instability. However, to adequately assess athletic injuries of the elbow, some familiarity with the imposed stresses of, and injuries unique to, the particular sport is necessary.

Treatment of elbow injuries continues to evolve, but most injuries are still treated nonsurgically. The basic principles of rest, ice, compression, and elevation for acute injuries or exacerbations apply, and should be followed with a carefully planned rehabilitation program. Indications for the use of elbow arthroscopy have been better defined as the understanding of the applied surgical anatomy has improved. Elbow arthroscopy has been beneficial in confirming difficult diagnoses and in identifying appropriate treatment for intra-articular bony lesions of the joint. Improved techniques for open surgery, including ulnar collateral ligament (UCL) reconstruction, distal biceps tendon repair, and ulnar nerve transposition, have recently been reported.

Biomechanics

Throwing

Injuries to the elbow in throwing athletes, regardless of the athlete's specific sport, are similar. The biomechanics of throwing has been best described in baseball players in general and pitchers specifically. Detailed biomechanical analysis of the pitching mechanism allows for the most comprehensive understanding of throwing mechanics. The pitching motion is divided into several phases, which include wind-up, cocking, acceleration, deceleration, and follow-through. Figure 1 shows the various phases, and Figure 2 outlines the muscle activities and torques present during each phase.

The acceleration phase occurs between cocking and ball release. Acceleration refers specifically to the ball and not the various arm segments because these may go through deceleration phases as the ball is accelerated. Over the course of approximately 50 to 80 ms, the ball is accelerated from a stationary position to over 80 miles per hour. This mechanism involves transfer of momentum, in a whiplike fashion, from the trunk to the shoulder, the humerus, the elbow, the forearm, the hand, and finally, the ball. During the first half of this phase, the pectoralis and subscapularis muscles contract to accelerate the humerus anteriorly along a horizontal plane. Also, the shoulder internal rotators (subscapularis, latissimus dorsi, and teres major) contract to start the internal rotation of the humerus. Tremendous forward forces are generated in the humerus at this time, with the hand and ball essentially left behind. This results in the elbow being placed in a position of extreme valgus, generating significant tensile forces across the medial side of the elbow and compressive loads on the lateral side of the joint. At the midway point of this phase, the rate of humeral adduction decreases by imposition of a deceleration from the teres minor, infraspinatus, and the supraspinatus muscles. Thus, momentum is transferred to the forearm, adding to the rate of internal rotation and further accelerating the ball. With forearm and wrist acceleration, centrifugal forces impose an extension moment across the elbow. The rate of elbow extension is regulated by the elbow flexors, particularly the biceps and brachialis muscles. A large degree of torque is generated at this point and is coupled with a high rate of extension, creating large shear forces on the articular surface. It is these shear forces that can initiate articular surface degeneration in the joint. The forearm, hand, and

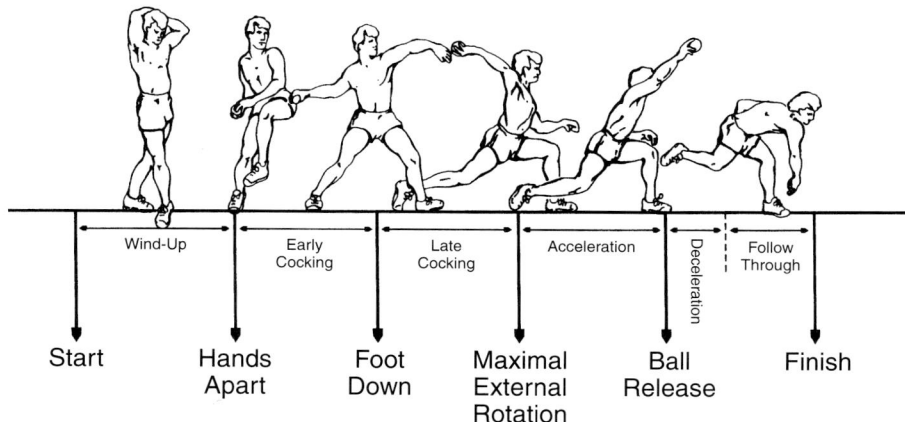

Fig. 1 The phases of the pitching motion. (Reproduced with permission from DiGiovine NM, Jobe FW, Pink M, et al: An electromyographic analysis of the upper extremity in pitching. *J Shoulder Elbow Surg* 1992;1:15-25.)

ball reach their maximum speed at the end of the acceleration phase. The grip on the ball is loosened, and the ball leaves the hand over the next 6 to 10 ms. This is called the release point, after which the arm motion must be decelerated.

The arm momentum thus developed places an outwardly directed force of about 300 lb on the arm upon entering the deceleration phase. The forces that must be counteracted through deceleration include humeral internal rotation, glenohumeral distraction, and elbow extension. At the elbow, the biceps, brachioradialis, and brachialis all contract to prevent hyperextension. If deceleration does not occur rapidly enough, hyperextension injuries can occur. If deceleration occurs too rapidly, high flexion forces can overstress the long head of the biceps muscle and its tendon.

During follow-through, the body moves forward with the arm, reducing the distraction forces applied to the shoulder and decreasing the tension in the rotator cuff muscles.

Electromyographic (EMG) analysis combined with high-speed photography has shown that measurable muscle activity about the elbow is only mild to moderate throughout all phases of the throwing motion. It appears that the elbow musculature acts to position the elbow and forearm so that maximum transfer of momentum generated by the muscles of the shoulder and trunk can be achieved. Also, forceful contractions of muscles about the elbow as a means of altering ball delivery (eg, a curve ball) do not occur. Rather, the ball grip and minor changes in position of the wrist and elbow appear to be all that is necessary to create different types of pitches. It has been theorized that forceful firing of the flexor-pronator mass leads to medial elbow morbidity. However, based on the abovementioned EMG data and the knowledge of forces generated across the elbow, it is more likely that medial elbow morbidity is secondary to the forceful passive distraction during the acceleration phase of throwing.

Racquet Sports

Biomechanically, the overhead tennis serve is essentially the same motion as the overhand pitch in baseball. Tennis ground strokes are somewhat different mechanically and are generally described as having three phases: preparation, acceleration, and follow-through. Muscle activities during the various phases have been documented with EMG analysis.

Faulty mechanics in competitive tennis players with lateral epicondylitis have been documented by EMG analysis. Excessive activity of the extensor digitorum communis, extensor carpi radialis longus and brevis, flexor carpi radialis, and pronator teres was found in affected individuals versus normals during the backhand stroke. Through video analysis, a characteristic "leading elbow" backhand and open racquet face were also identified among the affected players.

Golf

The golf swing is usually divided into four phases: takeaway, forward swing, acceleration, and follow-through. Medial epicondylitis in the dominant or trailing arm is a common injury in golf, and muscle activity has been documented by EMG in this arm in asymptomatic and symptomatic golfers. In players affected with medial epicondylitis, studies of the wrist flexor and extensor activities with surface electrodes showed greater flexor activity during the takeaway and forward swing phases.

Other Sports

Weight lifting and gymnastics are sports in which the elbow is often used in a weightbearing position that generates compressive and valgus forces on the elbow. The stresses on the elbow are range-of-motion dependent, with the greatest resultant force occurring at about 30° of flexion. A simple two-handed push-up produces peak compressive forces of

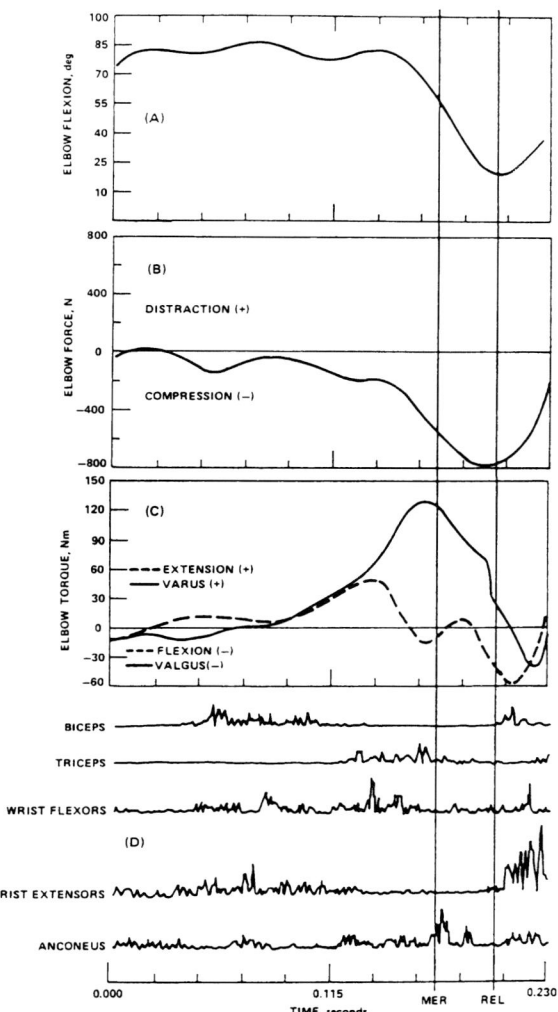

Fig. 2 Time-matched measurements during the baseball pitch: (A) elbow flexion, (B) force applied at the elbow, (C) torque applied at the elbow, and (D) EMG muscle activity. (Reproduced with permission from Werner SL, Fleisig GS, Dillman CJ, et al: Biomechanics of the elbow during baseball pitching. *J Orthop Sports Phys Ther* 1993;17:274-278.)

45% body weight, but peak loads can exceed three times body weight with more vigorous exercises and higher weights.

Specific Injury Patterns

A familiarity with injuries associated with specific sports is important in the treatment of an athletic patient population. Table 1 gives a listing of common elbow injuries and the sports in which they are commonly seen.

Throwing injuries of the elbow refer to overuse syndromes caused by the act of throwing over many months or years. Cumulative pathologic changes occurring in the anatomic structures about the joint eventually exceed the body's ability to repair or compensate for these changes. Most elbow injuries in the throwing athlete fall into a continuum of diagnoses that represent the progression of a single injury termed valgus extension overload. These conditions have been classified and are presented in Table 2.

Medial Elbow Injuries

Ulnar Collateral Ligament Injury Rupture of the UCL in the throwing athlete often presents as acute onset of medial elbow pain during the act of throwing. The athlete will complain of pain at the medial elbow and will often have concomitant signs of ulnar nerve irritation. Pain on palpation along the course of the anterior bundle of the UCL is usually present, with tenderness more often at the distal than the proximal insertion, but differentiation of the injured structure is difficult because of the proximity of other structures. A high index of suspicion is important in the diagnosis of this injury.

If the injury is suspected, stress radiographs and some form of contrast imaging are helpful in confirming the diagnosis. Side-to-side opening of 0.5 mm on stress radiographs with the elbow flexed 25° and an applied 150 N (34 lb) valgus force has been shown to accurately differentiate normal and injured ligaments. However, stress radiographs should be correlated with the athlete's symptoms and other studies before diagnosing functional UCL instability.

Also, MRI and computed tomographic (CT) arthrography are important tools in confirming the diagnosis of UCL injury. A study comparing MRI and CT arthrography showed that the respective sensitivities and specificities of the two methods were 57% and 100% for MRI, and 86% and 91% for CT arthrography. This study also described a "T-sign" on CT arthrography that was present with undersurface tears of the UCL. There is no distal subligamentous potential space in the uninjured elbow, but with distal undersurface tearing, dye leaks under the distal ligament and creates the image of a "T". Saline magnetic resonance arthrography gives excellent visualization of the soft tissues and also exhibits the "T-sign" for partial thickness tears.

A series of undersurface tears of the UCL in baseball players was recently reported. These players had persistent medial elbow pain with throwing and valgus stress tests. Six of the seven patients had normal preoperative MRI studies, with one MRI showing degeneration within the ligament. Preoperative CT arthrograms showed the "T" sign without extravasation of dye outside of the joint capsule in five of the seven patients. Arthroscopic evaluation showed medial elbow instability with valgus stress at 70° of flexion in all seven patients. Medial elbow dissection performed prior to UCL reconstruction demonstrated an intact external layer, but the deep layer was torn from its insertion into the ulna. The authors also dissected ten cadaver elbows and demonstrated that the anterior bundle of the UCL consistently inserts within 1 to 2 mm of the articular margin of the ulna. The authors concluded that undersurface tears of the anterior bundle of the UCL are associated with medial elbow instability, and a diagnosis can be

Table 1. Sports commonly producing elbow injuries

Sport	Common Elbow Injuries
Racquet sports	Lateral epicondylitis with backhand
Golf	Medial epicondylitis on downswing (trailing arm)
	Lateral epicondylitis at impact (leading arm)
Basketball	Posterior compartment problems with follow-through on jump shot
Waterskiing	Valgus extension overload of posterior compartment with trick skiing
Bowling	Flexor-pronator soreness
Baseball	Valgus stress of pitching yields medial traction, lateral compression, and posterior abutment
Volleyball	Valgus stress at instant of spiking
Football	Valgus stress when passing
	Hyperextension and dislocation with direct trauma
Weight training	Ulnar collateral ligament sprain, ulnar nerve irritation
Canoeing, kayaking	Distal bicipital tendinitis
Archery	Extensor muscle fatigue, lateral epicondylitis of bow arm

(Reproduced with permission from Whiteside JA, Andrews JR: Common elbow problems in the recreational athlete. *J Musculoskeletal Med* 1989;6:17-34.)

Table 2. Valgus extension overload syndrome

Medial tension injury
  Type I: UCL injury
    UCL subacute injury with inflammation
    UCL partial rupture
    UCL complete rupture
  Type II: Posterior-medial impingement
    Chondromalacia
    Osteophyte formation
    Olecranon stress fractures and loose bodies
  Type III: Flexor-pronator injury
    Medial epicondylitis
    Partial rupture of flexor-pronator muscle type
  Type IV: Ulnar nerve entrapment
    Cubital tunnel syndrome
    Ulnar nerve subluxation

Lateral compression injury
  Type V: Radiocapitellar overload syndrome
    Lateral elbow pain
    Capitellum and radial head chondromalacia
    Capitellum and radial head osteochondritis dissecans

made by visualization of distal dye leakage along the ulna with CT arthrogram (the "T"-sign).

Extensive study of the anatomy and biomechanics of the UCL have been performed. The anterior bundle of the UCL is very important in resisting valgus loads to the elbow. Three functional portions of the anterior bundle have been reported, with differing tensions in each bundle depending on the degree of flexion. The average length of the anterior bundle has been found to be 20 mm, with an average width of 8 mm. The average load to failure has been reported to be 260 N. In comparison, the average load to failure of the most common substitute, the palmaris longus, was 360 N. The contribution to elbow stability has also been studied. At full extension, valgus stability is equally divided between the UCL, the anterior capsule, and the bony articulation. At 90° of flexion, the UCL provides 55% of valgus stability. A cadaver study showed that transection of the anterior bundle of the UCL resulted in maximum valgus and internal rotation instability at 70° of elbow flexion.

Direct repair of the UCL is done in a minority of ruptures caused by throwing injuries because these ligaments have undergone attrition with long-term use and are no longer normal tissue. Acute rupture of healthy tissue does occasionally occur in the teenage thrower, and some of these injuries may be appropriate for repair. However, the more usual case involves chronic attenuation of the ligament with or without an acute event, in which reconstruction is the procedure of choice. A recent report, with over 6 years of follow-up, of repairs and reconstructions for medial elbow instability showed that 50% of the repairs and 68% of the reconstructions allowed players to return to their previous level of competition. Twelve of 16 major league players who had reconstructions were able to return to major league play. Reconstructions were performed with a free tendon graft, either palmaris longus, plantaris, Achilles, or long toe extensor. The authors noted that since 1987, reconstruction, not isolated repair, has been used for the treatment of the incompetent UCL. A negative prognostic factor was a previous operation on the involved elbow. Ulnar neuropathies were common following surgery (15 of 68 patients), but only 3% of players were likely prevented from returning to play secondary to ulnar nerve problems. The ulnar nerve was routinely submuscularly transposed in this series. Published techniques for UCL reconstruction vary mainly in whether the ulnar nerve is transposed subcutaneously (with or without fascial slings), submuscularly, or not transposed at all.

Prior to open surgery, arthroscopy is often performed to rule out coexisting intra-articular pathology. Also, the medial instability can be confirmed by performing an intraoperative valgus stress test at 70° of flexion. Medial joint openings can be directly visualized with the arthroscope (Fig. 3). Both repairs and reconstructions can be approached through a curvilinear medial or posterior incision using a technique similar to that described in the above study. The ulnar nerve is carefully mobilized and routinely subcutaneously transposed. A fascial sling is made to loosely secure the nerve over the flexor pronator mass. Reconstructions are done in a figure-of-8 fashion through drill holes in the ulna and medial epicondyle, and a free tendon autograft is used for the reconstruction (palmaris longus, plantaris, or long toe extensor) as shown in Figure 4. Postoperative rehabilitation is extremely important. Motion is started in the first

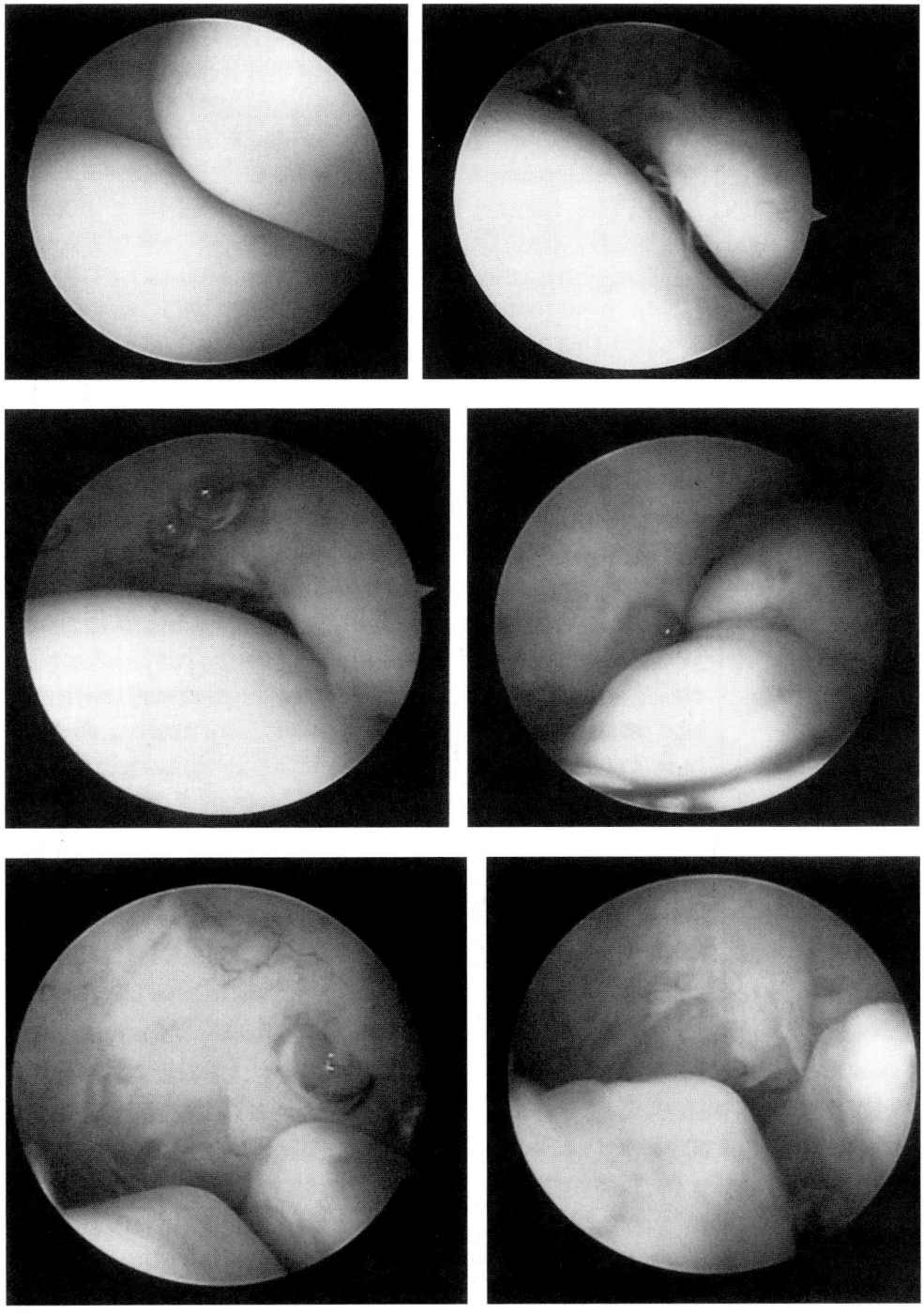

Fig. 3 The ulnar collateral ligament (UCL) stress test is performed at 70° of elbow flexion under direct arthroscopic visualization of the ulnar-humeral joint. **Top left,** Normal UCL; no stress applied. **Top right,** Full stress applied; no joint opening, confirming the presence of a normal UCL. **Center left** and **right,** Grade I UCL injury. **Center left,** No stress applied. **Center right,** Full stress applied; 1.5 mm of opening, indicating a low grade UCL injury and trace elbow instability. **Bottom left** and **right,** Grade III UCL injury. **Bottom left,** No stress applied. **Bottom right,** Full stress applied; 3.0 mm of opening, indicating a complete UCL tear with gross elbow instability. (Reproduced with permission from Joyce ME, Jelsma RD, Andrews JR: Throwing injuries to the elbow. *Sports Med Arthroscopy Rev* 1995;3:225-236.)

postoperative week in a brace between 30° and 90° of flexion, progressing from 0° to 110° by week 4, and 0° to 130° at week 6, at which time the brace is discontinued. Resistive exercises are started at week 4, a gentle throwing program is initiated at 4 months, and return to play occurs between 6 and 12 months postoperatively.

Acute rupture of the anterior band of the UCL can occur in contact injuries in many sports when a large valgus load is placed on the elbow. Examples include a quarterback who is struck in the arm during cocking or acceleration, or a baseball infielder struck in the arm while tagging out a runner. In these situations, acute repair of the injured UCL may be considered.

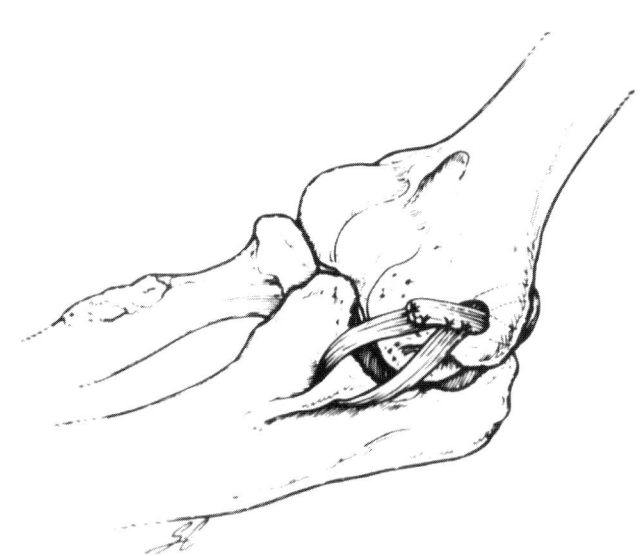

Fig. 4 An example of figure-of-8 reconstruction of chronic ulnar collateral ligament insufficiency using an autogenous tendon graft. (Reproduced with permission from Andrews JR, Schemmel SP, Whiteside JA, et al: Evaluation, treatment, and prevention of elbow injuries in throwing athletes, in Nicholas JA, Hershman EB, Posner MA (eds): *The Upper Extremity in Sports Medicine.* St. Louis, MO, CV Mosby, 1990, pp 781-826.)

At the time of surgery, potential injury to other soft tissues should be evaluated. These include avulsion of the flexor-pronator mass from its insertion, intrasubstance musculotendinous tears, and destabilization of the ulnar nerve in the cubital tunnel.

Medial Epicondyle Fractures Like most injuries on the medial aspect of the elbow in the throwing athlete, medial epicondyle fractures, although occurring acutely, are likely the result of chronic tensile overload. The forces applied to the medial epicondyle through the flexor-pronator muscle mass and the UCL result in adaptive changes within the epicondyle. These changes may be represented by overgrowth or fragmentation of the apophysis. These same forces are present throughout the player's career, and when these forces exceed the body's ability to repair itself, fractures occur. Fusion of the medial epicondylar apophysis occurs at about age 14 in girls and as late as age 17 in boys. Fractures in this age group usually enter the growth plate with displacement of the entire fragment. Anatomic reduction and internal fixation with K-wires or screws is recommended in this age group. There is a paucity of literature regarding the medial epicondyle fracture in the skeletally mature age group. Open reduction and internal fixation is recommended for displacements ranging from 1 cm to as little as 2 mm.

Flexor-Pronator Strain Throwing athletes can injure the flexor-pronator group at the musculotendinous junction, which is most commonly a partial rupture. These injuries are easier to prevent than to treat, and all throwing athletes should undergo preseason conditioning to improve the strength and flexibility of these muscle groups. Most of these injuries respond to a period of rest, followed by motion and strengthening exercises and return to their sport as symptoms permit. Flexor-pronator complete ruptures have been reported but are believed to be a rare injury. A report of two cases of complete tears in a group of 100 players with flexor-pronator strains showed that primary surgical repairs were unsuccessful, with players unable to return to an effective asymptomatic level of throwing.

Occasionally, ossification, which is usually asymptomatic, will occur in the muscle belly near its origin. If ossification is symptomatic, excision is usually successful without injury to the adjacent structures.

Medial Epicondylitis Medial epicondylitis, a common injury in golf and racquet sports, also occurs in throwing athletes. In these situations, the etiology is related to repetitive high tensile forces being placed on the flexor-pronator group at its insertion. The flexor burst in golf may play a role in the creation of this injury in golfers, but a study using EMG analysis showed increased activity in affected versus unaffected golfers during portions of the swing in which this group of muscles is usually quiescent (ie, takeaway and forward swing). Also, oversized grips and counterforce bracing, interventions often used to treat medial epicondylitis, did not lead to significant reductions in muscle activity in this study; thus, the use of these treatment modalities is questionable. Medial epicondylitis usually responds to a physical therapy program that includes eccentric stretching and strengthening. Should conservative measures fail, surgery may be necessary, with good results expected from surgical release and debridement of abnormal tissue. In a recent series, 34 of 35 patients experienced good to excellent results with this procedure.

Nerve Injuries Nerve injuries in general are discussed elsewhere in this volume. However, the ulnar nerve is commonly a source of pathology in the throwing athlete and deserves discussion here. Valgus extension overload results in injury to the UCL and tension-compression injury to the ulnar nerve, with the two conditions often coexisting. With repetitive use, inflammation followed by eventual formation of fibrotic scar tissue on the medial aspect of the elbow further compromises the ulnar nerve. Early treatment with rest and gentle mobilization will usually temporarily alleviate symptoms, but once scar tissue has formed, symptom recurrence is high.

Over 15% of the general population has hypermobility of the ulnar nerve, a risk factor for recurrent subluxation and injury. Examination demonstrates subluxation of the nerve over the medial epicondyle, and patients complain of snapping with throwing. These athletes have symptoms from friction alone and a concomitant UCL injury is usually not found. These patients respond well to ulnar nerve transposition alone. One study showed 40% of throwing athletes had symptoms of ulnar nerve entrapment. Injury to the ulnar nerve was found to be secondary to three factors: friction, traction, and compression. Traction injuries result from valgus stress loading, especially in the presence of medial instability. Compression on the nerve develops from the presence of bony spurs, fibrous tissue, scar tissue, adhesions, and calcifications in proximity to the nerve. An important clinical entity that is routinely missed is medial triceps subluxation. This is commonly the cause of compression of a subluxating ulnar nerve.

A series of ulnar nerve transpositions in 20 athletes, eight of whom were throwers, was recently reported. Preoperatively, patients had an average 16-month duration of elbow pain and paresthesias. Surgical technique emphasized protection of the medial antebrachial cutaneous nerve, resection of the arcade of Struthers, anterior stabilization with fascial slings, and good hemostasis. All patients had good or excellent results at 6-month follow-up.

Ulnar nerve transposition is recommended in throwing athletes with persistent ulnar nerve symptoms and nerve compression or subluxation. EMG studies may be normal, but this does not preclude surgical treatment. Subcutaneous transfer with one or two stabilizing fascial slings is the treatment of choice, because a submuscular transfer disrupts the integrity of the flexor-pronator mass.

Lateral Elbow Injuries

Lateral Epicondylitis The lateral aspect of the elbow is the most common location of pain in the general population, with lateral epicondylitis (often called tennis elbow) being the most common diagnosis. This condition tends to occur in the nondominant elbow of the golfer and dominant elbow of the tennis player. In golf, the leading elbow is brought into full extension as the ball is contacted, with the forearm undergoing supination into the follow-through, both of which stress the wrist extensor origin. As noted in the biomechanics discussion, faulty backhand swing mechanics and inappropriately high EMG activity of the wrist and finger extensors, pronator teres, and flexor carpi radialis have been documented in affected tennis players. Histopathologic studies have shown that the lesion is located in the origin of the extensor carpi radialis brevis. Tendon injuries are discussed in chapter 37.

Radiocapitellar Overload Syndrome: Radiocapitellar Chondromalacia, Degeneration, Osteochondral Fractures, and Loose Bodies In the skeletally mature throwing elbow, lateral compression syndrome follows the development of posteromedial impingement and UCL injury and is, therefore, considered a late finding in valgus extension overload syndrome. Increased load transmission across the radiocapitellar joint will lead to chondromalacia of the articular surfaces followed by more severe traumatic degeneration and, ultimately, osteochondritis dissecans. In the arthroscopic treatment of pitchers with valgus extension overload, the radiocapitellar joint is routinely visualized and the articular surfaces are pristine in the majority of cases even in the face of severe posteromedial impingement and/or UCL rupture. In general, development of pathology in this compartment occurs near the end of a pitching career.

In comparison to the conservative treatment of skeletally immature athletes with osteochondritis dissecans, skeletally mature athletes with osteochondral lesions are sometimes treated with arthroscopic debridement early, before loose bodies are generated. Debridement of the articular defects with chondroplasty and the pick-fracture technique is employed to stimulate a fibrocartilaginous healing response. These patients usually present with significant flexion contractures that are also released, and an aggressive range-of-motion program is pursued immediately after surgery.

Other Sources of Lateral Elbow Pain: Posterolateral Rotatory Instability, Radial Nerve Entrapment, and Plica Band Syndrome Pain referable to the lateral collateral ligament complex is infrequent because the lateral structures are rarely stressed in athletics. However, subtle posterolateral rotatory instability may cause elbow pain. An incompetent lateral ulnar collateral ligament, probably caused by previous injury such as a fall on the outstretched hand, has been implicated as the cause of this pain. Patients complain of painful clicking, snapping, clunking or locking in the extension half of the arc of motion when the forearm is supinated. Physical examination is only remarkable for a positive lateral pivot shift or posterolateral rotatory apprehension test. Surgical treatment reattaches the avulsed lateral ulnar collateral ligament or reconstructs it with a free tendon graft. This is more fully discussed in the chapter on instability.

Synovial tissues lining the joint on the lateral side of the elbow can undergo fibrosis from repetitive injuries. A synovial plica band is a normal finding in the lateral gutter of many patients. However, the repetitive compression in the radiocapitellar joint can lead to synovial hypertrophy and plica band fibrosis. At arthroscopy, the extent of pathology of this plica band must be determined. Associated radial head or capitellar chondromalacia lend support to the diagnosis of a pathologic plica, but in their absence, other more common diagnoses should be sought. Treatment is arthroscopic debridement with a shaver, taking care not to resect the normal annular ligament. Resection of this ligament could lead to instability.

Radial nerve entrapment must be included in the differential diagnosis of lateral elbow pain. This topic is discussed in detail in the chapter on nerve injuries and neuropathies.

Posterior Elbow Injuries

Posteromedial Impingement: Chondromalacia, Osteophytes, Stress Fractures, and Loose Bodies When the natural history of elbow injury in throwing athletes was first described in the 1960s, it was reported that 50% of pitchers have flexion contractures and about 30% have concomitant cubitus valgus deformity. Radiographs and surgical exploration revealed that hypertrophy of the olecranon process and decreased volume of the olecranon fossa lead to the formation of these osteophytes. Referred to as posteromedial impingement syndrome, the evolution of this injury pattern is now better understood.

The history and physical examination are important in making the diagnosis of posterior-medial impingement. Details of when pain occurs during the pitching cycle, level of competition, and recent performance provide helpful information; history of loss of control during pitching may be the first clue to the diagnosis. The valgus extension overload test is used to test for posterior-medial impingement pain. The forearm is fully supinated, a valgus stress is placed on the elbow, and the elbow is forcibly brought into full extension. The test is positive when pain is produced with this maneuver. Palpation of crepitus in the posterior-medial elbow while performing this test also lends support to the diagnosis.

The first stage in posterior-medial impingement is development of chondromalacia on the medial aspect of the trochlear groove. Erosion of articular cartilage to subchondral bone is often seen when olecranon osteophytes are just beginning to form (Fig. 5). In young throwers with increased joint laxity, this finding may precede significant olecranon pathology. Therefore, radiographs are normal and the diagnosis is easily missed. Typically, these patients have pain that continually recurs after a period of rest. Arthroscopic evaluation is diagnostic. Treatment is debridement of the olecranon tip, with light abrasion chondroplasty of the damaged cartilage.

The second stage of posterior-medial impingement is the generation of osteophytes on both the olecranon and medial humeral trochlear groove. Laxity of the UCL may be slight or nonexistent at the time of presentation. The patient will complain of posterior and medial elbow pain during the cocking and acceleration phases of throwing. The valgus extension overload test will be positive and radiographs will show joint degeneration and osteophytes at the posterior and medial aspects of the olecranon, along with a kissing lesion on the medial trochlear groove. Treatment consists of arthroscopic debridement with an aggressive postoperative rehabilitative course (Fig. 6).

Stress fractures arise in the proximal third of the olecranon tip in patients presenting with isolated posterior elbow pain associated with both the acceleration and deceleration phases of throwing. Radiographs are usually normal, so the diagnosis is made with a bone scan followed by CT or MRI evaluation. The lesion may arise from a previous olecranon apophysis that never underwent complete ossification. Treatment is immobilization and rest until the bone heals. However, if this regimen fails, surgical treatment consists of drilling the lesion and/or bone grafting.

Loose bodies within the elbow joint are common in high-caliber throwing athletes who have extensive throwing experience. Most loose bodies are either broken spurs that formed initially by the impingement at the posterior aspect of the olecranon and trochlea, or osteocartilaginous lesions of the capitellum. When loose bodies become symptomatic, arthroscopic removal is the treatment of choice. The incidence of elbow loose bodies in the general throwing population is unknown, but they have been reported in 39% of professional baseball players at the time of surgery. A review of 72 professional baseball players who underwent elbow surgery indicates that preoperative radiographs are poor predictors of the presence of loose bodies at surgery, being positive in only 29% of this patient population. Unpublished data from our institution (American Sports Medicine Institute, Birmingham, AL) indicates that CT arthrograms improved preoperative detection to 72%, but this is still far short of optimal.

Treatment of these athletes is complicated by the difficulty of finding and removing all loose bodies at the time of surgery. A systematic inspection of the elbow, use of multiple portals, and a realization that loose bodies float around are all important factors to consider. Whenever a loose body is found, the presence of other loose bodies should be assumed until arthroscopy proves otherwise. Intraoperative radiographs are of little help and patients should be advised preoperatively of the possibility of not finding all loose bodies in a single arthroscopic procedure.

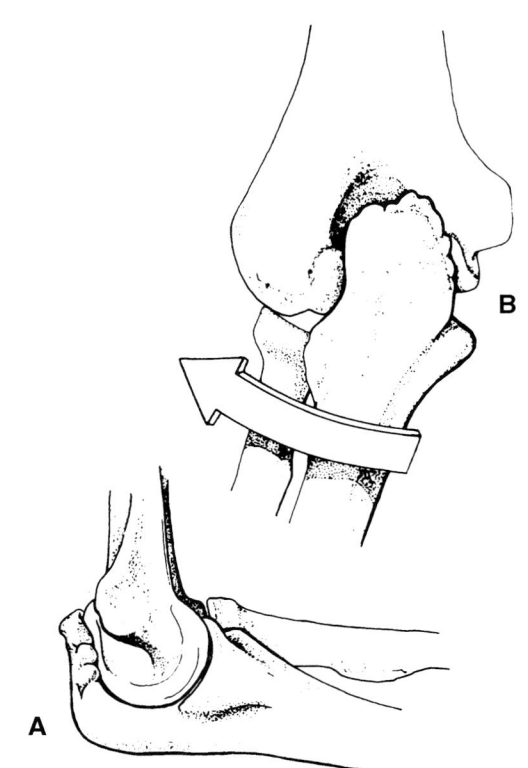

Fig. 5 Posterior medial impingement. **A,** Lateral view of elbow shows medial olecranon osteophytes with impingement along the humeral medial trochlea groove. **B,** Posterior view of the elbow showing extent of posterior and posteromedial osteophytes as elbow impinges into the olecranon fossa. Arrow indicates direction of dynamic stress generated in valgus extension overload syndrome and the resulting impingement of the olecranon process in olecranon fossa. (Reproduced with permission from Wilson FD, Andrews JR, Blackburn TA, et al: Valgus extension overload in the pitching elbow. *Am J Sports Med* 1983;11:83-88.)

Traction Apophysitis Similar to Osgood-Schlatter disease of the tibial tubercle, olecranon apophysitis can occur secondary to chronic stress, musculotendinous imbalance, and rapid growth. The condition has been described with the separated ossification center persisting into adulthood. Patients with olecranon apophysitis will have pain on resisted extension and tenderness over the olecranon. Radiographs may show widening of the olecranon apophysis. Initial treatment is conservative, but persistence past skeletal maturity may result in a painful nonunion requiring internal fixation and possible bone grafting.

Triceps Tendinitis and Rupture Triceps tendinitis, an uncommon cause of posterior elbow pain, can be caused by intrinsic muscle overload such as that occurring during the throwing motion. Patients will usually have distal triceps pain with resisted extension or full passive flexion. The condition can occur as an acute or chronic problem. If chronic, radiographs may show calcific deposits within the tendon. Treatment is usually conservative, and steroid injections are not

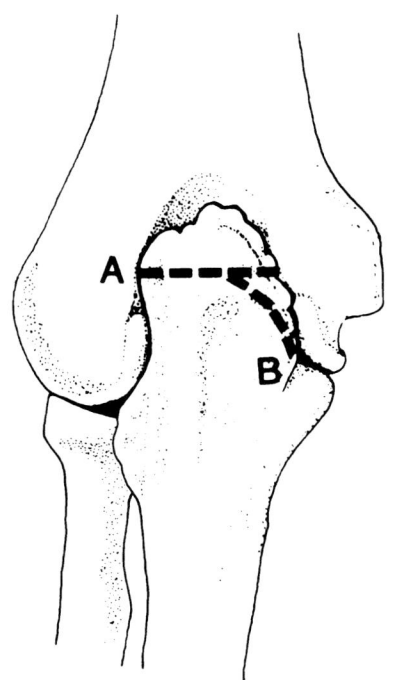

Fig. 6 Posterior view of olecranon—first cut made straight across (**A**). Second cut made with curved osteotome (**B**). (Reproduced with permission from Wilson FD, Andrews JR, Blackburn TA, et al: Valgus extension overload in the pitching elbow. *Am J Sports Med* 1983;11:83-88.)

recommended because they may precipitate tendon rupture. If the symptoms do not respond to nonsurgical measures, and if calcific deposits are present, surgery may be warranted.

Anterior Elbow Injuries

Anterior Capsular Tear, Brachialis Tendinitis, and Biceps Tendinitis Anterior elbow pain is usually caused by stretch or tear of the anterior capsule, distal biceps, or brachialis tendons. An anterior capsular sprain can result from a hyperextension injury to the elbow. This injury can be sustained in football when the outstretched arm is "run through" by the ball carrier or when the fatigued gymnast hyperextends the elbow during walkover or handstand stunts. For treatment, rest and early motion are indicated, with gradual return to resistive exercise as symptoms resolve.

Brachialis tendinitis has been referred to as climber's elbow and results from repeated use of the forearms in a pronated and semiflexed position. Electromyographic analysis has shown that the brachialis has the greatest activity in this position, but some still argue that this pain is related to the anterior capsule or distal biceps tendon. Biceps tendinitis may result from friction and inflammation caused by motion at the bicipital tuberosity of the radius. Treatment is almost always conservative for these conditions, with emphasis on early range of motion.

Coronoid Impingement Syndrome Elbow flexion contractures in throwing athletes do not always occur from the development of olecranon spurs and posterior-medial impingement; infrequently, the pathology is anterior. The deceleration phase of throwing produces large distraction forces that can lead to hypertrophy of the coronoid process. The repetitive motion of throwing will produce impingement of this enlarged coronoid process in the coronoid fossa. This scenario leads to scar tissue formation throughout the anterior capsule and subsequent anterior capsule contracture. Treatment is arthroscopic capsular debridement with a motorized shaver. The neurovascular structures in the cubital fossa are protected by debriding the capsule off the humerus at the bony surface, not in the midportion of the capsule. Finally, the bur is used to osteotomize the hypertrophied coronoid and reform the coronoid and radial fossae.

Arthroscopy

Information about the use of the arthroscope in the elbow has increased in recent literature. Much has been published regarding surgical anatomy, technique, indications, and potential pitfalls.

Anatomic Approach and Technique

Several studies regarding the anatomy of portal placement and proximity of neurovascular structures have been published over the last decade. The anterolateral and anteromedial portals were shown to be precariously close to neurovascular structures. In one study in a cadaveric dry joint, the anterolateral portal averaged 4 mm from the radial nerve (range, 3 to 10 mm). The anteromedial portal averaged 4 mm (range, 3 to 10 mm) and 9 mm (range, 8 to 13 mm) from the median nerve and brachial artery, respectively. Distention of the joint capsule with 35 to 40 cc of fluid increased these distances by 5 to 10 mm. Distention of the joint, a position of 90° of elbow flexion, and avoidance of local anesthesia were recommended during routine arthroscopy. Other cadaveric studies showed that these distances could be improved with more proximal placement of the portals. Based on the greater distances from the major neurovascular structures, it was recommended that the anteromedial portal be the initial site of joint entry. Anteromedial, anterolateral, straight lateral, posterolateral, and straight posterior portals are routinely used for elbow arthroscopy.

Indications and Results

Common indications for elbow arthroscopy in athletes include loose body removal; evaluation of valgus instability; debridement of chondral or osteochondral injuries; osteophyte debridement (coronoid fossa/process, olecranon fossa/process); posttraumatic pain and stiffness; posttraumatic arthritis; inflammatory arthritis; primary degenerative arthrosis; posterolateral rotatory instability; and diagnostic dilemma. Figures 7 and 8 demonstrate some common findings during elbow arthroscopy.

A series of 71 elbow arthroscopies in 70 patients provided information on indications for maximizing diagnostic and therapeutic benefit. A technique with the patient positioned in the lateral decubitus position was recommended. Examination began in the anterior compartment of the elbow through an anterolateral portal. Strict criteria were used to select patients for the study and identify indications for arthroscopy of the elbow. Fifty-one (73%) patients benefited in some way from the procedure: 22 (31%) of these benefited diagnostically; 17 (24%) benefited both diagnostically and therapeutically, and 12 (17%) benefited therapeutically. In patients with subjective complaints and no objective findings, arthroscopy provided little benefit. Arthroscopic examination allowed identification of a causal relationship in 11 of 12 patients with unexplained snapping and three of five patients with unexplained contracture. Patients with indications for removal of loose bodies realized the most benefit from arthroscopy. However, arthroscopy was of benefit to patients with symptomatic posttraumatic arthritis, inflammatory arthritis, osteochondritis dissecans, primary degenerative arthrosis, and undiagnosed subtle instability. Complications, all minor, occurred in 10%; these included persistent drainage from portal site and transient radial nerve palsy, both of which resolved without sequelae. One patient developed a flexion contracture in which 10° of flexion was lost.

A recent study of the use of arthroscopy in the treatment of posttraumatic elbow pain and stiffness showed that 79% of patients achieved good to excellent results. Nineteen patients who developed arthrofibrosis after previous fracture or fracture-dislocation were treated with arthroscopic debridement and manipulation. A 100-point scoring system was used to assess subjective and objective outcomes. The subjective scores improved from 39 preoperatively to an average of 91 postoperatively. The objective score averages improved from 46 preoperatively to 81 postoperatively. Both of these improvements were statistically highly significant. Eleven of 14 patients who had preoperative sports limitations were able to return to preinjury levels of activity.

According to a recent retrospective study of elbow surgery, both arthroscopic and open, in baseball players, the most common diagnoses were posteromedial olecranon osteophyte (65%), UCL injury (25%), and ulnar neuritis (15%). Loose bodies were found in 39% of the patients at the time of surgery. Minimum follow-up was 24 months (average, 42 months). One third of the patients required two or more surgical procedures; 25% of the reoperations were UCL reconstructions after removal of posteromedial olecranon osteophyte. Eighty percent were able to return to play for at least one season, and 73% returned at the same or higher level of play.

Rehabilitation

A four-phase approach to the rehabilitation of the injured or postsurgical elbow has been suggested. In phase 1 (the immediate postoperative period), regaining full elbow motion, decreasing pain and inflammation, and retarding muscular atrophy are stressed. Phase 2, the intermediate phase, is initiated after the acuteness of the injury or surgery has subsided, and emphasizes mobility, strengthening, and endurance. Phase 3, advanced strengthening, is initiated after reacquisition of full, painless range of motion, and at least 70% of strength. This phase involves strengthening and preparation of the entire extremity for a return to normal activity. Much of the first three phases can be accomplished in the first 3 weeks with progression of the protocol tempered according to the pathologic or surgical condition. Phase 4, the return to activity phase, involves functional drilling and an interval throwing program with a gradual return to unrestricted activity. Specific rehabilitation programs for UCL reconstruction, subcutaneous nerve transposition, and routine elbow arthroscopy are part of this approach.

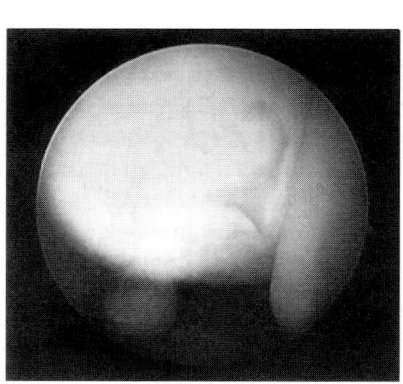 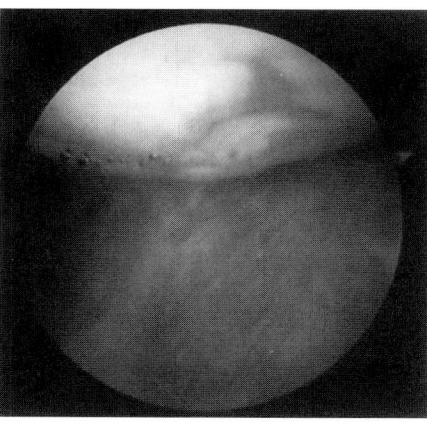 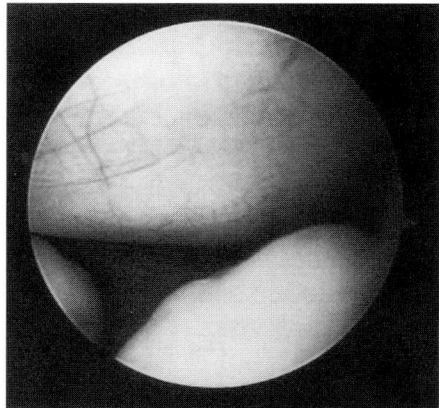

Fig. 7 Posterior medial impingement: chondromalacia. **Left,** Arthroscopic view of the humeral medial trochlea groove opposed to the olecranon tip. Grade III chondromalacia is demonstrated. When a valgus stress is placed on the elbow, the olecranon impinges at the lesion. **Center,** Same lesion viewed through the posterior portal further illustrating the damaged articular cartilage. **Right,** Posterior medial impingement: olecranon osteophyte. Arthroscopic view of posterior elbow from the posterior-lateral portal with a 30° scope. An olecranon spur is demonstrated on the inferior aspect of the field in a patient with advanced posterior medial impingement. (Reproduced with permission from Joyce ME, Jelsma RD, Andrews JR: Throwing injuries to the elbow. *Sports Med Arthroscopy Rev* 1995;3:225-236.)

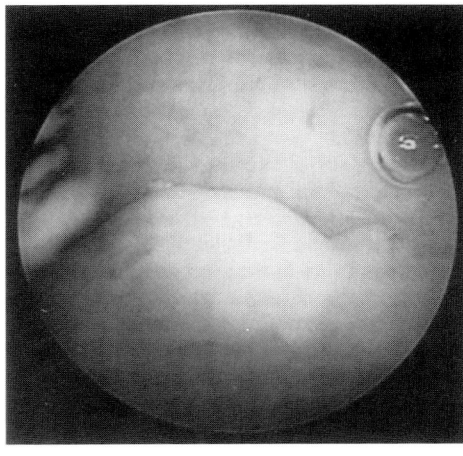 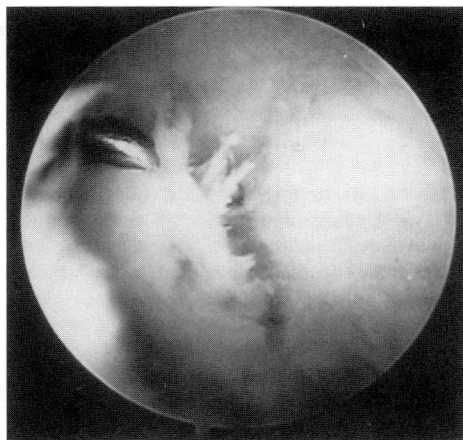
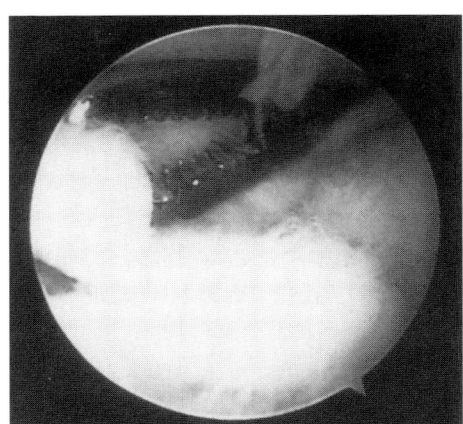 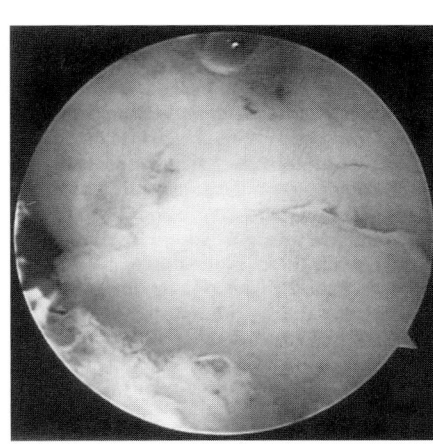

Fig. 8 Posterior medial impingement: olecranon osteophyte with fragmentation. Arthroscopic view of posterior elbow from the posterior-lateral portal with a 30° scope. **Top left,** An olecranon spur is demonstrated on the inferior aspect of the field in a patient with advanced posterior medial impingement. **Top right,** Same view in the same patient demonstrating fragmentation at the medial (left) aspect of a spur that was loose and easily pulled off the olecranon with a probe. **Bottom left,** Posterior medial impingement: loose body. Arthroscopic view of posterior elbow from the posterior-lateral portal with a 30° scope. Removal of loose bodies off the olecranon in the most advanced stage of posterior medial impingement is demonstrated. **Bottom right,** Posterior medial impingement: olecranon osteotomy. Arthroscopic view of posterior elbow from the posterior-lateral portal with a 30° scope. Osteotomy of the proximal olecranon tip relieves impingement that was present when the elbow was placed into a valgus extension overload position. (Reproduced with permission from Joyce ME, Jelsma RD, Andrews JR: Throwing injuries to the elbow. *Sports Med Arthroscopy Rev* 1995;3:225-236.)

Conclusion

The elbow is commonly injured during participation in sports in which the elbow is subjected to repetitive valgus and extension load, and in sports in which the elbow is subjected to heavy weightbearing loads. Acute trauma occurs but, more commonly, elbow pathology in sports is an overuse phenomenon. Progress is being made in the prevention and treatment of elbow injuries because of improved understanding of the elbow's underlying biomechanics and pathophysiology in sports. Improved understanding of instability patterns in sports, especially UCL instability and posterolateral rotatory instability, is leading to increased success in reconstructions for treatment of these lesions. Better imaging techniques, such as CT arthrography and saline-enhanced MRI, have led to more accurate preoperative diagnoses. Also, more experience with arthroscopic techniques has led to better definitions of appropriate indications, better arthroscopic techniques, and improved safety. The arthroscopist should be ever-mindful of the close proximity of neurovascular structures to arthroscopic portals and intra-articular structures. Rehabilitation continues to play a crucial role in the nonsurgical and perioperative treatment of elbow injuries.

Selected Bibliography

Biomechanics

Fleisig GS, Andrews JR, Dillman CJ, et al: Kinetics of baseball pitching with implications about injury mechanisms. *Am J Sports Med* 1995;23:233-239.

Elbow and shoulder kinetics for 76 highly skilled healthy adult pitchers were studied. Two critical instants were identified in which shoulder and elbow forces were maximal: shortly before maximal shoulder external rotation and shortly after ball release. Kinetics and force data are reported for pitching motion.

Glousman RE, Barron J, Jobe FW, et al: An electromyographic analysis of the elbow in normal and injured pitchers with medial collateral ligament insufficiency. *Am J Sports Med* 1992;20:311-317.

Decreased muscle activity in the flexor carpi radialis and pronator teres muscle was found in the medial collateral ligament-deficient pitchers. This pattern of asynchronous muscle action in the presence of medial collateral ligament linjury may lead to further injury. Understanding of the pathomechanics was stressed to provide a sound basis for treatment and rehabilitation of the injured elbow.

Kibler WB: Clinical biomechanics of the elbow in tennis: Implications for evaluation and diagnosis. *Med Sci Sports Exerc* 1994;26:1203-1206.

The clinical biomechanics of the elbow in tennis was reviewed, and implications for evaluation of the injured tennis player were discussed.

Werner SL, Fleisig GS, Dillman CJ, et al: Biomechanics of the elbow during baseball pitching. *J Orthop Sports Phys Ther* 1993;17:274-278.

Joint motion, loads, and muscle activity that occur during baseball pitching were quantified by studying seven healthy adult pitchers with synchronized high-speed video digitalization and surface electromyography. Implications for preventative and rehabilitative programs for pitchers were discussed.

Pathophysiology

Andrews JR, Whiteside JA: Common elbow problems in the athlete. *J Orthop Sports Phys Ther* 1993;17:289-295.

Common elbow problems and their relationship to specific sports were reviewed. General guidelines for initial treatment were discussed.

Ilfeld FW: Can stroke modification relieve tennis elbow? *Clin Orthop* 1992;276:182-186.

Fifty-seven tennis players with painful elbows were treated by modification of faulty stroke mechanics and the usual conservative measures. Ninety percent of patients who had symptoms for less than 6 months had excellent or good results.

King J, Brelsford HJ, Tullos HS: Analysis of the pitching arm of the professional baseball pitcher. *Clin Orthop* 1969;67:116-123.

Rettig AC, Patel DV: Epidemiology of elbow, forearm, and wrist injuries in the athlete. *Clin Sports Med* 1995;14:289-297.

The epidemiology of athletic injuries of the elbow, forearm, and wrist are reviewed.

Medial Elbow Injuries

Andrews JR, Schemmel SP, Whiteside JA, et al: Evaluation, treatment, and prevention of elbow injuries in throwing athletes, in Nicholas JA, Hershman EB, Posner MA (eds): *The Upper Extremity in Sports Medicine.* St Louis, MO, CV Mosby, 1990, pp 781-826.

Conway JE, Jobe FW, Glousman RE, et al: Medial instability of the elbow in throwing athletes: Treatment by repair or reconstruction of the ulnar collateral ligament. *J Bone Joint Surg* 1992;74A:67-83.

Seventy-one patients underwent operations for valgus instability of the elbow because of an incompetent ulnar collateral ligament. Ten of 14 patients in whom direct repair was performed and 45 of 56 patients in whom ulnar collateral ligament reconstruction was performed had excellent or good results. Follow-up averaged 6.3 years. Major league pitchers had a better rate of return to major league pitching when treated with reconstruction. Nine of 15 patients with postoperative ulnar neuropathy were able to return to sports.

Joyce ME, Jelsma RD, Andrews JR: Throwing injuries to the elbow. *Sports Med Arthrosc Rev* 1995;3:224-236.

The syndrome of valgus extension overload in the throwing athlete was classified and reviewed. Arthroscopic findings are discussed and nicely demonstrated with a series of arthroscopic photographs.

Rettig AC, Ebben JR: Anterior subcutaneous transfer of the ulnar nerve in the athlete. *Am J Sports Med* 1993;21:836-840.

Twenty athletes underwent 21 anterior subcutaneous ulnar nerve transfers with a fascial sling. Elbow rating scores averaged 9/10 with subjective scores of 84/100. Average return to full activity was 12.6 weeks.

Smith GR, Altchek DW, Pagnani MJ, et al: A muscle-splitting approach to the ulnar collateral ligament of the elbow: Neuroanatomy and operative technique. *Am J Sports Med* 1996;24:575-580.

The neuroanatomy and operative technique for reconstruction of the ulnar collateral ligament through a muscle-splitting approach without transposition of the ulnar nerve was described. The neuroanatomy was investigated by dissection of 15 cadaveric elbows and a "safe zone" was defined. Twenty-two ulnar collateral ligament reconstructions were performed with this technique, and no adverse neurologic sequelae were noted at 1 year follow-up.

Timmerman LA, Andrews JR: Undersurface tear of the ulnar collateral ligament in baseball players: A newly recognized lesion. *Am J Sports Med* 1994;22:33-36.

Seven baseball players were found to have undersurface tears of the ulnar collateral ligament, which was associated with persistent medial elbow pain with throwing. At surgery, all ligaments were intact externally, but had undersurface detachments from the ulna or humerus. Study of cadaveric dissections confirmed that this lesion was not an anatomic variant.

Vangsness CT Jr, Jobe FW: Surgical treatment of medial epicondylitis: Results in 35 elbows. *J Bone Joint Surg* 1991;73B:409-411.

Lateral Elbow Injuries

Bauer M, Jonsson K, Josefsson PO, et al: Osteochondritis dissecans of the elbow: A long-term follow-up study. *Clin Orthop* 1992;284:156-160.

Thirty-one patients with osteochondritis dissecans of the elbow were followed for 23 years. About half of the elbows were symptomatic, and over half had radiographic signs of degenerative joint disease.

Jackson DW, Silvino N, Reiman P: Osteochondritis in the female gymnast's elbow. *Arthroscopy* 1989;5:129-136.

Safran MR: Elbow injuries in athletes: A review. *Clin Orthop* 1995;310:257-277.

The author provides an excellent comprehensive review of elbow injuries in athletes.

Posterior Elbow Injuries

Andrews JR, Craven WM: Lesions of the posterior compartment of the elbow. *Clin Sports Med* 1991;10:637-652.

Ireland ML, Hutchinson MR: Upper extremity injuries in young athletes. *Clin Sports Med* 1995;14:533-569.

This is an excellent review of upper extremity injuries in the skeletally immature athlete.

Maffulli N, Chan D, Aldridge MJ: Overuse injuries of the olecranon in young gymnasts. *J Bone Joint Surg* 1992;74B:305-308.

Overuse injuries in 14 elbows of ten elite young gymnasts were reported. Radiographic abnormalities varied and were similar to the Osgood-Schlatter lesion of the knee. Conservative management was successful except in one 18-year-old patient with a stress fracture that required internal fixation.

Micheli LJ: The traction apophysitises. *Clin Sports Med* 1987;6:389-404.

Arthroscopy

Andrews JR, Timmerman LA: Outcome of elbow surgery in professional baseball players. *Am J Sports Med* 1995;23:407-413.

A retrospective review of open and arthroscopic elbow surgery in 72 professional baseball players showed 80% were able to return to play at least one season; 73% returned to the same or higher level of competition. The most common diagnoses were olecranon osteophytes (65%), loose bodies (39%), ulnar collateral ligament injury (25%), and ulnar neuritis (15%).

Lynch GJ, Meyers JF, Whipple TL, et al: Neurovascular anatomy and elbow arthroscopy: Inherent risks. *Arthroscopy* 1986;2:190-197.

O'Driscoll SW, Bell DF, Morrey BF: Posterolateral rotatory instability of the elbow. *J Bone Joint Surg* 1991;73A:440-446.

O'Driscoll SW, Morrey BF: Arthroscopy of the elbow: Diagnostic and therapeutic benefits and hazards. *J Bone Joint Surg* 1992;74A:84-94.

The results of 71 arthroscopies were analyzed to determine the benefits and hazards of elbow arthroscopy. Seventy-three percent of the patients benefited either diagnostically (31%), therapeutically (17%), or both diagnostically and therapeutically (24%). Arthroscopy provided the least benefit in patients with subjective complaints and no objective findings. Loose body removal was the most beneficial of treatments, although several diagnostic categories benefited significantly. Minor complications occurred in 10%.

Timmerman LA, Andrews JR: Arthroscopic treatment of posttraumatic elbow pain and stiffness. *Am J Sports Med* 1994;22:230-235.

Seventy-nine percent of patients with posttraumatic elbow pain and stiffness achieved good or excellent results after arthroscopic debridement and manipulation. Eleven of 14 patients with preoperative sports limitations returned to their previous level of activity. Outcomes were evaluated by both subjective and objective scoring scales.

Timmerman LA, Andrews JR: Histology and arthroscopic anatomy of the ulnar collateral ligament of the elbow. *Am J Sports Med* 1994;22:667-673.

A histologic and arthroscopic study of cadaveric specimens was conducted. The ulnar collateral ligament was found to have two distinct bands: the anterior bundle, which has a superficial and a deep component, and the posterior band, which is a distinct thickening within the capsule. Only a small portion of the anterior band was visible at arthroscopy. Sectioning of the anterior band showed that ulnar collateral ligament instability could be diagnosed with an arthroscopic valgus stress test.

Verhaar J, van Mameren H, Brandsma A: Risks of neurovascular injury in elbow arthroscopy: Starting anteromedially or anterolaterally? *Arthroscopy* 1991;7:287-290.

Rehabilitation

Ellenbecker TS: Rehabilitation of shoulder and elbow injuries in tennis players. *Clin Sports Med* 1995;14:87-110.

Wilk KE, Arrigo C, Andrews JR: Rehabilitation of the elbow in the throwing athlete. *J Orthop Sports Phys Ther* 1993;17:305-317.

Imaging

Rijke AM, Goitz HT, McCue FC, et al: Stress radiography of the medial elbow ligaments. *Radiology* 1994;191:213-216.

Forty-two injured athletes and four control patients underwent stress radiography. The diagnosis of all complete and large partial tears was made with a side-to-side opening of greater than 0.5 mm. Side-to-side differences of less than 0.5 mm were found in all patients with normal ligaments and small partial tears.

Timmerman LA, Schwartz ML, Andrews JR: Preoperative evaluation of the ulnar collateral ligament by magnetic resonance imaging and computed tomography arthrography: Evaluation in 25 baseball players with surgical confirmation. *Am J Sports Med* 1994;22:26-32.

This prospective study comparing nonenhanced magnetic resonance imaging (MRI) and computed tomography arthrography (CTA) for diagnosis of ulnar collateral ligament tears found the CTA to have a sensitivity of 86% and specificity of 91%. MRI was 57% sensitive and 100% specific. A newly described "T-sign" was found to be diagnostic of undersurface ulnar collateral ligament tears.

35

Stiffness and Ankylosis of the Elbow

Graham J.W. King, MD, MSc, FRCSC

Introduction

The primary function of the elbow is to position and stabilize the hand in space. Unlike that of the shoulder and wrist, stiffness of the elbow is poorly tolerated because of a lack of compensatory motions in adjacent joints. The range of motion of the elbow in regard to performing activities of daily living has been studied extensively. Morrey and associates demonstrated that an arc of elbow flexion from 30° to 130° was required to perform most activities of daily living. Patients with elbow stiffness from any cause have varying degrees of impairment in functional abilities, depending on the location of stiffness in the arc of motion and the magnitude of the contracture. In one recent study, volunteers who were fitted with an elbow brace to restrict motion were able to adapt to an arc of 70° to 120° for 12 activities of daily living. Despite the marked stiffness that can be tolerated when adjacent joints are normal, most patients complain of functional disability and request treatment when flexion contractures approach 40°. The indications for treatment of an established elbow contracture are primarily based on patient complaints of functional impairment as a consequence of decreased elbow motion. Pain is sometimes an additional factor. Patients who have an arc of motion from 30° to 130° rarely require surgery unless their vocation or avocation specifically requires terminal elbow flexion and/or extension.

Etiology

Contractures of the elbow are either congenital or acquired. Congenital contractures of the elbow are rare, with arthrogryposis being the most frequent cause, followed by cerebral palsy. Acquired contractures are most frequently encountered as a consequence of previous elbow fractures, dislocations, and surgery. Varying degrees of elbow contractures are also seen in patients with inflammatory, degenerative, or septic arthritis. Paralytic contractures are most frequently seen in older patients following a cerebral vascular accident and in younger patients with cerebral palsy. Burns are now an infrequent cause of elbow contractures because of rapid joint mobilization in the upper limbs.

Incidence

The frequency of elbow contractures is difficult to determine from current literature. Mohan reported on 200 patients with elbow ankylosis. Fracture-dislocations accounted for 38% of this patient population, dislocations for 20%, and isolated fractures for 30%. The severity of elbow contractures following elbow dislocations is reportedly highly correlated with the time of immobilization following reduction. In one series in which simple elbow dislocations were studied, 15% of the patients treated with closed reduction had a residual flexion contracture of greater than 30°. In recent years, it has become more common to treat displaced elbow fractures in adults with open reduction and internal fixation and early postoperative mobilization. Although this approach may have reduced the incidence of symptomatic elbow contractures, some residual loss of extension is common, regardless of the elbow disorder or its treatment.

Outline 1. Classification of heterotopic ossification

Class I	Heterotopic ossification without functional limitation
Class II	Heterotopic ossification with functional limitation
IIA	Limited flexion-extension
IIB	Limited prosupination
IIC	Limited flexion-extension and prosupination
Class III	Ankylosis

(Adapted with permission from Hastings H, Graham TJ: The classification and treatment of heterotopic ossification about the elbow and forearm. *Hand Clin* 1994;10:417-437.)

Classification

Elbow stiffness can be classified according to the etiology, pathology, and location of stiffness within the arc of motion. A new classification for heterotopic ossification has recently been developed for the elbow (Outline 1). Only ankylosis or a functional loss of flexion-extension and/or prosupination requires treatment. Contractures are classified on the basis of the underlying pathology as extrinsic, intrinsic, or mixed. Extrinsic contractures arise in the soft tissue, bone, or both. Intrinsic contractures involve intra-articular adhesions with articular cartilage destruction. Almost all stiff elbows, regardless of cause, have a contracted capsule. Thickening of the anterior and posterior elbow capsule commonly occurs following elbow injuries. With the development of elbow stiffness, secondary contractures of the collateral ligaments and muscles around the elbow also occur. Other extrinsic causes include heterotopic ossification following closed head injuries, burns, or elbow fracture-dislocations. Patients with an osseous ankylosis usually have a concomitant contracture of the elbow capsule, ligament, and muscles about the elbow. All contributing tissues need to be considered when deciding on the optimal treatment of contractures of the elbow.

Evaluation

Patients with elbow stiffness should be carefully evaluated with appropriate history, physical examination, and imaging prior to proceeding with treatment. In the course of this evaluation it is imperative that the surgeon assess the patient's understanding of his or her disability and the potential for patient compliance should treatment be initiated.

When obtaining the history, the duration of the contracture and any possible progression should be determined. The etiology is usually clear from the history. The functional impact of the contracture on the patient's vocation and avocations should be determined as well as any limitation of activities of daily living. Any previous treatment of the contracture should be noted, including duration, type, and appropriateness of physical therapy or surgery. The presence of residual internal fixation devices and the history of any remote infection should be considered when planning treatment.

Physical examination should include a general assessment as well as a focused examination of the involved upper extremity. The skin should be inspected to evaluate its quality and evidence of any previous incisions, skin grafts, or areas of wound breakdown. An adequate soft-tissue envelope is vital before considering surgical release of an elbow contracture. Active and passive motion should be measured with a goniometer and compared where appropriate. The valgus, varus, and rotational stability of the elbow should be carefully tested. Motor strength of the muscles around the upper limb should be carefully evaluated because a joint without adequate motor strength is unlikely to maintain motion following an elbow release. In fact, the patient may become more disabled as a result of the consequent weakness induced in the upper limb. A careful neurologic examination should be performed because many patients with traumatic and inflammatory elbow contractures often have associated involvement of the ulnar nerve that may require treatment at the time of surgery. A careful evaluation of the remaining joints in both upper limbs should be completed.

Directed imaging studies of the elbow should be performed prior to proceeding with treatment. Routine anteroposterior, lateral, and oblique radiographs of the elbow provide most of the information as to the cause and appropriate management of the contracture. Additional imaging studies are necessary in selected cases. Spiral tomography and/or computed tomography (CT) scanning should be employed to evaluate the extent of articular congruity, where appropriate, and in some cases to evaluate the extent and location of heterotopic ossification or loose bodies in the elbow. Recently, magnetic resonance imaging (MRI) assessment has proved useful in identifying soft-tissue causes for the contracture. Nerve conduction studies and electromyography should be performed in selected patients if there is associated neurologic involvement of the upper limb. Technetium bone scans have not been found useful in predicting the chances of recurrence of heterotopic ossification following excision. Most physicians rely on the time elapsed since injury and the radiographic maturity of the heterotopic bone. The persistence of cognitive deficits following a brain injury has been correlated with the risk of recurrence of heterotopic bone.

Nonsurgical Management

The nonsurgical treatment of elbow stiffness should be considered up to 1 year after onset of the contracture. In general, contractures of more recent onset respond more favorably to nonsurgical treatment. On physical examination, contractures with a firm end range are generally less likely to respond to nonsurgical treatment than those with a springy end range.

The principles of nonsurgical treatment are to gradually gain motion and at the same time minimize pain and elbow inflammation. The generous use of ice and anti-inflammatory agents can be helpful. Mild nonnarcotic analgesics are often required so that patients can tolerate wearing splints through the night. Although manipulation of stiff elbows has reportedly been successful, passive stretching of the elbow in the operating room is not recommended because of the risk of heterotopic ossification and periarticular fractures. Physical therapy should be active-assisted. Therapy that is too aggressive will result in increasing stiffness, swelling, pain, and possibly heterotopic ossification. The warning signs of elbow inflammation should be heeded by edema control, nonaggressive therapy, and avoidance of passive manipulation.

The key to nonsurgical management of elbow stiffness is the generous use of splinting. Static progressive resting splints in the flexed and extended positions should be used between therapy periods (Fig. 1). At night, it is imperative that the patient wear a splint that positions the elbow in the direction in which motion is most lacking. Dynamic hinged splinting can be useful; however, these splints are often less well tolerated than static progressive splints because the tension in the tissue is continuous.

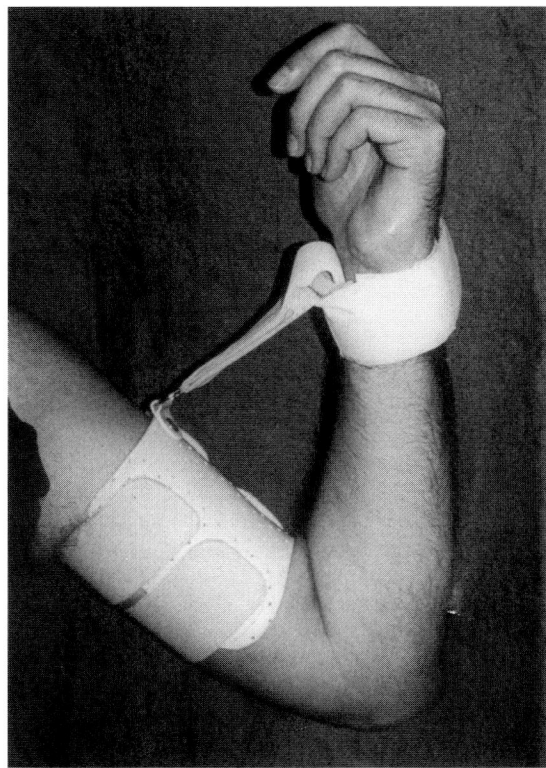

Fig. 1 Static progressive flexion splint. Velcro strap on the two-part flexion splint is adjusted by the patient to provide a gentle passive stretch to the elbow.

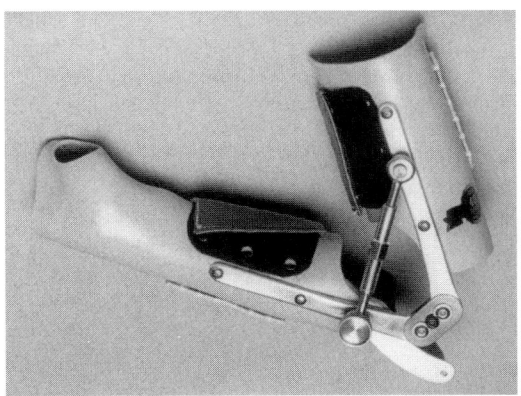 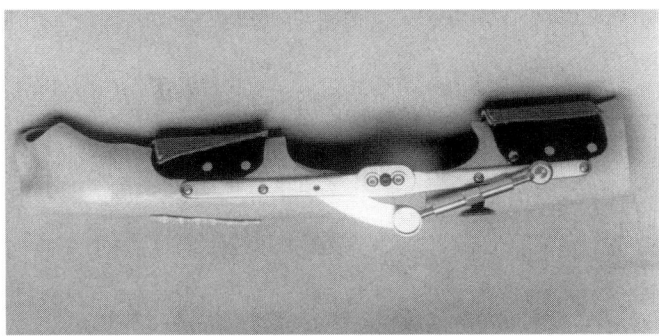

Fig. 2 Turnbuckle splint. Custom turnbuckle orthosis has an adjustable bolt to provide patient-controlled passive stretching of the elbow. The device is used both for elbow flexion **(left)** and extension **(right)** by changing the attachment site of the bolt.

Static progressive splinting with the use of a turnbuckle orthosis has reportedly been useful in the treatment of established elbow contracture not responsive to traditional therapy (Fig. 2). The force in the turnbuckle is controlled by the patient to allow gradual, progressive stretching of the elbow joint. It is important to keep in mind that as patients gain motion in one direction, they often lose motion in another direction. Therefore, treatment of any elbow contracture must focus on range of motion in both directions to achieve an optimal result. A 20-hour wear cycle is recommended, alternating flexion with extension splinting. Nighttime splinting is performed in the direction in which motion is most deficient.

Green and McCoy reported on the effectiveness of turnbuckle splinting using a custom orthosis in 15 patients. The average increase in the arc of motion was 43°. In three patients with articular damage the splint could not be tolerated because of excessive pain, and the treatment was unsuccessful. In a more recent series reported by Bonutti and coworkers, 20 patients were treated using a noncustom commercially available splinting system. The Joint Active System (JAS, Effingham IL) uses a static progressive stretch to achieve motion in 30-minute periods of therapy. The device is said to reduce joint compression using a tripod system of force application. The average gain in arc of motion was 31° in patients with both recent and long-standing elbow contractures.

Surgical Management: Extrinsic Contracture

Arthroscopic Capsular Release
Arthroscopic release of a posttraumatic elbow flexion contracture was first reported in 1992. Subsequent studies involving larger series of patients have been reported. In one study of 12 patients treated with arthroscopic capsular release, the mean flexion contracture improved from 38° to 3°. Unfortunately, one patient in this series sustained a permanent posterior interosseous nerve palsy from an iatrogenic nerve injury at the time of arthroscopic release. A more recent study reported on 19 patients with arthroscopic debridement and manipulation for posttraumatic elbow pain and stiffness. No neurovascular injuries were reported; however, there was an improvement in the mean flexion contracture from 29° to 11°.

Numerous studies have reported the proximity of neural structures to arthroscopic portals and joint capsule. The decreased capsular volume with elbow contractures reduces the ability of capsular distention to displace the neurovascular structures from the portal sites, increasing the risk of injury. Arthroscopic capsular release exposes the nerves to further potential injury as the anterior and/or posterior capsule is divided from its bony attachment. The exact role of arthroscopic capsular release is evolving. Clearly, this is a difficult surgical procedure, even in the hands of surgeons skilled in elbow arthroscopy. Further experience with this technique is needed before it can be recommended for widespread use.

Open Capsular Release
The surgical management of patients with elbow contractures, although rewarding, is fraught with potential complications. Adequate surgical exposure is the key to successful outcome. Consideration should be given to all potential structures that may impede motion, and all relevant pathology must be addressed at the time of elbow release. For example, if the elbow will not extend following an anterior capsular release, it may be possible that posterior structures such as an olecranon osteophyte or loose body are preventing elbow extension. An important principle is that the range of motion after surgery is almost never greater and is usually less than that achieved in the operating room.

Although most patients undergoing surgery for symptomatic elbow contractures lack motion in both directions, some patients lack either extension or flexion. Therefore, the treatment approach must be individualized to address all relevant pathology based on preoperative physical examination and imaging studies. In general, the anterior and/or posterior elbow capsule needs to be excised. Internal fixation may be removed at the time of elbow contracture release; however, it has been suggested that this procedure leads to a higher risk of stiffness and recurrent heterotopic ossification. Removal of the internal fixation should only be done at the end of the release to avoid an intraoperative fracture as a consequence of the stress riser effect of empty screw holes and the cortical atrophy under the plates.

Portions of the collateral ligaments are released when this must be done in order to achieve elbow motion, particularly in patients with more severe contractures. The posterior band of the medial collateral ligament is not isometric and often needs to be released in patients with limited elbow flexion. Controlled partial surgical release of the collateral ligaments is preferable to intraoperative disruption by manipulation. Subchondral impression fractures can occur in manipulated joints as a result of high joint reactive forces in patients with disuse osteoporosis. In rare cases of severe contractures and ossified collateral ligaments, a complete ligament release may be necessary to achieve a functional arc of elbow motion intraoperatively. In such cases, an articulated external fixator may be beneficial, allowing immediate elbow mobilization postoperatively. The triceps and brachialis are often scarred down to the distal humerus and subperiosteal elevation of these muscles is often necessary to achieve improved joint motion. Only rarely are fractional lengthening or stepcut lengthening of the elbow musculature required to achieve motion in post-traumatic contractures. All heterotopic bone should be excised. Commonly the tip of the olecranon or coranoid needs to be removed to allow full extension or flexion respectively. Bone wax is used on exposed cancellous surfaces to minimize bleeding, and suction drains are routinely used postoperatively to prevent hematoma formation.

Surgical Technique

There are no studies comparing surgical techniques used for open capsular release of the elbow. Each has its proponents, with good results reported in all series. For uncomplicated extrinsic contractures, a lateral ligament sparing approach is preferred. The results of this technique have recently been reported by Hastings and Cohen. In patients with associated heterotopic ossification, a more flexible philosophy should be considered such that the surgical approach chosen allows all relevant pathology to be addressed. The isolated use of one approach may not be the best choice in all patients. The use of a midline posterior skin incision can be helpful in patients with more significant elbow contractures. The skin flaps can be elevated on the deep fascial plane to protect adjacent cutaneous nerves while allowing wide exposure of both the medial and lateral aspects of the elbow joint, avoiding the need for both a medial and lateral incision.

Anterior Approach Urbaniak described an anterior capsulotomy for release of elbow flexion contractures using an anterior (Henry) approach. Partial release of the anterior portions of the lateral and medial collateral ligaments can be performed, if necessary, to achieve adequate extension. Lengthening of the biceps and release of the brachialis can be considered in selected cases of more severe contractures. This approach provides only partial access to the anterior portions of the collateral ligaments and does not allow posterior pathology to be addressed. In the initial report by Urbaniak and associates, the mean flexion contracture improved from 48° to 19° in 15 patients treated with this technique. Eight of the 15 patients lost flexion when treated with this method. In a second series of 18 patients treated with this technique and postoperative continuous passive motion, flexion was diminished in only one of the patients. Because of the limited exposure afforded by this approach, this technique has only limited clinical usefulness and is generally not recommended except in patients with isolated flexion contractures resulting from anterior capsular scarring.

Lateral Approach A number of authors have reported good results of elbow contracture release through a lateral approach. Initially, the lateral ligament complex was divided as part of the surgical approach. More recently, the approach has been modified to allow preservation of the lateral collateral ligament complex while permitting exposure of both the anterior and posterior aspects of the elbow so that all relevant pathology can be addressed (Fig. 3). For isolated flexion contractures, this can be done using a limited approach developing the interval between the extensor carpi radialis longus (radial nerve) and the extensor carpi radialis brevis (posterior interosseous nerve) to expose the anterior aspect of the elbow joint and the anterior capsule. If greater exposure is required, the extensor carpi radialis longus and brachioradialis can be elevated off the lateral supracondylar ridge. The posterior aspect of the elbow can be exposed, when necessary, using the Kocher approach between the anconeus and extensor carpi ulnaris without the need for a second skin incision. The posterior capsule, olecranon, osteophytes, and loose bodies in the olecranon fossa can be excised while preserving the origin and insertion of the lateral collateral ligament complex.

In a recent report by Hastings and Cohen, 22 patients treated with this technique improved their average flexion contracture from 42° to 7°, while flexion improved from 110° to 140°. The Mayo elbow performance index, a measure of pain, motion, function, and stability, improved from 43 to 90 points. This technique allows improvement in elbow flexion and extension by providing exposure of both the anterior and posterior aspects of the elbow. If a lateral skin incision is used rather than a midline posterior one, a supplementary medial incision will be required to allow concomitant treatment of an associated ulnar neuropathy.

Medial Approach Hotchkiss and associates have reported the successful use of the medial approach in the treatment of patients with established elbow contracture. After isolation of the ulnar nerve, excellent exposure of the anterior aspect of the elbow can be achieved using the interval between the flexor carpi ulnaris and the pronator teres (Fig. 4). The posterior aspect of the elbow can be visualized by elevation of the triceps, and the posterior capsular tissues removed under direct vision. This approach is particularly useful in cases requiring excision of medial heterotopic bone, particularly if there is an associated ulnar neuropathy or calcification of the medial collateral ligament. Hotchkiss and associates have reported using this technique in seven patients with severe elbow contractures and associated heterotopic ossification. In this series, the patients were mobilized in an elbow distraction device in the postoperative period. The average flexion contracture improved from 45° to 13° while elbow flexion improved from 70° to 130°.

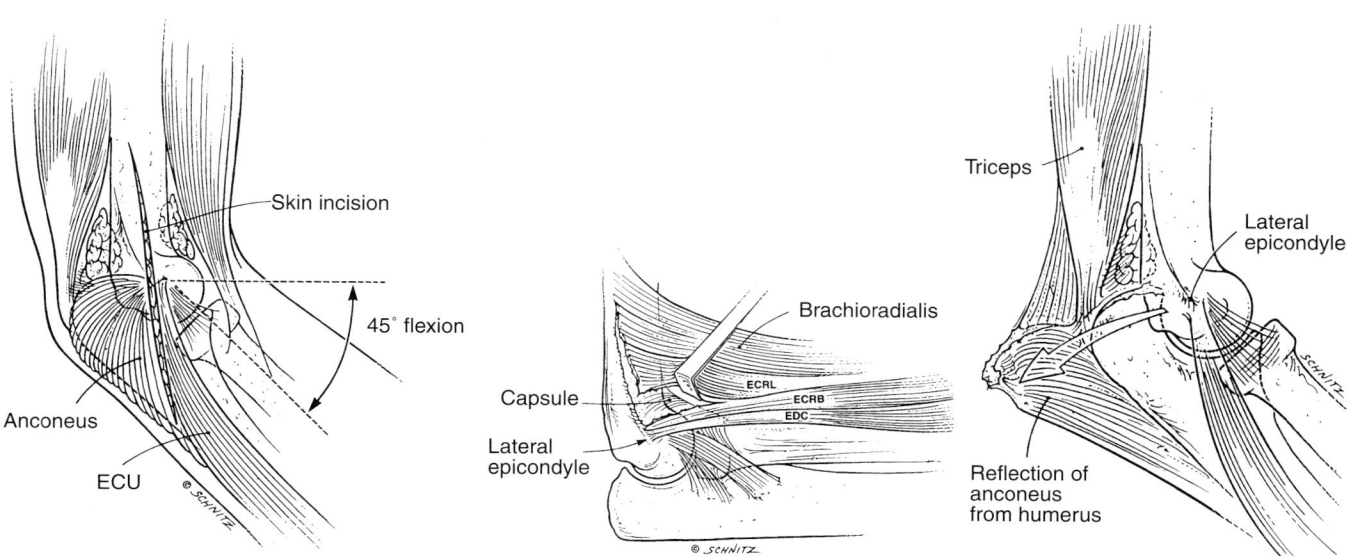

Fig. 3 Lateral approach. **Left,** A lateral incision is made with the elbow in 45° of flexion. The incision is marked parallel to the humerus, along the supracondylar ridge, across the lateral epicondyle, and onto the subcutaneous border of the ulna. This line identifies the interval between the anconeus and the extensor carpi ulnaris (ECU). **Center,** The interval between the extensor carpi radialis longus and brevis (ECRL, ECRB) is developed and the extensor carpi radialis longus and brachioradialis are elevated off the lateral supracondylar ridge. Anterior retraction of these muscles allows the anterior capsule to be excised. EDC = extensor digitorum communis. **Right,** The interval between the extensor carpi ulnaris and anconeus is developed to expose the posterior aspect of the elbow. The anconeus and triceps tendon are elevated along with the posterior fat pad and a posterior capsulectomy is performed. Excision of the olecranon tip may be required to gain extension in some patients. (Reproduced with permission from Hastings H: Elbow contractures and ossification, in Peimer CA (ed): *Reconstructive Surgery of the Upper Extremity.* New York, NY, McGraw-Hill, 1996, pp 516-517.)

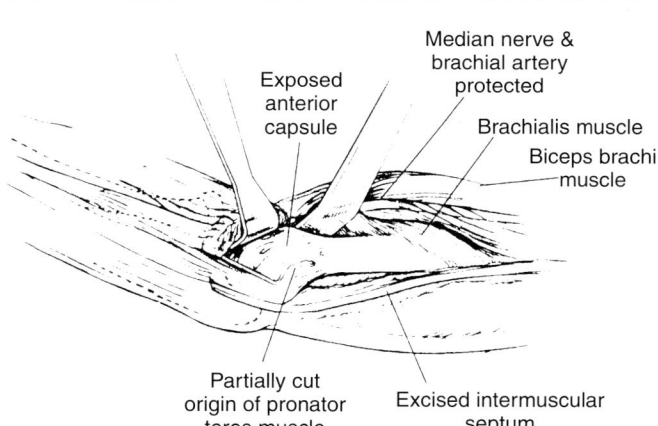

Fig. 4 Medial approach. The anterior aspect of the elbow is exposed by developing the interval between the flexor carpi ulnaris and pronator teres. The biceps and brachialis are retracted anteriorly while the ulnar nerve is protected. The posterior aspect of the elbow is exposed by elevating the triceps posteriorly. (Reproduced with permission from Hotchkiss R: *Compass Elbow Hinge.* Memphis, TN, Smith and Nephew Richards, 1993.)

Postoperative Care

The optimal management of patients following the surgical release of an elbow contracture is unknown. Edema must be controlled to allow joint mobilization. The judicious use of ice and anti-inflammatory agents is beneficial in the postoperative period. The analgesic properties of indomethacin have been well documented. In addition, it may be a useful adjunct in the prevention of heterotopic ossification as has been reported following total hip replacement. Continuous brachial plexus blockade may be helpful in controlling postoperative pain and may facilitate early mobilization of the elbow. There is some evidence that continuous passive motion may be helpful in obtaining and maintaining elbow motion after surgery. Alternatively, early active motion can be considered with a resting flexion and extension splinting program. The flexion and extension splints are alternated during the day and the extension splint is usually worn at night because this is the motion that is usually hardest to maintain postoperatively. After postoperative swelling and pain have subsided, turnbuckle splinting can be used about 4 to 6 weeks following an elbow release.

Although the risk of recurrent heterotopic ossification is low, some patients may be candidates for postoperative radiation, including those with a short duration from the development of the heterotopic bone to its excision, the need for repeated surgery, and poorer preoperative cognitive function. Although there is significant evidence in the literature to support the efficacy of postoperative radiation in patients with acetabular fractures and hip replacement arthroplasty, its use in heterotopic ossification of the elbow remains undefined. Because many patients undergoing surgical treatment of elbow contractures are young, the risk of teratogenicity makes its use rarely indicated.

Surgical Management: Intrinsic Contracture

Preoperative clinical and radiographic assessment is helpful in defining the extent of articular pathology in patients with intrinsic or combined elbow contractures. The decision to proceed with an interposition arthroplasty, however, is often only made at the time of surgical inspection of the joint following elbow release. Interposition arthroplasty is an established procedure for the treatment of joints damaged by posttraumatic arthritis. It has been suggested that if less than half of the articular surface of the joint is covered with hyaline cartilage, interposition arthroplasty is indicated. In addition, patients who require reshaping of the articular surface because of a malunion are also candidates for interposition arthroplasty. A number of interposition materials have been used historically to resurface damaged joints. Whereas dermal arthroplasty was frequently used in the past, fascia lata has been used in recent studies.

As with any surgical procedure, adequate exposure of the elbow joint is required for interposition arthroplasty. Division of the humeral origin of the lateral collateral ligament complex has been recommended to obtain adequate exposure. This ligament is repaired back to bone through drill holes at the end of the surgical procedure. Hinging the elbow open on the intact medial collateral ligament allows the articular surface of the distal humerus and ulna to be reshaped as necessary. Radial head excision should be avoided, if possible, because of the increased instability that can occur following this procedure. Debridement and retention of the radial head is preferred in all but the most advanced cases.

Fascia lata is obtained from the ipsilateral extremity using a lateral incision over the proximal thigh; a fascial strip measuring approximately 4 × 15 cm in size is harvested. The graft is trimmed and the joint surface of the distal humerus is resurfaced using a three-ply graft (Fig. 5). The graft is carefully sutured in place through drill holes in bone to prevent postoperative graft detachment.

In recent years, improved elbow distraction devices have been used to allow early postoperative mobilization in patients undergoing interposition arthroplasty. The distal humerus has been demonstrated to approximate a hinge joint with a locus of centers of rotation less than 4 mm in size. The Mayo distraction device (Howmedica, Rutherford, NJ) has one pin that is placed at the axis of rotation of the elbow joint. Laterally the landmark is at the center of the radius of curvature of the capitellum while medially the pin is placed just anterior and inferior to the medial epicondyle (Fig. 6). Care must be taken to isolate and protect the ulnar nerve while placing a small drill bit through the axis of rotation. After confirming the correct position of the axis with fluoroscopy, a transfixion pin is placed through the distal humerus. The lateral collateral ligament complex is then repaired by reattaching it to the lateral epicondyle through drill holes after the elbow has been reduced. Two more pins are placed in the ulna, and the distraction device is applied to the elbow. The joint is distracted approximately 3 to 5 mm by the device and the wound is then closed in layers. In six patients treated with interposition arthroplasty using the Mayo distraction device, a decrease in the average fixed flexion contracture from 65° to 28° was reported. Flexion improved from 92° to 135°.

Recently, the compass elbow hinge (Smith and Nephew Richards, Memphis, TN) has become available. This device also relies on the concept of a small locus of centers of rotation in the distal humerus; however, fixation pins are placed remote to the joint. A small axis pin is placed through the distal humerus while centering the device on the elbow. Fluoroscopy is used to ensure appropriate placement of the hinge axis. Three pins are placed in the humerus and two to three pins are placed in the ulna. After the hinge is placed, the distal humeral axis pin is then removed. The compass elbow hinge can also be used in a distraction mode similar to the Mayo device.

There are no studies comparing the Mayo device (Fig. 7) with the compass elbow hinge (Fig. 8). The compass hinge is

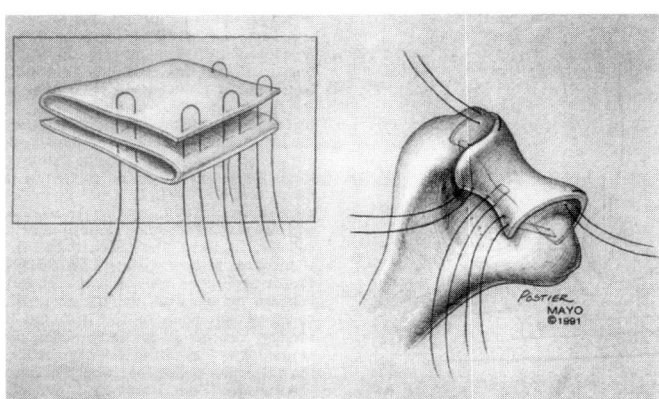

Fig. 5 Three-ply interposition graft. **Left,** Fascia lata graft is sutured into three layers. **Right,** Graft is secured to the distal humerus through drill holes placed along the margins as well as centrally. (Reproduced with permission from The Mayo Foundation, Rochester, MN.)

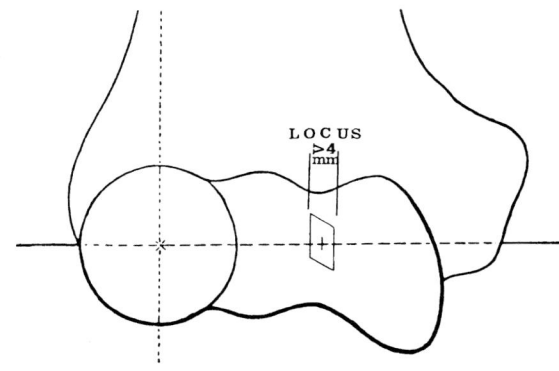

Fig. 6 Distraction device axis. The locus of instant centers of rotation is smaller than 4 mm. The center of the capitellum is used as the lateral landmark, while the pin is placed just anterior and inferior to the medial epicondyle. (Reproduced with permission from Morrey BF: Post traumatic stiffness and distraction arthroplasty, in Morrey BF (ed): *The Elbow and Its Disorders,* ed 2. Philadelphia, PA, WB Saunders, 1993.)

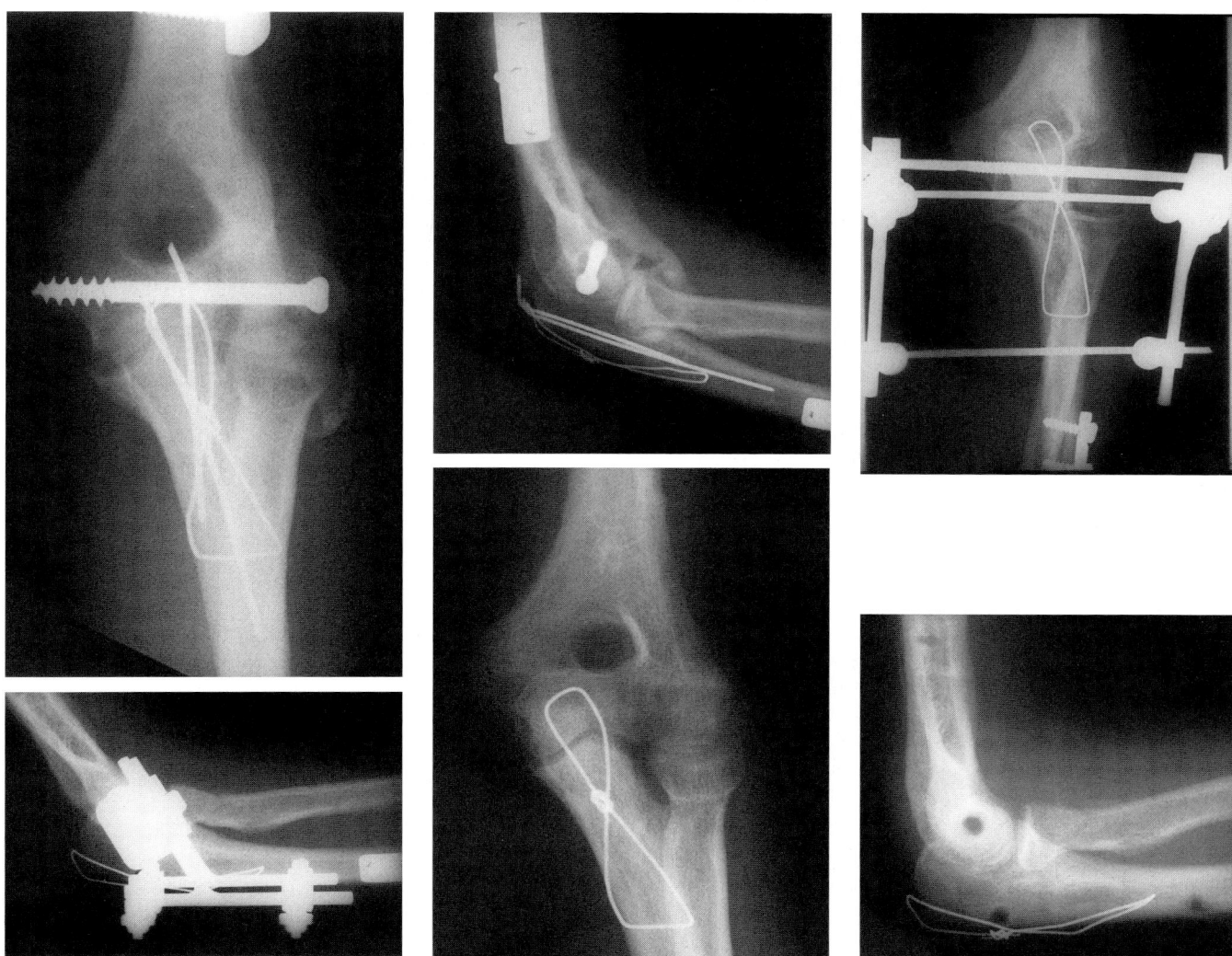

Fig. 7 Mayo distraction device. **Top left,** Anteroposterior radiograph of a 21-year-old man involved in a motorcycle accident 1 year ago. The patient has no flexion-extension or prosupination of the elbow and forearm. **Top center,** Lateral radiograph demonstrating extensive heterotopic ossification. **Top right,** Postoperative anteroposterior radiograph following excision of heterotopic bone and application of Mayo distraction device to control posterolateral rotatory instability induced by the surgical release. **Bottom left,** Lateral radiograph following excision of heterotopic bone and debridement of the radial head. **Bottom center,** Appearance of anteroposterior radiograph following removal of distraction device 6 weeks postoperatively. **Bottom right,** Lateral radiograph after removal of distraction device.

significantly more bulky than the Mayo device and is more difficult to apply. Unlike the Mayo device, it is recommended for single use. The Mayo device seems to be more amenable than the compass hinge to use with continuous passive motion. The compass hinge has a significant advantage in that no axis pin is left in the distal humerus. In older patients with age-related osteoporosis or patients with disuse osteoporosis as a result of long-standing severe elbow contractures, the distal humerus axis pin of the Mayo distractor may loosen. With the Mayo device, a pin tract infection is likely to result in deep sepsis of the elbow; in contrast, the compass device has its fixation pins placed remote to the joint. In addition, the compass hinge allows for gradual, progressive, patient-controlled stretching of the joint due to its worm gear mechanism, which can also be disengaged for active range of motion exercises. More study of these devices will clarify their ultimate place in the management of elbow contractures.

Postoperative Care

In patients with mixed or intrinsic contractures, general principles of treatment of extrinsic elbow contractures are followed. With the application of the distraction device, continuous brachial plexus blockade is used for pain control after surgery and continued for 2 to 4 days. Use of a continuous passive motion machine is sometimes recommended in an attempt to gain early motion. Patients are discharged with

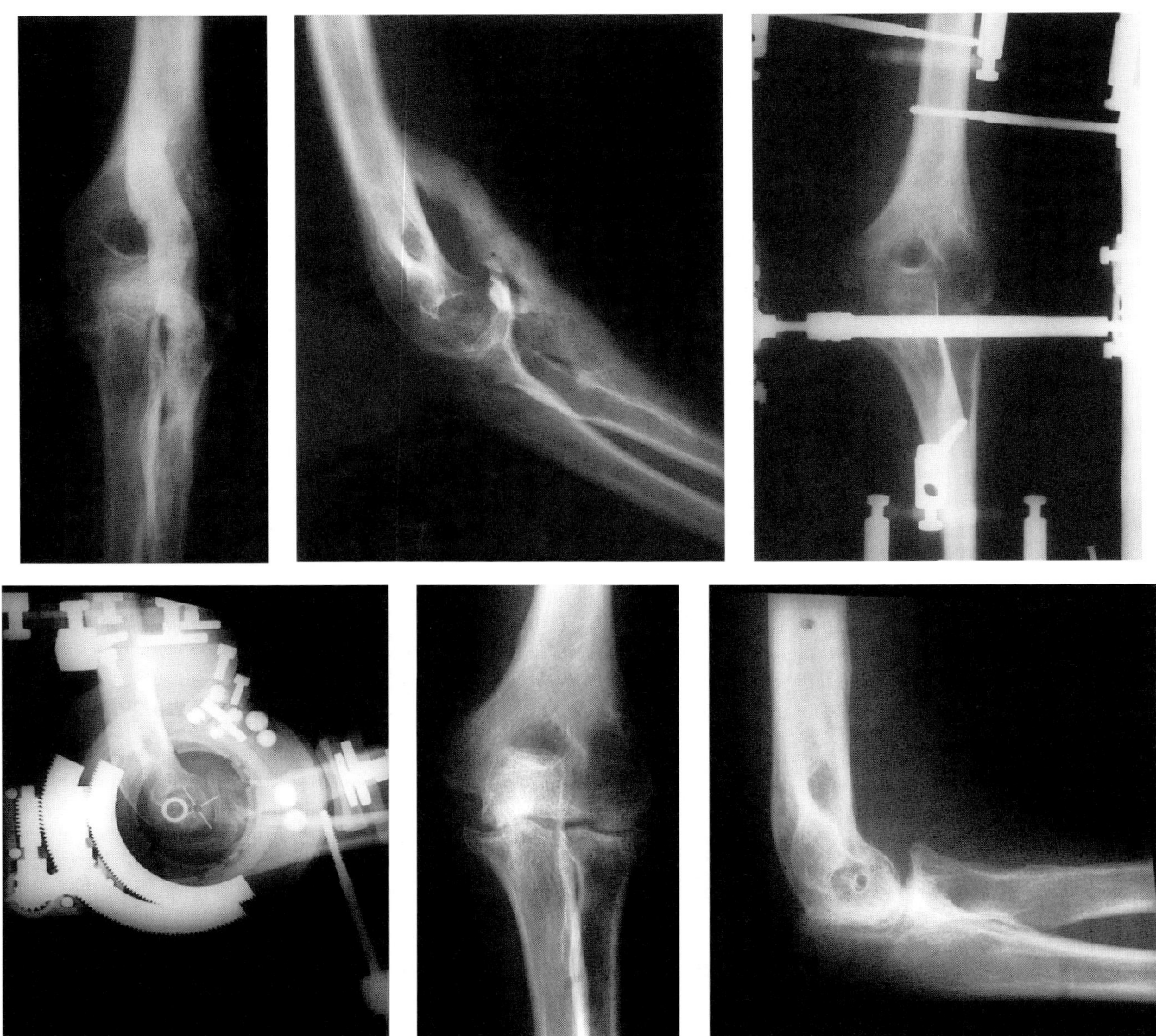

Fig. 8 Compass hinge distraction device. **Top left,** Anteroposterior radiograph of a 24-year-old man involved in a motorcycle accident 18 months ago. The patient has no flexion-extension or prosupination of the elbow and forearm. **Top center,** Lateral radiograph demonstrating extensive heterotopic ossification. **Top right,** Postoperative anteroposterior radiograph following excision of heterotopic bone and application of compass elbow hinge to control posterolateral rotatory instability induced by the surgical release. Bar from worm gear mechanism that is projected across the elbow joint permits passive stretching of the elbow joint in the flexion-extension plane postoperatively. **Bottom left,** Lateral radiograph following excision of heterotopic bone. Cross hairs on device ensure proper replication of axis of rotation. **Bottom center,** Appearance of anteroposterior radiograph following removal of distraction device 6 weeks postoperatively. **Bottom right,** Lateral radiograph after removal of distraction device.

a home continuous passive motion machine to be used for 20 hours per day, with active exercises performed during the remainder of the 24-hour period. At 4 to 6 weeks the distraction device is removed and a flexion-extension splinting program is then initiated, as previously described for patients with extrinsic contractures.

Results

The outcome of elbow contracture release has been rewarding. All series, regardless of the surgical approach and specific technique, have reported an overall improvement in motion following the surgical release of a stiff elbow. Surgical release of a stiff elbow results in improved motion in 95% of patients. Approximately 80% of patients achieve a functional arc of motion (30° to 130°) and 90% achieve within 10° of this goal. Patient satisfaction is high. Studies report that patients with greater restriction of elbow motion preoperatively have greater improvement in the arc of motion postoperatively. Pain usually decreases following the release of an intrinsic elbow contracture with interposition arthroplasty. About half of the patients report some residual mild discomfort; however, more significant pain is uncommon. Stability of the elbow is usually maintained with adequate ligament preservation intraoperatively or postoperative protection with an articulated external fixator when indicated.

Complications

Numerous complications have been reported following elbow contracture release. Recent literature has reported that the incidence of these complications has decreased, probably as a consequence of a better understanding of the pathoanatomy of elbow contractures and improved surgical approaches for their treatment. Local skin complications are occasionally seen in patients having previous traumatic causes for their elbow stiffness. The surgeon should use a previous incision whenever possible in order to avoid flap necrosis. Pressure over the posterior incision should be avoided postoperatively by careful splinting. Deep infections are occasionally seen as a result of extensive surgical exposures and prolonged operating times in more severe elbow contractures. Prophylactic antibiotics should be used routinely. Pin tract infections are frequently seen with the use of elbow distraction devices and are usually controlled with care of the local pin site and oral antibiotics. Permanent neurologic injury is uncommon if appropriate precautions are taken at the time of surgery. Neurapraxias are occasionally encountered as a result of nerve dissection and retraction; however, they usually resolve with time. Vessel injury is rarely a result of direct trauma, but can occur in older patients with long-standing flexion contractures resulting from intimal tears. Periarticular fractures can occur through the site of previous hardware both intraoperatively and postoperatively.

With a compliant patient and experienced therapist to assist with postoperative splinting and active motion, recurrence of the contracture is unusual. Heterotopic ossification can recur; however, this is uncommon as long as the previous elbow injury that caused the contracture is remote. As in any upper limb procedure, reflex sympathetic dystrophy can occur. This condition is often associated with an intraoperative nerve injury and should be treated with aggressive sympathetic blocks and supervised physiotherapy. Ligament instability is occasionally seen following elbow contracture release, particularly if an interposition arthroplasty is performed. This condition is usually responsive to splinting and activity modification; however, ligament reconstructions are occasionally required. A neurotrophic joint can occur following an elbow contracture release because of the extensive soft-tissue stripping and denervation of the elbow joint. Elbow weakness is a potential risk if the patient's motor groups were inadequate before surgery.

Selected Bibliography

Boerboom AL, de Meyier HE, Verburg AD, et al: Arthrolysis for post-traumatic stiffness of the elbow. *Int Orthop* 1993;17:346-349.

Bonutti PM, Windau JE, Ables BA, et al: Static progressive stretch to reestablish elbow range of motion. *Clin Orthop* 1994;303:128-134.

Twenty patients with elbow contractures were treated with static progressive stretch using a commercially available noncustom splint. The arc of motion improved an average of 31° with no complications and no loss of motion at 1 year follow-up.

Cullen JP, Pellegrini VD Jr, Miller RJ, et al: Treatment of traumatic radioulnar synostosis by excision and postoperative low dose irradiation. *J Hand Surg* 1994;19A:394-401.

Four patients with traumatic radioulnar synostosis were treated by excision and postoperative low dose radiation. Two of these patients had their synostosis removed less than 1 year postinjury. The radiation was well tolerated and there was no recurrence of the heterotopic bone.

Dowdy PA, Bain GI, King GJW, et al: The midline posterior elbow incision: An anatomical appraisal. *J Bone Joint Surg* 1995;77B:696-699.

Duke JB, Tessler RH, Dell PC: Manipulation of the stiff elbow with patient under anesthesia. *J Hand Surg* 1991;16A:19-24.

Eleven patients underwent 13 manipulations of the elbow under general anesthesia to improve a dysfunctional range of motion. Motion was improved in six of these patients (55%). Two transient sensory ulnar neuropathies were the only complications.

Engber WD, Reynen P: Post-burn heterotopic ossification at the elbow. *Iowa Orthop* 1994;14:38-41.

In this retrospective review of six elbow releases for heterotopic ossification, excellent results were achieved with excision of heterotopic bone an average of 8.3 months after burn. The arc of motion improved from an average of 6° preoperatively to over 121° postoperatively. Excision was recommended when the heterotopic bone appears mature and the skin is completely healed and stable.

Evans EB: Orthopaedic measures in the treatment of severe burns. *J Bone Joint Surg* 1966;48A:643-669.

Fortier MV, Forster BB, Pinney S, et al: MR assessment of posttraumatic flexion contracture of the elbow. *J Magn Reson Imaging* 1995;5:473-477.

Twelve patients with flexion contracture of the elbow were studied using magnetic resonance imaging (MRI). The MRI was better able than plain films to demonstrate loose bodies. Abnormalities in the capsule and collateral ligaments were demonstrated.

Gallay SH, Richards RR, O'Driscoll SW: Intraarticular capacity and compliance of stiff and normal elbows. *Arthroscopy* 1993;9:9-13.

Garland DE, Hanscom DA, Keenan MA, et al: Resection of heterotopic ossification in the adult with head trauma. *J Bone Joint Surg* 1985;67A:1261-1269.

Garland DE, O'Hollaren RM: Fractures and dislocations about the elbow in the head-injured adult. *Clin Orthop* 1982;168:38-41.

Gates HS III, Sullivan FL, Urbaniak JR: Anterior capsulotomy and continuous passive motion in the treatment of post-traumatic flexion contracture of the elbow: A prospective study. *J Bone Joint Surg* 1992;74A:1229-1234.

Thirty-three patients who had a posttraumatic flexion contracture were managed with an elbow contracture release through an anterior approach, with or without the use of postoperative continuous passive motion. The use of continuous passive motion resulted in a greater improvement in flexion; however, it did not influence the residual flexion contracture.

Green DP, McCoy H: Turnbuckle orthotic correction of elbow-flexion contractures after acute injuries. *J Bone Joint Surg* 1979;61A:1092-1095.

The effectiveness of turnbuckle splinting using a custom orthosis was studied in 15 patients. The average increase in the arc of motion was 43°. In three patients with articular damage the splint could not be tolerated because of excessive pain, and the treatment was unsuccessful.

Hastings H: Elbow contractures and ossification, in Peimer CA (ed): *Reconstructive Surgery of the Upper Extremity.* New York, NY, McGraw-Hill, 1996, pp 507-534.

Hastings H, Cohen MS: Post-traumatic contracture of the elbow: Operative release using a new surgical approach. *Trans ASES* 1996;13:32.

Twenty-two patients with posttraumatic elbow contractures were treated with surgical release through a ligament-sparing lateral approach. Extension improved from 42° ± 8° to 7° ± 10° at an average 26-month follow-up. Elbow flexion improved from 110° to 140° following surgery. Total elbow motion increased an average of 65°. The Mayo elbow performance index, which includes motion, function, pain, and stability increased from 43 to 90 points.

Hastings H II, Graham TJ: The classification and treatment of heterotopic ossification about the elbow and forearm. *Hand Clin* 1994;10:417-437.

The authors propose a new classification for heterotopic ossification that may be useful in managing heterotopic ossification of the upper limb. This article is an excellent review of the treatment considerations for heterotopic ossification of the upper limb.

Hedley AK, Mead LP, Hendren DH: The prevention of heterotopic bone formation following total hip arthroplasty using 600 rad in a single dose. *J Arthroplasty* 1989;4:319-325.

Hotchkiss RN, An KN, Weiland AJ, et al: Treatment of severe elbow contractures using the concepts of Ilizarov. Proceedings of the American Academy of Orthopaedic Surgeons 61st Annual Meeting, New Orleans, LA. Rosemont, IL, American Academy of Orthopaedic Surgeons, 1994, p 61.

Seven patients with severe contractures and heterotopic ossification were treated with an open anterior and posterior capsular release and the application of the compass elbow hinge device. The average arc of motion improved from 25° to 117° postoperatively.

Husband JB, Hastings H II: The lateral approach for operative release of post-traumatic contracture of the elbow. *J Bone Joint Surg* 1990;72A:1353-1358.

Seven patients had a surgical release of a posttraumatic elbow contracture through a lateral approach. The average arc of motion improved from 71° to 117°. Six of seven patients achieved a functional arc of motion.

Jones GS, Savoie FH III: Arthroscopic capsular release of flexion contractures (arthrofibrosis) of the elbow. *Arthroscopy* 1993;9:277-283.

Twelve patients with flexion contractures of the elbow were treated with arthroscopic anterior capsular release and posterior debridement of the olecranon fossa. The mean flexion contracture improved from 38° preoperatively to 3° postoperatively. One patient sustained a permanent posterior interosseous nerve palsy.

Jupiter JB: Heterotopic ossification about the elbow, in Eilert RE (ed): *Instructional Course Lectures XL.* Park Ridge, IL, American Academy of Orthopaedic Surgeons, 1991, pp 41-44.

Karachalios T, Maxwell-Armstrong C, Atkins RM: Treatment of post-traumatic fixed flexion deformity of the elbow using an intermittent compression garment. *Injury* 1994;25:313-315.

Lamine A, Fikry T, Essadki B, et al: Arthrolysis of the elbow: Apropos of 70 cases. *Acta Orthop Belgica* 1993;59:352-356.

Ljung P, Jonsson K, Larsson K, et al: Interposition arthroplasty of the elbow with rheumatoid arthritis. *J Shoulder Elbow* 1996;5:81-85.

Interposition arthroplasty with processed bovine collagen was performed in 35 elbows in patients with rheumatoid arthritis. At 6-year follow-up pain relief was good; however, the elbows had only fair results with regard to mobility and stability. Radiographically, elbow destruction progressed and made subsequent procedures difficult. The authors recommended total elbow replacement as the first choice in management of the painful rheumatoid elbow with cartilage destruction.

Lynch GJ, Meyers JF, Whipple TL, et al: Neurovascular anatomy and elbow arthroscopy: Inherent risks. *Arthroscopy* 1986;2:190-197.

Mehlhoff TL, Noble PC, Bennett JB, et al: Simple dislocation of the elbow in the adult: Results after closed treatment. *J Bone Joint Surg* 1988;78A:244-249.

Fifty-two adults were reviewed an average of 34 months following a simple elbow dislocation treated with closed reduction. A flexion contracture of greater than 30° was documented in 15% of patients. The longer the period of immobilization after reduction, the greater the residual stiffness and pain.

Mih AD, Wolf FG: Surgical release of elbow-capsular contracture in pediatric patients. *J Pediatr Orthop* 1994;14:458-461.

Nine pediatric patients with elbow flexion contractures were treated by surgical release using a lateral approach. The total arc of motion improved from 55° to 108°.

Modabber MR, Jupiter JB: Reconstruction for post-traumatic conditions of the elbow joint. *J Bone Joint Surg* 1995;77A:1431-1446.

This article is a good review of treatment approaches for the stiff elbow.

Mohan K: Myositis ossificans traumatica of the elbow. *Int Surg* 1972;57:475-478.

Moore TJ: Functional outcome following surgical excision of heterotopic ossification in patients with traumatic brain injury. *J Orthop Trauma* 1993;7:11-14.

The average arc of motion following the excision of heterotopic ossification in seven ankylosed elbows was 65°. One patient had recurrent heterotopic ossification. Prerequisites to a successful surgical excision in patients with traumatic burn injuries were believed to include a delay of at least 18 months following brain injury, a radiographically mature ossification, a relatively high patient cognitive level, and selective control of the involved extremity.

Morrey BF (ed): *The Elbow and Its Disorders,* ed 2. Philadelphia, PA, WB Saunders, 1993.

Morrey BF: Post-traumatic contracture of the elbow: Operative treatment, including distraction arthroplasty. *J Bone Joint Surg* 1990;72A:601-618.

Twenty-six patients were treated with surgical release of a posttraumatic elbow contracture through a lateral approach, with or without fascial interposition arthroplasty and the use of an elbow distraction device. The arc of motion improved from 30° preoperatively to 96° postoperatively. The management of these patients during and after surgery is outlined in detail.

Morrey BF, Askew LJ, An KN, et al: A biomechanical study of normal functional elbow motion. *J Bone Joint Surg* 1981;63A:872-876.

Thirty-three normal volunteers performed 15 activities of daily living while their elbow motion was recorded with an electrogoniometer. Most of the activities of daily living could be performed with a range of flexion-extension from 30° to 130°, and pronation-supination from 50° to 50°.

Nowicki KD, Shall LM: Arthroscopic release of a posttraumatic flexion contracture in the elbow: A case report and review of the literature. *Arthroscopy* 1992;8:544-547.

O'Driscoll SW, Shankland SW, Beaton D: Patient-adjusted static elbow splints for elbow contractures: A preliminary report. *J Shoulder Elbow Surg* 1996;5:S73.

Six patients with elbow contractures in whom conventional physical therapy had failed were treated with patient-adjusted static elbow splints and followed for 8 months. The average arc of motion improved from 73° to 103°.

Roberts JB, Pankratz DG: The surgical treatment of heterotopic ossification at the elbow following long-term coma. *J Bone Joint Surg* 1979;61A:760-763.

Rymaszewski L, Glass K, Parikh R: Post-traumatic elbow contracture treated by arthrolysis and continual passive motion under brachial plexus anaesthesia. *J Bone Joint Surg* 1996;76B:S30.

Eighteen patients were treated with arthrolysis followed by continuous passive motion for established posttraumatic elbow contractures. The average arc of motion improved from 42° to 100°. Pain decreased following the procedure.

Segstro R, Morley-Forster PK, Lu G: Indomethacin as a postoperative analgesic for total hip arthroplasty. *Can J Anaesth* 1991;38:578-581.

Seth MK, Khurana JK: Bony ankylosis of the elbow after burns. *J Bone Joint Surg* 1985;67B:747-749.

Timmerman LA, Andrews JR: Arthroscopic treatment of posttraumatic elbow pain and stiffness. *Am J Sports Med* 1994;22:230-235.

Nineteen patients with posttraumatic arthrofibrosis were treated with arthroscopic debridement and manipulation. Extension improved from 29° to 11° and flexion improved from 123° to 134°. Good to excellent results were reported in 79% of these patients without any major complications.

Urbaniak JR, Hansen PE, Beissinger SF, et al: Correction of post-traumatic flexion contracture of the elbow by anterior capsulotomy. *J Bone Joint Surg* 1985;67A:1160-1164.

Vasen AP, Lacey SH, Keith MW, et al: Functional range of motion of the elbow. *J Hand Surg* 1995;20A:288-291.

Fifty normal volunteers who were fitted with a brace that limited elbow motion were asked to perform 12 activities of daily living. Forty-nine of the subjects were able to perform these tasks with the arc of elbow motion limited to between 75° and 120°.

Zander CL, Healy NL: Elbow flexion contractures treated with serial casts and conservative therapy. *J Hand Surg* 1992;17A:694-697.

Tendon Injuries and Tendinopathies About the Elbow

Bernard F. Morrey, MD

Epicondylitis

Tennis elbow, or lateral epicondylitis, is much more common (9:1 ratio) than medial involvement; thus, most information about this condition focuses on the lateral lesion. However, causative factors, pathology, and treatment are similar for both sites.

Etiology

Epicondylitis is caused by a variety of overuse activities. The eccentric repetitive overload seen during the backhand stroke in tennis, for example, is the classic mechanism. However, a host of other occupational or recreational activities that cause similar loads are even more common. Acute direct and even indirect trauma to the lateral and, less commonly, the medial epicondylar prominences are also causative factors. A correlation between fluoroquinolone antibiotics and tendinous inflammation has also recently been established, with two cases of acute onset tennis elbow confirmed by clinical assessment and magnetic resonance imaging.

Pathology

Certain pathologic conditions have been attributed to lateral epicondylitis, which histologically is not inflammatory but is a degenerative process. Although microscopic evidence of neovascularization is commonly present, inflammatory cells are not, and the histologic features of the tissue are best characterized as hyaline degeneration (Fig. 1). The role of prior injection of steroid as a cause of the histologic findings has not been established.

Anatomic Involvement

It is generally recognized that the extensor carpi radialis brevis (ECRB) is probably the most common specific site of extensor mechanism involvement. However, the other tendons of the common extensor origin can be involved more often than is typically recognized. Confusion and difficulty in distinguishing tennis elbow from posterior interosseous nerve (PIN) irritation is ongoing, which may possibly be explained by recognizing the anatomic feature of a fascial arcade. This arcade is present at the deep surface of the common extensor tendon, serving as a source of attachment for this complex. Hence, careful examination of the entire extensor mechanism origin, as well as an awareness of the role and possible concurrent involvement of the PIN, is required to confirm the diagnosis and determine proper treatment of this condition. A detailed clinical and anatomic study documented coincident involvement of the PIN and lateral epicondylitis in 5% of patients. If the presentation includes pain or aching of the extensor forearm musculature, PIN entrapment should be considered as an isolated or concurrent diagnosis. Examination consists of specifically palpating the entry site of the PIN at the arcade of Frohse. Because this is normally a sensitive area, comparison with the uninvolved extremity is important. Pain on resisted supination is probably the most sensitive test. Pain from resisted extension of the middle finger is not specific for PIN entrapment and often reproduces pain from lateral epicondylitis.

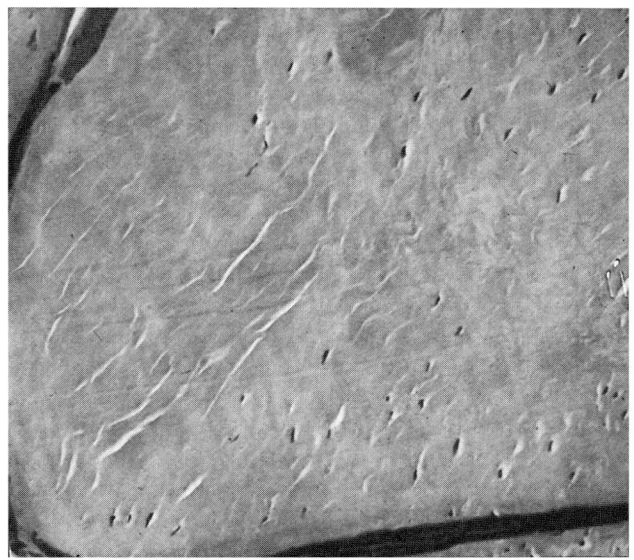

Fig. 1 Histologic section from extensor carpi radialis brevis demonstrating hyaline degeneration, which is indicative of a degenerative rather than an inflammatory process.

Nonsurgical Treatment

A host of nonsurgical treatments alone or in combination have been recommended, including activity modification, forearm bands and other orthoses, anti-inflammatory agents, oral, topical, or injectable steroids, various "modalities," splinting, cast immobilization, manipulation, radiotherapy, acupuncture, and vitamins. In a recent meta-analysis of 185 articles involving lateral epicondylitis, only 18 were believed to have had sufficient data to be considered legitimate controlled studies. Of these 18, only six were believed to provide data regarding therapy from which valid expectations could be drawn. It was concluded that the literature did not clearly establish the importance or the central role of any one nonsurgical treatment modality over the other. Specifically, in two reports ultrasound was found to relieve symptoms, but it was of no benefit over the control group in two additional studies. Likewise, iontophoresis was found to be superior to control in one but no better than the control population in two additional studies. In three randomized investigations, nonsteroidal anti-inflammatory agents were documented to be of no advantage over the control population. Cortisone injections were observed to be helpful in a consistent fashion but the exact dose or type of steroid did not seem to influence outcome. Shock wave therapy has recently been added to this list. A recent investigation found significant improvement in a controlled random study with good or excellent results in 48% of patients with shock wave treatment compared to only 24% improvement in the control group.

Surgical Treatment

The surgical treatment for tennis elbow continues to most popularly involve a direct surgical approach to the lateral epicondyle under a variety of anesthetics, including local, regional, or general. Most commonly the ECRB is exposed and the pathologic degenerative tissue is removed according to the technique of Nirschl or Coonrad, or a variation of these two. Management of the lesion may be partial excision with repair or release and "slide" of the extensor origin.

The most popular procedure still consists of a direct limited exposure over the lateral epicondyle under a local or general anesthetic. The common extensor tendon is incised longitudinally at its anterior third. The tissue is retracted, exposing the ECRB origin and generally revealing the pathology. The degenerative tissue is removed in an elliptical fashion until the "shiny silver fibers" of normal common extensor tendon are observed. A loose superficial closure of the common extensor is then carried out. The extremity is protected and the patient restricted from activity for approximately 2 weeks postoperatively. Gradual increase in functional use beginning at 3 weeks is followed by return to normal activity at about 3 months.

In addition to open surgery, open or percutaneous release is also advocated. An impressive success rate with percutaneous release as an office procedure under local anesthesia has been reported in 19 consecutive patients. A significant implication of this particular report is an estimated savings of over $4,000 with the office procedure compared to that done in a hospital setting. A thought-provoking and innovative surgical treatment for this condition is extra-articular endoscopic-assisted common extensor tendon release. The German report is primarily directed toward description of the technique with minimal discussion of the clinical outcome. Intra-articular releases are also being performed, but the technique and data have not yet found their way into the literature. Obviously, no definitive statement can be made at this time, but it would seem prudent to await confirmation of the value of percutaneous release over other options.

Expected Results

Review of the literature suggests that lateral epicondylitis will spontaneously resolve in 90% of patients; the process may be intermittent, with symptoms waxing and waning for 1 year or longer. In general, surgical release is offered to the approximately 10% whose condition does not resolve after 1 year of nonsurgical treatment. Of these patients, most surgical techniques are reported to be about 90% successful.

For those patients complaining of aching discomfort in the forearm with marked localizing signs over the PIN, a diagnostic cortisone injection is performed. If there is definite evidence of a concurrent lesion based on clinical evidence and response to the diagnostic injection, the PIN is explored through a slightly more anteriorly based and extended excision. If the clinical assessment implicates the PIN, electromyographic confirmation is not considered necessary before exploration is carried out. The interval between the extensor carpi radialis longus and common extensor tendon is developed, readily exposing the PIN at the arcade of Frohse. It is relatively uncommon that this procedure is indicated, and exposure of the PIN is not routinely performed for tennis elbow procedures.

Chronic Refractory Tennis Elbow Following Failed Surgical Intervention

Surgical failure poses a particularly difficult problem to the surgeon because its interpretation can be confused by issues related to workers' compensation or secondary gain. The assessment begins by determining that an adequate duration of time has elapsed since surgery—a minimum of 6 months, and preferably 1 year. If this is the case, it must be determined whether the symptoms are the same as or different from those present before surgery. If the symptoms are the same, then it can be concluded that the pathology was not addressed, either because the procedure was not performed correctly or the proper diagnosis was not made. If the symptoms differ from those before surgery, ligamentous deficiency from an aggressive release or possible herniation of synovial fluid from a pseudocapsular rent of the lateral capsule should be considered. In a series of 13 consecutive reoperations, 11 of the 13 were benefited by a second procedure directed by the above logic and as depicted in more detail in Figure 2. Note that it would be expected that in the majority no additional surgery is recommended because the criteria favorable to surgery are not met.

Medial Epicondylitis

Although for years relatively little has been known about medial epicondylitis, two recent reports have demonstrated surprisingly similar and optimistic outcomes. Although it was generally considered that surgical treatment for medial epicondylitis is much less successful than that for the lateral lesions, both studies report satisfactory results approaching those attributed to lateral epicondylitis. The procedure is analogous to that performed on the lateral side, with direct exposure over the point of maximum tenderness and an elliptical excision of the degenerative tissue concluded by a loose closure of the tendon remnants. Great care is taken to localize the precise point of maximum tenderness as the focal point of the incision. One study emphasized that those individuals

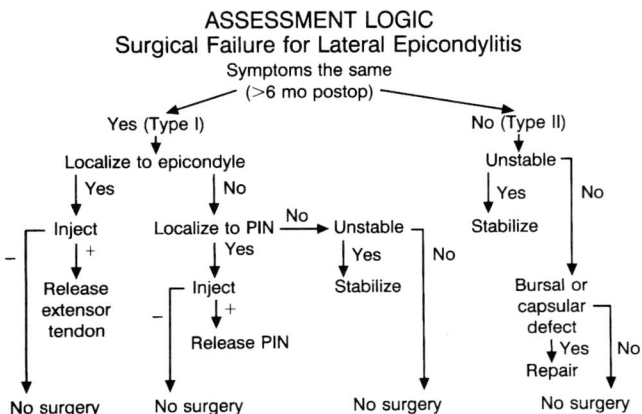

Fig. 2 Assessment logic as an approach to the management of patients with failed surgical procedures for the treatment of lateral epicondylitis. (Reproduced with permission from the Mayo Foundation, Rochester, MN.)

with associated ulnar nerve irritation have a prognosis of about 70%, compared to 90% in patients without ulnar nerve involvement.

Distal Biceps Tendon Injury: Classification

Although rupture of the distal biceps has been considered an uncommon if not a rare injury in the past, there have been a number of reports on this entity in the recent literature, indicating that either there is an increased awareness of its occurrence or possibly a true increased incidence. As the prognosis is dramatically altered by timely treatment, enhanced awareness of this particular tendon injury and its diagnosis is appropriate.

There are three distinct types of distal biceps tendon injury: strain, partial rupture, and complete avulsion from the tuberosity. The mechanism for each of these three is identical: sudden resistance opposing an abrupt flexion force of the biceps mechanism, that is, sudden eccentric biceps muscle contraction. This mechanism may possibly occur in a tendon already altered by microtrauma or repetitive stress.

Strain

A strain of the biceps tendon is characterized by a history of a forced flexion against resistance causing acute pain in the region of the antecubital space. Chronic use may elicit a similar symptom complex; thus, the diagnosis of overuse syndrome is distinguished from strain by the history of an acute event with an acute strain. The patient is not aware of a snap or pop that accompanies a complete disruption. Flexion and supination strengths are near-normal but are painful. There is, of course, no change in the contour of the biceps with flexion, and subcutaneous ecchymosis and bleeding into the deep structures do not occur. There has not been a similar problem with repeated use but this is also a possible cause.

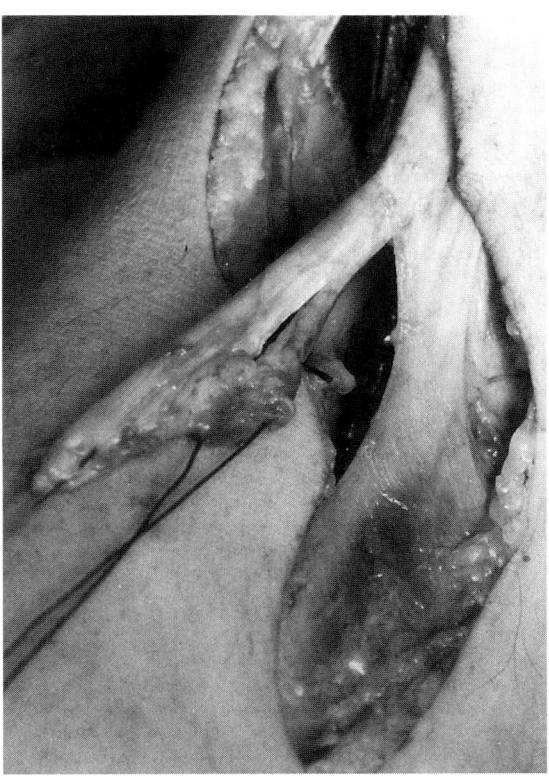

Fig. 3 Surgical exposure of a partial rupture of the biceps tendon. The long suture is in the portion of the tendon that had ruptured and proximally migrated. The remaining portion of the tendon was detached prior to the entire portion being trimmed and reattached. Note the stretched lacertus fibrosus, which helped to maintain the integrity of the flexor mechanism.

Treatment Strain may be treated symptomatically, although there are not sufficient data to clearly define the natural history of such an injury. Current recommended treatment is immediate immobilization for approximately 3 weeks followed by protected use for an additional 3 to 6 weeks. Although clinical experience is limited, this treatment has proved effective enough that subsequent surgery is not usually required.

Partial Rupture

Partial rupture of the distal flexor mechanism may also be categorized into one of three types: 1) partial avulsion at the tuberosity; (2) tear of the biceps tendon in continuity; and (3) injury of the musculotendinous junction (Fig. 3).

Partial Detachment Of the three types of partial injury, partial detachment is the most common. The patient will frequently have heard a sound or snap, or felt a searing pain that suggests an acute event. The initial pain subsides but the patient has persistent weakness on flexion and supination that is most notable with repetitive activity. Fatigue pain is a most common presentation. The patient may also notice crepitus deep in the antecubital space with pronation and supination.

Pain is localized to this area. Soft-tissue imaging, such as magnetic resonance imaging (MRI), can be helpful but may be difficult to interpret. A high level of suspicion is necessary to make the diagnosis. Injection of a local anesthetic into the region of insertion of the biceps tendon to the tuberosity is confirmatory for a lesion in this area. The history of strength degradation with time and aching discomfort that does not improve over 6 to 12 months is highly suggestive of this entity.

There is little evidence to anticipate marked improvement in a partial detachment treated nonsurgically for more than 6 months. These patients are best treated by surgical repair. After detachment of the remaining fibers, the degenerated end of the tendon is debrided and then reattached into the tuberosity as is done for the acute lesion as described below. The prognosis for this injury and repair is good and approaches that following treatment of an acute rupture.

In Continuity Disruption of the Biceps Tendon This condition is suspected with symptoms as described above, but the pain is clearly along the palpable biceps tendon, proximal to its insertion. There is inadequate experience to offer a definitive recommendation for surgical treatment. Plication would seem less reliable than some form of augmentation as with a ligament augmentation device (LAD™) or possibly tendon autograft/allograft. The nonsurgical approach is acceptable. However, if restoration of a person to gainful employment is a consideration, the surgical option is favored.

Disruption of the Musculotendinous Junction This is a very rare entity, which is fortunate because its prognosis is guarded. Few have been identified with this lesion following a confirmatory operation. Typically the pathology consists of scar tissue with obvious signs of attenuation at the musculotendinous junction. Efforts to reinforce this junction with the Bunnell suture placed across the site of injury have been unrewarding. The use of an augmentation device with strong tensile strengths such as an LAD™ has been an appropriate option. The prognosis must be clearly explained to the patient, making it clear that surgical intervention might offer improvement but not completely relieve symptoms.

Complete Rupture From the Tuberosity
This is by far the most common of this family of lesions and, as noted above, is becoming more recognizable.

Etiology and Pathology The classic histologic description of the avulsion of the biceps tendon from the tuberosity is that of a degenerative process. The position of the forearm at the time of disruption may be either in full supination or in neutral rotation, but the condition is rarely seen when the forearm is fully pronated. The histologic appearance of the torn tendon reveals a degenerative process that is devoid of blood vessels. According to the literature, this injury is seen almost exclusively in males. The use of anabolic steroids in bodybuilders has also been implicated in the etiology of this injury.

Diagnosis A clearly audible pop or a snap and proximal retraction of the biceps are diagnostic indicators of complete rupture. In some instances, retraction of the biceps may not be as notable becaused of tethering of the lacertus fibrosus. In this instance, definite weakness in flexion is present, but

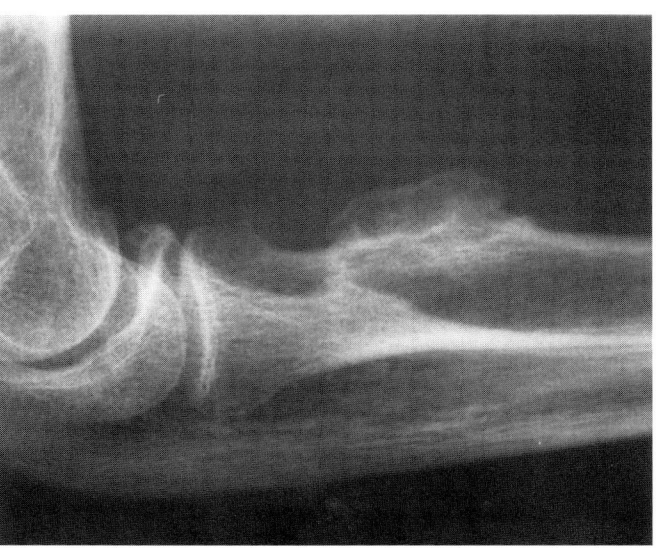

Fig. 4 Lateral radiograph of a patient with ruptured distal biceps tendon showing marked hypertrophic changes at the tuberosity.

marked weakness and pain with resisted supination is a more sensitive indicator. Careful palpation may demonstrate tenderness in the region of the biceps tendon at its site of osseous attachment. The lacertus fibrosus is also palpated and may or may not be intact. A radiograph sometimes reveals the indicative lesion of a hypertrophic radial tuberosity (Fig. 4). MRI can be of benefit because it can accurately demonstrate the expected pathologic changes. However, because of the obliquity of the tendon, equivocal or inaccurate MRI interpretation is possible. For this reason, this test need not be ordered to confirm the diagnosis if all other elements are present. However, accurate diagnosis is important because the prognosis for chronic detachment is poor, with moderate flexion weakness and marked supination weakness. Furthermore, the lesion is quite amenable to immediate or early reattachment. MRI is indicated if the diagnosis is suspected clinically but the signs and symptoms are equivocal or inconclusive.

Treatment Early immediate repair to the tuberosity is the accepted treatment for patients with distal biceps tendon avulsion. There are two basic exposures: the preferred is the two-incision technique, which simply first identifies the tendon through a limited antecubital incision, and then, through a safe muscle-splitting exposure on the dorsal aspect of the forearm, the tuberosity is exposed (Fig. 5). The tendon is readily reattached. The other is the modified anterior Henry approach that follows the biceps tendon down to the tuberosity identifying and protecting the PIN. Both of these approaches have been well described. The use of suture anchoring techniques has been reported. The potential benefits of metal suture anchors are outweighed by factors such as cost, decreased repair strength, and the potential for hardware complications. There is some concern that nerve injury is possible if these devices become dislodged.

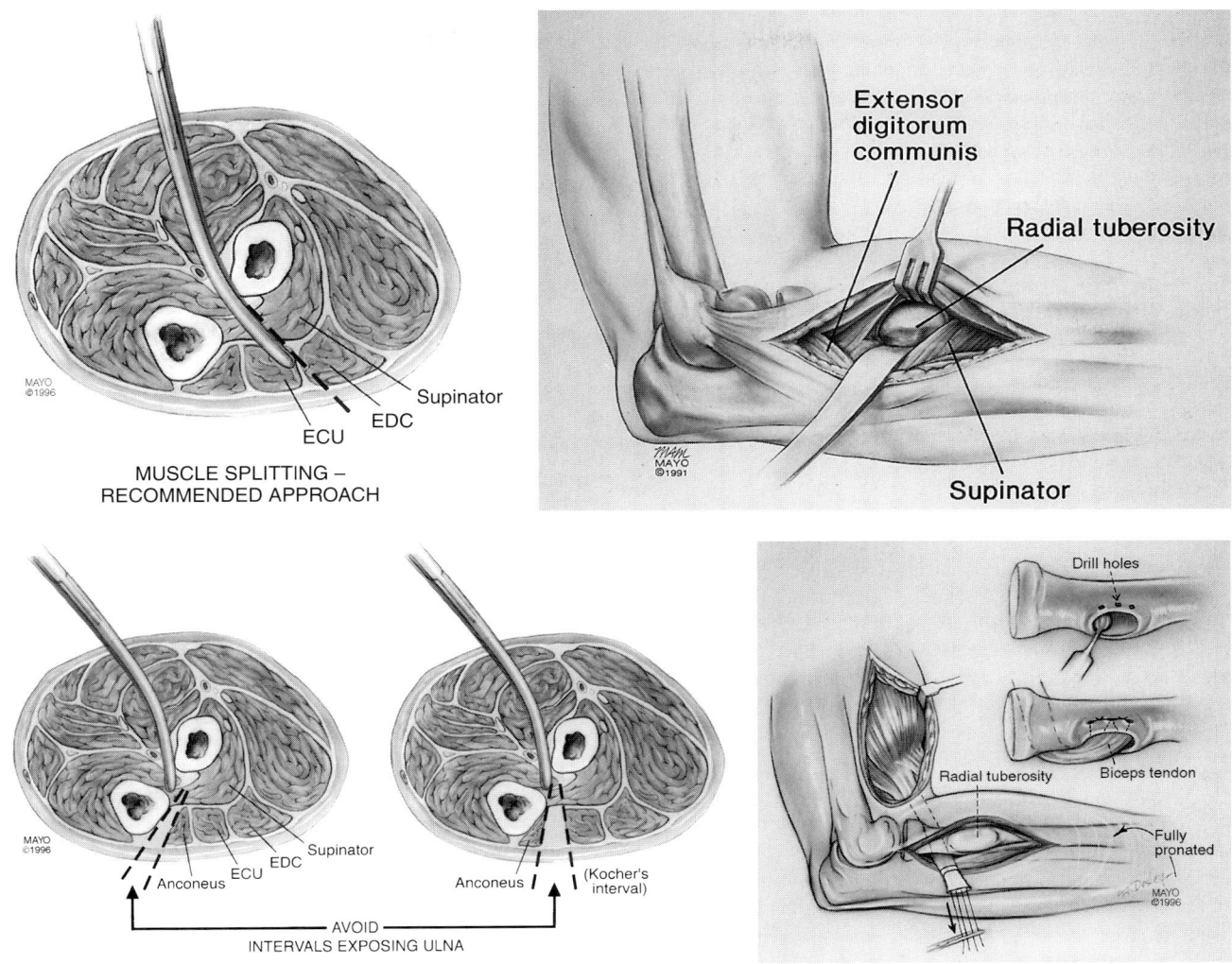

Fig. 5 Technique of surgical reattachment. The interval between the radius and the ulna is identified through the cubital incison. **Top left,** The blunt, curved instrument is directed through the extensor muscle mass, generally between the extensor carpi ulnaris and the extensor digitorum communis. **Top right,** This interval has been split and with full pronation the radial tuberosity is identified. **Bottom left,** Special attention should be paid to avoid heterotopic ossification. The intervals to be avoided are those between the anconeus and extensor carpi ulnaris, which also exposes the margin of the ulna. **Bottom right,** Two grasping sutures are placed in the distal tendon, which is brought through the abovementioned interval and placed into an excavated portion of the tuberosity. ECU, extensor carpi ulnaris; EDC, extensor digitorum communis. (Reproduced with permission from the Mayo Foundation, Rochester, MN.)

Delayed Reconstruction In some instances in which the diagnosis is not accurately made or the decision to operate is deferred, a delayed reconstruction might be considered. Typically, the golden period for immediate reattachment without requiring a detailed and sometimes difficult dissection in the antecubital space is approximately 2 weeks. After this period of time, scarring will occur in the region occupied by the biceps tendon and, more importantly, the muscle and tendon begin to retract. However, there have been occasions on which reattachment of the recoiled biceps tendon to the tuberosity has occurred as late as 3 months after the initial injury. For those seeking reconstruction more than 1 year after the event to improve flexion strength, a surgical option consists of attaching the biceps to the brachialis, which will improve flexion but of course has no influence on supination weakness. The other option to be considered if enhanced supination strength is required is an augmentation procedure, typically using a tendon autograft or the LAD™. This procedure has been effective in the few instances in which it was indicated.

Results Following acute repair, biomechanical studies have demonstrated that flexion and supination strength approach normal. However, it has been suggested that if the nondominant extremity is involved, residual weakness of 15% to 25% may be expected. If surgery is not performed, it has been shown that a residual flexion weakness of about 15% to 20%, but, more importantly, residual supination weakness of 30% to 50%, is regularly present.

Rehabilitation After surgical repair the extremity is placed in a protective splint for 1 to 2 weeks. The splint is then removed and gradual resumption of stretching and use of the extremity for activities of daily living are allowed. By the end of 3 to 4 weeks, normal motion and sedentary functions are present. A gradual increase in loading is begun, starting with 1 to 2 lb and progressing to about 80% strength over the next 3 months. At 6 months, full activity is allowed. After the patient is experienced in using the surgical reattachment, this process may be altered somewhat. However, the virtual lack of reavulsion with this procedure and postoperative program would seem to favor a more conservative program if a selection between an aggressive or more protected course is required.

Complications Radial nerve palsy is seen in as many as 5% of patients undergoing the anterior approach in the classic report by Dobbie. With "a two-incision technique," proximal radioulnar synostosis has been observed, but the incidence of its occurrence depends on the specific technique (Fig. 6). In the two-incision technique that splits the supinator and extensor musculature and does not expose the ulna, proximal radiulnar synostosis is rare to nonexistent. Any dissection that exposes the surface of the proximal ulna, as suggested by the original description of Boyd and Anderson, increases the risk of synostosis formation between the ulna and radial tuberosity. Rerupture, although it appears to be quite uncommon, is a distinct possibility that must be discussed with the patient.

Triceps Tendon Injury

Rupture of the triceps tendon is probably one of the rarest of tendinous injuries, especially about the elbow. Disruption of the triceps tendon may occur either following trauma or spontaneously. Spontaneous rupture is sometimes seen as with biceps tendon ruptures in laborers, or those involved with heavy activity, such as weight lifters. A traumatic event such as a laceration is one of the most common causes of triceps dysfunction, and the diagnosis is rather straightforward. However, the indirect causes of injury to this tendon result in a much more subtle diagnosis and a more difficult examination. A history of steroid use or a chronic inflammatory process are helpful when determining underlying etiologies that may raise a certain level of suspicion.

Diagnosis
The most common diagnosis is complete rupture, although partial tears of the triceps may also occur. The most consistent

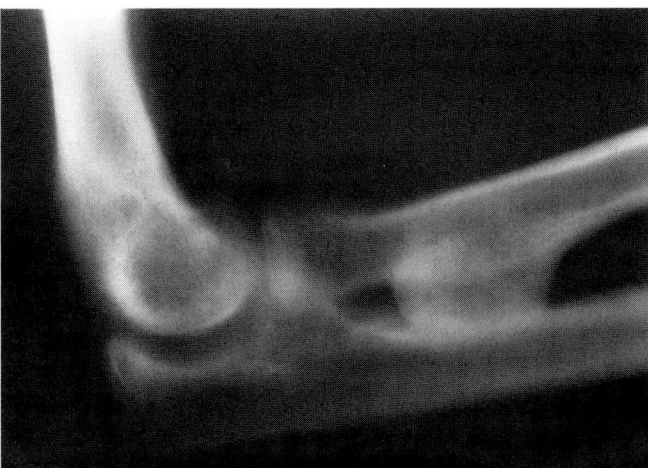

Fig. 6 Extensive ectopic bone bridging the radius and the ulna. In this particular instance the exposure was through an interval that exposed a portion of the ulna.

finding on the physical examination is a palpable defect in the posterior aspect of the elbow with demonstrable weakness of extension. It is of some interest to note that a radiograph may be helpful for triceps avulsion injuries because a flake of bone is sometimes present.

Treatment
Immediate surgery is the treatment of choice for a complete rupture because spontaneous healing of these injuries does not occur. With an early diagnosis, a direct suture technique through drill holes placed in the olecranon is employed, which is similar to the technique performed to reattach the triceps muscle after it has been released. A fascial turn-down technique to reinforce the reattachment may be beneficial in those with systemic disease. The postoperative management consists of immobilization in approximately 90° of flexion for about 3 weeks. Gentle active motion is then begun.

The results of immediate or delayed repair have generally been satisfactory. As a matter of fact, surprisingly good results have been observed even in those who have had a delayed reconstruction up to 1 year after the injury. However, as with any such injury, immediate repair is more effective than delayed reconstruction.

Selected Bibliography

Epicondylitis

Gabel GT, Morrey BF: Operative treatment of medical epicondylitis: Influence of concomitant ulnar neuropathy at the elbow. *J Bone Joint Surg* 1995;77A:1065-1069.

   Detailed results of surgical intervention for medial epicondylitis that demonstrated 90% successful without and 70% successful with concurrent ulnar nerve involvement are presented.

Grifka J, Boenke S, Krämer J: Endoscopic therapy in epicondylitis radialis humeri. *Arthroscopy* 1995;11:743-748.

   This article describes a technique with little clinical data.

Labelle H, Guibert R, Joncas J, et al: Lack of scientific evidence for the treatment of lateral epicondylitis of the elbow: An attempted meta-analysis. *J Bone Joint Surg* 1992;74B:646-651.

   A thorough assessment of the literature is presented. The lack of basis for nonsurgical treatment is probably overstated as injections are shown to be consistently effective.

LeHurc JC, Schaeverbeke T, Chauveaux D, et al: Epicondylitis after treatment with fluoroquinolone antibiotics. *J Bone Joint Surg* 1995;77B:293-295.

   The relationship of tendinitis with this family of antibiotics is defined.

Morrey BF: Reoperation for failed surgical treatment of refractory lateral epicondylitis. *J Shoulder Elbow Surg* 1992;1:47-55.

   A scheme for assessment and treatment is provided. Using this logic, 11 of 13 (80%) successful reoperations are reported.

Regan W, Wold LE, Coonrad R, et al: Microscopic histopathology of chronic refractory lateral epicondylitis. *Am J Sports Med* 1992;20:746-749.

   In this first study of blinded random histologic material, the pathologic lesion is shown to be degenerative rather than inflammatory in nature.

Rompe JD, Hope C, Küllmer K, et al: Analgesic effect of extracorporeal shock-wave therapy on chronic tennis elbow. *J Bone Joint Surg* 1996;78B:233-237.

   In this recent carefully performed clinical study, the value of shock wave therapy is documented.

Savoie FH III: Percutaneous release for lateral epicondylitis: An office procedure. Proceedings of the American Shoulder and Elbow Surgeons 11th Annual Meeting, Manchester, VT. Rosemont, IL, American Shoulder and Elbow Surgeons, 1994, pp 55-56.

   The clinical effectiveness and the cost containment of 19 conservative percutaneous releases done as office procedures are reported.

Vangsness CT Jr, Jobe FW: Surgical treatment of medial epicondylitis: Results in 35 elbows. *J Bone Joint Surg* 1991;73B:409-411.

   A surprisingly high rate of success is reported after 35 procedures. A mean of 7 years after surgery, approximately 90% were deemed satisfactory.

Distal Biceps Tendon Injury

Barnes SJ, Coleman SG, Gilpin D: Repair of avulsed insertion of biceps: A new technique in four cases. *J Bone Joint Surg* 1993;75B:938-939.

   The technique and recommendations for using metallic suture anchors for biceps tendon repair are reported.

Bourne MH, Morrey BF: Partial rupture of the distal biceps tendon. *Clin Orthop* 1991;271:143-148.

   This article documents experience with and treatment for partial disruption. Detachment and reattachment are recommended.

D'Alessandro DF, Shields CL Jr, Tibone JE, et al: Repair of distal biceps tendon ruptures in athletes. *Am J Sports Med* 1993;21:114-119.

   Good results are observed with reattachment, but objective strength studies show injuries to the nondominant elbow may result in residual weakness of 15% to 20%.

Davis WM, Yassine Z: An etiological factor in tear of the distal tendon of the biceps brachii: Report of two cases. *J Bone Joint Surg* 1956;38A:1365-1368.

   This article presents the first histologic analysis providing the description of a degenerative process at the tendinous attachment.

Dobbie RP: Avulsion of the lower biceps brachii tendon: Analysis of 51 previously unreported cases. *Am J Surg* 1941;51:662-683.

   This article presents the classic and first detailed report of presentation and treatment. The high frequency of radial nerve injury by the anterior approach is documented.

Fitzgerald SW, Curry DR, Erickson SJ, et al: Distal biceps tendon injury: MR imaging diagnosis. *Radiology* 1994;191:203-206.

   The surgical changes seen with distal biceps injury are described, and MRI recommended to help confirm diagnoses.

Failla JM, Amadio PC, Morrey BF, et al: Proximal radioulnar synostosis after repair of distal biceps brachii rupture by the two-incision technique: Report of four cases. *Clin Orthop* 1990;253:133-136.

   Etiology and successful excision of this complication are described. The muscle-splitting dorsal forearm approach is emphasized.

Koch S, Tillmann B: The distal tendon of the biceps brachii: Structure and clinical correlations. *Anat Anz* 1995;177:467-474.

   Presented here is further histologic evidence that biceps attachment failure is a degenerative process involving the tendon at its site of attachment.

Rokito AS, McLaughlin JA, Gallagher MA, et al: Partial rupture of the distal biceps tendon. *J Shoulder Elbow Surg* 1996;5:73-75.

   A case report and literature review are presented.

Seiler JG III, Parker LM, Chamberland PD, et al: The distal biceps tendon: Two potential mechanisms involved in its rupture: Arterial supply and mechanical impingement. *J Shoulder Elbow Surg* 1995;4:149-156.

The mechanical component of the pathology is implicated as contributing to the degenerative process.

Visuri T, Lindholm H: Bilateral distal biceps tendon avulsions with use of anabolic steroids. *Med Sci Sports Exerc* 1994;26:941-944.

According to this article, distal biceps tendon avulsion is seen in association with body building and the regular use of anabolic steroids.

Triceps Tendon Injury

Morrey BF: Tendon injuries about the elbow, in Morrey BF (ed): *The Elbow and Its Disorders,* ed 2. Philadelphia, PA, WB Saunders, 1993, pp 492-504.

Presentation and treatment are reviewed.

Sherman OH, Snyder SJ, Fox JM: Triceps tendon avulsion in a professional body builder: A case report. *Am J Sports Med* 1984;12:328-329.

Effective delayed repair with a direct suture technique is discussed.

Elbow Instability

Shawn W. O'Driscoll, MD, PhD, FRCSC

Epidemiology

A Swedish study has documented an annual incidence of six acute elbow dislocations per 100,000 population. The median age is 30, but the mode is in the late teens in both men and women. This injury typically occurs during sports activities and results from falls on the outstretched hand. Disruption of both collateral ligaments (and often the common flexor and extensor origins as well) is common.

Recurrent instability has confounded physicians for years, but has recently become better understood. It is probably more common than previously believed, and indeed, two long-term studies reported symptoms of recurrent instability in 15% and 35%, respectively, of their patients, although the instability could not be demonstrated on examination, possibly because the diagnosis of recurrent instability of the elbow has only recently been clarified.

Recent clinical and basic research has helped in the understanding of the pathoanatomy, mechanism of injury, kinematics, symptoms and signs, and management of elbow instability.

Etiology

It had been traditionally taught that the mechanism of dislocation is hyperextension, but this is not likely correct, and is not substantiated by data. Elbow dislocations or subluxations typically occur as a result of falls on the outstretched hand (Fig. 1). As the body approaches the ground, the elbow extends to place the hand on the ground. Upon contact with the ground, the elbow immediately begins to flex. This flexion causes eccentric loading of the triceps, principally the medial head, which produces an external rotation moment at the ulnohumeral joint. Contraction of the adductors and internal rotators of the abducted shoulder internally rotates the humerus against the forearm and hand, which are stabilized by the ground. Further internal rotation torque develops as the body rotates internally with respect to the hand (that is, the forearm rotates externally on the humerus). A valgus moment results from the fact that the mechanical axis is medial to the elbow. This combination of supination or external rotation torque, along with valgus and axial compression during flexion, is precisely the mechanism that results in a posterolateral rotatory subluxation or dislocation of the elbow and can be reproduced clinically by what is referred to as the "lateral pivot shift test," which is described below. This clinical mechanism has been confirmed by video analysis of a college wrestler during an actual elbow dislocation.

The pathoanatomy can be thought of as a circle of soft tissue and/or bone disruption from lateral to medial in three stages (Fig. 2). In stage 1 the lateral collateral ligament (LCL) is partially or completely disrupted (the ulnar part is dis-

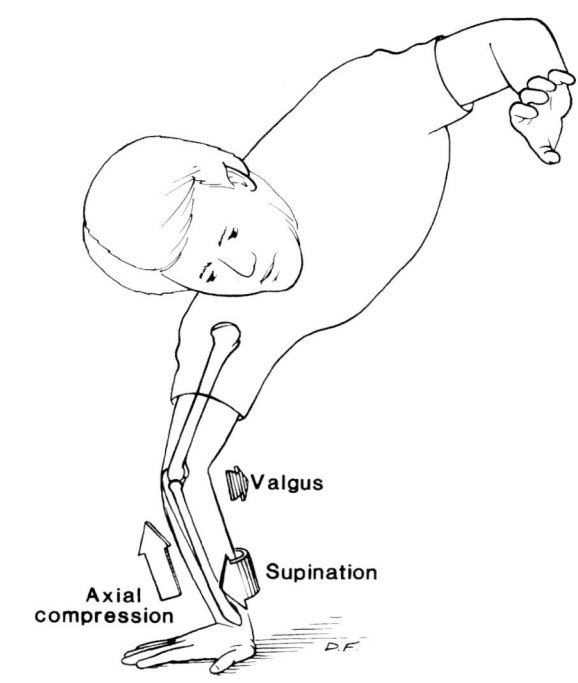

Fig. 1 The mechanism of elbow dislocation is a fall on the outstretched hand. (Reproduced with permission from O'Driscoll SW, Morrey BF, Korinek S, et al: Elbow subluxation and dislocation. *Clin Orthop* 1992;280:195.)

rupted). This injury results in posterolateral rotatory subluxation of the elbow, which reduces spontaneously. With further disruption anteriorly and posteriorly, the elbow in stage 2 instability is capable of an incomplete posterolateral dislocation in which the concave medial edge of the ulna rests on the trochlea such that a lateral radiograph gives the impression of the coronoid being perched on the trochlea. This injury can readily be reduced with minimal force or by manipulation of the elbow by the patient. Stage 3 is subdivided into three parts. In stage 3A, all the soft tissues are disrupted, around and including the posterior part of the medial collateral ligament (MCL), leaving the important anterior band intact. This permits posterior dislocation by the previously described posterolateral rotatory mechanism. The elbow pivots around on the intact anterior band of the MCL. Reduction is accomplished by gentle manipulation of the elbow in supination and valgus, temporarily recreating the deformity. The intact anterior medial collateral ligament (AMCL) provides valgus stability provided that the elbow is kept in pronation to prevent

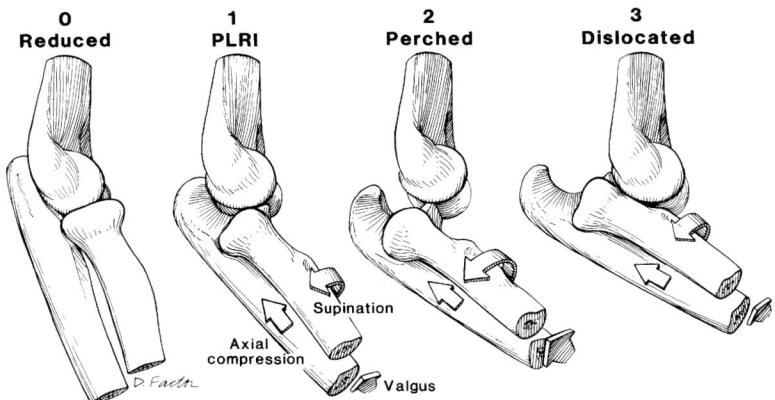

Fig. 2 Elbow instability is a spectrum from subluxation to dislocation. The three stages illustrated here correspond with the pathoanatomic stages of capsuloligamentous disruption in Figure 3. Forces and moments responsible for displacements are illustrated. PLRI = posterolateral rotatory instability. (Reproduced with permission from O'Driscoll SW, Morrey BF, Korinek S, et al: Elbow subluxation and dislocation. *Clin Orthop* 1992;280:195.)

posterolateral rotatory subluxation during valgus testing. This stage of instability is most commonly seen in the presence of radial head and coronoid fractures. In stage 3B, the entire medial collateral complex is disrupted. Varus, valgus, and rotatory instability are present following reduction. In stage 3C, the entire distal humerus is stripped of soft tissues, producing severe instability such that the elbow will dislocate or subluxate even in a cast at 90° of flexion. Reduction can be maintained usually only by flexing the elbow past 90° to 110°. The flexor/pronator and common extensor muscle origins are important secondary stabilizers of the elbow. These pathoanatomic stages all correlate with clinical degrees of elbow instability.

Thus, dislocation is the final of three sequential stages of elbow instability resulting from posterolateral ulnohumeral rotatory subluxation, with soft-tissue disruption progressing from lateral to medial. In each stage, the pathoanatomy correlates with the pattern and degree of instability. This theory has been confirmed in cadaver elbows; in 12 of 13, the elbow could be dislocated posteriorly with the AMCL intact. This circle of disruption is referred to as the "Horii circle" and is analogous to the Mayfield spiral of soft-tissue and/or bony disruption in carpal instability (Fig. 3). As disruption progresses from lateral to medial it may pass through the soft tissues and/or bone, that is, the capsule is normally torn but may be intact if the coronoid is fractured. Similarly, the anterior bundle of the MCL is often intact when the radial head and coronoid are both fractured.

Thus, the spectrum of instability is explained, from posterolateral rotatory instability to perched dislocation, to posterior dislocation without or with disruption of the AMCL, which occurs with further posterior displacement. Such a posterolateral rotatory mechanism for dislocation would be compatible with those suggested in the 1960s by Osborne and Cotterill, and Roberts.

Recurrent posterolateral rotatory instability usually is posttraumatic because of inadequate soft-tissue healing following elbow subluxation, dislocation, or fracture-dislocation. It can be iatrogenic, and is caused by violation of the lateral collat-

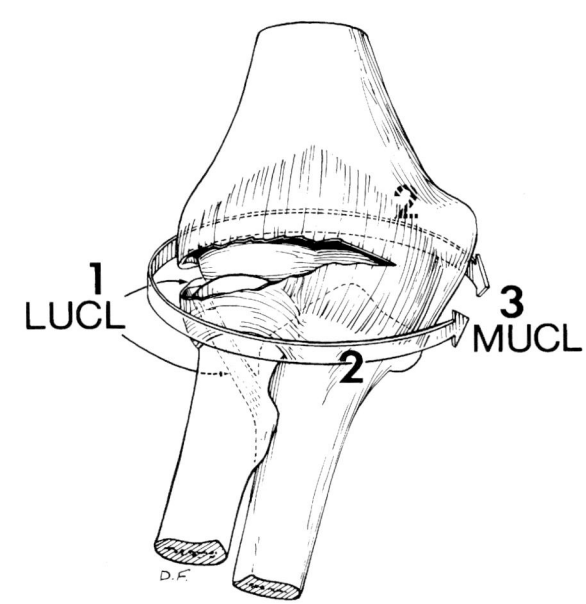

Fig. 3 Soft-tissue injury progresses in a "circle" from lateral to medial in three stages correlating with those in Figure 2. In stage 1, the ulnar part of the lateral collateral ligament, the lateral ulnar collateral ligament (LUCL), is disrupted. In stage 2, the other lateral ligamentous structures and the anterior and posterior capsule are disrupted. Stage 3, disruption of the medial ulnar collateral ligament (MUCL), can be partial with disruption of the posterior MUCL only (3A), or complete (3B). The common extensor and flexor origins are often disrupted as well. (Reproduced with permission from O'Driscoll SW, Morrey, BF, Korinek S, et al: Elbow subluxation and dislocation. *Clin Orthop* 1992;280:194.)

eral ligament (LCL) complex during release for tennis elbow. This type of instability also can result from chronic soft-tissue overload in patients with long-standing cubitus varus deformity from childhood supracondylar malunions. It is also seen in patients who bear weight on the upper extremities (paralysis caused by polio, paraplegia, etc) and in those with connective tissue disorders such as Ehlers-Danlos syndrome. For several reasons other mechanisms such as hyperextension need not be implicated to explain these clinical observations. A posterolateral rotatory mechanism would be consistent with the observation that some patients experience recurrent dislocations requiring reduction and also have a positive lateral pivot-shift test. Furthermore, such patients with recurrent dislocations typically do very well with surgical reconstruction of the LCL complex alone, without any attention paid to the medial side, which suggests that the essential lesion of such instability is on the lateral side. Finally, it has not been shown that the results of surgical repair of the AMCL following acute dislocations are superior to those of nonsurgical treatment. On the other hand, the above observations do not preclude hyperextension as a cause of elbow dislocation in some instances.

Constraints to Elbow Instability

The elbow has both static and dynamic constraints. There are three primary static constraints to elbow instability: the ulnohumeral articulation, the MCL, and the LCL, especially the ulnar part of the LCL (also referred to as the lateral ulnar collateral ligament). The secondary constraints include the radial head, common flexor and extensor origins, and the capsule. Dynamic stabilizers include the muscles that cross the elbow joint and produce compressive forces at the articulation. The anconeus, triceps, and brachialis are the most important in this regard. Originating near the lateral epicondyle and inserting broadly on the ulna in a fan shape, the anconeus is perfectly designed to serve its major function as a dynamic stabilizer preventing posterolateral rotational displacement of the elbow. A word of caution: the nerve to the anconeus, which enters the muscle proximally, is divided with the traditional olecranon osteotomy for distal humeral fractures.

An elbow with its three primary constraints intact will be stable. If the coronoid is fractured or lost, the radial head becomes a critical stabilizer. The radial head must not be removed from dislocated elbows in which the coronoid is fractured, unless the coronoid and ligaments can be securely fixed.

An important concept in elbow stability is that an elbow with intact joint surfaces (that is, no fractures or bone defects) requires only two ligamentous structures for functional stability. These are the anterior band of the MCL and the ulnar part of the LCL. Both are conceptually simple bands of tissue with attachments to bone at each end and can be reconstructed.

Classification of Elbow Instability

Elbow instability can be classified according to five criteria: (1) articulation(s) involved; (2) direction of displacement; (3) degree of displacement; (4) timing; and (5) presence or absence of associated fractures.

Articulation(s) Involved
Elbow instability can be categorized according to the articulation(s) involved: the "elbow joint" itself and the proximal radioulnar joint. The displacement can be of the radial head (proximal radioulnar joint), of the forearm from the humerus (ulnohumeral and radiohumeral joints), or both.

Elbow Joint A discussion of elbow instability usually refers to that involving the "elbow joint" itself (ulnohumeral and radiohumeral joints). This condition can be congenital or acquired, though the former is exceedingly rare. It is subclassified according to the direction and degree of displacement, chronicity, and presence of associated fractures.

Proximal Radioulnar Joint Instability at the elbow can also involve the proximal radioulnar joint, with subluxation or dislocation of the radial head from the ulna, and can be congenital or acquired. The latter is usually traumatic and can be acute or chronic.

Elbow and Proximal Radioulnar Joints (Divergent) This injury is usually traumatic and represents a combination of the previous two. Functionally speaking, this injury can be thought of as a variant of elbow dislocations.

Direction of Displacement
Previous descriptions of elbow dislocations have unnecessarily distinguished medial and lateral dislocations from posterior or other dislocations. The pathology of such medial or lateral dislocations is not different from that of complete posterior dislocations (stage 3B dislocations). A pure medial or lateral dislocation/subluxation is most commonly seen following incomplete reduction of a posterior dislocation; that is, only the posterior displacement has been corrected, as seen on the lateral radiograph, and the medial or lateral displacement remains. Therefore, the reduction must be complete in the coronal plane (medial to lateral on the anteroposterior film) and not just the sagittal plane.

Valgus Valgus instability is seen in one of two varieties: posttraumatic or chronic overload. Posttraumatic valgus instability implies rupture of the MCL. It is usually associated with disruption of the other soft tissues on the medial side of the elbow, including the common flexor/pronator origin, and is usually found in patients with radial head fractures that are associated with tears of the MCL, or severe elbow instability such as following a dislocation that has disrupted the lateral ligament complex as well. The MCL usually heals following an elbow dislocation, perhaps because of the vascularized muscles that surround it. However, if the radial head is excised, the elbow is at high risk of remaining permanently unstable in valgus.

Valgus instability can also occur from repetitive microtrauma or overload. Attenuation or rupture of the anterior band of the MCL, which is the pathology responsible for this pattern of instability, is usually seen in baseball players (typically pitchers).

Varus Varus instability is caused by disruption of the LCL complex and is present acutely in elbow dislocations and recurrently or chronically in those in whom this ligament fails to heal. The biomechanics of the elbow are such that it is not often subjected to varus stress, except in those who use their arms as weightbearing extremities (for example, post-polio patients and other crutch walkers). This pattern of instability may not be as apparent as posterolateral rotatory instability, which is always present when the LCL is disrupted. Patients are more likely to complain of the symptoms of posterolateral rotatory instability than those of varus instability.

Anterior Anterior instability of the elbow is typically seen in association with fractures, especially of the olecranon. The collateral ligaments are sometimes intact when the olecranon fracture is comminuted and extends close to the coronoid.

Posterolateral Rotatory Instability This is the most common pattern of elbow instability. It is usually posterolateral rather than directly posterior so that the coronoid can pass inferior to the trochlea. It is essentially a rotational displacement of the ulna on the humerus (the radius moving with the ulna) such that the ulna supinates, or externally rotates, away from the trochlea (Figs. 1 through 3).

Degree of Displacement
As described in detail above in the section on etiology, elbow instability can be considered a spectrum consisting of three stages (Fig. 2). Each stage has specific clinical, radiographic, and pathologic features that are predictable and have implications for treatment. The pathology can be predicted from the degree of instability.

Timing
Elbow instability can be acute, chronic, or recurrent.

Associated Fractures
Elbow subluxations and dislocations can be associated with fractures about the elbow. Some fractures, such as intra-articular supracondylar fractures of the humerus and comminuted fractures of the olecranon and coronoid, can cause elbow instability without disruption of the collateral ligaments. However, the majority of unstable elbows also have disruption of one or both ligaments, even in the presence of fractures. Radial head fractures do not cause clinically significant instability unless the MCL is disrupted. These fractures can have a strong influence on prognosis and treatment and, in many cases, are the main indication for surgery.

An important feature to recognize in elbow injuries is that the small "flake" fracture of the coronoid so commonly seen in elbow dislocations is not an "avulsion" fracture, because nothing attaches to the tip of the coronoid (Fig. 4). The brachialis inserts further distally on the ulna. Indeed, the tip can be clearly seen arthroscopically. This fracture is a shear fracture and is likely pathognomonic of an episode of elbow subluxation or dislocation, analogous to the bony Bankart lesion of anterior shoulder instability.

The most dreaded injury seen by orthopaedic surgeons with some degree of regularity is the triad of an elbow dislocation with fractures of the coronoid and radial head. Recommendations for treatment are presented below. The coronoid is the critical element in such an injury.

Evaluation

Acute Elbow Dislocations
Dislocated elbows must be evaluated for stability after reduction of the dislocation. Instability is assessed by gently moving the elbow through a range of motion.

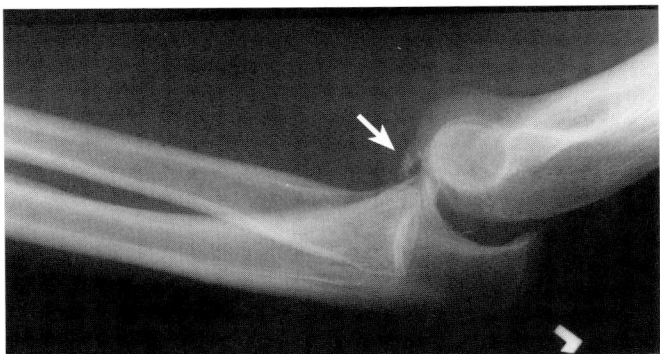

Fig. 4 Lateral stress radiograph (as described in Figure 5) of a patient with stage 2 posterolateral rotatory instability. The coronoid is "perched" on the trochlea. Note the small shear fracture of the coronoid (*arrow*), which is probably pathognomonic for elbow subluxation or dislocation.

Instability may need to be assessed with the patient under general anesthetic; this is sometimes the only way to adequately do so. Assessment of instability is easiest to perform and interpret with the arm in the overhead position (resembling a leg), and the elbow resembling a knee. The elbow is examined for valgus, varus, and posterolateral rotatory instability. Valgus testing is performed with the elbow fully pronated so that posterolateral rotatory instability is not mistaken for valgus instability, which occurs because the ulna and radius as a unit rotate away from the humerus in response to valgus stress when the LCL is disrupted. Forced pronation prevents this from happening by using the intact medial soft tissues as a hinge or fulcrum, just as the periosteum is used for this purpose during the reduction of a supracondylar fracture in a child. Varus testing is easiest to perform with the shoulder fully internally rotated. Both valgus and varus testing are performed with the elbow in full extension and several degrees of flexion to about 30° to unlock the olecranon from the olecranon fossa. Posterolateral rotatory instability is diagnosed by the lateral pivot-shift test of the elbow, which is described in the next section on recurrent instability. If there is severe soft-tissue disruption, this test can be falsely negative. A positive test is manifested by a clunk that is seen and felt when the ulna and radius reduce on the humerus. With severe soft-tissue disruption, the elbow can sometimes remain dislocated even when flexed past 90°. This situation can be avoided when dislocation is suspected by using the examiner's thumb to prevent the elbow from fully dislocating (or limiting the degree of subluxation during pivot-shift testing).

Stress radiographs are performed in the anteroposterior plane in valgus and varus with the arm overhead as described above. With the shoulder in 90° of abduction and full external rotation, stress radiographs are also performed in supination and pronation to detect posterolateral rotatory instability and to determine if the medial side opens up with pronation (indicating disruption of the medial soft tissues).

Recurrent Instability

Recurrent instability of the elbow, once enigmatic, is now understood to involve a common pathway of posterolateral rotatory subluxation. In virtually all cases, the ulnar part of the LCL is detached or attenuated. The MCL is usually intact, though it remains unclear why the lateral ligament is less likely to heal than the medial one. Posterolateral rotatory instability is being diagnosed with increasing frequency since its discovery, probably because of increased awareness of the condition. Patients typically present with a history of recurrent painful clicking, snapping, clunking, or locking of the elbow, and careful interrogation reveals that this occurs in the extension half of the arc with the forearm in supination. Unless the patient has a severe abnormality of the connective tissue, a preceding history of trauma or surgery is present unless there is a connective tissue disorder or chronic stretching caused by crutch-walking. The typical cause is a previous dislocation, but it can be as subtle as a "sprain" resulting from a fall on the outstretched hand. Surgical causes include radial head excision and lateral release for tennis elbow (caused by violation of the ulnar part of the LCL).

The physical examination is typically unremarkable except for a positive lateral pivot-shift apprehension test or posterolateral rotatory apprehension test (Fig. 5). With the patient in the supine position and the affected extremity overhead, the wrist and elbow are grasped as the ankle and knee are held when examining the leg. The elbow is supinated with a mild force at the wrist and a valgus moment is applied to the elbow

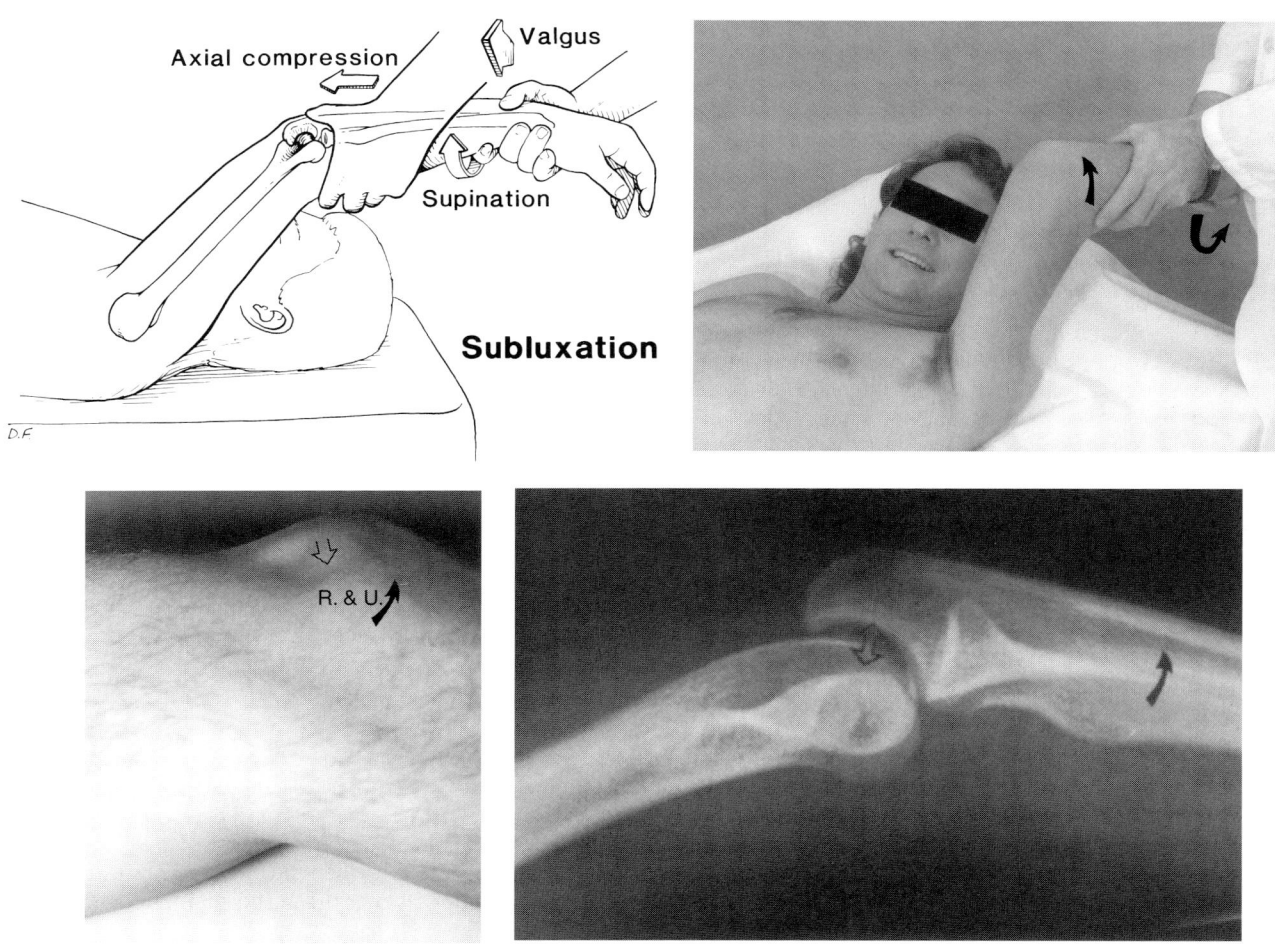

Fig. 5 Top left, The lateral pivot-shift test of the elbow for posterolateral rotatory instability is performed with the patient supine and the arm overhead. A supination/valgus moment is applied during flexion, causing the elbow to subluxate maximally at about 40° of flexion. **Top right,** This maneuver creates apprehension in the patient and is highly sensitive. **Bottom left,** If the patient is able to relax adequately, or is under general anesthesia, the elbow can be observed to subluxate so that the radius and ulna (R and U) rotate off the humerus (*dark arrow*). The skin is sucked in (*hollow arrow*) behind the radial head. Further flexion produces a palpable visible clunk as the elbow reduces if the patient is able to relax enough to permit that part of the examination. Unfortunately, the subluxation/reduction maneuver usually is not possible in the awake patient. **Bottom right,** A lateral stress radiograph obtained during the lateral pivot shift test reveals the radius and ulna to have supinated away from the humerus (*dark arrow*), leaving a gap in the ulnohumeral articulation (*hollow arrow*) and the radial head posterior to the capitellum. (Top left and bottom right, reproduced with permission from O'Driscoll SW, Bell DF, Morrey BF: Posterolateral rotatory instability of the elbow. *J Bone Joint Surg* 1991;73A:440-446. Top right and bottom left, reproduced with permission from Frymoyer JW (ed): *Orthopaedic Knowledge Update 4.* Rosemont, IL, American Academy of Orthopaedic Surgeons, 1993, pp 335-352.)

during flexion. This action results in a typical apprehension response with reproduction of the patient's symptoms and a sense that the elbow is about to dislocate (Fig. 5, *top right*). Reproducing the actual subluxation and the clunk that occurs with reduction can usually only be accomplished with the patient under general anesthetic, or after injecting local anesthetic into the elbow joint. The lateral pivot-shift test performed in that manner results in subluxation of the radius and ulna from the humerus, which causes a prominence posterolaterally over the radial head and a dimple between the radial head and the capitellum (Fig. 5, *bottom left*). As the elbow is flexed to approximately 40° or more, reduction of the ulna and radius together on the humerus occurs suddenly with a palpable, visible clunk. It is the reduction that is apparent. A lateral stress radiograph taken prior to the clunk can be helpful to demonstrate the rotatory subluxation (Fig. 5, *bottom right*). Arthroscopic examination will confirm excessive opening of the ulnohumeral articulation and posterior subluxation of the radial head with supination stress applied to the elbow.

Valgus Instability

This condition has been extensively documented by Jobe and others. Chronic valgus overload with rupture or attenuation of the MCL is diagnosed with patient history, physical examination, and stress radiographs. With a history of repetitive valgus loading, as in pitchers, the patient typically complains of medial elbow pain and may have actually heard and/or felt a "pop" at the time of ligament rupture. Physical examination confirms tenderness over the MCL just anterior to the ulnar nerve and distal to the epicondyle. In contrast to medial epicondylitis, MCL insufficiency is more commonly tender at the ulnar insertion of the ligament. Valgus stress is painful. The valgus instability can often be confirmed by a valgus stress radiograph, although Jobe emphasizes that a normal stress radiograph does not rule out symptomatic ligament attenuation; the diagnosis is thus more dependent on the history and physical examination. Stress testing can be performed manually with the elbow flexed 30° or with the "gravity stress radiograph." Manual stress testing is most reliably performed by fully pronating the forearm, internally rotating the shoulder, and directing the x-ray beam from posterior to anterior, which permits better control of humeral rotation. The arthroscopic valgus stress test, performed with the elbow flexed 70°, is specific for MCL injuries, and one cadaver study showed that any opening of more than 1 mm indicates damage to at least the anterior band of the MCL.

Treatment

Acute Dislocations

The initial treatment of a dislocation that is not complicated by the presence of fractures is closed reduction, which should be done in supination to clear the coronoid under the trochlea, thereby minimizing additional trauma to the medial soft tissues that have not yet been disrupted. Essentially, the deformity is "recreated" to make reduction possible and easy. A simple principle to follow in managing the patient after reduction is that the elbow should be splinted briefly (for 3 to 5 days), then motion started unless subluxation or dislocation are noted. Subluxation or dislocation must be detected by careful examination throughout the comfortable range of motion and with anteroposterior and lateral radiographs initially and every 5 to 7 days for the first 3 weeks. If at any time subluxation or dislocation is detected clinically or radiographically, a change of treatment is required. If the elbow subluxates or dislocates in extension or is noncongruent on the radiograph, it should be placed in pronation and reassessed. If stability is restored, a hinged brace or cast brace with the forearm in full pronation is applied. An extension block of 30° is sometimes necessary. If the elbow requires more than 30° to 45° of extension block, surgery should be considered. Extension blocks should be eased gradually so that by 3 weeks full motion is permitted by the brace.

Treatment is dictated by the stage, or degree of instability, as previously outlined. Valgus stability following reduction is present when the forearm is fully pronated in stages 1 to 3A. Treatment is immediate unlimited flexion and extension in a cast brace that is applied with the forearm in full pronation. If the elbow feels stable in any position of forearm rotation, a cast brace is not necessary. Such stability is usually caused by the dynamic stabilizing effects of the muscles crossing the elbow joint. In stages 3B or 3C, the elbow is unstable in extension and a cast brace (usually in neutral rotation) is applied with an extension block incorporated to prevent extension beyond the point of instability. Use of the extension block is gradually extended during the healing phase. A total of 3 to 6 weeks of protected motion is adequate. The reason that stage 3B and 3C dislocations are not pronated is that the medial soft-tissue disruption is sufficient to permit the medial side to open up with forearm pronation.

Fractures

The presence of fractures usually changes the management of the instability. These options are discussed in detail elsewhere in this book. Fractures of the olecranon usually do not cause clinical instability if less than 50% of the joint surface is involved. However, there is a measurable decrease in stability that is proportional to the percentage of the olecranon that is lost or fractured. Fractures that involve the joint surface anteriorly toward the coronoid or insertion of the ligaments on the ulna are unstable. An unstable elbow associated with a fracture of the olecranon should be treated by open reduction and internal fixation of the olecranon. This procedure can be accomplished by plating the ulna posteriorly with an 8-hole 3.5 dynamic compression plate bent at an angle of 80° between the last two holes at the tip of the olecranon. This method permits excellent fixation on the proximal fragment and acts as a buttress to prevent anterior subluxation.

The coronoid is a vital part of the force-bearing surface of the elbow and important for stability. Fractures of the coronoid have been classified by Regan and Morrey. Type I fractures are small shear fractures that are caused by subluxation or dislocation as the coronoid passes beneath the trochlea. (They are not actually avulsion fractures as previously thought; nothing is attached to the tip of the coronoid.) They do not destabilize the joint, but signify the soft ligamentous disruption that has occurred. Type II fractures (less than 50% of the coronoid) should be fixed if the joint is subluxated or dislocated. Type III fractures (more than 50% of the coronoid) cause instability and should be fixed. Type III fracture-dislocations have a poor prognosis. In general, the approach to the unstable elbow is to fix the bones so that the only limitation is the ligaments and then to repair them if the elbow is not stable enough to permit early motion. Malunion or nonunion of the coronoid sometimes cause recurrent instability and must be reduced and fixed in such cases.

Fractures of the radial head associated with an elbow dislocation or subluxation are best managed by internal fixation where possible. If the radial head is comminuted and has to be excised, prosthetic replacement is indicated if the elbow is unstable and cannot be rendered stable by ligament reconstruction alone.

Intra-articular fractures and supracondylar fractures of the distal humerus with intra-articular extension are sometimes accompanied by severe displacement of the joint surfaces. This displacement is not necessarily caused by ligamentous disruption. The soft-tissue and ligament attachments should be preserved, which will permit the elbow to be stable when the bones are reduced and rigidly fixed.

Acute Ligament Repair

The indication for acute ligament repair is instability that does not permit early protected motion in a cast brace, usually the case when associated fractures are present. In such cases, the ligament(s) may have been avulsed and can be repaired directly to bone with heavy sutures. In some cases, the tissue can be repaired but not strongly enough to stabilize the joint. In such cases the repair is augmented by passing a heavy absorbable suture (# 2 PDS) through the same course as for a ligament reconstruction (see below) and fixing it to the normal ligament attachments on the epicondyle and ulna.

Recurrent Dislocations or Subluxations

Surgical correction is performed by reattaching the avulsed lateral ulnar collateral ligament or reconstructing it with a tendon graft such as that of the palmaris longus or the semitendinosus (Fig. 6). The reconstruction technique that is currently employed involves isometric placement of the origin on the lateral epicondyle and fixation to bone at either end. Surgery is performed in young patients in such a way as to prevent violation of the epiphyseal plate on the lateral side of the humerus. Patients with valgus as well as posterolateral rotatory instability must have the anterior band of the MCL reconstructed as well. Typically, motion in a cast brace can be commenced in the first week following surgery with the forearm in full pronation (unless the AMCL was also reconstructed). An extension block is sometimes used. In patients with severe instability or in revision cases, the elbow is sometimes immobilized in a cast for 3 weeks. In children, and in those patients who have previously undergone prolonged immobilization for up to 6 weeks without developing contractures, immobilization might be continued for 6 weeks.

Valgus Instability

The treatment for MCL injuries includes anterior transposition of the ulnar nerve and reconstruction of the anterior band of the MCL with a palmaris longus tendon graft.

Chronic Instability

Because all that is required for valgus, varus, and rotatory stability of the elbow is the presence of a normal articular surface, anterior band of the MCL, ulnar part of the LCL, and

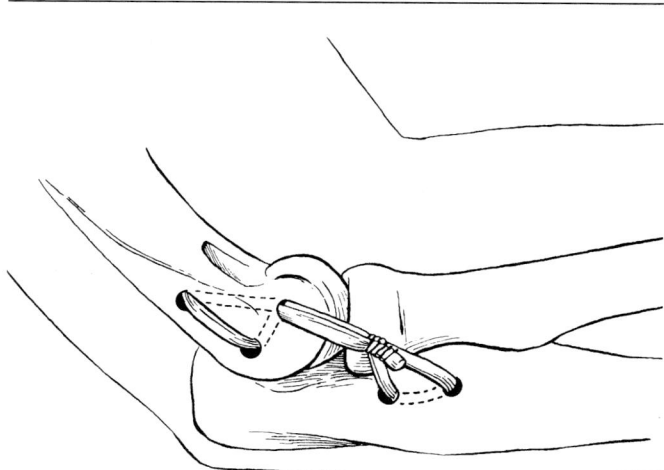

Fig. 6 Reconstruction of the ulnar part of the lateral collateral ligament for posterolateral instability or recurrent dislocations. The tendon graft is fixed to the ulna near the tubercle on the supinator crest (which is felt by stressing the elbow in varus or supination) just at and distal to the annular ligament. The tendon graft is then passed through the isometric point on the lateral epicondyle (this point is usually more anterior than might be thought), out through a proximal hole posteriorly, and back into bone distally to reemerge at the isometric origin. It is then overlapped and sutured to itself. The capsule is imbricated and closed beneath the tendon graft to prevent it from rubbing on the side of the joint. (Reproduced with permission from Gino Maulucci, Ontario, Canada, © 1992.)

annular ligament, there is no need for unusual, nonanatomic procedures for ligament reconstruction in recurrent or chronic instability. Also, transarticular pinning of the elbow for subluxation is no longer indicated. Thus, the approach to chronic dislocation of the elbow is to reconstruct the bony articulation and then the medial and lateral ligaments. Active and passive motion in a cast brace are commenced immediately. If the joint surface itself is destroyed, it is resurfaced with periosteum for cartilage regeneration in young patients or fascia lata as an interposition arthroplasty in older patients whose periosteum does not have adequate chondrogenic potential. The articulation is held stable by use of a hinged external fixator when the bony anatomy is inadequate.

Results of Treatment

Because treatment is varied, the interpretation and predictability of the long-term results of closed treatment of dislocations not complicated by associated fractures merits scrutiny. Motion should be commenced early. The large majority of patients appear to regain excellent function and strength unless they are immobilized and become stiff, or develop recurrent instability, as discussed in conjunction with the complications outlined in the following paragraphs.

The results of treating fracture dislocations, especially those involving both the radial head and coronoid, have been poor enough to intimidate most surgeons. However, early clinical results from aggressive ligament reconstruction in combination with internal fixation in complex fracture dislocations of the elbow have been very promising. Immediate motion is possible and stability has been maintained. The current approach is to start motion immediately in all injured and operated elbows; those in which this is not possible are reconstructed to permit such early motion. Future studies will be necessary to validate these observations. Further, the role of hinged external fixators is evolving.

Clinical outcomes of ligament reconstruction for recurrent instability of the elbow in patients from age 4 to 46 years have been successful. The authors who described the technique reported success in 10 of 11 patients whose clinical presentations included recurrent subluxations and/or dislocations.

Complications

The two main complications of simple dislocations (no fractures) are contractures and recurrent instability. Stiffness can be minimized by starting early motion. Mehlhoff and associates, in a long-term study of 52 patients with dislocations not complicated by associated fractures, showed that 60% of patients had some symptoms at final follow-up. These included pain or stress pain in 45% and significant flexion contractures of more than 30° in 15%. Stiffness was directly related to the duration of immobilization, and predictable if the elbow was immobilized for 3 weeks or more.

Summary

Elbow instability is a spectrum of conditions ranging from subluxation to dislocation, with corresponding clinical or pathologic features and therapeutic implications. Posterolateral rotational displacement of the ulna (with the radius) on the humerus appears to be the common mechanism. The three prerequisites for stability of the ulnohumeral articulation are an intact joint surface, anterior MCL, and ulnar part of the LCL. Recurrent instability is usually caused by insufficiency of the LCL complex. Reconstruction of the ulnar part of the LCL typically corrects the problem.

Selected Bibliography

Abe M, Ishizu T, Morikawa J: Posterolateral rotatory instability of the elbow after posttraumatic cubitus varus. *J Shoulder Elbow Surg* 1997;6:405-409.

This article is a case report describing recurrent posterolateral rotatory instability in a 16-year-old patient who had a supracondylar varus malunion resulting from a fracture at age 5. The mechanism is chronic overload of the lateral soft tissues.

An KN, Morrey BF, Chao EY: The effect of partial removal of proximal ulna on elbow constraint. *Clin Orthop* 1986;209:269-279.

Cage DJ, Abrams RA, Callahan JJ, et al: Soft tissue attachments of the ulnar coronoid process: An anatomic study with radiographic correlation. *Clin Orthop* 1995;320:154-158.

This article confirms that small flake fractures are not "avulsion" fractures, but are shear fractures caused by instability.

Cobb TK, Morrey BF: Use of distraction arthroplasty in unstable fracture dislocations of the elbow. *Clin Orthop* 1995;312:201-210.

A hinged external fixator is a salvage option for unstable fracture-dislocations that cannot be repaired. Though not a problem in this series, deep sepsis from the pin across the distal humerus is a serious risk.

Cohen MS, Hastings H II: Rotatory instability of the elbow: The anatomy and role of the lateral stabilizers. *J Bone Joint Surg* 1997;79A:225-233.

Pure rotational laxity was evaluated in cadaver elbows before and after sequential release of the lateral soft tissues. The common extensor tendon and the lateral collateral ligament complex (including the annular ligament) were interdependent in stabilizing the elbow. True posterolateral rotatory instability, a three-dimensional displacement, was not studied in the model.

Conway JE, Jobe FW, Glousman RE, et al: Medial instability of the elbow in throwing athletes: Treatment by repair or reconstruction of the ulnar collateral ligament. *J Bone Joint Surg* 1992;74A:67-83.

This article is an extensive review of 68 patients followed for an average of over 6 years following medial collateral ligament repair or reconstruction. Direct repair permitted half of the patients to return to sport, whereas two thirds returned to their same level of participation following reconstruction, typically with a palmaris longus tendon graft. This procedure was performed primarily in throwers. Fifteen patients had postoperative ulnar neuropathy and nine of these required additional surgery. The authors recommend reconstruction rather than repair.

Field LD, Altchek DW: Evaluation of the arthroscopic valgus instability test of the elbow. *Am J Sports Med* 1996;24:177-181.

In seven cadaver elbows, the athroscopic valgus stress test was evaluated before and after medial collateral ligament sectioning and valgus loading. No opening of the ulnohumeral articulation was observed in any normal specimen, 1 to 2 mm was seen after releasing the anterior band of the medial collateral ligament, and gross opening after complete medial collateral ligament division.

Hamilton CD, Glousman RE, Jobe FW, et al: Dynamic stability of the elbow: Electromyographic analysis of the flexor pronator group and the extensor group in pitchers with valgus instability. *J Shoulder Elbow Surg* 1996;5:347-354.

Twenty-six baseball pitchers with chronic medial collateral ligament injuries were compared to noninjured pitchers with high speed cinematography and electromyography. The flexor carpi radialis demonstrated significantly decreased firing during early cocking and deceleration compared to that in the controls. The medial dynamic stabilizers are not necessarily sufficient to stabilize the elbow in the absence of the medial collateral ligament.

Jobe FW, ElAttrache NS: Diagnosis and treatment of ulnar collateral ligament injuries in athletes, in Morrey BF (ed): *The Elbow and Its Disorders,* ed 2. Philadelphia, PA, WB Saunders, 1993, pp 566-573.

Jobe FW, ElAttrache NS: Treatment of ulnar collateral ligament injuries in athletes, in Morrey BF (ed): *Master Techniques in Orthopaedic Surgery: The Elbow.* New York, NY, Raven Press, 1994, pp 149-168.

The technique of medial collateral ligament reconstruction is illustrated and described in detail.

Jobe FW, Stark H, Lombardo SJ: Reconstruction of the ulnar collateral ligament in athletes. *J Bone Joint Surg* 1986;68A:1158-1163.

Josefsson PO, Gentz CF, Johnell O, et al: Surgical versus non-surgical treatment of ligamentous injuries following dislocation of the elbow joint: A prospective randomized study. *J Bone Joint Surg* 1987;69A:605-608.

This is one of several articles dealing with prospective investigation of elbow ligament injuries with dislocation. In all cases treated surgically, both ligaments were found to be disrupted. The results of the treatment were similar whether the ligaments were operated on or treated nonsurgically. Only half of the patients with completely disrupted medial and lateral ligaments demonstrated lateral instability, but this is understandable considering the fact that this study was conducted before an awareness of the posterolateral rotatory mechanism of instability or the proper method for clinical examination of patients with this problem.

Josefsson PO, Johnell O, Gentz CF: Long-term sequelae of simple dislocation of the elbow. *J Bone Joint Surg* 1984;66A:927-930.

This article discusses long-term follow-up data of 52 children and adults with dislocation of the elbow. One third of patients had slight or moderate flexion contractures. Instability was seen in about 15%, and was the most common complication other than heterotopic ossification, which was not described to be related to the loss of extension. Heterotopic ossification was primarily in the collateral ligaments.

Josefsson PO, Johnell O, Wendeberg B: Ligamentous injuries in dislocations of the elbow joint. *Clin Orthop* 1987;221:221-225.

Josefsson PO, Nilsson BE: Incidence of elbow dislocation. *Acta Orthop Scand* 1986;57:537-538.

Linscheid RL, O'Driscoll SW: Elbow dislocations, in Morrey BF (ed): *The Elbow and Its Disorders,* ed 2. Philadelphia, PA, WB Saunders, 1993, pp 441-452.

Mehlhoff TL, Noble PC, Bennett JB, et al: Simple dislocation of the elbow in the adult: Results after closed treatment. *J Bone Joint Surg* 1988;70A:244-249.

This is a landmark article on the long-term results following elbow dislocation in 52 patients.

Morrey BF, Tanaka S, An K-N: Valgus stability of the elbow: A definition of primary and secondary constraints. *Clin Orthop* 1991;265:187-195.

Using sophisticated aerospace technology to map the position and orientation of a body in a three-dimensional space using a highly accurate electromagnetic tracking system, the authors demonstrated with sequential cutting and resection that the anterior band of the MCL is the primary constraint to valgus instability, and the radial head is a secondary constraint.

Nestor BJ, O'Driscoll SW, Morrey BF: Ligamentous reconstruction for posterolateral rotatory instability of the elbow. *J Bone Joint Surg* 1992;74A:1235-1241.

Clinical outcomes of ligament reconstruction for recurrent instability of the elbow in patients from age 4 to 46 years were successful in 10 of 11 patients whose clinical presentations included recurrent subluxations and/or dislocations.

O'Driscoll SW: Elbow instability. *Hand Clin* 1994;10:405-415.

O'Driscoll SW: Classification and spectrum of elbow instability: Recurrent instability, in Morrey BF (ed): *The Elbow and Its Disorders,* ed 2. Philadelphia, PA, WB Saunders, 1993, pp 453-463.

Clinical, radiographic, and pathologic features, along with the implications for treatment, are presented based on scientific laboratory data and clinical experience.

O'Driscoll SW: Technique for unstable olecranon fracture-subluxations. *Op Tech Orthop* 1994;4:49-53.

O'Driscoll SW, Bell DF, Morrey BF: Posterolateral rotatory instability of the elbow. *J Bone Joint Surg* 1991;73A:440-446.

Posterolateral rotatory instability of the elbow is a condition that has not previously been described. The clinical and radiographic characteristics of this condition are described in detail, and this report is the first of a series that describes the anatomy, pathology, kinematics, surgical technique, and results of surgery for this condition.

O'Driscoll SW, Horii E, Morrey BF, et al: Anatomy of the ulnar part of the lateral collateral ligament of the elbow. *Clin Anat* 1992;5:296-303.

This anatomic study advances knowledge of and corrects misunderstandings about the anatomy of the lateral collateral ligament.

O'Driscoll SW, Morrey BF: Surgical reconstruction of the lateral collateral ligament, in Morrey BF (ed): *Master Techniques in Orthopaedic Surgery: The Elbow.* New York, NY, Raven Press, 1994, pp 169-182.

The technique of lateral collateral ligament reconstruction for recurrent instability of the elbow is described and illustrated in detail in 12 steps.

O'Driscoll SW, Morrey BF, Korinek S, et al: Elbow subluxation and dislocation: A spectrum of instability. *Clin Orthop* 1992;280:186-197.

Elbow subluxation and dislocation are part of a spectrum of instability with a common mechanism of posterolateral rotatory displacement. This spectrum occurs by a combination of axial load, valgus, and supination moments as the elbow flexes. Soft-tissue disruption starts on the lateral side and progresses in a "circle" anteriorly and posteriorly to the medial side in 3 stages that have anatomic, clinical (symptoms and signs), and radiographic correlations that also predict treatment. This applies to acute, recurrent and chronic instability.

Olsen BS, Vaesel MT, Sojbjerg JO, et al: Lateral collateral ligament of the elbow joint: Anatomy and kinematics. *J Shoulder Elbow Surg* 1996;5:103-112.

This cadaver study confirmed previous anatomic descriptions of the lateral collateral ligament complex, including the ulnar part of the lateral collateral ligament called the lateral ulnar collateral ligament. Three-dimensional kinematic analysis also confirmed that the lateral collateral ligament prevents varus or external rotatory displacement of the elbow.

Osborne G, Cotterill P: Recurrent dislocation of the elbow. *J Bone Joint Surg* 1966;48B:340-346.

This is a classic article describing the presentation, pathology, and treatment of recurrent elbow dislocation.

Regan W, Morrey B: Fractures of the coronoid process of the ulna. *J Bone Joint Surg* 1989;71A:1348-1354.

The classification of coronoid fractures is presented. Type I (small flake fractures) are really shear fractures from elbow subluxation or dislocation, not avulsion fractures, as nothing attaches to the tip of the coronoid. Type III fractures (> 50%) carry a grave prognosis.

Schwab GH, Bennett JB, Woods GW, et al: Biomechanics of elbow instability: The role of the medial collateral ligament. *Clin Orthop* 1980;146:42-52.

Stormont TJ, An KN, Morrey BF, et al: Elbow joint contact study: Comparison of techniques. *J Biomech* 1985;18:329-336.

38
Loose Bodies of the Elbow
Shawn W. O'Driscoll, MD, PhD, FRCSC

Etiology

Loose bodies usually result from osteoarthritis, osteochondritis dissecans, or acute or repetitive trauma, but they can be idiopathic, presenting as isolated entities causing mechanical symptoms. Repetitive microtrauma, such as that to which the elbow is subjected in high-level baseball players (especially pitchers and catchers), can cause fragmentation of the articular surface of the capitellum. Loose pieces of cartilage are capable of growing in size in the joint, and subsequently becoming calcified.

Classification

No classification system has been generally applied, but loose bodies can be considered idiopathic or secondary to associated pathology. Isolated loose bodies occur, but are more commonly secondary. This is an important factor because if arthritis is present, simple loose body removal alone does not help the patient; the joint must be debrided of impinging osteophytes as well.

Evaluation

In a patient with a history of joint snapping, locking, or catching, the diagnosis of a loose body is usually suspected. Impingement pain is also common. Osteoarthritis should be suspected in patients with a history of pain on terminal extension, which might be limited. Primary osteoarthritis of the elbow is most commonly seen in men with a history of heavy use of the arm, weightlifters, and throwing athletes. Patients range in age from 30 to 80 years, although athletes and those with arthritis secondary to osteochondritis dissecans present while still young. There is a characteristic history of mechanical impingement pain at the extremes of motion, classically more in extension than in flexion. Carrying an item, such as a briefcase, with the elbow extended can cause pain. Pain in the mid arc of motion is present only in the late stage. A flexion contracture of approximately 30° is typical and may be associated with some loss of flexion as well. There may be crepitus in the elbow, but the characteristic finding is pain on forced extension or flexion. Radiographs show osteophytes on the olecranon and coronoid, osteophytes filling in the olecranon and coronoid fossae, and usually loose bodies (which may not be loose) (Fig. 1). In advanced stages, the radioulnar joint and finally the radiohumeral joint may become involved.

Together with the history and physical examination, which are so predictable, standard anteroposterior and lateral radiographs are usually sufficient. However, it should be realized that loose bodies are not always detected radiographically, and they are often multiple, usually in both the anterior and posterior compartments (Fig. 2). In a series of 23 patients with loose bodies, the preoperative radiographs did not

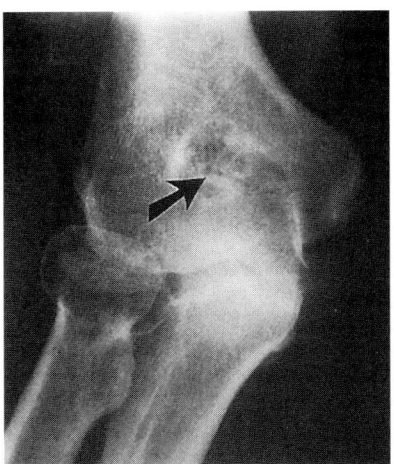
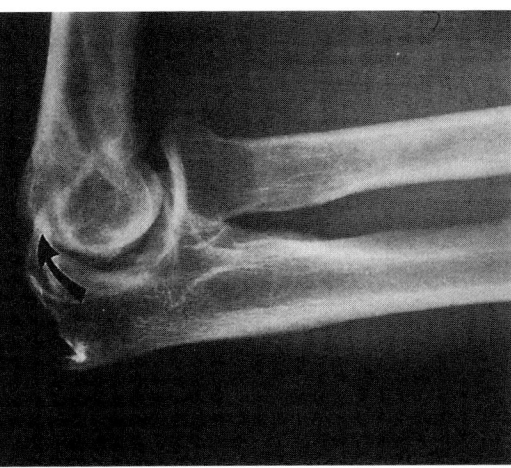
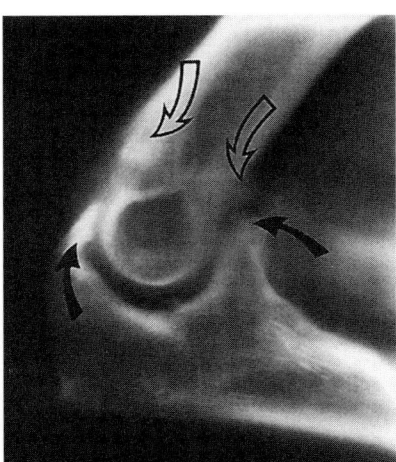

Fig. 1 Radiographic findings in osteoarthritis of the elbow. **Left,** Anteroposterior radiograph reveals loss of definition of the coronoid and olecranon fossae due to thickening of the bone in this region and osteophyte formation (*arrow*). **Center,** Lateral radiograph demonstrates the osteophytes on the olecranon (*arrow*). The anterior osteophytes are sometimes more difficult to distinguish. **Right,** Lateral tomograms are the imaging study of choice to visualize the osteophytes on the olecranon and coronoid (*dark arrows*) as well as those in and around the olecranon and coronoid fossae (*hollow arrows*).

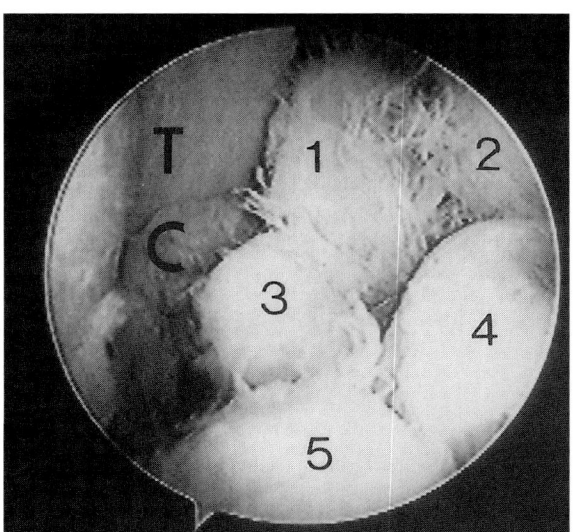

Fig. 2 Loose bodies are often multiple, as seen here in the coronoid (C) and trochlea (T), and more numerous than that counted on radiographs.

confirm the diagnosis in seven. All of these loose bodies were in the posterior compartment.

Lateral tomograms are usually quite helpful in delineating the osteophytes and clarifying the deformity of the olecranon and coronoid fossae (Fig. 1, *right*). Magnetic resonance imaging, computed tomography, and arthrotomography are not usually necessary in confirming the diagnosis. As with all elbow arthroscopies, it must ascertained preoperatively whether or not the ulnar nerve subluxates or dislocates anteriorly. If it does, which has been found to be the case in 16% of the population, it is at risk for injury when the anterior medial portal is established.

Treatment

The treatment of loose bodies brings the techniques of arthroscopy into discussion. With the advances in technical skill and experience that have occurred in recent years, an arthrotomy is rarely needed to remove loose bodies, regardless of their number or size. Furthermore, the treatment of loose bodies introduces the management of other pathologies, because, as previously discussed, loose bodies are usually secondary to arthritis or another condition.

Surgical Technique

A standard 4-mm, 30° arthroscope with a wide-angle lens is used. It is important that the sheath be specifically designed for the 30° arthroscope with no openings or slots near the tip, because these permit fluid extravasation into the soft tissues (because of the short distance the scope is inserted into the joint). A variety of hand-held graspers, power shaver blades and burs, and osteotomes must be available. The role of light amplification by stimulated emission of radiation has not been established. A sharp 4-mm Steinmann pin that has been smoothed off at the end is useful for the switch-stick technique. Long, blunt periosteal elevators placed through accessory portals serve as retractors. Additional plastic cannulae are necessary. A pump system is preferable to gravity pressure

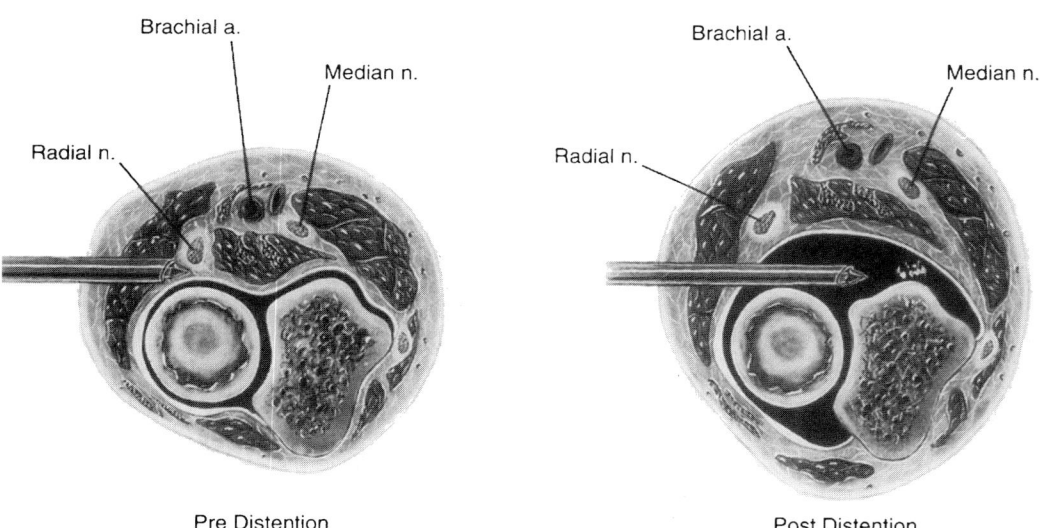

Fig. 3 When establishing the anterior portals, the neurovascular structures are displaced away and protected by distending the joint capsule with the elbow flexed 90°. The radial nerve, which can lie right on the capsule, is an average of only 4 mm from the arthroscope trocar as it enters the *undistended* joint, but about 11 mm away when the joint capsule is *distended* (**left**). The anteromedial portal is established using a switching stick. It must be confirmed before surgery that the ulnar nerve does not subluxate or dislocate anteriorly or this procedure would put the nerve at serious risk (**right**). (Reproduced with permission from C. Lichaa, Rochester, MN.)

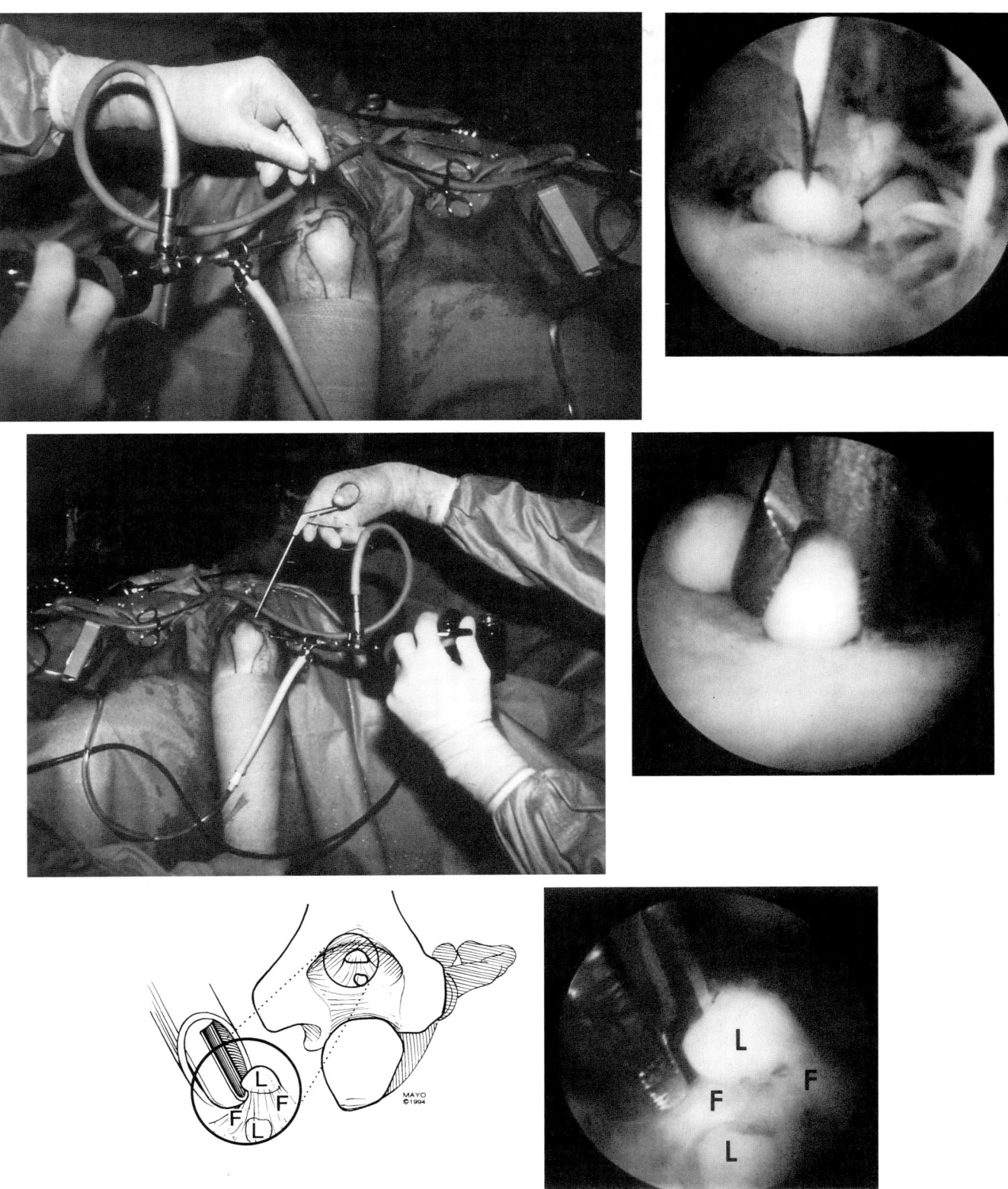

Fig. 4 Locating and removing posterior loose bodies. **Top left and right,** A needle is inserted into the joint under direct vision to confirm ideal portal placement. **Center left and right,** The grasper is inserted through the portal at the same site. **Bottom,** Loose bodies that are not loose are typical of osteoarthritis. What appear as loose bodies (L) on the radiograph are often stuck in the fibrous tissue (F) and synovium in the olecranon fossa. They can be missed if the fibrous tissue is not cleared from the fossa. (Bottom left, reproduced with permission from the Mayo Foundation, Rochester, MN.)

alone. The patient is placed in the lateral decubitus or prone position, which offers the best access posteriorly and good access to the front of the elbow.

Many different portals have been described for elbow arthroscopy but there are eight with which to be familiar (two lateral, two posterior, and four anterior): direct and accessory lateral (midlateral), posterolateral, posterior, anterolateral, high anterolateral, anteromedial, and high anteromedial. These portals are used interchangeably for removal of loose bodies, synovectomy, debridement and removal of osteophytes. To avoid cutaneous nerve injury, the cut should be made just through the skin with the knife, then dissected bluntly down to the capsule or down on the switch-stick as it emerges under the skin.

Approximately 25% to 30% of loose bodies are not detected on preoperative plain radiographs. These loose bodies are found mainly in the posterior fossa; therefore, posterior as well as anterior arthroscopy should be performed in patients undergoing arthroscopy for removal of anterior loose bodies.

The elbow is flexed 90° and the capsule fully distended. Lynch and associates showed that this displaces the anterior neurovascular structures as much as 10 mm away from the scope and instruments in the anterior portals (Fig. 3). Most authors recommend that the high (also called superior or proximal) anteromedial portal be established first, then the anterolateral and the retrograde switch-stick technique for safety reasons. The latter is in the sulcus that can be felt between the radial head and capitellum anteriorly. It should be recognized that entry must not be distal to this point, which is only about 1 cm distal and 1 cm anterior to the lateral epicondyle, not 3 cm distal as had been previously recommended by some authors.

Osteophyte and Loose Body Removal

The technique for loose body removal is shown in Figure 4. It is best to start in the posterior compartment, viewing initially from the direct lateral portal. From this portal the entire lateral joint can be seen, posterolaterally, and into the posterior fossa. It may not be possible to see all the way around to the posteromedial region from this portal. A posterolateral or direct posterior portal is then established and the loose bodies removed from the posterior fossa with appropriate-sized graspers. Many times the loose bodies are not loose, but are stuck or even embedded in the synovium. A shaver is useful to debride the surrounding synovium from such loose bodies.

Posterior osteophytes are removed with a bur and/or osteotome. There are two techniques for removing osteophytes anteriorly. One is to work only through the anterior portals; the other is to create a fenestration in the olecranon fossa through to the coronoid fossa and work directly through the elbow into the front as is done with the open procedure known as the Outerbridge-Kashiwagi arthroplasty.

Finally, the need of the surgeon to work quickly and efficiently to minimize edema cannot be overemphasized. Adequate training as well as a clear step-by-step plan of action can eliminate frustration and save time, enabling the surgeon to remove multiple loose bodies (Fig. 5).

There are some valuable techniques to be aware of when performing this surgery anteriorly. Large loose bodies and fragments of osteophyte can best be removed by firmly grasping them in a longitudinal alignment. Large anterior loose bodies (up to 2 cm) can best be removed through arthroscopic portals after being firmly grasped by uncoupling the scope and retracting it a few millimeters into the sheath, advancing the scope sheath up against the loose body, and pushing the loose

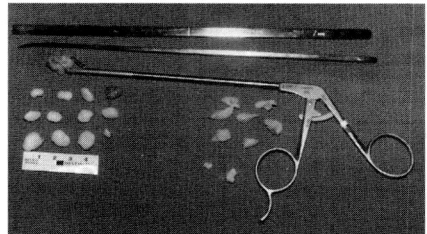
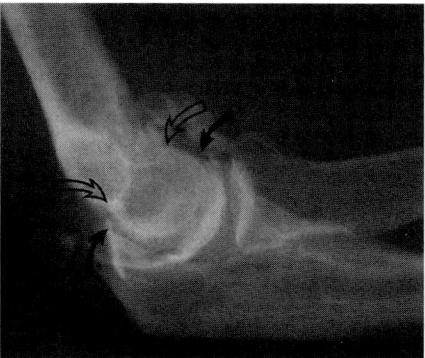
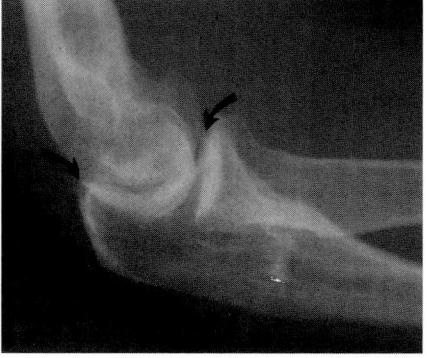

Fig. 5 **Left,** Different size graspers were needed to remove multiple loose bodies from a patient. On the right side of the picture are the osteophyte fragments that were removed using the osteotome and graspers. **Center,** Preoperative radiograph of the same patient. Multiple loose bodies are seen anteriorly and posteriorly. In addition, osteophytes (*dark arrows*) are seen on the olecranon and coronoid. The trochlea has osteophytes at the bottom of the olecranon and coronoid fossae (*hollow arrows*), so that the trochlea has become U-shaped rather than O-shaped. These osteophytes must be removed to eliminate impingement and gain motion. **Right,** Postoperatively, the osteophytes and loose bodies are not seen.

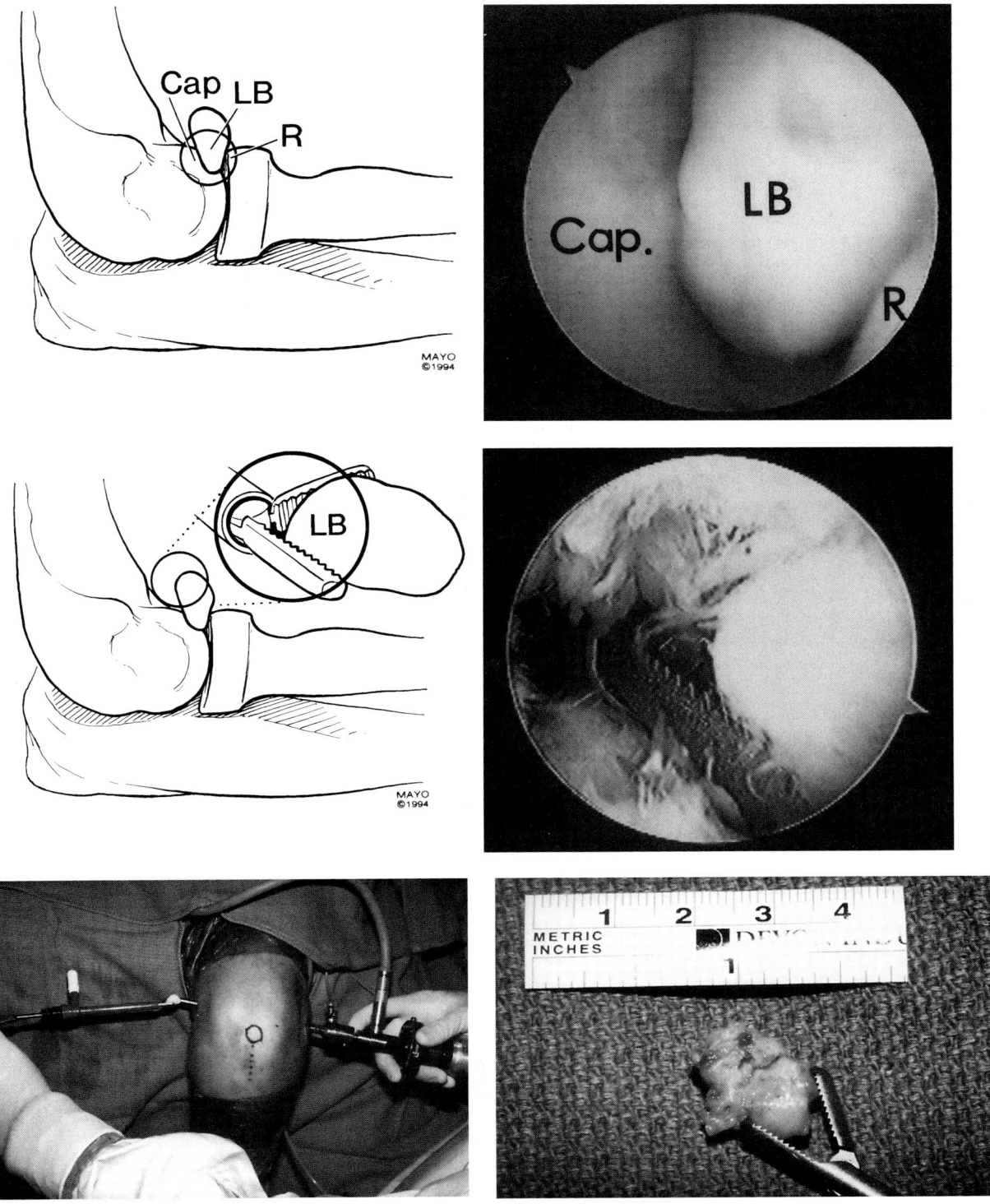

Fig. 6 Techniques for removing large anterior loose bodies up to 2 cm. **Top,** Very large loose body (LB) between the capitellum (Cap.) and radial head (R). **Center,** A grasper (preferably large, with teeth) is inserted from the medial side. **Bottom left,** As the grasper is withdrawn against the cannula, the scope is advanced against the loose body, uncoupled from the sheath, and the scope sheath used to push the loose body out while it is pulled by the grasper. The cannula of course exits with the loose body, but is simply reinserted over the scope sheath. The cannula acts as a dilator ahead of the loose body, and also helps to prevent prominences such as those seen on this loose body **(right)** from catching up in the soft tissues. (Top left and center left reproduced with permission from the Mayo Foundation, Rochester, MN.)

body out through the opposite portal together with the plastic cannula in that portal while pulling with the grasper. This procedure prevents loss of the loose body in the soft tissues. The cannula is then reinserted over the scope sheath, the scope coupled in the sheath, and redrawn back into the joint. Presence of the cannula is helpful because it keeps the soft-tissue track dilated ahead of the loose body during its removal (Fig. 6).

If an anterior portal is loosened by withdrawing an instrument too far, the instrument should be advanced in the opposite portal across the elbow and out the empty portal, and a cannula inserted over it, or a blunt Steinmann pin inside it to allow reinsertion of the appropriate instrument.

A small curved osteotome can be escorted into the elbow by first advancing the scope out the opposite portal, uncoupling the scope from its sheath, backing the scope out somewhat, and placing the osteotome partly into the sheath, then advancing them all back into the elbow as a unit. Similarly, a large 5.5-mm bur can be introduced into the anterior compartment after the scope (in its sheath) has been advanced out the other side, by taking the bur out of its own sheath, placing the sheath over the scope sheath into the elbow, withdrawing the scope out of the sheath of the bur, and inserting the bur back into its sheath. A quicker way is to advance the scope out the other portal, withdraw the scope into the sheath a few millimeters, place the bur against the end of the sheath and use the sheath as a guide, which the bur follows into the elbow as the two are moved together.

A word of caution: simple removal of loose bodies does not help these patients. An initial diagnosis of loose bodies is made in many of these patients, and the presence of osteophytes or their significance is missed. The only indication for simple loose body removal would be in a patient with full range of motion, no impingement pain at the extremes of motion, and mechanical symptoms only referable to a loose body.

Results

A very high success rate is seen when the loose bodies are not caused by an underlying disorder such as arthritis. Simple loose body removal in the presence of degenerative arthritis of the elbow does nothing to improve the patient's condition, and should not be performed.

In one series of 23 patients with loose bodies, those with isolated loose bodies, as well as three in whom the primary diagnosis was osteochondritis dissecans and a loose body, were all improved by arthroscopic removal of the bodies. However, those with posttraumatic arthritis, degenerative joint disease, or other pathology were not improved, because osteophytes were not removed from the arthritic elbows.

Arthroscopic treatment of primary degenerative arthritis in the early stages has entered the realm of standard treatment by experienced arthroscopists. In a series of 35 athletes in whom loose bodies and/or osteophytes were removed arthroscopically, improvement in pain and function was documented in 90% of patients.

In another series of 34 patients with loose bodies, pain was improved in 85% of patients, locking in 92%, and swelling in 71%. However, crepitus was improved in only 47% of patients. There were two transient symptoms of numbness of the forearm but no permanent complications. Arthroscopic treatment was possible provided that the osteophytes and not just the loose bodies are removed.

In one study, removal of osteophytes yielded symptomatic improvement in all 12 patients studied. Abundant anecdotal experience is being collected to support the usefulness of this procedure.

Osteochondritis dissecans can lead to arthritis and is often seen and treated arthroscopically in the early stages. This method can be very successful if the symptoms are primarily related to loose bodies. However, Jackson and associates found that return to full painless elbow function is unlikely in high-level female gymnasts once the main fragment has become detached.

Complications

Complications of arthroscopy occur in fewer than 10% of cases and are usually minor. They include iatrogenic cartilage damage, instrument failure, tourniquet complications, transient nerve palsies lasting a few hours because of local anesthetic extravasation from the anterolateral portal, persistent drainage from the portals, and stiffness and injuries to either the major or the cutaneous nerves.

Nerve injury is a serious concern. There have been few reports giving definite information regarding the frequency of this complication. According to a retrospective review from the members of the Arthroscopy Association of North America, one radial nerve injury (less than 0.01%) was reported in 1,569 elbow arthroscopies. The radial nerve is the most likely to be injured because of its proximity to the anterolateral portal. Stiff elbows have capsular contractures that limit the intra-articular capacity. Displacement of the nerves anteriorly away from the portals is accomplished by capsular distention with saline, but the average intracapsular capacity of stiff elbows was reduced by half to two thirds of normal. Therefore, the space available in which to work in the anterior elbow is reduced and adequate distention might not be possible, increasing the risk of nerve injury. One recent report on arthroscopic release of elbow contractures included a permanent nerve injury. The median nerve has also been injured during anterior synovectomy with a shaver.

Selected Bibliography

Adolfsson L: Arthroscopy of the elbow joint: A cadaveric study of portal placement. *J Shoulder Elbow Surg* 1994;3:53-61.

    This article describes a detailed cadaveric dissection of the proximity of the deep and superficial nerves to the portals used in elbow arthroscopy.

Andrews JR, Craven WM: Lesions of the posterior compartment of the elbow. *Clin Sports Med* 1991;10:637-652.

Baker CL Jr, Shalvoy RM: The prone position for elbow arthroscopy. *Clin Sports Med* 1991;10:623-628.

Boe S: Arthroscopy of the elbow: Diagnosis and extraction of loose bodies. *Acta Orthop Scand* 1986;57:52-53.

Gallay SH, Richards RR, ODriscoll SW: Intraarticular capacity and compliance of stiff and normal elbows. *Arthroscopy* 1993;9:9-13.

    The intracapsular capacity of 11 stiff and ten normal elbows was compared in 11 patients undergoing surgery for elbow contractures. The average volume capacity of the stiff elbows was reduced to less than half of that of the normal elbows. The capsular compliance was reduced to 14% of normal, indicating that it was not as distensible either. The anterior neurovascular structures need to be displaced away from the arthroscopic instruments by capsular distention, which might not be possible in stiff elbows.

Jackson DW, Silvino N, Reiman P: Osteochondritis in the female gymnasts elbow. *Arthroscopy* 1989;5:129-136.

Jones GS, Savoie FH III: Arthroscopic capsular release of flexion contractures (arthrofibrosis) of the elbow. *Arthroscopy* 1993;9:277-283.

Kim SJ, Kim HK, Lee JW: Arthroscopy for limitation of motion of the elbow. *Arthroscopy* 1995;11:680-683.

    Twenty-five patients with contracture were treated with arthroscopic removal of loose bodies and osteophytes, and capsular release. Both extension and flexion improved, as did the elbow performance scores.

Lindenfeld TN: Medial approach in elbow arthroscopy. *Am J Sports Med* 1990;18:413-417.

    The major risks of arthroscopic instrumentation of the anterior aspect of the elbow are encountered during establishment of the anterolateral or anteromedial portals. In a study of six cadaver elbows, the author showed that the radial nerve was only an average of 3 mm away from the arthroscope in the anterolateral portal but the median nerve was on average at least 11 mm away from the scope in the anteromedial portal.

Lynch GJ, Meyers JF, Whipple TL, Caspari RB: Neurovascular anatomy and elbow arthroscopy: Inherent risks. *Arthroscopy* 1986;2:190-197.

Marshall PD, Fairclough JA, Johnson SR, Evans EJ: Avoiding nerve damage during elbow arthroscopy. *J Bone Joint Surg* 1993;75B:129-131.

Morrey BF: Primary degenerative arthritis of the elbow: Treatment by ulnohumeral arthroplasty. *J Bone Joint Surg* 1992;74B:409-413.

O'Driscoll SW: Elbow arthroscopy for loose bodies. *Orthopedics* 1992;15:855-859.

O'Driscoll SW, Morrey BF: Arthroscopy of the elbow: Diagnostic and therapeutic benefits and hazards. *J Bone Joint Surg* 1992;74A:84-94.

    This article details the risks and benefits of arthroscopy of the elbow from an overall viewpoint and describes the diagnostic and therapeutic roles of this procedure. The current techniques are described and illustrated and a detailed statistical analysis of a large series of patients provided.

O'Driscoll SW, Morrey BF: Arthroscopy of the elbow, in Morrey BF (ed): *Master Techniques in Orthopaedic Surgery: The Elbow.* New York, NY, Raven Press, 1994, pp 21-34.

    A detailed description with illustrations of the techniques in elbow arthroscopy is presented.

O'Driscoll SW, Morrey BF, An K-N: Intraarticular pressure and capacity of the elbow. *Arthroscopy* 1990;6:100-103.

    The average capacity of the elbow capsule is about 20 ml and rupture can occur at relatively low pressures (about 80 mm Hg). The capacity is maximum at 80° of flexion, which explains the position of comfort and also the typical position of a stiff elbow.

Ogilvie-Harris DJ, Schemitsch E: Arthroscopy of the elbow for removal of loose bodies. *Arthroscopy* 1993;9:5-8.

Papilion JD, Neff RS, Shall LM: Compression neuropathy of the radial nerve as a complication of elbow arthroscopy: A case report and review of the literature. *Arthroscopy* 1988;4:284-286.

Poehling GG, Ekman EF: Arthroscopy of the elbow. *J Bone Joint Surg* 1994;76A:1265-1271.

    This is an excellent and comprehensive review of elbow arthroscopy.

Redden JF, Stanley D: Arthroscopic fenestration of the olecranon fossa in the treatment of osteoarthritis of the elbow. *Arthroscopy* 1993;9:14-16.

    The authors describe their arthroscopic approach to the treatment of elbow osteoarthritis that permits debridement of the elbow joint together with the removal of intra-articular loose bodies. It is the arthroscopic equivalent of the open debridement procedure known as the Outerbridge-Kashiwagi arthroplasty. Twelve patients underwent the procedure and all had improvement in their symptoms.

Rodeo SA, Forster RA, Weiland AJ: Neurological complications due to arthroscopy. *J Bone Joint Surg* 1993;75A:917-926.

Small NC: Complications in arthroscopic surgery performed by experienced arthroscopists. *Arthroscopy* 1988;4:215-221.

Stothers K, Day B, Regan WR: Arthroscopy of the elbow: Anatomy, portal sites, and a description of the proximal lateral portal. *Arthroscopy* 1995;11:449-457.

    Proximal placement of the anterolateral portal ensures that the nerves are farther away and therefore less likely to be injured.

Timmerman LA, Andrews JR: Arthroscopic treatment of posttraumatic elbow pain and stiffness. *Am J Sports Med* 1994;22:230-235.

Verhaar J, van Mameren H, Brandsma A: Risks of neurovascular injury in elbow arthroscopy: Starting anteromedially or anterolaterally? *Arthroscopy* 1991;7:287-290.

Ward WG, Anderson TE: Elbow arthroscopy in a mostly athletic population. *J Hand Surg* 1993;18A:220-224.

This article addresses the early osteoarthritic changes typically seen in elbows subjected to repetitive heavy overuse, which results in olecranon and coronoid osteophytes, as well as osteophytes and often loose bodies in the olecranon and coronoid fossae. Thirty-five athletes were treated for loose bodies and/or osteophytes of the elbow by arthroscopic loose body removal and debridement. Improvement in pain and function occurred in approximately 90% of patients and 34 of 35 believed that the operation was worthwhile. Arthroscopic treatment is possible, provided that the osteophytes and not just the loose bodies are removed.

Ward WG, Belhobek GH, Anderson TE: Arthroscopic elbow findings: Correlation with preoperative radiographic studies. *Arthroscopy* 1992;8:498-502.

Osteochondritis Dissecans of the Elbow

Gary G. Poehling, MD

Osteochondritis dissecans of the elbow begins as a localized injury or condition affecting the articular surface of the capitellum that involves separation of a segment of cartilage and subchondral bone. The terminology used to describe this condition has led to much confusion. The terms osteochondritis dissecans, osteonecrosis, osteochondrosis, osteochondral fracture, Panner's disease, and hereditary epiphyseal dysplasia have been used interchangeably.

The removal of loose bodies, presumably osteochondral fragments, from joints was first described in a report published in 1840. In 1870, the condition was described as "quiet necrosis" leading to loose bodies of the knee. The term osteochondritis dissecans was first used in 1888, with 'osteochondritis' describing the inflammation of the osteochondral joint surface, and 'dissecans' originating from the Latin word "dissec," which means to separate. In a 1928 study of three boys aged 7 to 10 years who had osteonecrosis of the entire capitellum that resembled Perthes disease of the hip, the boys' conditions returned to normal following a protracted course over 3 years. In a study of 57 cases, no inflammation was reported in these lesions. Osteochondritis dissecans of the elbow has been divided into three groups by age range. Category I patients are those younger than 13 years of age. Category II patients are 13 years up to adulthood. Category III patients are adults. The younger patients had a better outcome with nonsurgical treatment.

Etiology

Few authors would disagree that repetitive microtrauma plays an important role in osteochondritis dissecans of the elbow. Two groups of patients are identified as being at high risk for this type of injury. The first group is throwing athletes, in whom "Little Leaguer's elbow" is most common in baseball pitchers. The compressive forces experienced by the radiocapitellar joint are believed to play an important role in the pathogenesis of osteochondritis dissecans in this group. These forces occur as a result of valgus loading of the elbow during the pitching motion. The second high-risk group is the female gymnast. Top-level female gymnasts are usually involved in an aggressive training program at a very young age, exposing their developing radiocapitellar joint to repetitive shear and compressive forces at an age when their maturing capitellar physes have a tenuous vascular supply.

In a study of the vascular anatomy of the capitellum, it was found that between the ages of 8 and 19 years, the capitellar ossific nucleus is supplied by isolated vessels traversing the epiphysis from posterior to anterior. There were no contributions from the metaphyseal vascular supply to either the ossified or nonossified portion of the epiphyses. It is presumed that a combination of this tenuous blood supply with repetitive trauma sets the stage for the clinical condition known as osteochondritis dissecans of the elbow.

The pathophysiology of osteochondritis dissecans, based on current knowledge, is likely caused by repetitive microtrauma leading to fatigue failure of the subchondral bone that, because of ongoing repetitive stress, does not heal. Bone resorption is followed by separation of the fragment from the underlying bed. The bone fragment becomes avascular because of the poor blood supply. The cartilage, although it remains viable through nutrition from the synovial fluid, breaks down into loose bodies because of insufficient underlying support.

Clinical Presentation

Osteochondritis dissecans of the elbow usually presents during adolescence and is characterized by lateral elbow pain, swelling, and limited range of motion. Plain anteroposterior radiographs usually reveal the characteristic rarefaction or radiolucency of a portion of the capitellum (Fig. 1). Loose

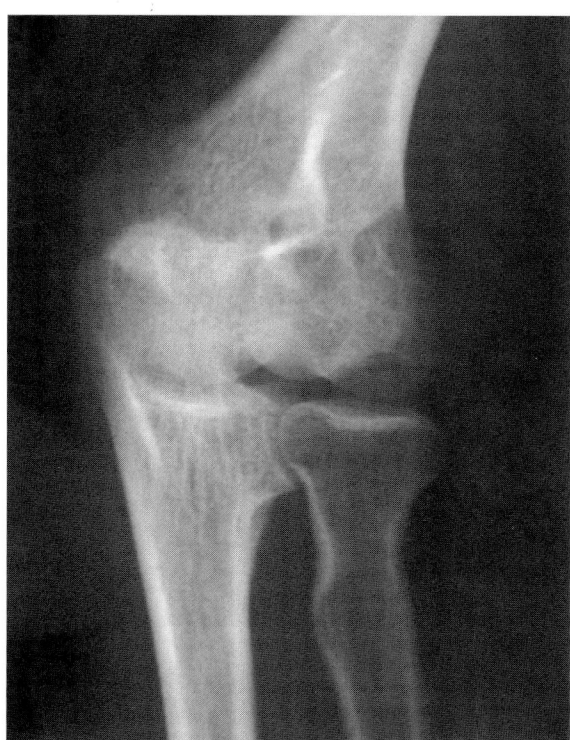

Fig. 1 Anteroposterior radiograph of elbow showing radiolucency of the capitellum.

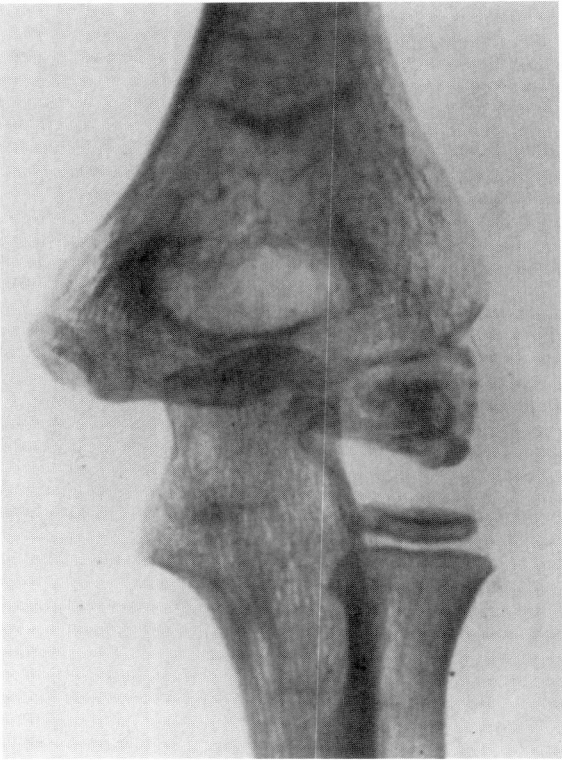 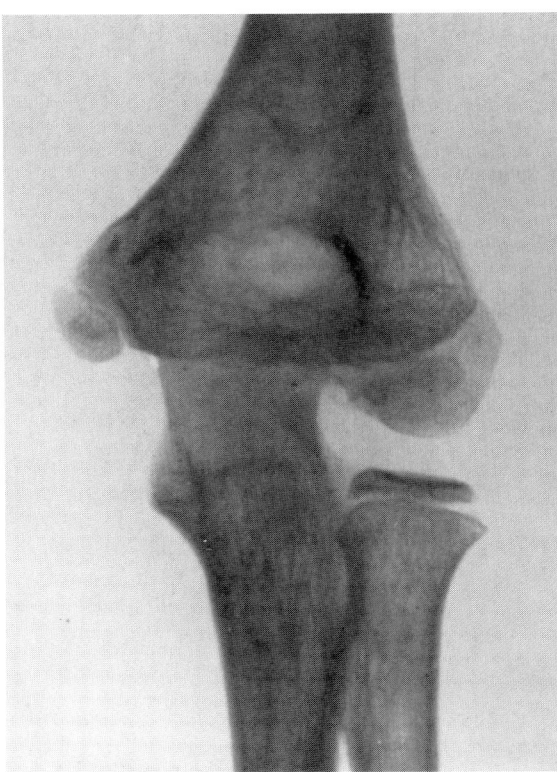

Fig. 2 Panner's disease. **Left,** Elbow radiograph of a 10-year-old boy, showing rarefaction and fragmentation of almost the entire ossific nucleus of the capitellum. **Right,** Same patient 1 year later, showing complete reconstitution of the capitellum. (Reproduced with permission from Panner HJ: A peculiar affection of the capitulum humeri, resembling Calvé-Perthes' disease of the hip. *Acta Radiol* 1929;10:234-242.)

bodies are seen in advanced stages as is radial head enlargement. If the entire capitellum is involved in a child between the ages of 4 and 10 years (Fig. 2), Panner's disease or osteochondrosis should be suspected.

A competent diagnosis of osteochondritis dissecans of the elbow can be made from the plain radiographs in about one half of cases. In questionable cases, a radiograph should be obtained tangential to the lesion. Rather than the usual position for an anteroposterior radiograph of the elbow, the elbow is flexed 45° so the forearm is still horizontal, but the humerus is at a 45° angle to the x-ray plate. Plain computed tomography (CT) accurately defines the site and extent of the osteochondral lesion. Arthrography combined with CT may add to the ability to make a preoperative diagnosis of a loose fragment of articular cartilage.

Arthrotomograms have been shown to have an accuracy of 89% for loose bodies and for joint surface abnormalities, whereas plain radiographs demonstrated 71% accuracy for joint surface abnormalities and 75% accuracy for loose bodies. Diagnostic arthroscopy adds additional information to preoperative studies. Magnetic resonance imaging of the elbow can confirm the diagnosis of osteochondritis dissecans and loose bodies. However, magnetic resonance imaging is not necessary if arthroscopy is being performed.

Natural History and Treatment

The true Panner's disease occurs in children between 4 and 10 years of age. These children may present with symptoms of pain on the lateral aspect of the elbow with a large area of rarefaction and fragmentation including most of the capitellum. This area is presumed to have a primary avascular origin similar to that seen in Perthes disease of the hip. These patients should avoid valgus stress and be treated symptomatically with a splint. A prolonged period of healing extending approximately 3 years is expected, with excellent long-term results with normal-appearing radiographs and little limitation of motion.

In adolescents, who generally present with mechanical symptoms in the elbow, it is presumed that this condition has a primarily mechanical origin. It is believed that the loose bodies should be removed, and that replacing the loose bodies is no more beneficial than removing them. Despite a slight decrease in range of motion and gradual degenerative changes, patients function without severe disability. Most reports of treatment in the literature involve arthrotomy. The difficulty is that loose bodies can be both in the anterior as well as the posterior compartments. Open exploration of both compartments can cause significant morbidity and a pro-

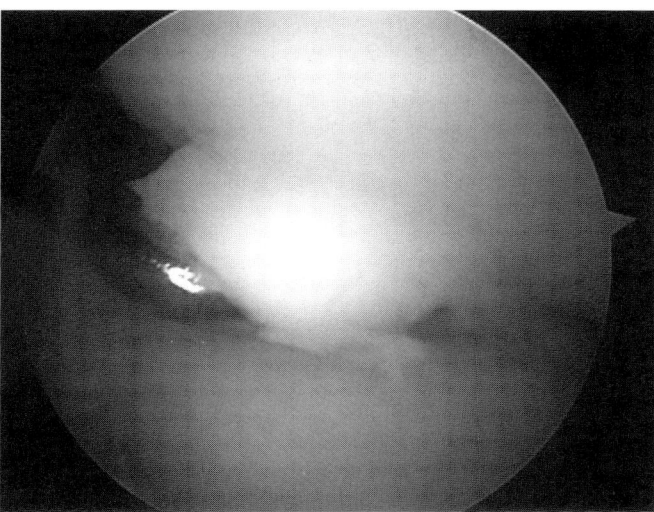

Fig. 3 Arthroscopic view of radial capitellum joint showing loose articular cartilage.

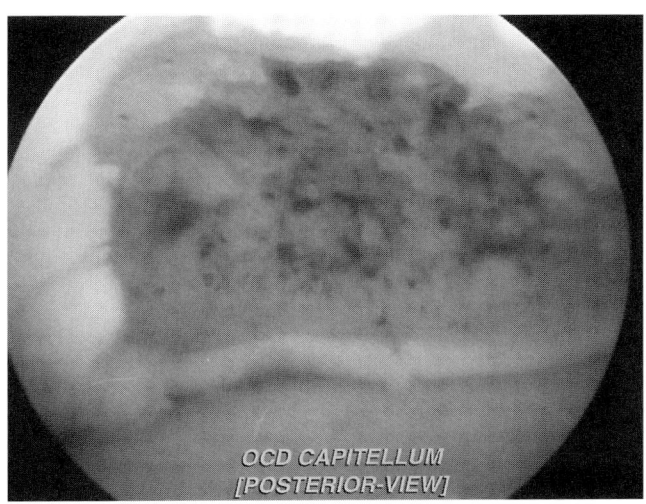

Fig. 4 Arthroscopic view of capitellum postdebridement showing good bone bleeding.

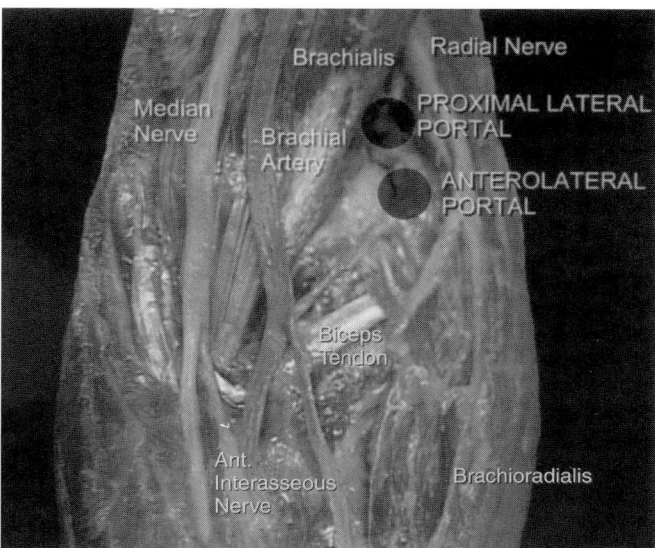

Fig. 5 Anatomy—anterolateral portal.

longed rehabilitation. With the advent of arthroscopy, easy and safe access to the anterior portion of the joint, as well as the posterior portion, allows for complete evaluation and treatment. Arthroscopy permits removal of loose bodies (Fig. 3) and cleaning of the bed of the fragment to bleeding bone (Fig. 4) with little morbidity. There are no long-term follow-up studies concerning arthroscopic treatment of osteochondritis dissecans in the literature. Short-term results of the arthroscopic treatment reveal more rapid and complete rehabilitation when compared to open treatment.

Treatment of osteochondritis dissecans depends on the clinical symptoms. If there is a loose body within the joint and the patient presents with diminished range of motion, locking, and catching, then removal of the loose body is indicated. It would be expected to relieve symptoms immediately; however, the range of motion gradually increases over a period of months to a year. Arthroscopic capsular release is also being performed in some centers. Procedures such as excision of the radial head, olecranon tip, and the lateral condyle, bone grafting of the capitellum, replacement of loose body, and osteotomy of the radial head have not been shown to be any better than loose body removal alone.

Any throwing athlete or gymnast presenting with pain on the lateral aspect of the elbow should be carefully evaluated by physical examination and radiograph. Rest is indicated until all symptoms have subsided, at which time the radiographs must be confirmed to still be normal. If abnormalities are present on radiographs, the current recommendation would be to refrain from sports for 6 to 8 weeks until all symptoms have cleared and radiographs show signs of improvement.

Results

In describing long-term results, the longest average follow-up was 23 years. It is agreed that, on the whole, the prognosis in patients with osteochondritis dissecans, after simple removal of the loose body, is good. Limitation of extension less than 20° was a consistent finding. The patients described little functional limitation. Fifty percent of the patients had diminished range of motion and pain with effort. The radiographs showed degenerative changes on greater than 50%, which correlated with diminished range of motion. Two thirds of the patients had an increase in radial head size.

There are conflicting data for the female gymnast. Five patients between 11 and 13 years of age were treated conservatively, with the exception of two who had arthroscopic removal of the loose body. Four of the five continued to compete in gymnastics at 3 years follow-up. Seven female gymnasts who ranged in age from 10 to 17 years (average, 13 years) had a 2.9-year average follow-up. All had surgery, but still suffered from loss of extension, and only one of the seven continued competing in gymnastics.

Complications

Anecdotal experience indicates that some patients may experience stiffness following open or arthroscopic surgery for osteochondritis dissecans. This stiffness might be secondary to an underlying inflammation or synovitis.

The only reported complication in patients is a compression neuropathy at the radial nerve following elbow arthroscopy in a patient who was placed in a supine position with an anterolateral portal established from the outside-in technique. Many arthroscopists believe that it is safer to establish the anterolateral portal from an inside-out direction, making for a more consistent portal approach in avoiding the radial nerve (Fig. 5).

Selected Bibliography

General

Jawish R, Rigault P, Padovani JP, et al: Osteochondritis dissecans of the humeral capitellum in children. *Eur J Pediatr Surg* 1993;3:97-100.

Thirteen cases of osteochondritis dissecans of capitellum humeri in 12 children (11 boys and one girl, ages 10 to 15 years) were studied. Surgical treatment was performed in seven out of 13 elbows for removal of loose bodies or excision of osteochondritis in situ with cartilage damage. Functional treatment was carried out in other cases. At long-term follow-up, ranging from 2 to 13 years, clinical examination demonstrated satisfactory results in nine cases; in three cases limitation of movement was related to fracture of the radial head or to delay in surgical treatment. Roentgenographically, changes related to growth disturbance were consistently observed; they involved the radial head, the olecranon, the trochlea and the proximal end of the ulna.

Nagura S: The so-called osteochondritis dissecans of König. *Clin Orthop* 1960;18:100-121.

On the basis of histologic as well as experimental investigations, König's osteochondritis dissecans was attributed to a succession of secondary destructive and constructive processes resulting from an original, but not very significant, interruption in the continuity of the subchondral bone tissue and its filling with cartilaginous callus. The significance of cartilaginous callus formation in human fractures in the etiology and the pathogenesis of what may be called osteochondritic disease and aseptic epiphyseal necroses is also emphasized.

Panner HJ: A peculiar affection of the capitulum humeri, resembling Calvé-Perthes' disease of the hip. *Acta Radiol* 1929;10:234-242.

This classic article is a report of three cases of elbow affection related to a definite trauma in boys 10 years old or younger. The clinical symptoms are mild, but the course of the disease may last 3 years or more. The radiographic picture is typical as only the capitulum humeri is affected. In the beginning there are only slight rarefactions resembling fissures with a certain blurring of the structural architecture. The osseous center becomes diminished, its contour flossy, irregular and fragmented, then resumes its normal shape and appearance.

Pappas AM: Osteochondrosis dissecans. *Clin Orthop* 1981;158:59-69.

Osteochondrosis dissecans is an osteochondrosis limited to the periphery of secondary ossification centers of diarthrodial joints. It is most frequently diagnosed in the second decade of life. The knee is the most frequently involved joint, followed by the ankle, hip, and elbow. Concepts of pathogenesis consist of reaction to mechanical trauma or spontaneous focal avascular osteonecrosis, but the etiology is not known; however there is a definite correlation between skeletal maturation and outcome. The objective of treatment should be to prevent the formation of a partially detached or free osteochondral fragment. The preferred treatment in younger individuals is primarily immobilization with bivalved casts or splints. Surgery is recommended infrequently in the younger age group but with relatively increasing frequency in older individuals. In older individuals, tomography, arthrography, and arthroscopy are helpful diagnostic aids.

Ruch DS, Poehling GG: Arthroscopic treatment of Panner's Disease. *Clin Sports Med* 1991;10:629-636.

Panner's disease, or osteochondrosis of the capitellum, may actually be a continuum of disorders ranging from idiopathic osteochondrosis of the capitellum to a frank lesion of osteochondritis dissecans with an associated loose body and articular cartilage defect. Previously, such lesions were treated conservatively and surgical therapy was used only as a last resort, often leading to an inability of the patient to resume high-performance athletics. Use of the arthroscope in the treatment of Panner's disease is, therefore, a realistic treatment option, and it may be associated with fewer complications and a speedier recovery.

Etiology

Haraldsson S: On osteochondrosis deformans juvenilis capituli humeri including investigation of intra-osseous vasculature in distal humerus. *Acta Orthop Scand* 1959;38(suppl):1-232.

This investigation reported on the clinical and roentgenologic features of osteochondrosis deformans juvenilis of the capitulum humeri against the background of literature studies. The investigation also includes an experimental study of the intraosseous and extraosseous vasculature of the distal end of the humerus with special reference to the capitulum, and is based on injection experiments on cadavers of children and adults. The investigation shed light on the nutrition and vasculature of the chondroepiphysis in growing and full-grown bones, as well as on the possible etiology of osteochondrosis deformans of the capitellum.

Poehling GG, Whipple TL, Sisco L, et al: Elbow arthroscopy: A new technique. *Arthroscopy* 1989;5:222-224.

Elbow arthroscopy is a useful and therapeutic tool for the orthopaedic surgeon. This study presents a modification of the original technique by placing the patient in a prone position and using a proximal medial portal. This treatment simplifies the treatment of a wide variety of elbow pathology, including loose bodies, osteochondritis dissecans, persistent synovitis, suspected cartilaginous lesions, posterior osteophytes, selected radial head fractures, and chronically undiagnosed painful elbows.

Schenck RC Jr, Goodnight JM: Osteochondritis dissecans. *J Bone Joint Surg* 1996;78A:439-456.

This current concepts comprehensive review has 163 references, with a two-page review of the elbow. Most authors have noted osteochondritis dissecans of the elbow as a result of repetitive overuse (microtrauma) in athletes who are involved in throwing activities.

Clinical Presentation

Jobe FW, Nuber G: Throwing injuries of the elbow. *Clin Sports Med* 1986;5:621-636.

With the increasing popularity of racquet and throwing sports in our society, an increasing awareness of the elbow injuries sustained with repetitive upper extremity activity is important. Particular attention should be paid to proper technique, equipment, and duration of activity, and preventative measures should be taken. It is imperative that the treating physician recognize the pathologic stage early in order to minimize the consequences of these activities.

Ward WG, Belhobek GH, Anderson TE: Arthroscopic elbow findings: Correlation with preoperative radiographic studies. *Arthroscopy* 1992;8:498-502.

Correlation between arthroscopic findings and preoperative radiographic studies was performed in a consecutive series of 37 elbows. Arthrotomograms added significant diagnostic information unavailable from plain radiographs alone, thereby improving the sensitivity, specificity, positive predictive value, negative predictive value, and diagnostic efficiency (accuracy) in the evaluation of the elbow joint surface changes, marginal spurs, and loose bodies.

Results

Bauer M, Jonsson K, Josefsson PO, et al: Osteochondritis dissecans of the elbow: A long-term follow-up study. *Clin Orthop* 1992;284:156-160.

Thirty-one patients with osteochondritis dissecans of the capitellum humeri were followed for an average of 23 years. Impaired motion and pain on effort were the most common complaints. Radiographic signs of degenerative joint disease were present in more than half of the elbows and correlated with a reduced range of motion. The diameter of the radial head increased in comparison with the contralateral elbow in two thirds of the patients.

Jackson DW, Silvino N, Reiman P: Osteochondritis in the female gymnast's elbow. *Arthroscopy* 1989;5:129-136.

Ten cases of osteochondritis dissecans of the humeral capitellum are reviewed in seven high-performance female gymnasts ranging in age from 10 to 17 years old. All but one were evaluated and treated with arthroscopy and/or arthrotomy with curettage of loose articular margins, drilling of the lesion, and removal of loose bodies. The average length of follow-up is 2.9 years, and includes interview, physical examination, and radiographic evaluation. Once the bony changes in the capitellum are detected, and pain remains despite conservative management, symptoms can be improved with surgery, but persist in female gymnasts.

Papilion JD, Neff RS, Shall LM: Compression neuropathy of the radial nerve as a complication of elbow arthroscopy: A case report and review of the literature. *Arthroscopy* 1988;4:284-286.

Arthroscopic surgery of the elbow was performed in a 14-year-old male athlete for diagnosis and treatment of osteochondritis dissecans of the capitellum. Postsurgical examination revealed an immediate and complete palsy of the posterior interosseous nerve. This complication was attributed to the manipulation of the arthroscope and instrumentation in close proximity to the radial nerve. Neuromuscular function returned to normal over a 6-month period. This case demonstrates the importance of portal placement and instrument manipulation in arthroscopic evaluation and treatment of the elbow.

Singer KM, Roy SP: Osteochondrosis of the humeral capitellum. *Am J Sports Med* 1984;12:351-360.

Seven cases of osteochondrosis of the capitellum occurring in five high-performance female gymnasts between the ages of 11 and 13 years are presented. Two of the patients were treated by surgical excision of the loose osteochondral fragment in three elbows. It was postulated that this condition represents a lateral compression injury because of repetitive valgus overload. Investigation of the capitellar blood supply indicates that the common factors in osteochondrosis of the capitellum are repetitive or prolonged trauma to a vulnerable epiphysis on a basis of vascular interruption.

Woodward AH, Bianco AJ Jr: Osteochondritis dissecans of the elbow. *Clin Orthop* 1975;110:35-41.

Clinical findings, radiographic findings, and results of various forms of treatment of osteochondritis dissecans in 50 elbows are reviewed in a study of the records of 42 male patients. Two thirds of the patients were between 9 and 15 years of age when they first had symptoms of pain, loss of motion, and locking and clicking. Radiographically, rarefaction and flattening of the capitellum were common features. Some form of surgical treatment was used for 38 elbows with removal of loose bone and curettage and trimming of the crater being the most frequent procedures. This review suggests that loose bodies should be removed and that, in most instances, no other procedures are indicated.

Complications

Holland P, Davies AM, Cassar-Pullicino VN: Computed tomographic arthrography in the assessment of osteochondritis dissecans of the elbow. *Clin Radiol* 1994;49:231-235.

Eleven cases of osteochondritis dissecans of the elbow are reviewed. Computed tomography (CT) accurately identified the abnormality, its extent and its precise location. Computed tomographic arthrography (CTA) allowed accurate delineation of the overlying cartilage in all cases, identifying cartilage defects in four patients, fissuring in two, and cartilage thinning in a further two. In those patients who had plain CT, four were shown to have loose bodies, one of which was obscured by contrast medium at subsequent CTA. Two further patients with loose bodies were identified using CTA alone.

40

Nerve Injuries and Neuropathies About the Elbow

Thomas W. Wright, MD

Introduction

Nerve injuries and neuropathies about the elbow are relatively common. This chapter will discuss the anatomy, etiology, evaluation, and treatment of specific nerve injuries and neuropathies involving all the major nerves crossing the elbow. A brief discussion of the pathophysiology of nerve injury, either secondary to acute trauma or chronic compressive neuropathy, will be presented, along with a general evaluation of nerve injuries prior to the specific discussions of the individual nerves.

Pathophysiology of Nerve Injury

Acute Trauma

Acute trauma (blunt or sharp penetrating) to peripheral nerves can be described according to Seddon's classification of nerve injury into (1) neurapraxia, (2) axonotmesis, and (3) neurotmesis. Neurapraxia occurs when the nerve experiences a local acute stretch injury but the fascicles and the epineurium remain intact. This injury corresponds to a local demyelinating block, and is resolved when the myelin is repaired. Complete recovery may occur in a few days or in 8 weeks or longer. Axonotmesis is characterized by internal topographic disruption of axons, with maintenance of the neural tube (endoneurium) and epineurium. The nerve undergoes wallerian degeneration and requires complete regrowth of axons, at a rate of approximately 1 mm per day, for recovery. Expectations of recovery from axonotmetic injury are based on distance from the injury to the end organ, with more proximal injuries having a worse prognosis. However, the overall results are reasonably good, and complete recovery is common. Neurotmesis is complete disruption of the neural tubes along with the epineurium. Recovery in this case is dependent on sprouting axons finding the distal neurotube. The outlook for recovery in patients with a neurotmesis is poor. Acute injuries are treated with surgical repair; chronic injuries are treated with nerve grafting. With repair, the outcome is dependent on the distance to the end organ, particularly the distance to motor endplates. Therefore, the more proximal injuries, along with mixed motor-sensory nerves, have a poor prognosis; other factors that impact recovery of these injuries include vascularity of the tissue bed, patient age, and smoking.

A more complete grading system has also been described: first degree, neurapraxia; second degree, axonotmesis; third degree, disruption of axon and endoneurium; fourth degree, disruption of axon, endoneurium, and perineurium; fifth degree, neurotmesis or disruption of axon, endoneurium, perineurium, and epineurium. Nerve injuries may be mixed, with different degrees of injury involving different axons in the same nerve.

Chronic Neuropathy

Compression, considered the primary contributor to chronic mechanical neuropathy, may decrease the performance of the nerve by a direct mechanical effect, a vascular effect, or possibly a combination of both. Compression magnitude and duration also have a significant impact on nerve function.

It has been shown that 30 mm Hg of compression will significantly retard blood flow in neural venules. Blood flow in the nerve has been shown to be completely arrested with pressures of 60 to 80 mm Hg. Concerning mechanical compression alone, 30 mm Hg has been shown to be the critical gradient for blocking axonal flow. With longer duration, pressures of only 20 mm Hg will produce the same effect. Pressure alters axoplasmic flow in both directions; therefore, a decrease in cytoskeletal elements is transported to the distal axon and a decrease in axolemma constituents for synaptic function is transported to the cell body. The double crush syndrome, which occurs when a proximal or, in cases of reverse double crush syndromes, more distal compression site makes a second site on the same nerve more susceptible to injury, has also been studied.

Large, myelinated sensory fibers are the most susceptible to compression, whereas non-myelinated fibers are most resistant to compression even at very high compressive levels. Small myelinated fibers are not as susceptible to compression as are large ones.

Compression has the greatest effect on the nerve at the edge of the compression, a phenomenon known as the "edge effect." The compressive gradient is responsible for the neurologic injury. Long-term compression results in the "tadpole lesion" seen in chronic compressive neuropathies. This lesion represents an area of retraction of myelin at the compressed area and accumulation of myelin at the internodal areas outside of the compressed area.

Certain diseases, such as diabetes, make patients more susceptible to compressive neuropathy. The exact mechanism of how diabetes affects nerve function is unclear, but it appears that its pathology may be similar to that of the double crush syndrome. Axonal transport in the diabetic rat has been studied. Accumulation of sorbitol, which is a metabolic product of glucose, may cause endoneural edema. Edema results in decreased axonal flow in the peripheral nerves of those with diabetes, making a second compressive injury more likely. Another explanation commonly used but currently less favored is the presence of a peripheral neuropathy secondary to microvascular lesions.

Another potential cause of chronic neuropathies is chronic low grade traction. The peripheral nerves about the elbow require a significant effort to move proximally and distally as the elbow moves through a full range of motion. The farther the nerve is from the center of rotation, the greater amount of excursion is necessary to accommodate upper extremity motion. Anything that will impede the excursion of the nerve will result in increased strain and traction, therefore potentially contributing to the neuropathy. This scenario may work in synergy with compression, but it has not been well studied to this point. Friction associated with excursion of a nerve, particularly in a tight compartment, has also been implicated in the production of chronic neuropathy.

It may be that compression, traction, and friction contribute to chronic neuropathies to some extent. Clearly, however, chronic compression is the factor that has been studied the most and is probably the major contributor to neuropathy.

Evaluation

In addition to the mechanism of injury (onset, duration), important symptoms include pain, dysesthesias, paresthesias, clumsiness, and weakness. Physical signs of neuropathy include atrophy, trophic changes of the skin, and altered sweat patterns in the hand. Palpation for areas of tenderness and the presence and location of Tinel's sign should be determined. It has been shown that the vibrometer is the most sensitive apparatus for determining the presence of a compressive neuropathy, and that testing with Semmes Weinstein monofilaments is a repeatable measure of sensory function. Two-point discrimination is a good test of sensory density function, but inconsistent application pressure may present a problem. Provocative tests for the different nerve lesions are specific to each nerve. Muscle strength is measured manually or with specific strength testing equipment, which may give some indication of patient cooperation as well as provide a baseline evaluation. Electrodiagnostic changes that should be sought include slowed conduction, fibrillation potentials, sharp waves, and reduced interference patterns.

Ulnar Neuropathy at the Elbow

Ulnar neuropathy can result in significant long-term morbidity. The incidence of ulnar neuropathy is probably related to its location on the posterior medial aspect of the elbow because of its course through a confined space and its need for significant excursion to accommodate unrestricted upper extremity motion.

Anatomy

The ulnar nerve is a terminal branch of the medial cord of the brachial plexus. It passes through the upper two thirds of the arm along the anterior aspect of the medial intermuscular septum in close proximity to the median nerve and brachial artery. At the distal third of the arm the nerve pierces the intermuscular septum and passes under the anterior medial edge of the triceps to the medial epicondyle. At the medial epicondyle the nerve passes through the cubital tunnel, which is formed by the cubital tunnel retinaculum joining the medial epicondyle to the olecranon. The floor of the tunnel is the joint capsule and posterior band of the medial collateral ligament. Considerable anatomic variability exists in the cubital tunnel retinaculum, which is sometimes called the arcuate ligament, or Osborne's band. This retinaculum could be absent, fibrous and tight with full elbow flexion, fibrous and tight at 90° to 120° of flexion, or muscular (called the anconeus epitrochlearis). Distal to the cubital tunnel the nerve passes between the ulnar and humeral heads of the pronator teres. Accompanying the nerve throughout its course in the distal arm is a large longitudinal blood vessel. This vessel is supplied by smaller segmental blood vessels at 1- to 2-cm intervals.

The ulnar nerve supplies no branches of clinical significance in the upper arm. The first branch noted is a sensory branch to the elbow joint that usually arises proximal to the medial epicondyle. On occasion, the branch to the flexor carpi ulnaris may arise proximal to the cubital tunnel and course in intimate relationship with the main nerve through the cubital tunnel. In the distal aspect of the cubital tunnel the ulnar nerve gives off two to three branches to the flexor carpi ulnaris, which must be mobilized and carefully protected during the course of anterior transposition of the nerve.

Both the medial brachial cutaneous and antebrachial cutaneous nerves pass through the area of the posterior medial arm and medial epicondyle, respectively, and they are susceptible to iatrogenic trauma during surgical treatment of the ulnar nerve. A neuroma of either of these nerves is a major cause of failure of ulnar nerve surgery and is often very difficult to identify. When a neuroma of the medial brachial cutaneous or antebrachial cutaneous nerve occurs, it may appear as though the pain is arising from the ulnar nerve, when, in fact, it is coming from one of these nerves. The anatomic course of the medial brachial cutaneous and medial antebrachial cutaneous nerves should be carefully protected in the course of ulnar nerve surgery. Injury to the terminal branches of these nerves can best be avoided by moving the surgical incision to a straight posterior incision just medial to the olecranon.

Etiology

The ulnar nerve is subcutaneous and passes between two compartments in the arm. It traverses a very strict path that changes its dimensions with elbow flexion and extension, and it requires a significant amount of excursion to accommodate a full range of motion of the upper extremity. Some of these unique properties are likely responsible for the ulnar nerve being the most commonly injured nerve about the elbow.

The ulnar nerve may be injured by compression, traction, friction, or direct trauma. Compression has been most extensively studied, and alone, or in combination with the other causes, it can produce the clinical entity known as cubital tunnel syndrome. It has been shown that intraneural pressure increases six times over resting levels when the elbow is flexed, wrist extended, and shoulder abducted. With full elbow flexion, the confines of the cubital tunnel become more restrictive and the retinaculum becomes taut and compresses the nerve. The five most common sites of ulnar nerve compression from proximal to distal are the arcade of Struthers, medial intermuscular septum, medial epicondyle, cubital tunnel, and deep flexor pronator aponeurosis (Fig. 1). Primary ulnar nerve compression rarely originates at the arcade of Struthers and the medial intermuscular septum, but these structures are common sites for compression in a failed ulnar nerve transposition. Other less common causes of ulnar nerve compression are cubitus valgus and cubitus varus, which are

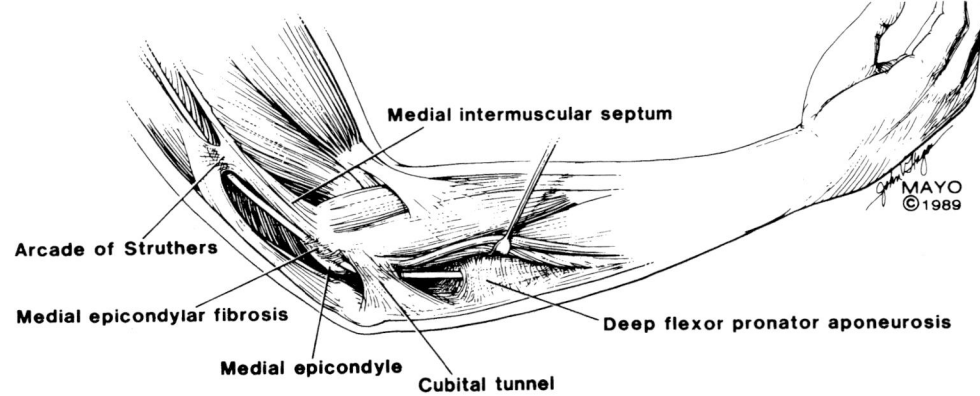

Fig. 1 Schematic drawing of the anatomic sites of ulnar nerve compression. (Reproduced with permission from the Mayo Foundation, Rochester, MN.)

sometimes associated with a hypertrophied subluxating medial head of the triceps—the snapping triceps syndrome.

It has been shown that the ulnar nerve elongates about 5 mm to accommodate upper extremity motion. Tethering of the nerve, which can occur with posttraumatic adhesions, will increase intraneural pressure twofold above normal. The relative role of traction in the pathophysiology of clinical neuropathy is not entirely understood. Clinically, traction becomes a significant cause of ulnar neuropathy, with increasing elbow valgus, and in association with medial collateral ligament insufficiency. Friction as a contributor to ulnar neuritis is seen with subluxation of the ulnar nerve, ossification of the medial collateral ligament, and with other osseous abnormalities along the course of the ulnar nerve. Childress found that subluxation occurs in 16% of ulnar nerves in the normal population. He described two types of subluxation: (1) type A (incomplete, subluxates to the medial epicondyle and is more prone to direct trauma); and (2) type B (complete, more prone to friction neuritis). Medial triceps subluxation must be ruled out in patients with ulnar nerve dislocation.

Direct minimal trauma causes temporary ulnar neuropathy, resulting in fleeting painful dysesthesias. Chronic or severe trauma may result in more profound ulnar nerve pathology. The most common chronic cause is working with the flexed elbow on hard surfaces.

Other significant factors contributing to ulnar neuritis include metabolic elements and the double crush phenomena. The most common metabolic problem seen in association with ulnar neuritis is diabetes. Patients with diabetes are more susceptible to compressive neuropathies. Sites of pathology that can produce symptoms in the ulnar nerve distribution or act in synergy with cubital tunnel syndrome include C8 radiculopathy, thoracic outlet syndrome, and compression of the ulnar nerve in Guyon's canal at the wrist.

Evaluation

Ulnar neuropathy presents with intermittent paresthesias or dysesthesias in the ulnar aspect of the hand and ulnar two digits. This may progress to constant numbness or a feeling of clumsiness and weakness. In the late stages patients will report severe weakness, constant anesthesia, inability to grasp large objects, and atrophy of the hand. A history may reveal that the patient works with the elbow hyperflexed (for example, holding a phone), with the elbow flexed on a hard surface, or has had a direct blow to the ulnar nerve. Throwers are particularly prone to ulnar neuritis. A recurrent history of ulnar nerve symptoms associated with late cocking or the early acceleration phase of throwing should raise the suspicion for ulnar neuritis associated with medial collateral ligament laxity.

A useful and practical grading system for ulnar neuropathy has been established: grade 1 (mild): paresthesias intermittent, positive Tinel's sign, subjective weakness; grade 2 (moderate): paresthesias, measurable weakness, positive Tinel's; and grade 3 (severe): constant paresthesias, weakness, atrophy.

Decreased sensation over the dorsal ulnar hand is a helpful factor in delineating an ulnar nerve injury proximal to Guyon's canal. Provocative tests include the elbow flexion test and elbow flexion with pressure over the ulnar nerve test. The elbow flexion test, with direct pressure applied over the cubital tunnel, appears to be the most sensitive and specific for locating the site of ulnar nerve compression. In advanced cases of ulnar neuropathy, the ulnar two digits (small and ulnar half of the ring) will have dry skin, atrophy of the hypothenar muscles, interossei and, occasionally, flexor carpi ulnaris. In severe cases, the patient may demonstrate clawing of the ulnar two digits (worse in low ulnar nerve palsies) and abduction of the little finger (Wartenberg sign). A positive Froment's sign (flexion of the interphalangeal joint of the thumb while attempting to pinch) is the best initial indication for a significant ulnar neuropathy.

Radiographic evaluation should include an anteroposterior, lateral, and cubital tunnel view. Radiographs may reveal ossification of the medial collateral ligament or ossification in the cubital tunnel. A valgus stress radiograph, anteroposterior radiograph of the elbow with valgus stress looking for medial joint widening, or arthrogram may show evidence of medial collateral ligament insufficiency in throwers. Electrophysiologic studies will be positive in moderate and severe cases but may be normal in patients with mild, intermittent symptoms. A nerve conduction delay of 10 ms or greater across the elbow when compared to the forearm is diagnostic of cubital tunnel syndrome. In more advanced cases, the electromyogram will show fibrillation potentials and sharp waves in ulnar nerve-innervated muscles.

Treatment

Initial treatment of ulnar neuropathy involves avoiding prolonged flexion of the elbow by using an extension splint or heel bow pad. Surgical treatment is initiated if nonsurgical management has failed and the diagnosis of cubital tunnel syndrome is confirmed. There are five main options for surgical treatment of cubital tunnel syndrome. No good randomized prospective study has been performed that clearly identifies one of these surgical options as superior to the other. Therefore, the indications for each are controversial and differ from surgeon to surgeon.

Release is performed by incising the cubital tunnel retinaculum and leaving the ulnar nerve in its normal bed. The advantages of cubital tunnel release are that it is relatively simple to perform; there is minimal need for manipulation of the nerve; there is no disruption of blood supply (vasa nervorum); and the elbow can be mobilized immediately. The disadvantages are the nerve may be left in a poor exposed bed, and more proximal and distal sites of compression are not necessarily addressed. Simple ulnar nerve release is generally reserved for patients with a mild ulnar neuritis who have a good nerve bed. This procedure is contraindicated in severe ulnar neuritis, in the presence of a scarred nerve bed or subluxating ulnar nerve, or when more proximal or distal pathology is suspected.

Medial epicondylectomy also leaves the ulnar nerve in situ. This procedure has many of the advantages of simple release and eliminates the medial epicondyle as a possible source of ulnar nerve compression. Medial epicondylectomy is recommended for mild grades of ulnar neuropathy with a good bed, and it can also be used as a somewhat controversial treatment of the symptomatic subluxating ulnar nerve. Contraindications include ulnar neuritis in throwing athletes because of concern over possible inadvertent injury to the medial collateral ligament. The important anterior band of the medial collateral ligament originates on the middle two thirds of the anterior-inferior surface of the medial epicondyle. Thus, more bone is removed posteriorly than anteriorly.

The remaining three surgical options for treatment of cubital tunnel syndrome involve transposition of the ulnar nerve to an anterior location and extensive mobilization and manipulation of the ulnar nerve. The important technical point is that the nerve is fully mobilized so as to avoid any acute angulation and compression when the elbow is in complete extension. In order to do this, the nerve is released from the arcade of Struthers to the motor branch of the flexor carpi ulnaris, including release of the pronator fascia. The vasa nervorum should be preserved, with ligation of segmental vessels so as to mobilize the vessel with the nerve. Complete resection of the distal medial intermuscular septum should be performed so as not to create a secondary site for compression. The nerve is then transposed anterior to the medial epicondyle. If the nerve is left subcutaneously, a fascial sling, or sutures from subcutaneous fat to the epicondyle, are created to keep it from subluxating posteriorly. If it is placed intramuscularly, a shallow trough is cut into the flexor pronator mass. In submuscular transposition (Learmonth) the entire humeral attachment of the flexor pronator mass is elevated extraperiosteally, with care taken to preserve the medial collateral ligament. The nerve is then transposed deep to the flexor pronator mass.

The advantages of anterior transposition of the ulnar nerve are as follows. The nerve is moved to a more protected anterior position, 2 to 3 cm of length is obtained, and all five potential sites of compression are addressed. The disadvantages of transposition are that a more extensive surgical procedure is required, neural blood supply is disrupted, and the ulnar nerve must be manipulated. No clear advantage has been shown for any of the three transposition procedures over the others. Subcutaneous transposition is recommended after treatment of distal humerus fractures, after total elbow arthroplasty, and after resection of heterotopic ossification because of disruption of the submuscular bed. Submuscular transposition is recommended when the anterior bed is scarred or during revision ulnar nerve surgery.

Results

The results of treatment of ulnar neuropathy are most consistent in mild to moderate grades of neuropathy and less consistent in severe neuropathy. Nonsurgical treatment of mild intermittent ulnar neuropathy has produced good results in 86% and 90% of cases. Good or excellent results were reported in 164 cases of mild ulnar neuropathy treated with simple release. In one study, subcutaneous transposition of the ulnar nerve was compared to in situ release and it was found that transposition gave better results in terms of return of sensation and muscle loss. In another study, there was no difference between anterior submuscular and subcutaneous transposition when compared to in situ release. Kleinman reported 87% good and excellent results in 47 anterior intramuscular transpositions with no reoperations. In a report on the treatment of 235 ulnar nerves treated with in situ release versus anterior subcutaneous or intramuscular transposition, there was an 82% improvement in both groups. Rettig reviewed the results of subcutaneous transposition in athletes with excellent results and return to sport in an average of 12.6 weeks. In Pasque's retrospective review of the results of 50 submuscular transpositions, subjective results were 92% satisfactory and 84% good and excellent. It is readily noted that controversy exists concerning the most appropriate surgical procedure to use in the treatment of cubital tunnel syndrome.

Complications of ulnar neuropathy can be severe. The most common complication associated with the greatest morbidity is persistent severe dysesthesias, which can often be difficult to treat. Other complications include reflex sympathetic dystrophy, hematoma, infection, neuroma of the medial brachial or medial antebrachial cutaneous nerves, persistent sensory deficit, and persistent weakness. Simple ulnar nerve release has been associated with the complication of nerve subluxation. Medial epicondylectomy has the potential complication of ulnar collateral ligament injury. Submuscular transposition has been associated with elbow flexion contractures. This complication can be minimized or negated with early motion.

Even after submuscular transposition has occurred, elbow motion can be initiated immediately because the flexor pronator mass has an extensive ulnar origin and will not migrate distally.

The treatment of recurrent or persistent ulnar neuropathy after previous failed ulnar nerve surgery is very difficult, with persistent significant symptoms reported in as many as two thirds of patients. Poor prognostic indicators for revision ulnar nerve surgery include: patient age older than 50 years, electromyographic evidence of denervation, and previous submuscular transposition. It has been demonstrated that implantable direct nerve electrical stimulation can be helpful, at least temporarily, when combined with a neurolysis.

Median Neuropathy at the Elbow

There are two neuropathies involving the median nerve at the elbow: the anterior interosseous neuropathy, a true motor neuropathy, and the pronator syndrome, which is primarily pain-related.

Anterior Interosseous Neuropathy

The anterior interosseous nerve (AIN) is a branch of the median nerve that separates from the main body of the median nerve just distal to the medial epicondyle. It can be injured by both traumatic and atraumatic causes, and is often a self-limited process.

Anatomy

The median nerve crosses the elbow medial to the brachial artery. It courses distally below the lacertus fibrosus and then penetrates the pronator teres. The AIN runs with the main body of the median nerve as a posterior fascicle at the level of the elbow and then separates from the median nerve at approximately 5 cm distal to the medial epicondyle. In an anatomic study, Beaton demonstrated the variable anatomy of the passage of the median nerve through the pronator teres.

Etiology

AIN neuropathy is of spontaneous onset in one third of cases. It can also be caused by trauma, mild or repetitive. Significant trauma associated with AIN neuropathy includes supracondylar humerus fractures. Anatomic causes of AIN neuropathy include a band in the deep head of the pronator (most common), or a band in the superficial head of the pronator (less common). AIN neuropathies have also been described following both-bone forearm fractures, proximal ulnar fractures, Monteggia fractures, Galeazzi fractures, iatrogenic after open reduction and internal fixation, and after treatment of elbow dislocations. Penetrating lesions, including placement of or cutdowns for intravenous lines and stab or gunshot wounds, are also responsible for AIN injury.

Evaluation

AIN neuropathy initially presents as a transient, painful, aching sensation in the proximal forearm. These complaints may have immediately predated the current complaints of weakness, clumsiness, and inability to pinch. Sensory examination is normal. The typical AIN neuropathy will demonstrate weakness of the flexor pollicis longus and flexor digitorum profundus to the index finger and, to a lesser extent, the long finger. However, atypical presentations can occur, including variability in weakness, ranging from complete paralysis to minor weakness. Pronator quadratus strength is tested by fully flexing the elbow and comparing pronation strength to the opposite side. Full flexion of the elbow removes the contribution of the pronator teres to pronation strength.

A tendon rupture can be differentiated from a partial AIN neuropathy by the tenodesis effect of wrist motion on finger position. With wrist extension and intact profundus and flexor pollicis longus tendons, the fingertips will flex in response to wrist extension; this mechanism will not occur with a tendon disruption in a relaxed hand.

Electromyographic evaluation after 3 weeks from the time of injury is confirmatory and will demonstrate fibrillation potentials and sharp waves in the affected muscles.

Treatment

Treatment of penetrating injuries in the antecubital fossa associated with AIN should include early exploration and repair. An exception is gunshot wounds; observation for a period of 3 months is indicated unless there are other reasons for open evaluation, such as a vascular repair.

Treatment of AIN secondary to a traction injury is nonsurgical. Complete recovery in the majority of patients is expected to occur in 3 to 4 months.

Treatment of AIN neuropathy occurring spontaneously or as a result of minimal trauma is controversial. Treatment recommendations have varied from early surgical intervention to nonsurgical treatment only. A 2- to 3-month period of observation is currently favored. Nonsurgical treatment includes rest, avoidance of stressful pronation of the elbow, and splint immobilization in 90° of flexion and neutral rotation. Surgical exploration is indicated if no recovery of function has occurred in 3 months.

Exploration should include an anterior incision and release of the lacertus fibrosus. Any vascular leash crossing the AIN is released as are any fibrous bands in the deep and superficial heads of the pronator. The pronator teres should not be completely released because the patient already has some weakness in pronation and complete release may further exacerbate this weakness. The distal path of the AIN through the flexor digitorum superficialis should be evaluated all the way to the interosseous membrane.

In the rare late cases that have not responded to observation, nonsurgical management, or surgical management, a tendon transfer of the brachioradialis to the flexor pollicis longus and side-to-side repair of the flexor digitorum profundus of the index and long fingers to the flexor digitorum profundus of the ring and small fingers are indicated.

Results

The reported treatment outcome of AIN neuropathy both nonsurgically or surgically has been good. Schantz reported on the surgical treatment of 15 patients with AIN; 11 showed satisfactory recovery and three required tendon transfers. Treatment outcome has been satisfactory in some isolated cases of exploration of AIN of several years' duration. Complications include a persistent AIN neuropathy, unsightly anterior elbow scar, and injury to the lateral antebrachial cutaneous nerve.

Pronator Syndrome

Pronator syndrome is a pain-mediated neuropathy involving the median nerve at the level of the elbow. It is a distant second to carpal tunnel syndrome as a cause of median neuropathy. In rare situations it may occur in conjunction with carpal tunnel syndrome.

Anatomy

The anatomy of the median nerve has been well described with the discussion of AIN neuropathy. The pronator teres syndrome, however, may have a compressive lesion more proximal than those associated with AIN neuropathy. The presence of a supracondylar process and ligament of Struthers may cause compression of the median nerve just proximal to the elbow.

Etiology

The causes of pronator teres syndrome are considered to be compressive in nature. The locations of compressive lesions to be considered from proximal to distal are: ligament of Struthers, lacertus fibrosus, fibrous band of the pronator teres and, finally, fibrous band in the flexor digitorum superficialis (Fig. 2).

Evaluation

Pronator syndrome presents as a dull, aching pain in the proximal anterior forearm that may radiate down to the volar wrist and occasionally radiate proximally. Dysesthesias in the radial three and a half digits and complaints of weakness and clumsiness may also be noted. History may reveal a direct blow to the forearm, repetitive trauma, or, in a majority of cases, no known cause. Pronator syndrome is four times more common in women than men and usually occurs in the fifth decade of life.

Physical findings include tenderness over the proximal edge of the pronator teres, a positive median nerve compression test at the elbow that reproduces the patient's symptoms, a Tinel's sign over the nerve at the elbow and reproduction of symptoms with resisted pronation (pronator teres as the culprit) or, less commonly, with supination (lacertus fibrosus as the culprit). Manual muscle testing may demonstrate some mild weakness, but gross weakness as seen with AIN neuropathy does not occur. Pronator syndrome may also be dynamic in character and only occur with activity, particularly with resisted repetitive pronation. Objective sensory evaluation is normal. Electrophysiologic testing is seldom helpful in diagnosing pronator syndrome.

Treatment

Initial treatment of pronator syndrome is rest, avoidance of precipitating activities, anti-inflammatory medication, splinting with the elbow in 90° of flexion and neutral rotation. Surgical intervention will require the same approach made to the AIN release with the exception that if a supracondylar process is present, the dissection should extend proximally in order to release the ligament of Struthers.

Postoperative management includes immobilization in flexion and neutral rotation until the skin is healed. Early motion can be initiated after suture removal. Once full active and passive range of motion has been obtained, a graduated resisted strengthening program is started.

Results

The majority of patients will respond to nonsurgical treatment. Hartz reported on six failures in 39 patients treated surgically. The results of surgical treatment in patients involved with workers' compensation and litigation have not been consistent. Patients with significant dysesthesias will note

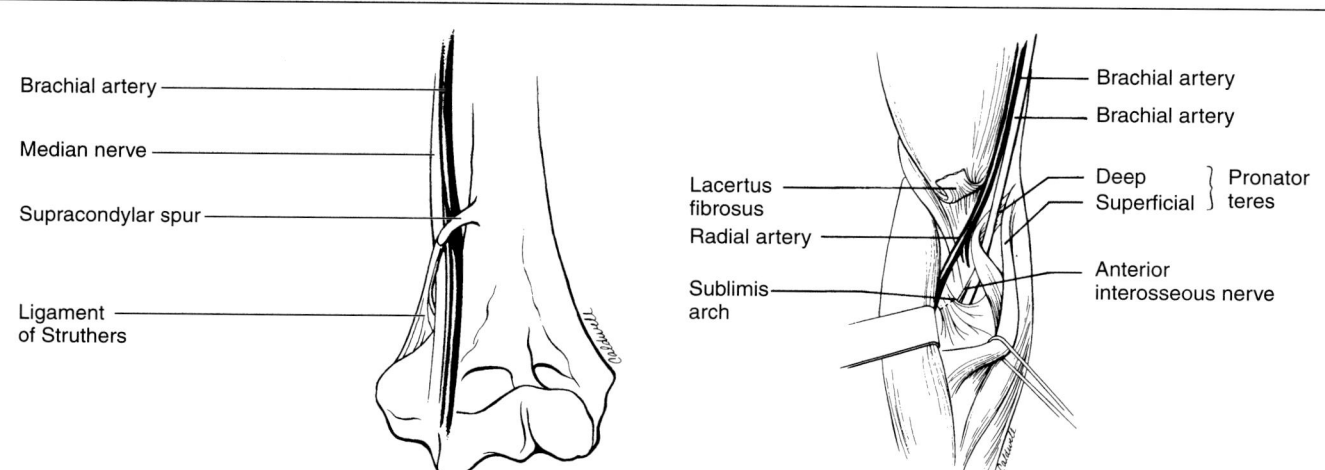

Fig. 2 Left, Schematic drawing showing a supracondylar process and the ligament of Struthers. **Right,** Schematic drawing demonstrating potential sites of median nerve compression at the elbow. (Reproduced with permission from Gelberman RH (ed): *Operative Nerve Repair and Reconstruction.* New York, NY, JB Lippincott, vol 2, 1991.)

improvement in the immediate perioperative period. The soreness in the proximal forearm resolves over a period of 1 to 3 months and complete recovery occurs in approximately 3 to 4 months.

Complications of treatment of pronator syndrome include persistence of pain, missed diagnosis, significant anterior elbow scar, and lateral antebrachial cutaneous neuritis. There are few good objective tests for pronator syndrome, which may result in an increased incidence of missed diagnosis. Missing a diagnosis of an associated carpal tunnel syndrome is another reason for failure.

Radial Nerve Neuropathy at the Elbow

There are two neuropathies involving the radial nerve or, more precisely, the posterior interosseous branch of the radial nerve at the elbow. The posterior interosseous nerve (PIN) syndrome is a motor neuropathy whereas the radial tunnel syndrome is pain-mediated.

Posterior Interosseous Neuropathy

Anatomy
The radial nerve, a terminal branch of the posterior cord of the brachial plexus, extends down the arm, wrapping around the posterior aspect of the humerus in the spiral groove. It then penetrates the lateral intermuscular septum in the distal one third of the arm. At this level the radial nerve extends distally between the brachioradialis and the brachialis. It will give motor branches in this area to the brachioradialis, and later the extensor carpi radialis longus (ECRL). At the level just proximal to the elbow, the nerve branches into two main nerves, the radial sensory nerve and the PIN. The radial sensory nerve then progresses distally deep to the brachioradialis, penetrating the forearm fascia in the distal third of the forearm between the brachioradialis and the ECRL. Pathology of the radial sensory nerve occurs predominantly in the distal third of the forearm and will not be discussed here. In pathologic states the PIN may be compressed by the leading edge of the extensor carpi radialis brevis (ECRB), a vascular leash of Henry, or, most commonly, the proximal edge of the supinator called the arcade of Frohse. There have been fibrous bands described in the supinator itself as well as its distal edge that may compress the PIN. The PIN at the distal end of the supinator branches extensively and is called the cauda equina.

Etiology
PIN neuropathy may occur after a direct traumatic event or secondary to a slow chronic compressive process. Traumatic causes of PIN neuropathy include a direct blow to the lateral aspect of the forearm, Monteggia fractures with anterior dislocation of the radial head, supracondylar humerus fractures, and iatrogenic causes. The PIN has been injured in treatment of radial head fractures, radial head excision, proximal radius fractures, and during elbow arthroscopy because of its close proximity to the radiocapitellar joint. The injury may result from a direct laceration or, more commonly, from traction or compression with a retractor. The PIN can be moved away from the elbow joint and the radial head by flexion and pronation. Supination moves the PIN closer to the radiocapitellar joint. The risk of PIN injury during elbow arthroscopy is decreased if the elbow capsule is insufflated and the elbow flexed to 80° to 90°. Chronic compressive causes of PIN neuropathy include radiocapitellar synovitis, ganglion, and lipoma.

Evaluation
Pain is variably present in the proximal dorsal forearm and may radiate to the wrist. The patient will demonstrate weakness or paralysis of the finger, thumb, and wrist extensors. Wrist extension may be possible but only with radial deviation. Sensory evaluation is normal. Tenderness over the proximal radial forearm, particularly at the leading edge of the supinator, is common.

In patients with inflammatory arthropathy, the PIN neuropathy must be differentiated from extensor tendon ruptures. The radiocapitellar joint and proximal forearm should be evaluated for a joint effusion or a mass, respectively. In these patients, radiographic workup will show the presence of an intra-articular process, including inflammatory arthritis. If a soft-tissue mass is anticipated or suspected, an MRI scan will confirm the diagnosis and identify it as a lipoma or ganglion. Electromyograms show denervation of the involved muscles.

Treatment
Treatment of PIN neuropathy secondary to a traction injury is nonsurgical; observation is recommended. The majority of these neuropathies will recover completely, first wrist extension, followed by finger extension, and finally, thumb extension. If at 3 months there is no evidence of wrist extension, surgical exploration should be performed.

Nonsurgical management of PIN includes rest, anti-inflammatory medication, and use of a long arm splint in supination and elbow flexion.

Treatment of sharp penetrating trauma, including iatrogenic causes, includes surgical exploration with repair of PIN versus nerve grafting. If the nerve was well visualized during the original surgical intervention, and was protected, then expectant management secondary to the traction injury will reveal good results.

In PIN neuropathy secondary to a compressive lesion in the area of the radiocapitellar joint, excision of this lesion and release of the PIN is indicated. In the case of rheumatoid arthritis, synovectomy (with or without radial head excision) is the treatment of choice.

The PIN can be approached from three main directions. The anterior approach develops the interval between the pronator teres and the brachioradialis. The transbrachioradialis route approaches the PIN straight anterolaterally. The dorsal approach of Thompson uses the interval between the extensor digitorum and the ECRB. The approach to the PIN is predicated on the etiology of the neuropathy and the surgeon's choice. Complete release of the nerve from proximal to distal starts at the radiocapitellar joint with release of any fibrous bands at the radiocapitellar joint, evaluation of the ECRB for any compression from its fibrous leading edge, and release of vascular leash of Henry, followed by release of the arcade of Frohse. Some surgeons will recommend complete release of the supinator all the way to its distal end.

If chronic PIN persists despite surgical management, the motor deficits can be salvaged with tendon transfers. The most common set of tendon transfers are the palmaris longus to a rerouted extensor pollicis longus, flexor carpi radialis to the extensor digitorum communis, and the pronator teres to the ECRB. If wrist extension is adequate, transfer of the pronator teres is not necessary.

Results

Kaplan reported satisfactory recovery of PIN neuropathy with nonsurgical treatment. The results of nonsurgical management of PIN nerve traction injuries are excellent with a majority experiencing no long-term sequelae. Complete recovery may take longer than 6 months, but recovery of wrist extension should be apparent within 3 months. The results of surgical management of PIN neuropathy, particularly if secondary to a known compressive lesion such as a ganglion, are also good except in situations in which there is a compressive lesion distal to the supinator where the nerve arborizes. Results of repair of a complete nerve laceration are good, because this is a pure motor nerve. If reinnervation does not occur, tendon transfers have a predictable excellent result.

Complications of PIN neuropathy include persistence of the neuropathy, or even progression of the neuropathy despite both surgical and nonsurgical management. Injuries at the distal end of the supinator have a particularly poor prognosis.

Radial Tunnel Syndrome

Radial tunnel syndrome, in contrast to PIN neuropathy, is a pain-mediated neuropathy.

Etiology

Radial tunnel syndrome is believed to be caused by compression of the PIN. This condition, which may be secondary to direct trauma or, more commonly, secondary to minor repetitive trauma, is often associated with lateral epicondylitis. The most common anatomic site of compression of the radial tunnel is the arcade of Frohse. Compressive sites from proximal to distal are: fibrous bands adjacent to the radiocapitellar joint, vascular leash of Henry, leading edge of the ECRB, arcade of Frohse (proximal edge of the supinator), and distal edge of the supinator (Fig. 3).

Evaluation

The history reveals a constant aching sensation of insidious onset in the dorsal radial aspect of the forearm. Direct or repetitive trauma may be the initiating event. The coexistence of lateral epicondylitis is extremely common. Repetitive supination will exacerbate the symptoms.

Physical findings include pain with resisted long finger extension and resisted supination, and tenderness over the course of the PIN in the supinator. Tenderness over the lateral epicondyle will be present if there is coexistent lateral epicondylitis. Sensory examination is normal. Weakness is secondary to pain and not the result of a motor neuropathy.

Electrodiagnostic studies are equivocal. There is no objective diagnostic test that can in itself confirm the presence of radial tunnel syndrome.

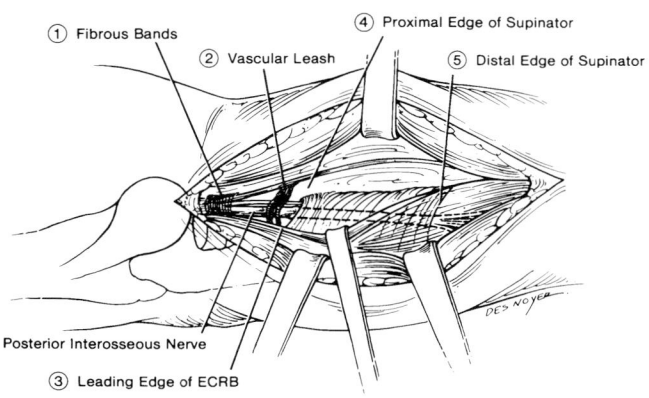

Fig. 3 Schematic drawing demonstrating the potential sites of neural compression of the posterior interosseous nerve. ECRB = extensor carpi radialis brevis. (Reproduced with permission from Gelberman RH (ed): *Operative Nerve Repair and Reconstruction*. New York, NY, JB Lippincott, vol 2, 1991.)

Treatment

Treatment of radial tunnel syndrome includes rest, avoidance of provocative activities, anti-inflammatory medication, supination splinting (elbow in 90° flexion and supination) and aggressive treatment of the lateral epicondylitis if present. The use of a counterforce brace in the treatment of lateral epicondylitis may exacerbate radial tunnel syndrome. Surgical management of radial tunnel syndrome is controversial. The same surgical approach as described for decompression of the PIN for neuropathy is used. Postoperative management of radial tunnel syndrome involves a compressive dressing and early motion after removal of sutures.

Results

Acute radial tunnel syndrome will usually respond to nonsurgical treatment. The results of surgical treatment for radial tunnel syndrome are mixed. In a series of 30 cases treated surgically, 70% good and excellent results were reported. Atroshi reported complications in 12 of 37 radial tunnel cases and believed that surgical decompression was very unreliable. Results of patients involved in workers' compensation claims have not been consistent. Full recovery takes up to 1 year.

Complications of treatment of radial tunnel syndrome are failed diagnosis (no objective tests to confirm the diagnosis), persistent or increased pain after surgical treatment, and a radial sensory neuritis. The anterior approach of Henry leaves an unsightly scar and can be complicated by a lateral antebrachial cutaneous neuritis.

Lateral Antebrachial Cutaneous Nerve

The lateral antebrachial cutaneous nerve is the terminal branch of the musculocutaneous nerve and is rarely injured. It exits below and lateral to the biceps tendon approximately

1 cm proximal to the elbow flexion crease. The lateral antebrachial cutaneous nerve gives sensation to the distal lateral aspect of the forearm and hand and has extensive overlap with the radial sensory nerve.

Entrapment neuropathy of the lateral antebrachial cutaneous nerve is exceedingly rare. The nerve, however, is at risk for injury during anterior approaches to the elbow and should be carefully protected during anterior approaches to the radial head, capsular releases, pronator release, and repair of distal biceps tendon ruptures.

Pediatric Supracondylar Elbow Fractures

Neurologic injury in association with displaced supracondylar humerus fractures is relatively common, occurring in 7% to 15% of patients studied. The radial and ulnar nerves were almost equally involved, with the median nerve being somewhat less frequently involved. The AIN with preservation of the rest of the median nerve can be injured because it is relatively tethered. In a study of 15 nerve injuries after supracondylar elbow fracture, 13 of these involved the AIN. Neurologic injury most often occurs from the initial injury but can occur with repeated forceful manipulations. A significant iatrogenic cause of ulnar nerve injury is nerve penetration from a medial percutaneous pin. This complication can be avoided if a small wound is created over the medial epicondyle with blunt dissection carried down to periosteum and use of a drill guide.

Nerve injuries associated with supracondylar fractures are invariably stretch injuries; most are neurapraxia lesions with an occasional axonotmetic injury. Observation is the recommended treatment. Indications for early or immediate open exploration include: inability to obtain an adequate reduction with known neurologic injury (nerve possibly interposed in fracture site), vascular injury requiring repair in association with a neurologic injury, and neurologic injury secondary to possible percutaneous pin insult. A neurologic deficit secondary to compartment syndrome is a significant complication that must be treated immediately with forearm fasciotomy.

Selected Bibliography

Atroshi I, Johnsson R, Ornstein E: Radial tunnel release: Unpredictable outcome in 37 consecutive cases with a 1-5 year follow-up. *Acta Orthop Scand* 1995;66:255-257.

According to this study, the symptoms and signs used as diagnostic criteria for radial tunnel syndrome may be unreliable and the results of posterior interosseous nerve decompression unpredictable.

Brown IC, Zinar DM: Traumatic and iatrogenic neurological complications after supracondylar humerus fractures in children. *J Pediatr Orthop* 1995;15:440-443.

In this retrospective review of 162 displaced supracondylar fractures, there were 23 neural injuries. Fifty-eight percent of these injuries were associated with a Holmberg type III fracture pattern and 42% with a type IV supracondylar fracture pattern. All of the injuries had resolved within 2 to 6 months.

Childress HM: Recurrent ulnar-nerve dislocation at the elbow. *Clin Orthop* 1975;108:168-170.

Cramer KE, Green NE, Devito DP: Incidence of anterior interosseous nerve palsy in supracondylar humerus fractures in children. *J Pediatr Orthop* 1993;13:502-505.

In a retrospective review of 101 supracondylar humerus fractures, there were 15 patients with neural lesions. Six of these lesions were isolated anterior interosseous nerve palsies, and four were anterior interosseous nerve injuries combined with another nerve injury.

Dahlin LB, Shyu BC, Danielsen N, et al: Effects of nerve compression or ischaemia on conduction properties of myelinated and non-myelinated nerve fibres: An experimental study in the rabbit common peroneal nerve. *Acta Physiol Scand* 1989;136:97-105.

Fardin P, Negrin P, Sparta S, et al: Posterior interosseous nerve neuropathy: Clinical and electromyographical aspects. *Electromyogr Clin Neurophysiol* 1992;32:229-234.

In 37 patients with posterior interosseous nerve neuropathy, origin was traumatic in five, iatrogenic in four, and nontraumatic in 28. In the nontraumatic cases with marked deficit, surgery gave the best results.

Hartz CR, Linscheid RL, Gramse RR, et al: The pronator teres syndrome: Compressive neuropathy of the median nerve. *J Bone Joint Surg* 1981;63A:885-890.

Johnson RK, Spinner M: Median nerve compression in the forearm: The pronator tunnel syndrome, in Szabo RM (ed): *Nerve Compression Syndromes: Diagnosis and Treatment.* Thorofare, NJ, Slack, 1989, pp 137-151.

Kaplan PE: Posterior interosseous neuropathies: Natural history. *Arch Phys Med Rehabil* 1984;65:399-400.

Kleinman WB, Bishop AT: Anterior intramuscular transposition of the ulnar nerve. *J Hand Surg* 1989;14A:972-979.

Lake PA: Anterior interosseous nerve syndrome. *J Neurosurg* 1974;41:306-309.

Lawrence T, Mobbs P, Fortems Y, et al: Radial tunnel syndrome: A retrospective review of 30 decompressions of the radial nerve. *J Hand Surg* 1995;20B:454-459.

In this report on 30 cases of release of the posterior interosseous nerve for radial tunnel syndrome, 70% of patients had good or excellent results; 13%, fair; and 17%, poor.

Nathan PA, Keniston RC, Meadows KD: Outcome study of ulnar nerve compression at the elbow treated with simple decompression and an early programme of physical therapy. *J Hand Surg* 1995;20B:628-637.

One hundred thirty-one patients underwent a simple release of the ulnar nerve at the elbow for mild or moderate cubital tunnel syndrome. Eighty-nine percent of these patients had good or excellent postoperative results. At an average of 4.3 years follow-up, 79% had good or excellent results.

Nemoto K, Matsumoto N, Tazaki K, et al: An experimental study on the "double crush" hypothesis. *J Hand Surg* 1987;12A:552-559.

Ogata K, Naito M: Blood flow of peripheral nerve: Effects of dissection, stretching and compression. *J Hand Surg* 1986;11B:10-14.

Pasque CB, Rayan GM: Anterior submuscular transposition of the ulnar nerve for cubital tunnel syndrome. *J Hand Surg* 1995;20B:447-453.

Forty-eight patients with cubital tunnel syndrome were treated with submuscular transposition of the ulnar nerve using a Z-lengthening of the flexor pronator mass. Eighty-four percent had excellent or good postoperative grades. Ninety-two percent were satisfied, or satisfied with some reservations.

Rettig AC, Ebben JR: Anterior subcutaneous transfer of the ulnar nerve in the athlete. *Am J Sports Med* 1993;21:836-839.

According to this article, anterior subcutaneous subfascial transfer of the ulnar nerve is a safe and effective way to treat cubital tunnel syndrome in athletes.

Rydevik B, Lundborg G, Bagge U: Effects of graded compression on intraneural blood flow: An in vivo study on rabbit tibial nerve. *J Hand Surg* 1981;6A:3-12.

Schantz K, Riegels-Nielsen P: The anterior interosseous nerve syndrome. *J Hand Surg* 1992;17B:510-512.

Verhaar J, Spaans F: Radial tunnel syndrome: An investigation of compression neuropathy as a possible cause. *J Bone Joint Surg* 1992;74A:539-544.

The data presented in this article do not support the hypothesis that signs and symptoms in most patients with radial tunnel syndrome are caused by compression of the posterior interosseous nerve.

41

Elbow Arthritis

Bernard F. Morrey, MD and Shawn W. O'Driscoll, MD, PhD, FRCSC

The three major types of arthritis that involve the elbow are, in order of frequency, rheumatoid, posttraumatic, and osteoarthritis. Although pain is the common complaint, patients with each type of elbow arthritis may experience stiffness, weakness, or instability. Because each of the three types has distinct characteristics and an array of treatment options with varying indications and expectations, they will be discussed in turn.

Rheumatoid Arthritis

An isolated presentation of rheumatoid arthritis of the elbow is uncommon and in our experience occurs in only about 5% of the patient population; approximately 90% of patients will have hand and wrist involvement, and another 80% will have involvement of the shoulder. However, rheumatoid arthritis affecting the elbow results in painful impairment of function that for years has been overlooked or minimized because of a general lack of awareness regarding treatment options and results. Patients who have had bilateral elbow involvement for an extended period of time on occasion do not realize the severity of their disability on the less involved joint until they have had one elbow replaced. These patients commonly request surgery on the contralateral side within a few months. The pattern of involvement of the elbow is similar to that of other joints, though significant loss of bone stock and periarticular soft-tissue damage can cause the elbow to become flail, with as much motion in the coronal as the sagittal plane.

Evaluation

The assessment must include the ipsilateral hand, wrist, and shoulder. However, it is important to recognize that the assumption that shoulder motion compensates for loss of elbow flexion and extension is invalid. Ball-and-socket and hinge motions are not complementary, as was recently demonstrated in a controlled experiment simulating function with such constraints. Using the analogy of the hand reaching into a sphere centered around the shoulder, the purpose of the elbow is to place the hand *within* that sphere, whereas the purpose of the shoulder is to place the hand *on the surface* of the sphere. The preoperative arc of motion is closely related to that obtained after surgery, so a stiff elbow will have less motion in the postoperative state as well. The only radiographs that are essential are the anteroposterior and lateral views of the elbow. If shoulder symptoms are apparent, these should be radiographically assessed and a shorter stemmed implant may be selected.

The radiographic presentation has four distinct stages: stage 1, normal radiograph, with the possibility of osteoporosis with active synovitis; stage 2, symmetric joint narrowing, normal architecture; stage 3, distinct alteration of subchondral architecture that may be relatively mild (type A) or extensive (type B); and finally, stage 4, gross destruction of most or all of the articular architecture. This stage is characterized clinically by instability and, sometimes, severe extensive pain.

Nonsurgical Treatment

The nonsurgical management of elbow arthritis includes the standard medical treatment and physical therapy for most other joints. Acetylsalicylic acid or nonsteroidal anti-inflammatory drugs are used unless precluded by gastrointestinal side effects. Other more potent agents, including antimalarials, gold salts, immunosuppressive drugs, and corticosteroids, are employed when necessary. Intra-articular injections of corticosteroids are easily performed and should be considered before surgery. Physical therapy includes pain control measures such as avoidance of activities that place excessive stresses on the elbow, intermittent periods of rest, and application of heat or cold. Also, splinting is sometimes useful. Lightweight hinged splints that permit active range of motion protect the elbow from varus-valgus stresses and minimize pain. Resting or night splints also can be helpful. Gentle exercises should be performed regularly to maintain mobility and strength in the muscles. Occupational therapy interventions with aids for activities of daily living are useful, including handle extensions to cope with elbow flexion contractures.

Surgical Treatment

Three viable surgical treatments for rheumatoid arthritis of the elbow are synovectomy, interposition arthroplasty, and joint replacement. The stage of the disease, age of the patient, and presence of other joint involvement are important determinants of treatment choice.

Synovectomy Not much has been published in the current literature regarding elbow synovectomy, although synovectomy with or without radial head excision is historically a well-recognized and accepted form of treatment for rheumatoid arthritis. Several fairly recent reports have helped provide some perspective. Arthrotomy and radial head excision may be effective for over 10 years in up to 80% of patients. Pain relief is common, but recurrences increase after 5 years. This treatment should be avoided in those with elbow instability (stage 3 or 4). There is controversy regarding the success of synovectomy in later stages after joint destruction has occurred. Also unclear is the role of radial head excision. Progressive articular destruction following synovectomy and radial head excision has been noted and is thought to be caused by increased ulnohumeral loading after radial head excision. Late valgus instability has been a problem in the experience of some surgeons. Performing a complete synovectomy arthroscopically without causing neurovascular

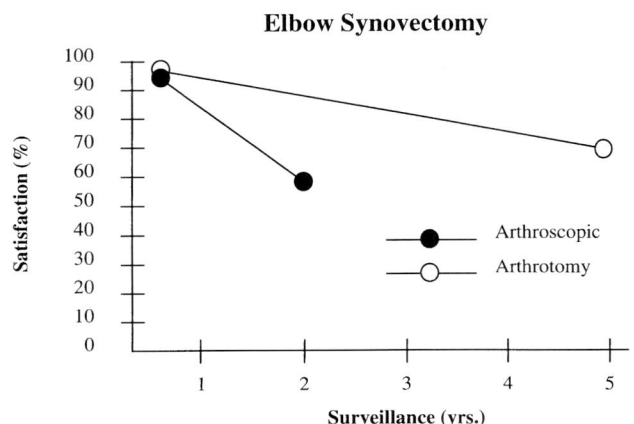

Fig. 1 The 2- and 5-year results of synovectomy carried out arthroscopically and by arthrotomy, respectively.

injury is a highly demanding procedure and, therefore, cumulative experience with it is still quite limited. One study of 14 arthroscopic synovectomies revealed an early success rate of 95%; however, at 3 years only approximately 60% were still considered satisfactory (Fig. 1). Hence, further data are required to define the role of arthroscopic synovectomy and to determine whether or not it is as effective as the open procedure. In general, surgeons experienced in both total elbow arthroplasty and synovectomy favor the former over synovectomy in the later stages of arthritis because of greater patient satisfaction and long-term functional improvement.

Interposition Arthroplasty There has been only a single report in the recent literature regarding interposition arthroplasty for rheumatoid involvement of the elbow. After a median follow-up of 6 years with 28 procedures from 1985 through 1991, 21 of the 28 patients (75%) experienced no or slight pain. Yet, the radiographs clearly demonstrated progression of the arthritis. These authors concluded that neither pain relief nor improved function are as satisfactory with interposition arthroplasty as with elbow joint replacement. Elbow joint replacement is recommended as the treatment of choice.

Joint Replacement Arthroplasty Advanced rheumatoid arthritis has emerged as the best indication for total elbow arthroplasty. Population statistics suggest that the utilization rate for total elbow arthroplasty is about 0.8 per 100,000 person-years, based on data from Olmstead County, Rochester, MN. These statistics are likely related to improvements in reliability and outcome. In fact, studies show that using linked or unlinked designs, the elbow can be treated as reliably with joint replacement for rheumatoid arthritis as can the hip or knee. There are two types of prosthetic joint designs in current use: unlinked (typically referred to as "unconstrained") surface replacements, and linked ("semiconstrained"). Some linked prostheses, such as the Coonrad-Morrey, are permanently linked so that they cannot dislocate, whereas others, such as the triaxial, snap together and can dislocate.

In several countries, reports discussing unlinked surface replacements have been encouraging. Of 34 consecutive Souter-Strathclyde procedures, approximately 85% were satisfactory, according to a European study. Three patients underwent revision because of instability, one because of loosening, and one because of infection. In the United States, the most definitive data are those reported by Ewald on the capitellar condylar design. Experience with 202 procedures with a mean follow-up of almost 6 years reveals a functional arc from 30° to 135° with 65° of supination and 70° of pronation. There was evidence of radiographic loosening in 4% of the humeral and 10% of the ulnar components, but few revisions. An uncemented option has been used in Japan in 32 elbows, with satisfactory results in 85%. Although it is a popular implant, the capitellar condylar design does require reasonable bone stock and ligamentous integrity for successful outcome. The insertion of unlinked implants can also be very challenging and tedious, requiring exact positioning and proper attention to the soft tissues. Instability (dislocation, subluxation, or maltracking) has been reported in 5% to 20% of unlinked total elbow arthroplasties, particularly in cases in which bone or soft-tissue destruction or loss is significant.

There was an initial trend to simply replace the articular surfaces of the distal humerus and proximal ulna, but these components without intramedullary stems had a tendency for loosening and displacement. Kudo reported five of 37 humeral implant displacements in a stemless design. The majority of components now available have intramedullary stems, which help prevent the rocking or tilting motion that causes loosening.

A number of linked semiconstrained sloppy-hinge prostheses allow for a degree of laxity that permits the soft tissues to absorb some of the stresses that would normally be applied to the prosthesis-bone interface. Though this design might theoretically be more likely to loosen than a minimally constrained design, this scenario has not yet been borne out in clinical experience. Over a 14-year period from 1978 to 1992 in Europe, 118 of 144 linked implants were placed in patients with rheumatoid arthritis. At an average follow-up of approximately 4.0 years, only 10 of the 118 patients required revision. These authors do, however, emphasize that the patient with rheumatoid arthritis is a more appropriate candidate for the procedure compared to those with posttraumatic afflictions. Similarly, in the United States, after 113 consecutive cases using the triaxial implant, a satisfactory result in 90% of patients has been reported after 5 years. On the other hand, in the same study, only 53% of patients with a posttraumatic condition were considered to have a satisfactory result. Using the Coonrad-Morrey total elbow arthroplasty, 91% of 58 consecutive patients with rheumatoid arthritis had a satisfactory result at a mean follow-up of approximately 4 years. No patient had undergone revision for loosening (Fig. 2). Thus, some consider a semiconstrained arthroplasty to be indicated in any patient requiring elbow replacement surgery. Other surgeons continue to employ minimally constrained types, especially for young patients.

It may be concluded that joint replacement arthroplasty has proved to be a successful option for the patient with rheumatoid arthritis, not only in this country but also in Europe and Asia. Depending on the degree of osseous and ligamentous

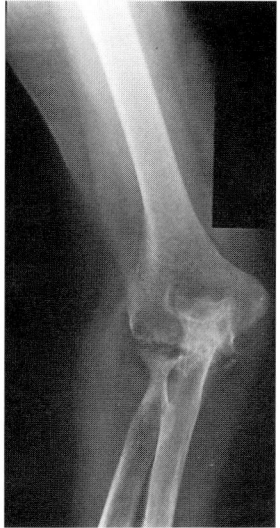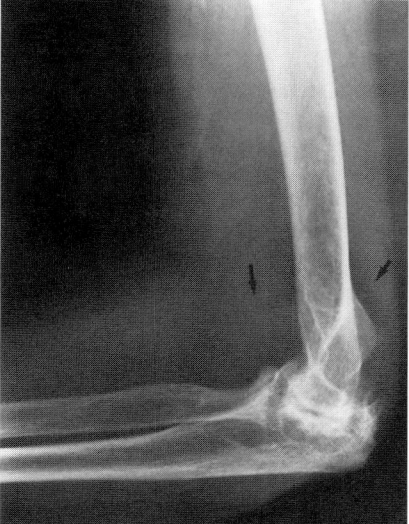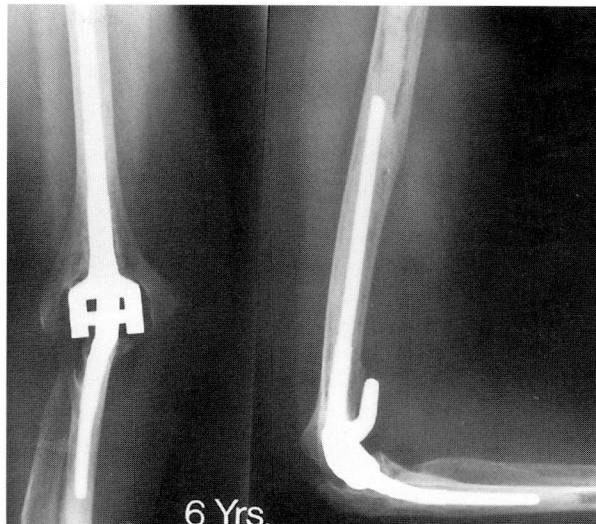

Fig. 2 **Left and center,** Type III rheumatoid involvement of the elbow. **Right,** Six-year satisfactory result following replacement.

integrity, either an unlinked resurfacing or a linked semiconstrained implant may be effective in experienced hands. The complication rate has decreased over the years.

An exhaustive analysis of the literature reporting the prior experience with complications after total elbow arthroplasty was recently presented. In this review, it was determined that from 1986 to 1992, 828 implants had an overall complication rate of 43% and a revision rate of 18%. This study did not include the more recent experience noted above. Still, the most common complications continue to include instability in patients with unlinked implants. Permanent ulnar nerve sensory damage also continues to be reported in 1% to 3%. These two problems underscore the need for surgical experience, as well as a proven implant design, when offering joint replacement for this patient population. Infection also continues to be a major problem for both designs, with rates of 2% to 5%. Loosening, however, is an uncommon complication in elbow joint replacement today with the newer semiconstrained and more established resurfacing implants.

Summary

Patients with rheumatoid arthritis are well managed today with disease-remitting agents such as chloroquine methotrexate, and D-penicillamine. If this treatment is unsuccessful, synovectomy is still considered a viable option, though arthroscopic techniques are yet to be of proven long-term value. Interposition arthroplasty is not considered a viable option except in select patients because of the unpredictability of pain relief and inferior functional result compared to prosthetic replacement. That both semiconstrained and resurfacing elbow joint replacements have a low loosening rate is particularly encouraging. In fact, data suggest that a patient with rheumatoid arthritis may be offered elbow joint replacement arthroplasty with approximately the same degree of confidence as a replacement of the hip and/or the knee for medium-term success. The long-term success rate will require continued follow-up studies.

Posttraumatic Arthritis

Posttraumatic arthritis at the elbow may present with the following symptoms: stiffness, pain, nonunion, or a combination of these. Treatment is dictated by the pathology, complaints, and age of the patient as discussed below.

As has been implied above, until recently, joint replacement arthroplasty has not provided a favorable experience in the management of patients with posttraumatic arthritis. In a European report, a complication rate of only 11% in patients with rheumatoid arthritis was in contrast to 34% in those with posttraumatic arthritis with the same surgeons using the same implant. The revision rate in patients with rheumatoid arthritis was only 8% compared to 31% in the posttraumatic group. Similarly, a report from New York indicates the 5-year survival rate using a semiconstrained implant in posttraumatic patients was only 53%. Experience with the Coonrad-Morrey total elbow replacement has recently been updated with 41 consecutive patients from 1981 through 1994 all receiving the same implant. Using the Mayo Elbow Performance Score (MEPS), 83% had a satisfactory result with a mean follow-up of almost 6 years. Subjectively, over 90% considered themselves improved following joint replacement. The most common problem was ulnar component fracture (10%) caused by increased use that came about largely because of the near-complete pain relief and functional restoration experienced after the joint replacement arthroplasty.

The major problems occur in patients with intra-articular pathology. In this setting, if the patient is younger than 60 years of age, an interposition arthroplasty is the treatment of choice. If this is performed, the elbow is often protected with some form of an external fixator that allows motion while the soft tissues are healing. The external fixation may be in the form of the Dynamic Joint Distractor™ (Rutherford, NJ) or the Compass Hinge.™ Experience with the distraction arthroplasty for posttraumatic stiffness reveals a mean arc of motion improvement of about 60°. Preoperatively the arc of motion averaged 60° to 90°. After surgery the arc of 30° to 120° was attained in a reliable and consistent fashion. The distraction arthroplasty is useful for patients with stiffness but less so for those with pain but good motion. There have been no reports in the recent literature of interposition arthroplasty for a painful but functional arc of motion. In fact, virtually all data on interposition arthroplasty are for patients with rheumatoid arthritis.

Joint replacement is emerging as a viable treatment option for some comminuted acute fractures and nonunions in the elderly, and in certain cases of ankylosis.

Complications
Typical complications include wound drainage and deep infection. Inadequate release or unattained goals occur in 10%. Hence, some form of surgical intervention in select patients is today considered a reliable option for those with posttraumatic stiffness.

For elderly patients with long-standing distal humeral nonunions, joint replacement arthroplasty is still considered the treatment of choice. Experience with 39 consecutive patients followed up more than 4 years reveals that 86% were objectively satisfactory and 91% were subjectively satisfied, experiencing no or minimal pain. The arc of motion is typically in the functional range: 20° to 135°. Further, it should be noted that the Coonrad-Morrey implant was employed in this setting without requiring the use of a custom device (Fig. 3).

As mentioned before, because of multiple prior surgical procedures, infection continues to be the most common complication, occurring in 6%. A total of 12% required reoperation, almost exclusively because of infection or particulate synovitis.

Arthrodesis
Arthrodesis of the elbow is incompatible with satisfactory function because range of motion of the elbow is essential for use of the hand. There is no single optimum position. It is indicated in the presence of intractable sepsis or when there is no possibility of reconstruction by total elbow revision. It is rarely indicated as a primary procedure, although its use in young males performing heavy labor is controversial. Fortunately, this situation is rare.

Osteoarthritis

Etiology and Presentation
Primary degenerative arthritis is becoming more recognizable as a distinct entity and is seen in patients, such as foundry workers, carpenters, and even athletes, who are known for heavy, repetitive use of the upper extremity.

The exact etiology of this condition is still not known, but repetitive use/overuse is a common link. The fact that both degenerative arthritis and osteochondritis dissecans are so prevalent in throwing athletes suggests a possible link between the two. Also, many patients with osteoarthritis have loose bodies, indicating that the loose bodies could potentially be causally related to the arthritis.

Although a number of problems or symptoms may be noticed, four predominate: (1) loss of motion; (2) catching or locking; (3) terminal or impingement pain; and (4) ulnar nerve irritation. These symptoms seem to vary depending on the stage of presentation or duration of involvement. In the early stages, patients commonly notice loss of full extension, which does not generally prompt medical attention until the loss is functionally disabling or until additional symptoms occur. Catching, caused by the presence of loose bodies, occurs in approximately 20%, and is the dominant feature prompting medical attention in about 10%. Terminal or impingement pain is most commonly noticed and is related to posterior osteophyte impingement as the elbow is forced into extension. Occasionally, anterior osteophytes will cause similar symptoms with full flexion. Pain during rest and in the mid-arc of motion is not usually apparent until later stages. Because the hypertrophic changes involve the medial ulnohumeral joint, irritation of the ulnar nerve is recognized in approximately 20% of patients.

Evaluation
The diagnosis is made with an anteroposterior and lateral projection showing the classic appearance of osteophytes on the lateral view of both the coronoid and tip of the olecranon. The anteroposterior view shows ossification of the olecranon and coronoid fossae. Radiohumeral involvement is observed in 25%; 20% to 25% have a loose body anteriorly or posteriorly, or both. Radiographs reveal osteophytes on the olecranon and coronoid, osteophytes filling in the olecranon and coronoid fossae, and usually loose bodies (which may not be "loose"). In the advanced stages the radioulnar and radiohumeral joints may be involved.

Treatment
The typical patient generally does not require anti-inflammatory agents and usually wants improved extension or relief from terminal extension pain. A spectrum of options is available and these are directed toward eliminating the pathology responsible for each component of the patient's symptoms: impingement pain, stiffness, catching/locking, and ulnar nerve symptoms.

Impingement Pain In patients who have pain on terminal extension or flexion, the anterior and posterior osteophytes are removed, usually through a lateral arthrotomy similar to that used to release the anterior and posterior capsule. The traditional procedure for this condition has been the Outerbridge-Kashiwagi or ulnohumeral arthroplasty, which consists of splitting and elevating the triceps, then removing the tip of the olecranon. A trephine is used to create a foramenectomy in the distal humerus; by flexing the elbow, the tip of the coronoid is visualized and removed, thus decompressing the joint from back to front (Fig. 4). More recently, however, it has been demonstrated that this debridement can be effectively performed arthroscopically. In one report of 12 patients, all had relief of pain and locking at follow-up of 3 to 30

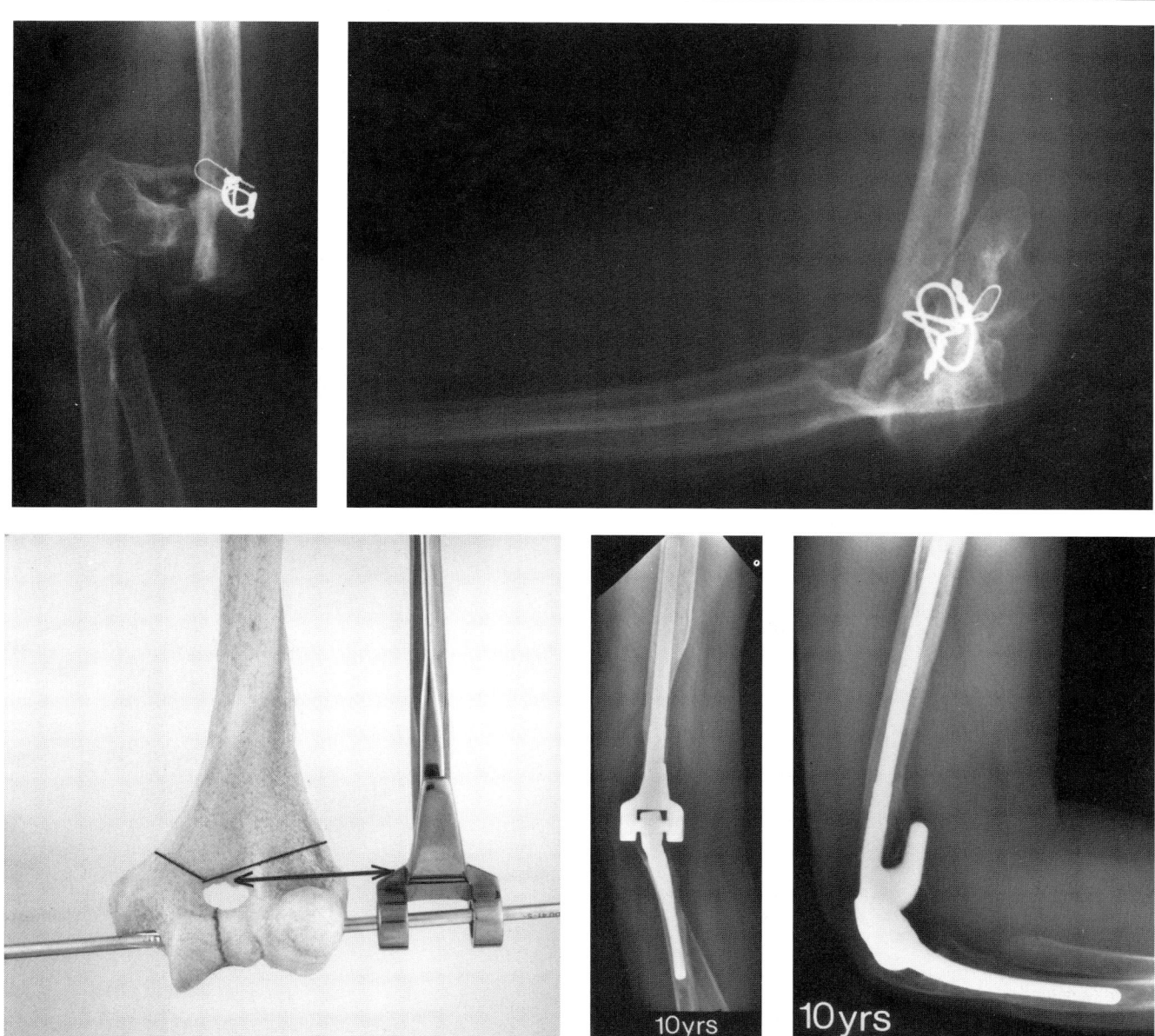

Fig. 3 **Top left and right,** Long-standing distal humeral nonunion with gross distortion. **Bottom left,** The absence of the distal humerus is accommodated by the noncustom device. **Bottom center and right,** Ten years after surgery, there is no evidence of loosening of the implant.

months. A similar experience has been reported with 21 patients in whom a debridement and removal of loose bodies were performed both in the anterior and posterior compartments. In this group with an average follow-up of almost 3 years, 84% were noted to have satisfactory outcomes. No complication was reported in either patient group.

Stiffness If stiffness is the primary complaint, a capsular release through the lateral exposure, discussed above, is quite effective. The osteophytes from the coronoid and olecranon can also be removed.

Catching/Locking Catching and locking are usually caused by loose bodies, but it should be realized that simple removal of a loose body does not help patients with osteoarthritis when stiffness and/or impingement pain are present. The latter require removal of the osteophytes.

Ulnar Nerve Symptoms In patients with ulnar nerve symptoms, the ulnar nerve is decompressed and, if necessary, transposed. The so-called ulnohumeral arthroplasty is then performed. This procedure has proved successful in approximately 85% of patients.

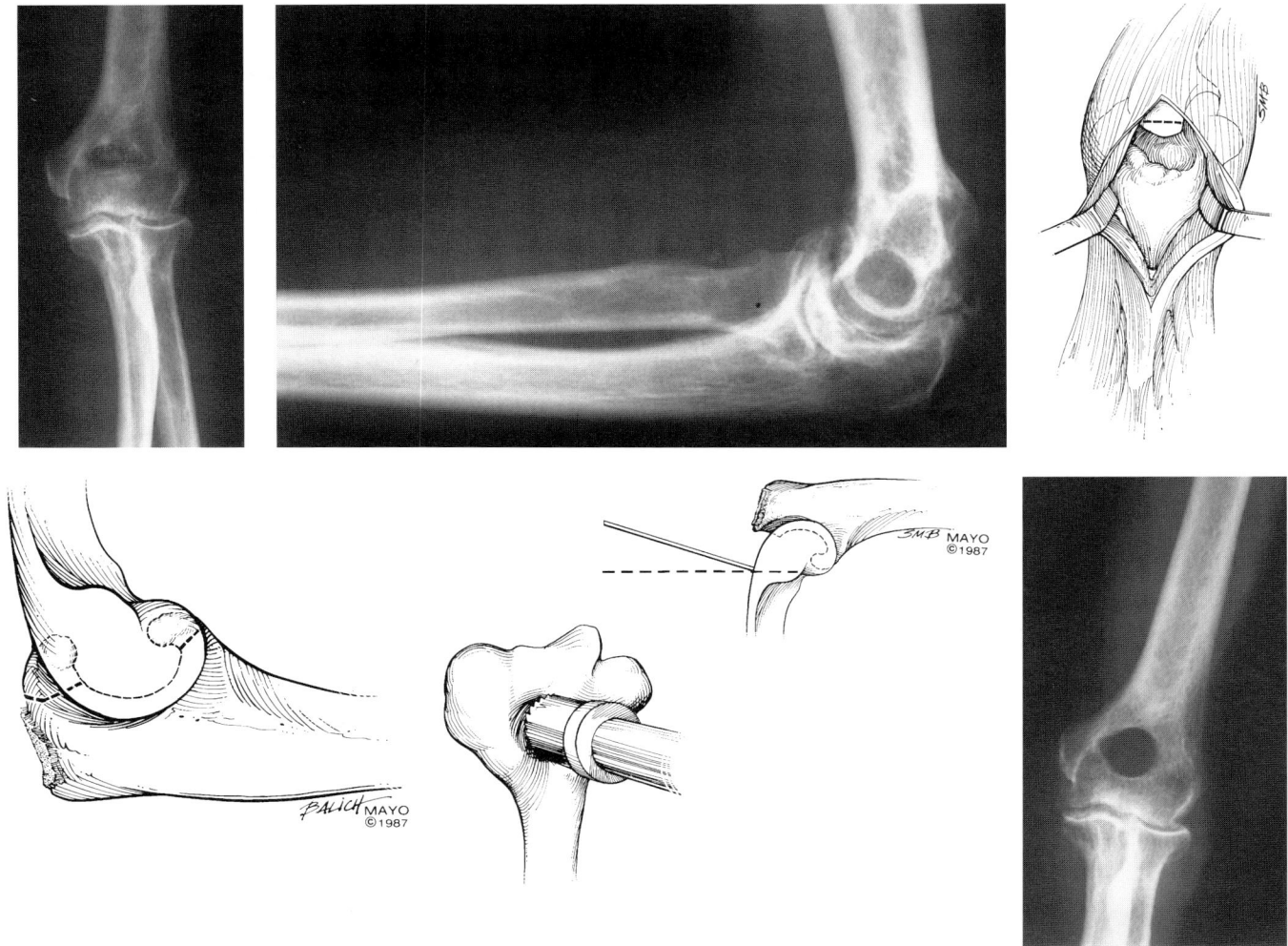

Fig. 4 **Top left and center,** Primary degenerative arthritis of the elbow. **Top right,** The debridement procedure consists of posterior exposure. **Bottom left,** Osteophyte of the olecranon is removed. **Bottom center,** The aggressive decompression procedure involves foraminectomy using a trephine across the olecranon fossa **(left).** Further removing the osteophytes on the tip of the olecranon, the coronoid completes the decompression **(right). Bottom right,** Long-term success reflected by the radiograph at 5 years. (Bottom left and bottom center figures are reproduced with permission from the Mayo Foundation, Rochester, MN. Top right figure is reproduced with permission from Morrey BF: Degenerative arthritis of the elbow, in Morrey BF (ed): *The Elbow and Its Disorders,* ed 2. Philadelphia, PA, WB Saunders, 1993.)

Results

In the majority of patients, improvement in motion of up to 35° and relief of pain are consistently achieved with few complications. Gradual recurrence of the symptoms can occur due to progression of the disease. Pain relief has been more reliable than motion restoration with the ulnohumeral arthroplasty.

Complications Probably the most common "complication" is recurrence of the disease, seen as an increasing flexion contracture and/or recurrence of impingement pain. Loose body formation and ulnar nerve irritation do not typically recur.

Summary

In summary, the treatment of elbow arthritis is conceptually similar to that for arthritis of other major joints. The reliability of total elbow replacement approaches that of total knee and hips, and is at least as successful as shoulder replacement. There remain a number of controversies and unanswered questions regarding prosthetic design that require further experience and longer follow-up for resolution. Finally, the role of arthroscopy in these conditions remains to be clarified. Although the indications are expanding, true efficacy remains to be determined.

Selected Bibliography

Rheumatoid Arthritis

Ewald FC, Simmons ED Jr, Sullivan JA, et al: Capitellocondylar total elbow replacement in rheumatoid arthritis. *J Bone Joint Surg* 1993;75A:498-507.

This article presents an excellent report of an experience with a resurfacing implant. There was a greater than 90% satisfactory result after over 200 procedures followed up for almost 6 years. Nonprogressive loosening was present in eight humeral and 19 ulnar components. Three were revised for aseptic loosening and three for dislocation. Recurrent dislocation occurred in five elbows and recurrent subluxation in ten.

Gschwend N, Simmen BR, Matejovsky Z: Late complications in elbow arthroplasty. *J Shoulder Elbow Surg* 1996;5:86-96.

In this review of the world's literature compared to the authors' experience with elbow replacement for both rheumatoid and posttraumatic conditions, satisfactory results are demonstrated in patients with rheumatoid arthritis using the semiconstrained implant. Those with posttraumatic conditions don't do as well with replacement.

Herold N, Schroder HA: Synovectomy and radial head excision in rheumatoid arthritis: 11 patients followed for 14 years. *Acta Orthop Scand* 1995;66:252-254.

This article reports excellent results in 10 of 12 procedures followed up for 14 years.

Kraay MJ, Figgie MP, Inglis AE, et al: Primary semiconstrained total elbow arthroplasty: Survival analysis of 113 consecutive cases. *J Bone Joint Surg* 1994;76B:636-640.

Of 113 cases, only 53% in 18 patients with traumatic arthrosis had a satisfactory outcome a mean of 5 years after surgery.

Kudo H, Iwano K, Nishino J: Cementless or hybrid total elbow arthroplasty with titanium-alloy implants: A study of interim clinical results and specific complications. *J Arthroplasty* 1994;9:269-278.

The uncemented titanium implant did not outperform the traditional cemented device because of a high incidence of humeral stem fracture.

Lee BP, Morrey BF: Arthroscopic synovectomy of the elbow for rheumatoid arthritis: A prospective study. *J Bone Joint Surg* 1997;79A:770-772.

Initial success of 93% after 14 elbow synovectomies at 6 months fell to 60% at 3 years' follow-up.

Ljung P, Jonsson K, Larsson K, et al: Interposition arthroplasty of the elbow with rheumatoid arthritis. *J Shoulder Elbow Surg* 1996;5:81-85.

After 35 elbows were followed up for a median of 6 years, these authors conclude that pain relief is not as predictable nor is the functional result as complete as that of joint replacement arthroplasty. They recommend prosthetic replacement as the treatment of choice rather than interposition arthroplasty for patients with rheumatoid arthritis.

Morrey BF, Adams RA: Semiconstrained arthroplasty for the treatment of rheumatoid arthritis of the elbow. *J Bone Joint Surg* 1992;74A:479-490.

This article reports that use of a semiconstrained implant in 58 patients with a follow-up of almost 4 years reveals satisfaction rates of greater than 91%. Complications occurred in 22% but necessitated reoperation in only 10%. These were for infection (four), triceps avulsion (one), and ulnar fracture (one). There were no cases of aseptic loosening and no progressive radiolucent lines. The Kaplan-Meier survivorship analysis revealed a 95% 7-year survival. This design concept is a reliable option for a broad spectrum of pathologic presentations.

Pöll RG, Rozing PM: Use of the Souter-Strathclyde total elbow prosthesis in patients who have rheumatoid arthritis. *J Bone Joint Surg* 1991;73A:1227-1233.

Thirty-one procedures followed for at least 2 years reveals that functional results are excellent if complications of irreducible dislocation (10%), loosening (3%), and infection (3%) are avoided.

Vahvanen V, Eskola A, Peltonen J: Results of elbow synovectomy in rheumatoid arthritis. *Arch Orthop Trauma Surg* 1991;110:151-154.

Mean surveillance of 7.5 years (range 1.5 to 22) after 70 procedures revealed marked (40%) or some (38%) relief of pain. Some instability existed in as many as 47%.

Tulp NJ, Winia WP: Synovectomy of the elbow in rheumatoid arthritis: Long-term results. *J Bone Joint Surg* 1989;71B:664-666.

In a long-term follow-up (mean 6.5 years), 50 patients who underwent 61 elbow synovectomies for rheumatoid arthritis had satisfactory results 70% of the time. The results did not deteriorate with time (more or less than 6 years) nor did they depend on radial head excision. The authors conclude that satisfactory long-term results can be expected with this procedure even in more advanced stages of arthritis.

Kudo H, Iwano K: Total elbow arthroplasty with a non-constrained surface-replacement prosthesis in patients who have rheumatoid arthritis: A long-term follow-up study. *J Bone Joint Surg* 1990;72A:355-362.

Madhok R, Lewallen DG, Wallrichs SL, et al: Utilization of upper limb joint replacements during 1972-1990: The Mayo Clinic experience. *Proc Inst Mech Eng [H]* 1993;207:239-244.

Traumatic Arthritis and Stiffness

Cobb T, Adams R, Morrey BF: Treatment of acute distal humeral fracture by a semi-constrained implant. *J Bone Joint Surg,* in press.

In elderly patients with comminution and osteoporosis, replacement has emerged as the treatment of choice proving successful in over 90% of 22 procedures followed up at least 2 years.

Froimson AI: Fascial interposition arthroplasty of the elbow, in Morrey BF (ed): *The Elbow.* New York, NY, Raven Press, 1994, pp 329-342.

The step-by-step surgical technique for executing the cutis interposition arthroplasty is detailed.

Husband JB, Hastings H II: The lateral approach for operative release of post-traumatic contracture of the elbow. *J Bone Joint Surg* 1990;72A:1353-1358.

The successful release of anterior contracture is reported in seven cases, with details of surgical technique. A separate medial incision is used to see and protect the ulnar nerve.

Jones GS, Savoie FH III: Arthroscopic capsular release of flexion contractures (arthrofibrosis) of the elbow. *Arthroscopy* 1993;9:277-283.

Arthroscopic release in 12 patients improved mean extension from 38° to 3° with one permanent posterior interosseous nerve palsy.

Jupiter JB, Goodman LJ: The management of complex distal humerus nonunion in the elderly by elbow capsulectomy, triple plating, and ulnar nerve neurolysis. *J Shoulder Elbow Surg* 1992;1:37-46.

Success in 85% is reported with essential adjuncts to surgical strategy: Arthrolysis and ulnar nerve decompression.

Morrey BF, Adams RA: Semiconstrained elbow replacement for distal humeral nonunion. *J Bone Joint Surg* 1995;77B:67-72.

With the semiconstrained device currently in use, approximately 90% had a satisfactory result with a mean surveillance of over 4 years. Complication rates decreased to 18% primarily because of reduction and wear debris synovitis.

Morrey BF: Post-traumatic contracture of the elbow: Operative treatment, including distraction arthroplasty. *J Bone Joint Surg* 1990;72A:601-618.

A detailed discussion of classification as intrinsic or extrinsic is accompanied by a rational and stepwise method of arthrolysis. The surgical technique described includes use of a distraction device and provided a satisfactory outcome in 90%.

Morrey BF, Adams RA, Bryan RS: Total replacement for post-traumatic arthritis of the elbow. *J Bone Joint Surg* 1991;73B:607-612.

This paper reports the experience over a course of a decade and a half and three sequential designs of prosthesis, ranging from the fully constrained to the currently used semiconstrained device in 53 patients with posttraumatic arthritis. The success rate was lower, and the complication rate higher, than in the treatment of rheumatoid or osteoarthritis. Replacement arthroplasty should be recommended only to patients over the age of 60 years.

Schneeberger A, Adams R, O'Driscoll S, Morrey BF: Semiconstrained joint replacement for posttraumatic arthritis. *J Bone Joint Surg,* in press.

Relatively long-term surveillance of 2 to 12 years (mean 62 months) of 41 patients reveals 95% subjective and 85% objective satisfactory results. There were no instances of mechanical loosening and most of the reoperations were for failure related to overuse: fracture of the ulnar component (12%) and worn bushings (5%).

Degenerative Arthritis

Morrey BF: Primary degenerative arthritis of the elbow: Treatment by ulnohumeral arthroplasty. *J Bone Joint Surg* 1992;74B:409-413.

Trephine decompression of the elbow was successful in about 90% of of the 15 patients reported in this paper and followed up for at least 2 years.

Ogilvie-Harris DJ, Gordon R, MacKay M: Arthroscopic treatment for posterior impingement in degenerative arthritis of the elbow. *Arthroscopy* 1995;11:437-443.

With a follow-up of almost 3 years, approximately 85% of patients with primary osteoarthritis benefited from arthroscopic decompression of the ulna and humeral osteophytes.

Redden JF, Stanley D: Arthroscopic fenestration of the olecranon fossa in the treatment of osteoarthritis of the elbow. *Arthroscopy* 1993;9:14-16.

Arthroscopic decompression was successful in all 11 patients in whom it was tried; however, follow-up averaged only 16 months.

Tsuge K, Mizuseki T: Debridement arthroplasty for advanced primary osteoarthritis of the elbow: Results of a new technique used for 29 elbows. *J Bone Joint Surg* 1994;76B:641-646.

In this detailed account of the pathology, it is revealed that most of the degenerative changes are on the radial side of the joint. With an average follow-up of over 5 years, a mean improvement motion of 30° is reported.

Ward WG, Anderson TE: Elbow arthroscopy in a mostly athletic population. *J Hand Surg* 1993;18A:220-224.

Thirty-five athletes with loose bodies and osteophytes of the elbow (90% had at least early osteoarthritis) were treated arthroscopically by loose body removal and debridement with excision of the osteophytes. Improvement in pain and function occurred in approximately 90%. Arthroscopic treatment is possible provided that the osteophytes, and not just the loose bodies, are removed.

42

Fractures of the Radial Head

Robert N. Hotchkiss, MD

Introduction

The treatment of fractures of the radial head continues to change and evolve with greater understanding of the basic mechanics of the elbow and improved techniques of internal fixation. Issues of major concern relate to the indications for surgical versus nonsurgical treatment, and for open reduction and internal fixation versus excision versus prosthetic replacement.

Evaluation and proper treatment of these injuries are based on the amount of displacement, the presence of significant mechanical incongruity, the practicality of stable internal fixation, and the stability of the elbow joint and radioulnar interosseous relationship. Thus, injuries to other tissues, especially the coronoid, ligaments, interosseous ligament, and distal radioulnar joint, must be considered. Excision after fracture, once regarded as merely an additional surgical procedure by some, is now viewed with more caution and circumspection. Metallic radial head replacement was first performed in the 1940s, then abandoned in favor of silicone replacement. As silicone replacement continued to demonstrate unpredictable mechanical behavior and fracture, both allograft replacement and metallic prostheses of titanium have been used in hopes of finding a material capable of withstanding repetitive load.

Because of increased recognition of the problems after radial head excision, there is growing emphasis on preservation of the radial head after fracture, using rigid internal fixation, if technically possible. Ligamentous injury in the elbow and forearm may also be associated with radial head fracture. The decision to employ excision or internal fixation may be influenced by the presence of concomitant ligamentous injury and its severity. With the advent of more suitable implants for internal fixation of the radial head and neck, excision is no longer the only surgical alternative to closed treatment. However, the ideal—an implant that provides secure fixation without interfering with motion—may be difficult to achieve. A simple fracture can be made worse with poorly executed surgery.

Biomechanics: The Mechanical Role of the Radial Head

The elbow's unique anatomy, combining two functionally independent articulations that share a synovial compartment, requires careful consideration after fracture of the radial head. The ulnotrochlear articulation directs flexion and extension, and the radiocapitellar joint governs forearm rotation in pronation and supination. The ulnohumeral articulation is highly constrained and approximates a hinge. Forearm rotation is centered about an axis from the center of the radial head to the center of the distal ulna. The mechanical role of the radial head is now better understood both in the uninjured elbow and after complex trauma. Considering that the elbow houses the two independent axes of movement, the radial head plays a role in both. Varus/valgus stability and the related potential for acute, catastrophic instability of the elbow with complete redislocation are influenced by the presence of effective mechanical contact at the radiocapitellar joint. Axial (longitudinal) stability of the forearm is directly affected by the load borne by the radial head. This particular role is greatly magnified and crucial after injury to the interosseous ligament of the forearm.

Elbow and Forearm Stability

The radial head potentially stabilizes the elbow and forearm in two ways. Radiocapitellar contact may resist valgus forces, preventing recurrent dislocation or excessive valgus displacement. In addition, the forearm and wrist are stabilized during gripping activity as a portion of load is transferred from the carpus to the radius to the radiocapitellar joint. Approximately 60% of the longitudinal force at the elbow is transmitted through the radiocapitellar joint.

Elbow Stability The presence of the radial head increases the moment arm, resisting valgus displacement of the ulnohumeral (hinge) joint, thereby decreasing the relative load on the medial ligaments (Fig. 1). However, if the medial and lateral ligaments are sectioned in the cadaveric specimen, the elbow becomes grossly unstable, whether the radial head is present or absent. Therefore, the radial head cannot function as a primary stabilizer, but rather as a secondary stabilizer of global elbow stability and especially of valgus load.

In the setting of gross acute instability, the importance of the radial head may be critical. When a complex fracture dislocation occurs, combining acute radial head and coronoid process fractures and complete elbow dislocation, gross instability with persistent and recurrent acute dislocation may occur. This complex injury is quite different from most uncomplicated radial head fractures. Concomitant injury to the medial and lateral collateral ligaments and a fracture of the coronoid are usually present. The fractured coronoid may represent a small piece of articular surface, but the injury reflects significant severity and potential for gross instability. In this setting, the destabilizing forces leading to recurrent dislocation are complex and basically those of posterolateral rotatory instability. In addition, the radiocapitellar joint is ineffective because the fracture itself leads to loss of lateral column resistance. The lateral side disengages and rolls out, either leaving the elbow perched or in complete posterior dislocation. The lateral and medial ligaments are often concomitantly injured, permitting posterior displacement, once the radiocapitellar contact is lost.

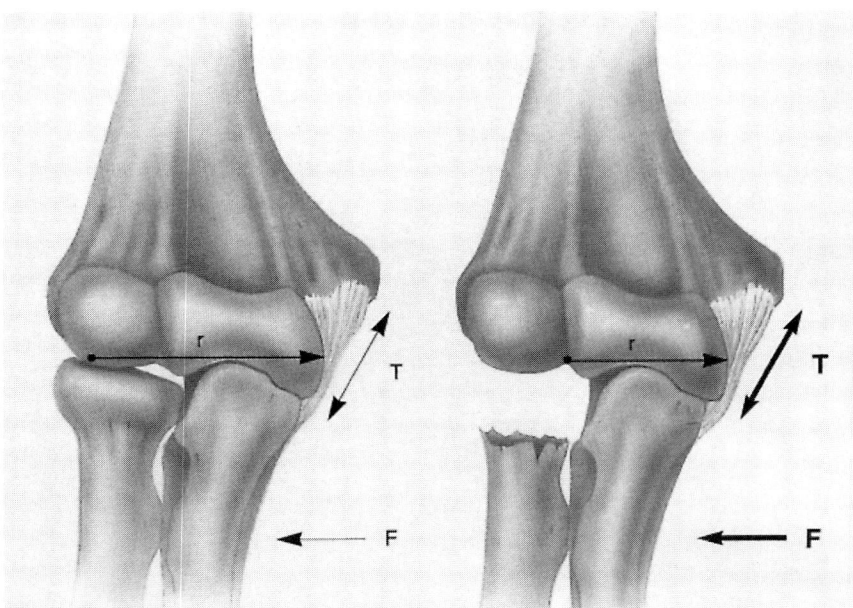

Fig. 1 Mechanical role of the radial head in valgus stability. F represents valgus force; T, tension that develops in the medial collateral ligament; r, distance from the fulcrum to the point of action of the ligament (level arm). With an intact radial head, the entire complex is stable (**left**). After excision of the radial head, the same force or torque results in increased tension on the ligament (**right**). (Reproduced with permission from Hotchkiss RN: Displaced fractures of the radial head: Internal fixation or excision? *J Am Acad Orthop Surg* 1997;5:1-10.)

The stability of the lateral side (column) is enhanced by a combination of tension in the posterolateral ligament complex and compression in the radiocapitellar joint. Radiocapitellar contact with an intact radial head, in combination with a functioning posterolateral ligament complex, will resist the posterolateral "rollout" (supination of both the ulna and radius) of the joint. During healing, it may be helpful to position the forearm in pronation to protect the repair and maximize the contact at the joint. The stability of the lateral side may be as critical to maintaining the reduction of the joint as repair of the ligaments on the medial side. Unfortunately, the radial head fracture itself may be too comminuted to accept internal fixation. In this setting, replacement using a silicone or metallic prosthesis may be an option, although these devices are not without potential complications. Other options include hinged external fixation with ligament repair and reconstruction.

There is little evidence in the living patient that loss of radial head contact in the otherwise normal elbow leads to excessive valgus laxity or instability over the long term. The valgus laxity, sometimes noted on physical examination, is more prominent after radial head excision, but does not seem to be clinically disabling. There are no reports in the literature of pathologic valgus laxity or late recurrent elbow dislocation secondary to radial head excision alone. If the patient is a throwing athlete, there may be a greater need to retain the radial head because the valgus load of the pitching arm may be quite high.

Forearm Stability After Radial Head Fracture From laboratory studies and clinical observation, the radial head bears a significant percentage (about 60%) of the axial load at the elbow joint, depending on the position of the forearm and elbow. Once the radial head is removed, this normal, physiologic load-sharing can no longer occur. If the main soft-tissue structures linking the interosseous ligament and the triangular fibrocartilage complex are disrupted, the radius will displace proximally relative to the ulna. Ascertaining the natural history and timing of the proximal translation has not been possible because most reports addressing "proximal migration" did not specify the status of the wrist and forearm ligaments at the time of injury. In addition, it is unclear whether the proximal translation of the radius occurred over the first few weeks, months, or years (Fig. 2). The principal injury is the loss of mechanical support from radiocapitellar contact and the associated compromise of the interosseous ligament of the forearm (Fig. 3). In contrast, if the radial head is intact, whether in the minimally displaced fracture or after internal fixation, proximal translation (migration) of the radius is precluded despite injuries to the soft tissue linking the radius and ulna.

In summary, the radial head serves as a secondary stabilizer in stability of the elbow and forearm. This role may become crucial if the primary supporting structures are also injured. Therefore, each patient with a fracture of the radial head must be evaluated for potential injury to the associated ligaments before treatment is considered.

Evaluation

Clinical evaluation includes inspection for a hematoma and tenderness on the medial side, in the interosseous area, and at

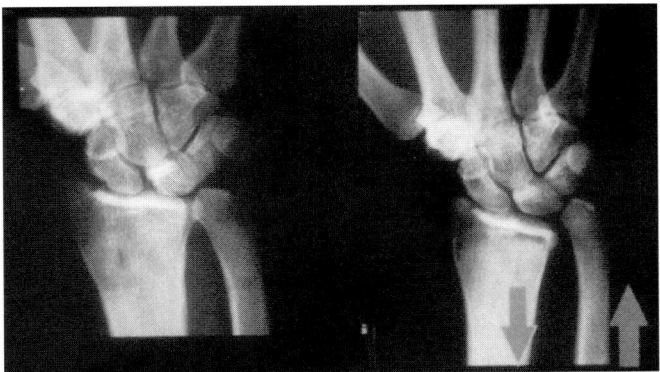

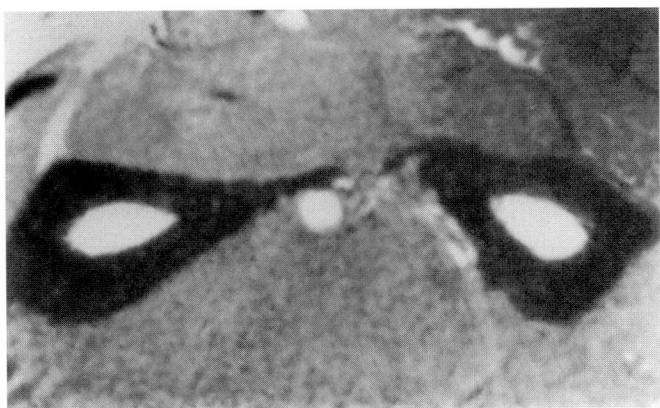

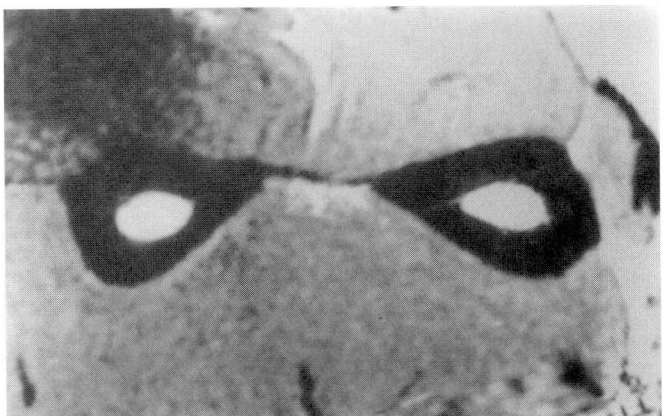

Fig. 2 **Top,** Two months after acute radial head excision, this patient was noted to have complete instability of the forearm. **Center,** Magnetic resonance imaging demonstrated a complete tear of the interosseous ligament of the forearm. **Bottom,** Normal scan.

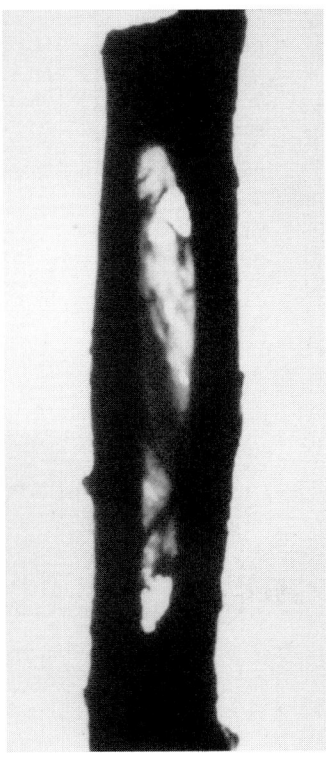 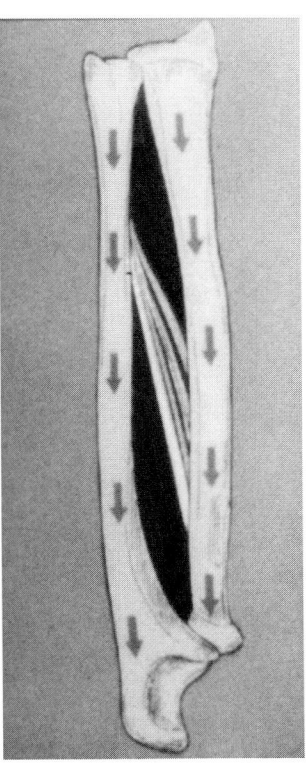

Fig. 3 The interosseous membrane demonstrating the central portion that behaves as a ligament, stabilizing the position of the radius relative to the ulna. (Reproduced with permission from Hotchkiss RN, An KN, Sowa DT, et al: An anatomic and mechanical study of the interosseous membrane of the forearm pathomechanics of proximal migration of the radius. *J Hand Surg* 1989;53:127.)

the distal radioulnar joint, which would indicate ligament injury and potential instability. Range of motion should be assessed after intra-articular local anesthetic injection if nonsurgical treatment is being considered.

Radiographic interpretation of radial head fractures may be confusing because of overlapping structures. Positioning of the patient may be challenging because of pain, but a true lateral view is essential. Associated fractures of the capitellum can occur, and the lateral view should be carefully examined. It is often difficult to judge the degree of comminution and the position of the fragments in displaced fractures. Radiographs of the wrist in the neutral posteroanterior view may also be needed if suspicion of a concomitant injury to the interosseous ligament is suspected (Essex-Lopresti). Comparison with radiographs of the uninjured side may be necessary.

Computed tomographic (CT) scans of the radial head in axial, sagittal, and coronal cuts can be quite helpful in estimating fracture size, degree of fragmentation, and amount of displacement (Fig. 4). Fractures being considered for open reduction and internal fixation are best visualized using a CT scan. The CT scan permits accurate assessment of the degrees of comminution and displacement.

Treatment Based on the Modified Mason Classification

As summarized in Outline 1, fractures of the radial head can be divided into three types. Those fractures that are minimally displaced and require no surgical treatment are type I. Those that require surgical intervention because of displacement and/or instability of the elbow or forearm and can be internally fixed

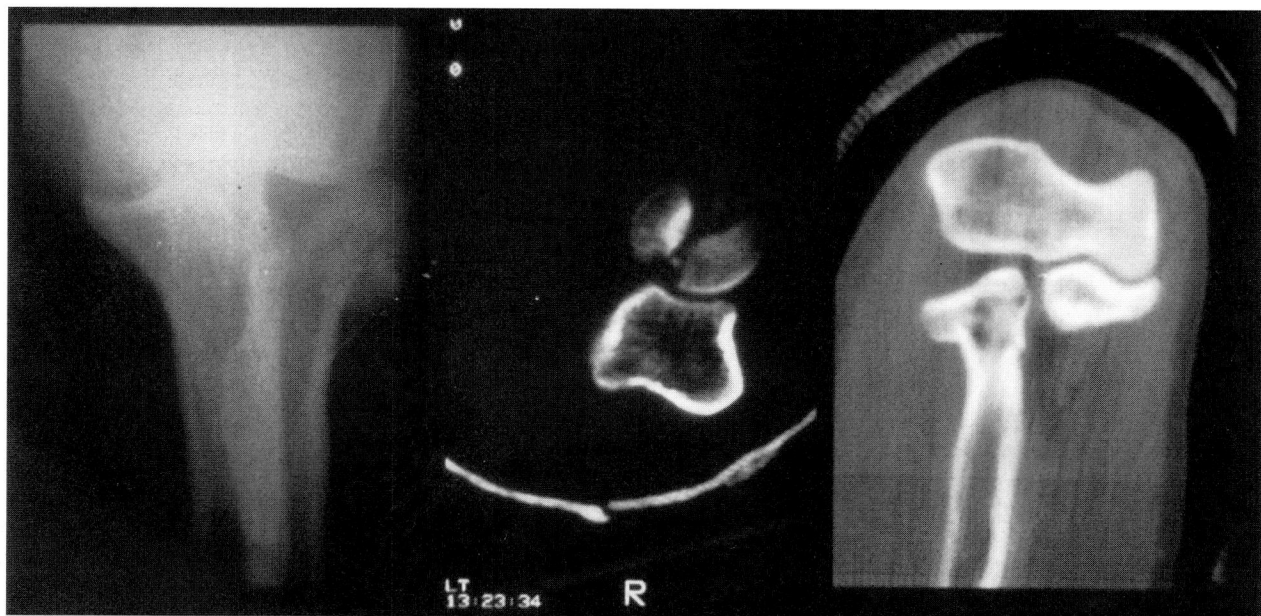

Fig. 4 These three different fractures represent different variants of type II radial head fractures. All can be potentially treated with open reduction and internal fixation. Head and neck (**left**); head only (CT scan, **center**); and neck only (CT scan, **right**) are shown.

Outline 1. Modified Mason Classification

Type I: Nondisplaced or minimally displaced fracture of head or neck
Forearm rotation (pronation/supination) is limited only by acute pain and swelling—no mechanical block
Intra-articular displacement of the fracture is usually less than 2 mm or a marginal lip fracture

Type II: Displaced (usually greater than 2 mm) fracture of the head or neck (angulated)
Motion may be mechanically blocked or incongruous
Without severe comminution (technically possible to repair by open reduction with internal fixation)
Fracture involves more than a marginal lip of the radial head

Type III: Severely comminuted fracture of the radial head and neck
Judged not reconstructable by radiograph or during surgery
Usually requires excision for movement

All of these fractures may have associated injuries with:
Elbow dislocation (usually posterior) with or without coronoid fracture
Interosseous ligament injury of the forearm
Injury to the triangular fibrocartilage complex of the wrist

(Adapted with permission from Hotchkiss RN: Displaced fractures of the radial head: Internal fixation or excision? *J Am Acad Orthop Surg* 1997;5:1-10.)

are type II. Those fractures that are so comminuted and displaced that internal fixation is technically impossible are type III. Excision is usually needed to permit forearm rotation in type III fractures.

Type I: Nondisplaced Fractures

Retrospective studies of radial head fractures since 1905 have concluded that nonsurgical treatment of type I fractures is usually successful. Although a few authors have favored cast immobilization for 2 to 4 weeks, most since the 1940s have advocated a sling and active motion as early as tolerated. Since then, few have questioned this practice. Most authors believe that early motion helps to shape and mold slight incongruities without substantial risk of greater displacement.

By definition, type I fractures are minimally or not displaced, require no reduction, and should not exhibit any mechanical block to passive forearm rotation. After intraarticular anesthesia is established using lidocaine or bupivacaine hydrochloride, the patient can be examined for the presence of crepitus or a mechanical block to forearm rotation. With the examiner's thumb or fingers over the radial head, gentle passive rotation of the forearm is attempted in several positions of elbow flexion. If there is a definite mechanical block, or severe crepitus, the fracture should be reduced and fixed. Substantial immediate relief of acute pain can be provided by aspirating the hematoma and injecting local anesthetic into the joint. The patient is given a sling, or the arm is splinted for a few days. Active forearm rotation is started as soon as tolerated. It is helpful to warn the patient that pain and stiffness can persist for some time and that fracture displacement may occur. If weekly gains in range of motion are not occurring, supervised physical therapy can be recommended. Patient-adjusted static splints are occasionally necessary to prevent contracture (see chapter 35).

Most patients with type I fractures can expect good to excellent function after 2 to 3 months of active-motion exercises. The most common complications are loss of extension

(10° to 15°) and pain. There are a few patients with type I fractures who do poorly. Contracture, pain, and radiocapitellar arthritis can occur, despite what appears to be a well-aligned, minimally displaced fracture. Capsular release and arthroscopic debridement have been reported to be successful in treating these complications (see chapter 35).

Type II: Displaced Fractures Amenable to Internal Fixation

The principal limitation of the original Mason classification is that it provides little guidance for patients with type II fractures and has not proved to be reliable in interobserver testing. For these fractures, one can find advocates for total excision, partial excision, open reduction with internal fixation, and nonsurgical care, each claiming good results. Unfortunately, these series are all retrospective, most affected by dropout bias, poor specificity of selection criteria, and inadequate measures of results. It is important to note that these fractures demonstrate significant displacement of a major segment of the head or neck. In modifying the Mason classification, type II fractures differ from type III because there is adequate potential to achieve rigid internal fixation (if indicated).

In general, every effort should be made to reduce and fix displaced fractures of the radial head. Preservation of the radial head becomes especially important with associated injuries to the interosseous ligament or collateral ligaments of the elbow, and is critical when the coronoid is fractured. Immediate excision should strongly be considered for those patients who are elderly (low-demand) and demonstrate a mechanical block. If this same patient has associated injuries to the interosseous ligament of the forearm or elbow dislocation, the radial head should be preserved if motion cannot be regained over the subsequent weeks; excision can be considered later. Some remolding of the displaced fragments may occur. If excision is delayed, those with interosseous ligament injury may experience proximal migration. In the low-demand patient, this phenomenon is usually less dramatic and much less disabling.

Internal fixation can be performed with screws (Herbert screws), and threaded or absorbable pins. Implants for internal fixation of the radial head are now more varied in size and permit rigid fixation of head and neck fractures (Figs. 5 and 6). Despite these improvements, great care must be taken to achieve rigid fixation without creating impingement in the proximal radioulnar joint. The "safe zone" for hardware placement along the radial head and neck has been identified (Fig. 5). It is a 110° arc on the lateral side of the radial head, extending 65° anteriorly and 45° posteriorly from the

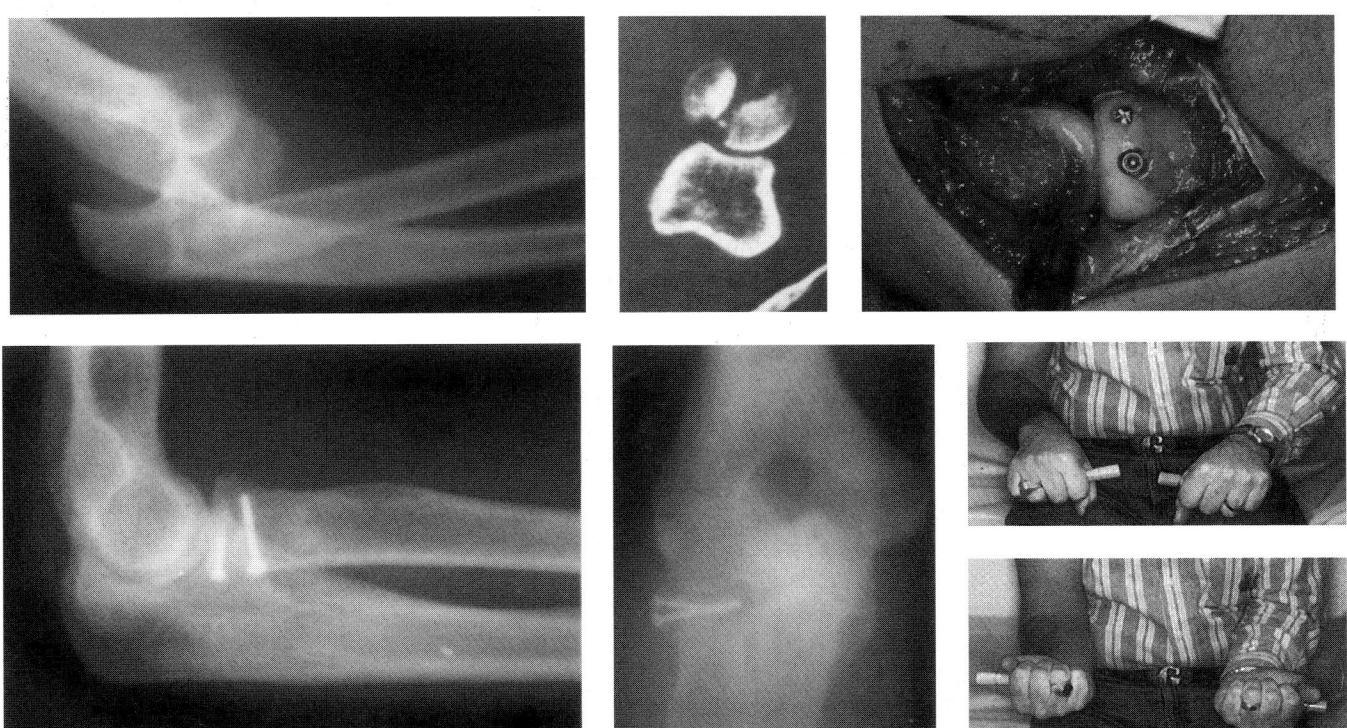

Fig 5 **Top left,** Dislocation of the elbow with a type II radial head fracture. **Top center,** Computed tomographic scan shows the displaced fracture with fragments amenable to internal fixation. **Top right,** Open reduction and internal fixation of radial head with two lag screws (one 2.0-mm and one 2.7-mm screw) in the "safe zone". **Bottom left** and **center,** Lateral and anteroposterior views obtained 5 months postoperatively. **Bottom right,** Pronation and supination approximately 1 year postoperatively. (Reproduced with permission from Hotchkiss RN: Displaced fractures of the radial head: Internal fixation or excision? *J Am Acad Orthop Surg* 1997;5:1-10.) (**Top right** and **bottom right,** © Robert N. Hotchkiss, MD.)

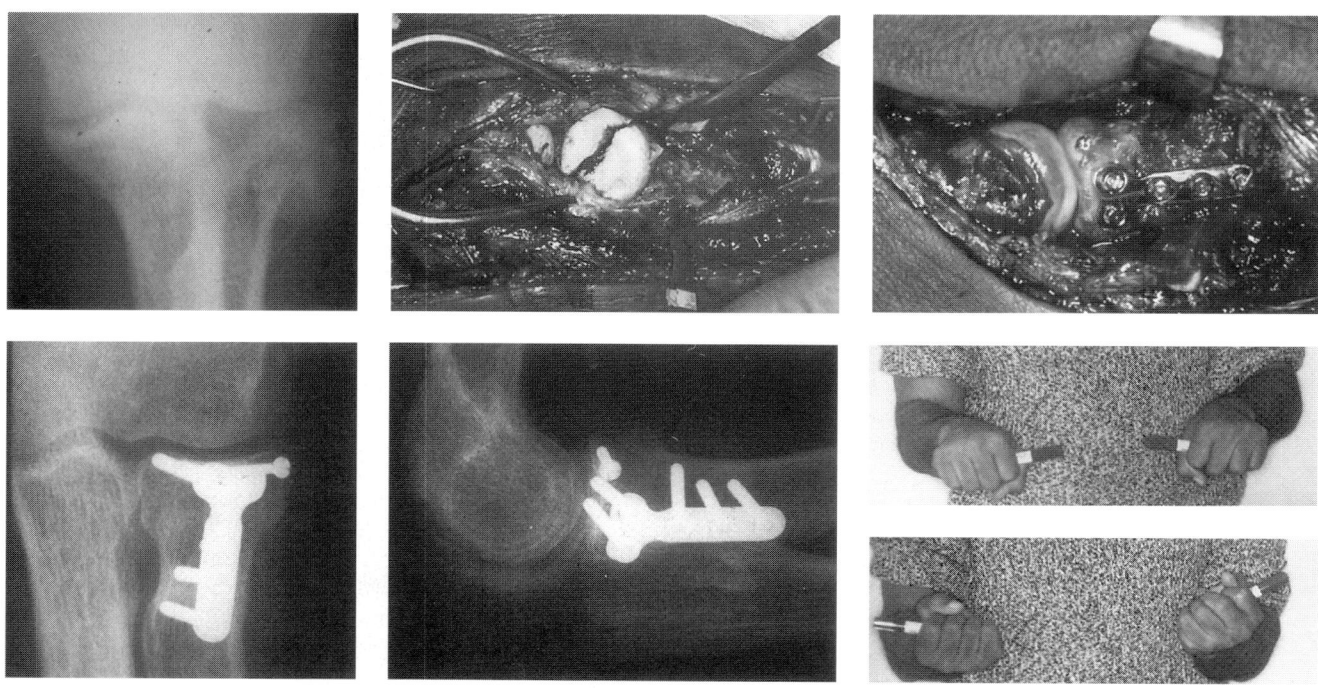

Fig. 6 Top left, Displaced fracture of the radial head and neck treated with open reduction and a contoured plate. **Top center,** Displaced fracture seen through the lateral approach. **Top right,** Contoured plate in place. **Bottom left** and **center,** Anteroposterior and lateral radiographs obtained after fixation. **Bottom right,** Motion after 1 year. (Reproduced with permission from Hotchkiss RN: Displaced fractures of the radial head: Internal fixation or excision? *J Am Acad Orthop Surg* 1997;5:1-10.)

midsection of the radial head when the forearm is in neutral rotation. Before attempting surgical repair, the surgeon should be fully prepared to excise the radial head at the time of surgery, and the patient should be forewarned of this possibility. Insecure fixation, or implants that protrude into the proximal radioulnar joint, will generally do more harm than good.

Type III: Displaced Fractures Not Amenable to Internal Fixation

For fractures with extensive comminution and displacement without concomitant dislocation or longitudinal dislocation, early excision remains the treatment of choice. Prosthetic replacement should not be performed routinely for this injury, unless there is elbow or forearm instability. After excision, the patient should begin early active motion with a passive assist as tolerated. Prolonged immobilization may lead to stiffness of the forearm and elbow.

For patients with associated elbow instability, prosthetic replacement is indicated if the collateral ligaments cannot be repaired or if the coronoid is fractured and cannot be fixed. Injury to the interosseous ligament of the forearm is an absolute indication for prosthetic radial head replacement.

Prosthetic Replacement of the Radial Head

Silicone radial head replacement began in the 1970s, and several reports of favorable results were published in a small number of patients. Problems with this prosthesis relate to inadequate biomechanical strength and wear. In one study, four of 16 patients demonstrated more than 4 mm of proximal translation of the radius. Other authors also reported several patients with continued proximal translation of the radius, despite the use of the silicone prosthesis. Others reported material failure and dislocation in addition to particulate synovitis. Silicone synovitis does not appear to be as common as with carpal implants.

The theoretical value of any radial head prosthesis is to improve elbow stability and prevent proximal translation of the radius. However, several independent biomechanical studies have demonstrated the lack of mechanical efficacy of the silicone replacement in resisting valgus stress and proximal translation of the radius.

A return to metallic prostheses, in an attempt to improve loadbearing, has also been attempted. The use of metallic prostheses for radial head replacement dates back to the 1940s, and the problems of loosening and capitellar wear with synovitis were reported. More recently a more compatible material and design were reported and the results were more encouraging in 21 patients. There is no evidence at this time to recommend the routine use of the metallic radial head implant. Others have begun to use allograft radial heads, but the indications for this are few, and more experience with each of these alternatives to the silicone prosthesis is needed (Fig. 7).

Indications for Prosthetic Radial Head Implants

At this time, radial head replacement should be considered for type III fractures with acute elbow dislocation and gross insta-

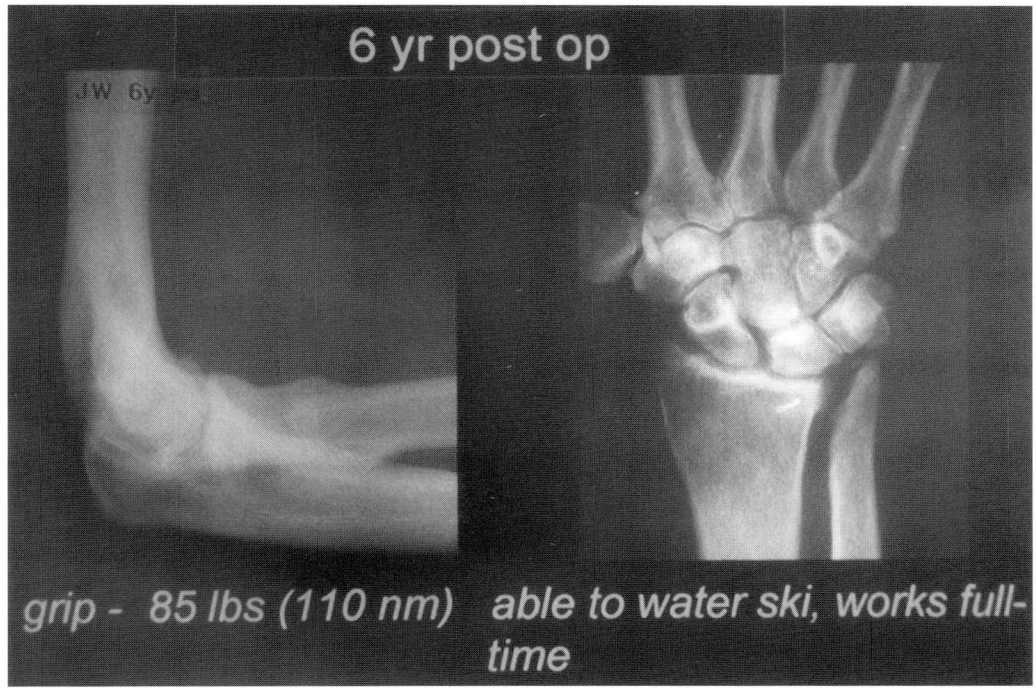

Fig. 7 Following frozen allograft radial head replacement for symptomatic proximal migration of the radius, wrist motion, grip strength, and forearm rotation have improved. The allograft is well incorporated 6 years after implantation (plate was removed because of prominence).

bility. However, radial head replacement will not suffice if the lateral collateral ligament is not securely repaired, or if a type II or III coronoid fracture is not fixed (see chapter 44). If the prosthesis is inserted without attention to this structure, the contact load is lost as the prosthesis dislocates posteriorly. The metallic prosthesis is more difficult to insert, but is mechanically better than the silicone material. Hinged external fixation may also be needed if a type III coronoid fracture has occurred.

For type III fractures with injury to the interosseous ligament, Essex-Lopresti prosthetic replacement is usually mandatory to prevent a fixed deformity. Although a metallic prosthesis affords better mechanical performance, the patient should be warned of potential dislocation, loosening, and capitellar wear. Frozen allografts have been used in reconstruction for this problem, but have not been used in the acute setting.

All of the implants must be considered for removal if they begin to show signs of mechanical failure, fragmentation, or pain due to wear. If a silicone prosthesis is used for elbow instability, it can be removed 6 to 12 months later.

Complications Following Fracture of the Radial Head

Radiocapitellar Arthrosis
For minimally displaced fractures that underwent closed treatment, the combination of displacement and initial impact may result in arthrosis at the capitellum. Arthroscopic debridement or excision is useful if the pain can be localized and attributed to degeneration of the joint.

Nonunion of the Radial Neck (Head)
Nonunion of the radial neck occurs infrequently; however, it may be symptomatic. Its treatment is dependent on the patient's symptoms and demands. Some symptoms are minimally bothersome and, if so, may be left untreated. Many of these patients become asymptomatic without evidence of secure bony union. If symptoms do persist, however, bone grafting and internal fixation or excision can be performed with the understanding that proximal migration of the radius may still occur.

Proximal Translation of the Radius After Radial Head Excision
Although every reasonable attempt should be made to preserve the radial head and prevent proximal migration, this complication may occur and not be recognized initially. The combination of radial head fracture and disruption of the interosseous ligament of the forearm may lead to loss of mobility at the wrist, forearm, and elbow because of excessive (> 1 cm) proximal translation of the radius (Fig. 2). The degree of disability is dependent on many factors, but most importantly on the amount of relative inequality between the radius and ulna at the distal joint. When mechanical dissociation of the forearm leads to radioulnar inequality exceeding 1 cm, the distal ulna sits in a position dorsal to the radius and carpus. In this position the ulna may block extension of the wrist. The mechanics of the forearm are also changed. Most

commonly, the forearm rests in pronation, with supination blocked by the relative dorsal position of the ulna as well as the contracture from injury.

In patients with less than 1 cm of proximal migration and distal inequality, the principal disability may be caused by pain at the ulnocarpal or distal radioulnar joints. It is also important to note that not all patients with proximal migration of the radius are symptomatic and many patients do not exhibit proximal migration following excision.

In patients with acute proximal translation (often referred to as the Essex-Lopresti lesion), there is little doubt that the interosseous ligament is torn. All attempts at radial head preservation should be made if this injury is suspected. Reliable repair of the interosseous ligament has not been reported. Cross-pinning the radius and ulna, hoping that the ligament could heal in the reduced position, has not been shown to be clinically reliable and may not be biologically possible.

The inability of the interosseous ligament to heal was also documented indirectly. In a study of metallic radial head replacement, one patient required removal of the metallic replacement months after implantation because of loosening. Despite having the radius held out to full length for several months by the metallic radial head replacement, within weeks of removal, proximal migration of the radius was evident and clinically significant, reaching a full centimeter of radioulnar inequality. Interestingly, significant displacement of the radius was not noted in this patient at the time of initial treatment, but the prosthesis was inserted to prevent that possibility.

In another study, the use of the silicone prosthesis with preemptive cross-pinning of the radius to the ulna was performed at the time of injury. Nonetheless, some of the patients continued to have proximal translation despite protection for several weeks. For those patients who seemed to have "settled" after proximal migration, shortening of the ulna, whether in the form of a Darrach procedure or segmental shortening, did not protect it from further symptomatic proximal migration.

A reliable solution to the problem of proximal translation remains elusive. Ligament reconstruction of the interosseous ligament is being investigated. The long-term results of metallic or allograft radial head replacement procedures are not yet available. Some patients may require the formation of a radioulnar synostosis to alleviate the pain.

Chronic Valgus Instability

The combination of medial collateral ligament deficiency and an absent radial head has received little attention in the literature, but is a problem for which there is no current solution. Attempts at ligament reconstruction have failed by chronic attenuation.

Summary

In summary, from both laboratory and clinical information, the radial head is both necessary and sufficient to prevent longitudinal proximal migration in the patient at risk. In the case of ulnohumeral dislocation, repair of the lateral collateral ligament and internal fixation of the radial head may be sufficient to prevent acute redislocation in the grossly unstable elbow. Excision in low demand patients without associated injuries is usually safe, well tolerated, and helps to optimize motion. In younger, active patients, the radial head should be preserved using newer techniques of internal fixation.

Selected Bibliography

Anatomy and Biomechanics

Hotchkiss RN, An KN, Sowa DT, et al: An anatomic and mechanical study of the interosseous membrane of the forearm: Pathomechanics of proximal migration of the radius. *J Hand Surg* 1989;14A:256-261.

Morrey BF, An KN, Stormont TJ: Force transmission through the radial head. *J Bone Joint Surg* 1988;70A: 250-256.

Morrey BF, Tanaka S, An KN: Valgus stability of the elbow: A definition of primary and secondary constraints. *Clin Orthop* 1991;265:187-195.

Although stability of the elbow can be defined in many ways, this set of experiments studied the interaction between the ligament and articulations with valgus stress. In order of importance, the anterior medial collateral ligament was defined as a primary stabilizer and the radial head a secondary stabilizer.

O'Driscoll SW, Bell DF, Morrey BF: Posterolateral rotatory instability of the elbow. *J Bone Joint Surg* 1991;73A:440-446.

This clinical-anatomic study defined a complex of ligaments stabilizing the lateral ulnohumeral joint. This concept of posterolateral stability must be understood in treating the unstable elbow after radial head fracture.

Rabinowitz RS, Light TR, Havey RM, et al: The role of interosseous membrane and triangular fibrocartilage complex in forearm stability. *J Hand Surg* 1994;19A:385-393.

This mechanical study confirmed the importance of the central portion of the interosseous membrane and also noted that with significant displacement, the triangular fibrocartilage complex must also be disrupted. The anatomic variability of the interosseous ligament was demonstrated as well.

Radial Head Fracture

Brockman EP: Two cases of disability at the wrist-joint following excision of the head of the radius. *Proc R Soc Med* 1931;24:904-905.

This article demonstrates early recognition of proximal migration of the radius following radial head fractures.

Lewis RW, Thibodeau AA: Deformity of the wrist following resection of the radial head. *Surg Gynecol Obstet* 1937;64:1079-1085.

Essex-Lopresti P: Fractures of the radial head with distal radio-ulnar dislocation: Report of two cases. *J Bone Joint Surg* 1951;33B:244-247.

Mason ML: Some observations on fractures of the head of the radius with a review of one hundred cases. *Br J Surg* 1954;42:123-132.

The original classification of Mason is outlined in this paper. With a more clear understanding of associated injuries and options for internal fixation, the original classification of this study should be modified.

Speed K: Ferrule caps for the head of the radius. *Surg Gynecol Obstet* 1941;73:845-850.

One of the first prosthetic replacements for the radial head is described.

Excision of the Radial Head and Prosthetic Replacement

Broberg MA, Morrey BF: Results of delayed excision of the radial head after fracture. *J Bone Joint Surg* 1986;68A:669-674.

Knight DJ, Rymaszewski LA, Amis AA, et al: Primary replacement of the fractured radial head with a metal prosthesis. *J Bone Joint Surg* 1993;75B:572-576.

A vitallium metallic radial head prosthesis was used in 31 comminuted fractures of the radial head, 21 associated with dislocation or ulnar fracture. At a mean follow-up of 4.5 years, there was reliable restoration of stability and prevention of proximal radial migration. There had been no dislocation or prosthetic failures, but two implants had been removed for loosening.

Judet T, Garreau de Loubresse C, Piriou P, et al: A floating prosthesis for radial-head fractures. *J Bone Joint Surg* 1996;78B:244-249.

An articulating radial head prosthesis was inserted in 12 patients—after acute radial head fractures in five, and for late reconstruction in seven. The initial results have been acceptable; however, the treatment of complex instability and long-term performance has not yet been documented.

Vanderwilde RS, Morrey BF, Melberg MW, et al: Inflammatory arthritis after failure of silicone rubber replacement of the radial head. *J Bone Joint Surg* 1994;76B:78-81.

This article represents one of many studies that has documented the mechanical failure and resultant fragmentation of the silicone radial head prosthesis. In this case, cartilage destruction was also noted.

Interosseous Ligament Injury (Essex-Lopresti)

Edwards GS, Jupiter J: Radial head fracture with acute distal radioulnar dislocation—Essex-Lopresti revisited. *Clin Orthop* 1988;234:61-69.

Sowa DT, Hotchkiss RN, Weiland AJ: Symptomatic proximal translation of the radius following radial head resection. *Clin Orthop* 1995;317:105-113.

Eight patients with symptomatic proximal translation of the radius were treated with a combination of immediate pinning of the radius to the ulna, silicone radial head replacement, or some form of ulnar shortening, including the Darrach procedure, formal ulnar shortening, or Suave-Kapandji fusion. Despite these measures, all of the patients remained disabled and exhibited positive ulnar variance of 3 mm or greater.

Szabo RM, Hotchkiss RN, Slater RR: The use of frozen allograft radial head replacement for treatment of established symptomatic proximal translation of the radius: Preliminary experience in five cases. *J Hand Surg* 1997;22A:269-278.

The treatment of the established forearm deformity after proximal translation of the radius is complex and difficult. Restoration of length of the radius relative to the ulna, as a first stage, is crucial before inserting the radial head allograft. The long-term performance of the allograft has not yet been documented.

Internal Fixation

Geel CW, Palmer AK, Ruedi T, et al: Internal fixation of proximal radial head fractures. *J Orthop Trauma* 1990;4:270-274.

Hotchkiss RN: Displaced fractures of the radial head: Internal fixation or excision? *J Am Acad Orthop Surg* 1997;5:1-10.

Radial head excision should be performed in patients with grossly comminuted fractures and in those with low demand on the upper extremities.

King GJ, Evans DC, Kellam JF: Open reduction and internal fixation of radial head fractures. *J Orthop Trauma* 1991;5:21-28.

Fourteen patients with displaced fractures of the radial head were reviewed. Excellent results were achieved in those patients without comminution and rigid fixation.

Smith GR, Hotchkiss RN: Radial head and neck fractures: Anatomic guidelines for proper placement of internal fixation. *J Shoulder Elbow Surg* 1996;4:113-117.

A cadaveric study of the radial head and neck was performed to determine a "safe zone" of approximately 110° of radial head and neck surface for internal fixation. An intraoperative method of finding this zone is described.

43

Fractures of the Distal Humerus

Jesse B. Jupiter, MD and David Ring, MD

Introduction

Fractures of the distal humerus remain among the most challenging to manage. Because this type of fracture is rare, the surgeon's experience is limited and the evaluation of large numbers of patients is hindered. The close proximity of a number of neurovascular structures about the elbow adds to the dangers related to surgical exposure and internal fixation in this region.

Anatomic reduction of the numerous, small articular fragments is necessary to maintain elbow stability and avoid arthrosis, but often proves technically difficult. The articular fragments consist of thin metaphyseal and epiphyseal bone, complicated by osteopenia in older patients. These bone fragments are often substantially displaced and comminuted. Furthermore, the anteroposterior dimension is narrow in the distal part of the humerus, particularly in the region of the coronoid, olecranon, and radial fossae, which must not be violated by the internal fixation if full motion is to be achieved. Obtaining secure fixation of small distal fragments in low columnar fractures can be extremely difficult. Contouring of the plates to match the complex anatomy of the distal humerus is an austere task.

Epidemiology/Etiology

Fractures of the distal humerus occur either in young adults following a high-energy traumatic injury or in elderly individuals following low or moderate energy injury. A typical gender distribution reflects both the preponderance of younger males to high-energy traumatic injury as well as the greater susceptibility of elderly women to osteoporosis-related fractures.

Fractures of the distal humerus most commonly involve both medial and lateral columns. Unicondylar fractures represent a mere 5% of distal humeral fractures in adults. Lateral condylar fractures are far more common than medial condylar fractures, which are extremely rare. Epicondylar fractures are also unusual following physeal closure. Coronal shearing fractures of the articular surface must be watched for because they are uncommon and occasionally difficult to recognize radiographically.

Evaluation

Younger patients with fractures of the distal humerus have typically experienced a high-energy injury and must be evaluated for serious head, chest, and abdominal injury as well as for other skeletal injury, particularly to the spinal column, pelvis, and ipsilateral upper extremity. In elderly individuals, a cardiac, pulmonary, or central nervous system condition may have been related to the cause of the fall, and careful evaluation may disclose the need for medical consultation. Evaluation for associated skeletal injuries, particularly other osteoporosis-related fractures, is also important in the elderly patient.

Open wounds are not uncommon among the high-energy fracture group. After preliminary evaluation, the wound should be dressed with a povidone-iodine dressing to inhibit wound colonization and further exposure should be avoided until definitive treatment is undertaken in the operating room. The upper extremity should be splinted for comfort and to minimize further soft-tissue and neurovascular injury. Appropriate tetanus and antibiotic prophylaxis should be administered in the emergency department.

Thorough evaluation of preoperative neurovascular deficits is important not only so that serious associated injuries can be addressed promptly, but also because surgical intervention is associated with the potential for neurologic injury.

Anteroposterior and lateral radiographs of the elbow will distinguish extra-articular from intra-articular injuries and bicolumnar from unicolumnar injuries. These studies usually provide an initial estimation of the fracture pattern and the number of fragments, their relative displacement, and associated comminution. However, upon surgical exposure, the injury is frequently more complex than the radiographs would suggest. Radiologic examinations that may assist with preoperative planning include radiographs taken with longitudinal traction applied to the upper extremity, tomograms, and computed tomography.

A single, perfect fracture classification scheme has yet to be developed for the distal humerus or for other anatomic regions. The classification of bicolumnar fractures of the distal humerus introduced by Mehne and Matta proves useful in the planning and execution of surgical fixation because it accounts for the height of the fracture through each column. The classification distinguishes high T and Y fractures from low T fractures and accounts for oblique fractures (medial and lateral lambda fracture) in which one column is fractured above the olecranon fossa and the other below it. The H fracture represents a complex fracture in which the medial column is fractured above and below its epicondyle and the trochlea is a free fragment at risk for osteonecrosis (Fig. 1). This classification reflects an improved understanding of the patterns of distal humeral fractures that has developed in the current trend toward routine surgical fixation of these fractures.

Separation of fracture patterns into types, groups, and subgroups according to the general principles of articular fracture classification used by the AO/ASIF group in the Comprehensive Classification of Fractures of Müller provides a relatively straightforward manner of organizing distal humerus injuries. The drawback of this classification in its current form is that

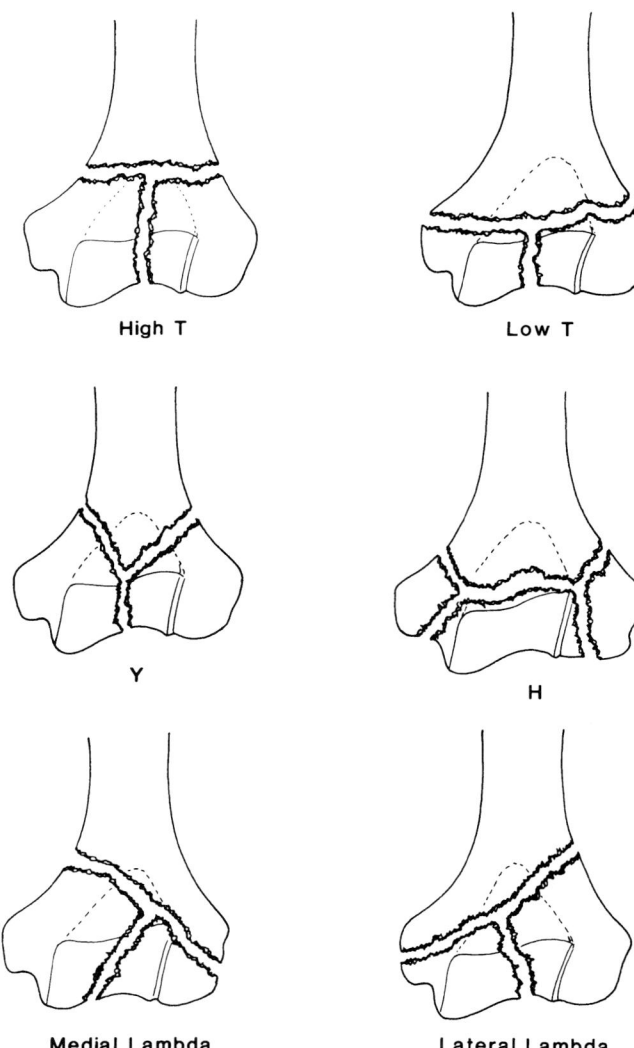

Fig. 1 The classification of bicolumnar fractures of the distal humerus developed by Mehne and Matta emphasizes fracture characteristics that influence surgical treatment and prognosis. **Top left,** In a high "T" fracture both columns are fractured above the olecranon fossa. **Top right,** In a low "T" fracture both columns are fractured through the olecranon fossa, just proximal to the trochlea. **Center left,** A "Y" fracture is characterized by oblique fracture lines that enter the olecranon fossa but divide the columns at a relatively high level. **Center right,** In an "H" fracture, the trochlea is a free fragment with disruption of both the medial and lateral columns. **Bottom,** Medial and lateral lambda fractures are characterized by a high fracture through one column and a low fracture through the other. (Reproduced with permission from Jupiter JB, Mehne DK: Fractures of the distal humerus. *Orthopedics* 1992;15:825-833.)

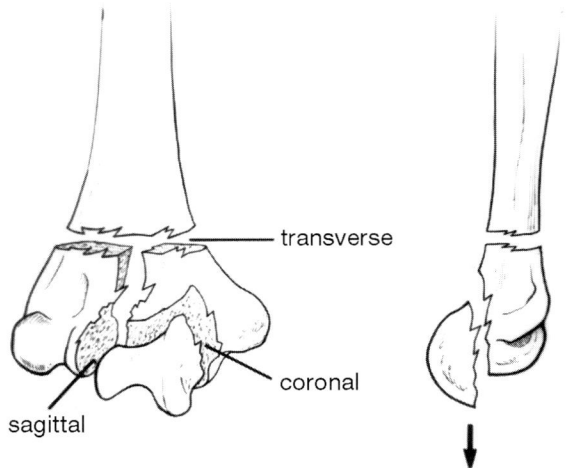

Fig. 2 An important fracture line is occasionally encountered in the coronal plane, particularly among complex bicolumnar fractures of the distal humerus. (Reproduced with permission from Jupiter JB, Barnes KA, Goodman LJ, et al: Multiplane fracture of the distal humerus. *J Orthop Trauma* 1993;7:216-220.)

it lacks the distinction of important elements such as the height of the columnar injury or the presence of a coronal component to the articular fracture, which will influence surgical tactic and possibly the prognosis.

Fractures of the lateral or medial column in isolation are distinguished by the presence or absence of associated elbow instability. This condition is more commonly related to associated collateral ligament damage than to loss of the stabilization afforded by the lateral wall (or lip) of the trochlear sulcus. Jupiter and Mehne choose to separate "high" fractures, which represent larger fragments that contain the bulk of the trochlea, are more easily fixed with a plate and screws, and are more frequently associated with cotranslation of the radius and ulna, from "low" fractures with the opposite characteristics.

The characterization of shearing fractures of the articular surface in the coronal plane has evolved with recent reports. It may be more appropriate to consider capitellum fractures as coronal shear fractures, because many of these fractures extend well into the trochlea. Furthermore, complex bicolumnar fractures on occasion contain a component of articular shearing injury in the coronal plane that must be sought and appropriately treated to assure an optimal result (Fig. 2).

Treatment

A thorough understanding of elbow anatomy and expertise in techniques of internal fixation are prerequisite in order for surgical fixation of a distal humerus fracture to be successful. One should therefore not hesitate to consult or refer to a surgeon with more experience treating these rare injuries.

Positioning of the patient in the lateral decubitus position with the involved arm draped over a bolster is safer than prone positioning and allows access to the posterior iliac crest when bone grafting is necessary. A sterile tourniquet is used.

A number of authors recommend curving the posterior incision of the skin slightly to the lateral or medial side to diminish the risk of wound breakdown and scar sensitivity over the tip of the olecranon. On the other hand, a number of elbow surgeons use a direct midline posterior incision—

analogous to that now popular for incisions about the knee—that falls between innervating cutaneous nerves and their associated angiosomes. The profuse cutaneous vascularity of the upper extremity allows for the creation of extensive medial and lateral skin flaps, permitting access to nearly the entire elbow.

The importance of isolation and protection of the ulnar nerve cannot be overemphasized. These measures help minimize ulnar nerve dysfunction, one of the most common iatrogenic complications encountered. Many skilled elbow surgeons strongly believe that routine subcutaneous transposition of the nerve should be performed. Subcutaneous transposition, although it prevents the nerve from becoming bound up in scar tissue and fracture callus and prevents irritation by internal fixation devices, is associated with a theoretical risk of injury caused by devascularization. Following transposition of the nerve, the groove below the medial epicondyle thereby becomes available for the placement of contoured plates and screws.

Medial and lateral triceps reflecting exposures have been advocated as a means of avoiding the complications associated with olecranon osteotomy. However, visualization and access to the entire distal humeral articular surface is not as apparent as that provided by a transolecranon exposure. When considering total elbow replacement in the acute setting, olecranon osteotomy should be avoided.

Careful attention to the detail of creation and fixation of the olecranon osteotomy will greatly reduce the incidence of complications. A chevron-shaped osteotomy with the apex pointing distally facilitates anatomic repositioning, enhances stability, and provides a broader interface of cancellous bone to encourage healing. The osteotomy should be located at the depth of the semilunar notch where there is little articular cartilage. This location is identified precisely under direct visualization following elevation of the anconeus muscle from its insertion on the olecranon. The osteotomy is initiated with a thin oscillating saw. The articular surface and subchondral bone is then cracked with a thin-blade osteotome, resulting in a rough interdigitating surface that further facilitates anatomic repositioning of the fragment.

When exposure is complete, the fracture is carefully assessed and the preoperative plan is modified according to the surgical findings. The order in which the various components of the injury are addressed may vary, but it typically proceeds from articular reconstruction to fixation of each column to the humeral shaft.

Provisional reduction is obtained by manipulation and held with smooth 0.045- or 0.062-in Kirschner wires and, occasionally, bone clamps. If there is no articular comminution, then the most stable reconstruction of the trochlear spool is with an interfragmentary lag screw. In the face of comminution, the trochlear sulcus must be carefully reconstructed in both depth and width, and fixation should be achieved with a screw threaded into both medial and lateral fragments in order to maintain these relationships. All resulting gaps are filled with cancellous autograft from the iliac crest.

When placing screws down the center of the trochlea, it is important to keep in mind that the diameter of the trochlea in the central sulcus area is one half that at the medial and lateral lips. To assure central location of the screw, retrograde drilling through one of the fracture fragments has been recommended.

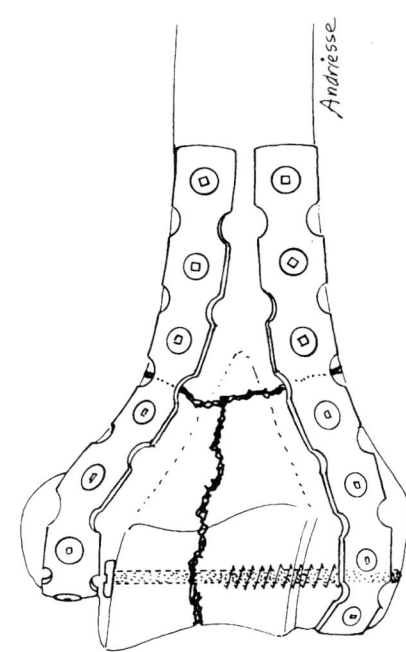

Fig. 3 Dual plate fixation of the distal humerus. The plates should converge upon one another because screw orientation as close to 90° as possible may enhance fixation strength. (Reproduced with permission from Jupiter JB, Mehne DK: Fractures of the distal humerus. *Orthopedics* 1992;15:825-833.)

A fracture of the articular surface in the coronal plane is not uncommon. These fractures can be addressed with Herbert screws that recess beneath the articular cartilage.

Fixation of the articular fragments onto the osseous columns has, historically, been the weak point of internal fixation of distal humeral fractures. The keys to success include the use of well-contoured plates; fixation with plates oriented as close to 90° to one another as possible; and adequate fixation to the distal fragments, frequently the most difficult aspect of fracture treatment.

A number of authors recommend 3.5-mm reconstruction plates because they are stout enough to resist the deforming forces in this region, and yet are easily contoured in three dimensions. This is particularly important in the distal humerus because the complex bony surfaces require equally complex and exacting contour of the plates (Fig. 3).

Some surgeons use a precontoured plate on the lateral column, claiming that it facilitates restoration of anatomy and more easily addresses fracture comminution. Another option in very distal or extremely comminuted fractures is the addition of a second plate onto the lateral column for a total of three plates.

A plate applied to the posterior aspect of the lateral column can extend distally to the posterior border of the capitellum. A stable hold on the distal fragment is enhanced by directing the most distal screws proximally so that they converge upon screws entering more proximally and engage the anterior cortex while avoiding the capitellum (Fig. 4).

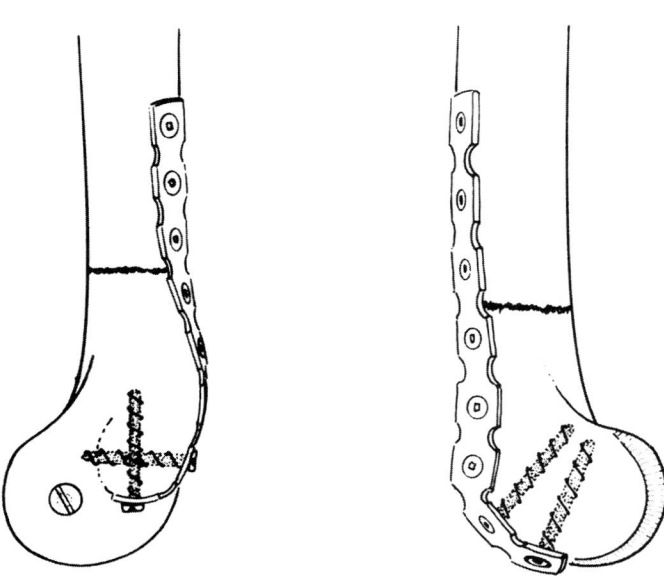

Fig. 4 The distal contour of the plates is crucial for secure fixation of low columnar fractures and osteoporotic ununited fragments. **Left,** Following subcutaneous transposition of the ulnar nerve, the medial epicondyle is available for plate and screw fixation. Contouring of the plate so that its most distal screw is directed superiorly results in a 90° interlocking relationship with more proximal screws, thereby enhancing fixation. **Right,** On the lateral column, although the distal extension of the plate is limited by the articular surface of the capitellum, a similar screw orientation is often possible. (Reproduced with permission from Jupiter JB, Mehne DK: Fractures of the distal humerus. *Orthopedics* 1992;15:825-833.)

For more proximal columnar fractures, a plate placed along the medial aspect of the medial column can gain adequate fixation in the distal fragment. When the fracture is more distal, the small articular fragment may only accept a single screw through a medially applied plate. Placement of the medial plate more posteriorly allows the distal end of the plate to be contoured so that it wraps around and cradles the medial epicondyle. The most distal screw is then inserted in a directly superior direction. This screw is thereby directed perpendicular to the more proximal screws, creating a mechanical interlocking construct (Fig. 4). Alternatively, a medially applied plate can be contoured to fit around the medial epicondyle so that the most distal screw can be a long screw directed up the medial column.

The anterior surface of the medial column is nonarticular. Screws entering through the medial plate can therefore gain purchase through the anterior cortex. Considering the triangular cross-sectional width of the columns, tapering into the olecranon and coronoid fossae, screws entering through a plate on the posterior aspect of the medial column should be directed anteromedially to enhance bony purchase. A corresponding relationship exists on the lateral column.

Enhanced fixation of screws with poor bony purchase can be achieved with the use of polymethylmethacrylate. Methylmethacrylate is prepared and injected in its liquid phase into loose screw holes. Extravasation of cement must be carefully avoided.

Once the fixation is in place, its stability should be evaluated through a full range of motion. If motion is observed at a fracture line, additional fixation should be provided. In the presence of severely osteopenic bone, a third plate can be placed on the lateral aspect of the lateral column (Fig. 5). Defects within the architecture of the distal end of the humerus are filled in with autogenous cancellous bone graft from the iliac crest.

The olecranon osteotomy is fixed with a tension band wire construct. The tips of the Kirschner wires are bent under the triceps insertion and impacted into bone. Hardware-related complications such as migration and symptomatic prominence are decreased by these measures.

Postoperative limb elevation is important to limit swelling. The dressing and splint are changed within 24 hours and a lightweight, removable thermoplastic splint is made for the patient to use as a resting splint for the first few days until the pain subsides. Because full extension of the elbow is often difficult to obtain, the patient is allowed to rest with the elbow in extension during the first week.

Early controlled motion is key to retention of elbow motion. Gravity is used to facilitate elbow flexion by placing the patient in the supine position with the shoulder flexed to bring the elbow overhead and the involved forearm supported by the uninjured arm. With the patient sitting upright, gravity is used to assist with extension.

Activities of daily living should be commenced within the first week. Muscle strengthening and endurance exercises are instituted by 8 to 12 weeks, when the surgeon is certain that osseous union has occurred. If residual stiffness is a problem following fracture healing, the use of turnbuckle splints may help to improve motion for as long as 6 to 12 months postoperatively.

A number of authors have suggested total elbow arthroplasty for fractures in osteopenic bone with extensive comminution. This procedure is indicated for elderly patients with low functional demands or fractures with excessive comminution and osteoporosis that precludes fixation. Total elbow arthroplasty represents a poor option for young adult patients.

Results/Outcome

Among a growing number of reported series, surgical intervention has consistently achieved approximately 75% excellent or good results. Södergård and associates documented a high rate of fixation failure (30%), primarily related to improper technique, in the early study period. Despite this, they achieved 65% excellent or good results following the primary intervention, which improved to 85% when operations for repeat fixation and reconstruction of nonunion were included.

Wang and associates, demonstrating an excellent understanding of the principles of sound surgical treatment in the treatment of 20 fractures of the distal humerus, found that a majority of fair and poor results occurred with the most complex fractures (group C3) and were related to associated

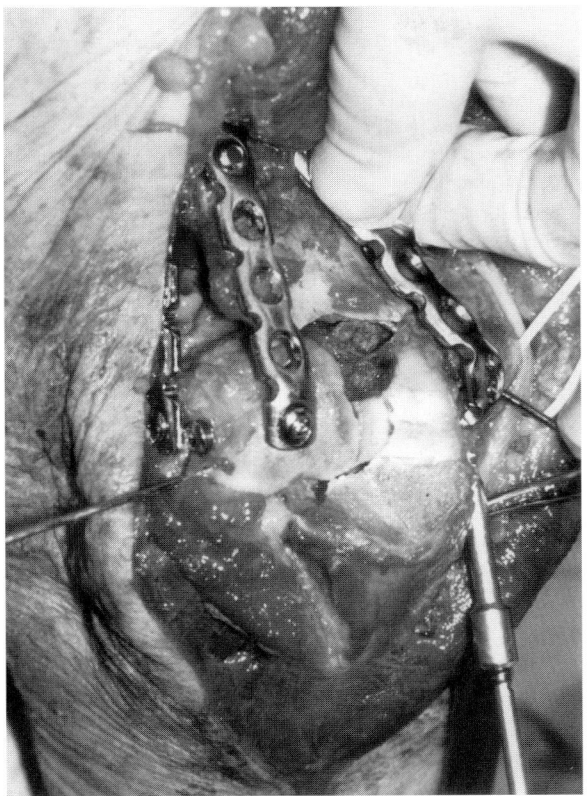 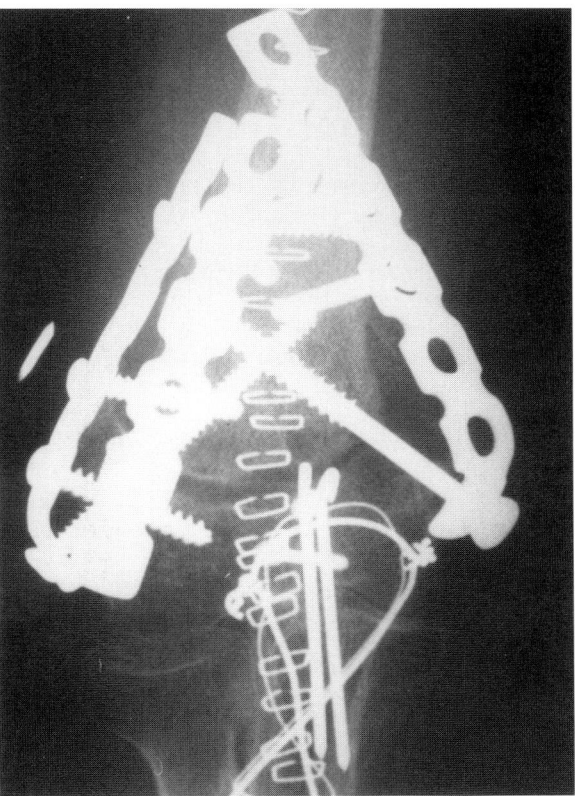

Fig. 5 Surgical stabilization of distal humeral nonunions often requires the placement of a third plate to enhance fixation. **Left,** This intraoperative photograph demonstrates the use of a third plate on the direct lateral aspect of the lateral column in addition to the posterolateral and posteromedial plates. Note the distal curvature of the medial plate about the medial epicondyle. **Right,** Anteroposterior radiograph depicting the early postoperative result.

injuries and complications: one nonunion, one malunion of the trochlear surface with arthrosis, and one deep infection in a patient with severe soft-tissue injury and a brachial artery laceration at the time of injury.

Complications

The most common complication encountered after surgical fixation of a fracture of the distal radius is elbow stiffness. This condition can be prevented by achieving stable fixation and starting motion almost immediately following surgery.

The majority of patients with an unsatisfactory result following surgical treatment of a fractured distal humerus have had one or more complications. Although some complications arise from factors such as severe soft-tissue injury or heterotopic ossification, most complications are the result of elements that are within the surgeon's control. Anatomic reduction and secure fixation of fracture fragments, proper handling of the ulnar nerve, and reliable fixation of a carefully performed olecranon osteotomy will substantially limit complications and thereby improve the results of surgical intervention.

Early failure of fixation has been related primarily to improper technique, but also to osteoporosis. Adequate fixation is almost always possible when proper technique is used, even in patients with moderate or severe osteoporosis. Prolonged postoperative immobilization must be avoided because even an excellent reduction will be compromised by the resulting stiffness.

Nonunion is usually the result of inadequate fixation. Surgical reconstruction of an ununited distal humerus fracture is a demanding procedure that involves mobilization and neurolysis of the ulnar nerve, resection of the nonunion site, anterior and posterior capsulectomy, and realignment and stabilization of the distal fragment, which is almost always small and osteoporotic. Using the techniques described above for fixation of low columnar fractures, including the use of a third plate when necessary, it is possible to gain stable fixation allowing immediate postoperative motion.

The addition of routine capsulectomy and ulnar nerve transposition and neurolysis to the surgical tactic for distal humeral nonunions as reported in previous series has improved the arc of flexion and extension to an average of nearly 100° following these reconstructive procedures. Elbow stability is restored, pain is relieved, and skeletal integrity is maintained.

The results of total elbow arthroplasty in the treatment of ununited fractures of the distal humerus have improved to the degree that this procedure can be considered an alternative for older patients with low functional demands. However, arthroplasty is relatively contraindicated for the younger, active individual. Allograft replacement has been attempted but is associated with numerous complications and its longevity is unproven.

Ulnar nerve dysfunction is one of the most common complications of surgical treatment of fractures of the distal humerus. Experience with reconstruction of nonunions and malunions of the distal humerus has revealed that fibrosis tends to occur, and the nerve adheres to the medial epicondylar region as a result of scar formation as well as the fracture healing response. We recommend adequate mobilization and anterior transposition at the initial surgery, because it has been shown to nearly eliminate the risk of this potentially disabling complication. Happily, the ulnar nerve has proven remarkably responsive to neurolysis and mobilization at the time of reconstruction.

Recent reports have noted little difficulty with heterotopic ossification about the elbow following distal humeral fractures; this may be the result of a number of factors including a trend toward timely surgical intervention, the institution of routine immediate postoperative mobilization, and an improved understanding of heterotopic ossification. Calcification of periarticular tissues, which is common and inconsequential, is distinguished from processes that form organized bone restricting joint mobility. This latter type of heterotopic bone is unusual in the absence of associated risk factors such as a burn or head injury. High-energy traumatic injuries, open injuries, and early repeat surgical intervention are also considered risk factors.

Nonsteroidal anti-inflammatory medications, low-dose radiation therapy, and continuous passive motion have been considered as prophylactic measures against the formation of heterotopic bone in high-risk cases, based on analogy with documented experience with trauma and reconstructive procedures of the hip. Continuous passive motion must be distinguished from forcible passive manipulation, which has been condemned as a risk factor for the development of heterotopic ossification.

In the absence of central nervous system injury, excision of disabling heterotopic bone should be considered within 6 to 9 months of the injury. Early intervention limits the degree of both capsular and ligamentous contracture as well as degeneration of articular cartilage. Excision of heterotopic bone and capsular release are performed through a medial and/or lateral approach, although existing scars are always incorporated in the approach when possible. A single posterior skin incision permits deep exposures on both the medial and lateral sides. In this setting, prophylaxis with both continuous passive motion and indomethacin is used.

The risk of recurrence is higher in patients with associated head injury. In at least one study, improvement in motion and function following excision of heterotopic ossification of the elbow in patients with head trauma correlated with minimal cognitive deficits, low levels of serum alkaline phosphatase, and the appearance of mature bone on radiographs of the elbow.

Conclusion

The high proportion of excellent and good results in recent series that document the surgical fixation of distal humerus fractures reflects the dramatic influence of advances in implant design and technique, but at the same time should reflect that experience with these techniques and a sound understanding of both the normal and pathologic anatomy in this region are essential for achieving good results while avoiding complications. When faced with a challenging fracture of the distal humerus, a surgeon who rarely treats such injuries should seek the assistance of a more experienced colleague.

Function is optimized when the fracture heals in good alignment following a program of early mobilization. Nonunion and elbow stiffness often respond to repeat fixation with autogenous bone grafting and capsulectomy. Alternative salvage procedures, including arthrodesis, allograft replacement, and arthroplasty, are poor alternatives for post-traumatic elbow conditions in healthy, active patients. Maintenance of skeletal integrity is the best option for patients with the prospect of many years with high functional demands.

Selected Bibliography

Ackerman G, Jupiter JB: Non-union of fractures of the distal end of the humerus. *J Bone Joint Surg* 1988;70A:75-83.

This earlier series from the Massachusetts General Hospital demonstrated that union was necessary, but not sufficient for a good functional result. Addition of routine elbow capsulectomy and ulnar nerve neurolysis to the surgical treatment of nonunions improved the results in later series.

Caja VL, Moroni A, Vendemia V, et al: Surgical treatment of bicondylar fractures of the distal humerus. *Injury* 1994;25:433-438.

A combined clinical and radiographic rating scale was used to evaluate a series of 22 patients with bicondylar (type C) distal humeral fractures. This combined scale is actually a step backward because it makes it difficult to relate the quality of the reduction determined radiographically to the functional result. This series is consistent with others in that stable, anatomic reduction and the avoidance of complications are the most important factors influencing outcome.

Figgie MP, Inglis AE, Mow CS, et al: Salvage of non-union of supracondylar fracture of the humerus by total elbow arthroplasty. *J Bone Joint Surg* 1989;71A:1058-1065.

Total elbow arthroplasty for the treatment of distal humeral nonunion represents a technically demanding procedure that should be reserved for salvage situations.

Helfet DL, Hotchkiss RN: Internal fixation of the distal humerus: A biomechanical comparison of methods. *J Orthop Trauma* 1990;4:260-264.

The first of many laboratory investigations regarding the biomechanical characteristics of different methods of distal humeral fixation, this study documented the clear superiority of double plating techniques over weaker plate designs.

Jupiter JB: Complex fractures of the distal part of the humerus and associated complications. *J Bone Joint Surg* 1994;76A:1252-1264.

This article is a recent comprehensive review of the topic.

Jupiter JB, Goodman LJ: The management of complex distal humerus nonunion in the elderly by elbow capsulectomy, triple plating, and ulnar nerve neurolysis. *J Shoulder Elbow Surg* 1992;1:37-46.

It is possible to achieve stable fixation of the distal humerus, even when the distal fragment is small and osteopenic as in these six patients with nonunion. Addition of autogenous bone graft resulted in stable union and pain relief in all cases, with persistent mild exertional discomfort in four patients. Capsulectomy and initiation of active motion in the immediate postoperative period resulted in an average of 102° of motion. These results are comparable to those achieved with total elbow arthroplasty in the same clinical setting.

Jupiter JB, Neff U, Holzach P, et al: Intercondylar fractures of the humerus: An operative approach. *J Bone Joint Surg* 1985;67A:226-239.

This study is one of the early series to report the use of stable internal fixation in the treatment of intercondylar fractures of the distal humerus. Duplication of these excellent results by subsequent authors has made surgical fixation the treatment of choice for these fractures.

McKee MD, Jupiter JB, Bamberger HB: Coronal shear fractures of the distal end of the humerus. *J Bone Joint Surg* 1996;78A:49-54.

The entire capitellum and a large portion of the trochlea may be sheared off as a unit in the coronal plane. Experience with this fracture in six patients emphasizes the importance of early recognition as a more extensive surgical exposure is required. Stable fixation, aided by the use of Herbert screws, allows early motion and reliable functional restoration. Osteonecrosis of the articular fragment was not observed.

McKee M, Jupiter J, Toh CL, et al: Reconstruction after malunion and nonunion of intra-articular fractures of the distal humerus: Methods and results in 13 adults. *J Bone Joint Surg* 1994;76B:614-621.

Thirteen patients with distal humeral malunions or nonunions achieved healing in adequate alignment with restoration of stability and an average 97° motion arc following stable internal fixation and autogenous bone grafting. Addition of routine elbow capsulectomy and ulnar neurolysis to the surgical tactic have improved the results as compared with the series of Ackerman and Jupiter reported 6 years previously. This procedure represents the best alternative for active patients with distal humeral nonunion.

Morrey BF, Adams RA: Semiconstrained elbow replacement for distal humeral nonunion. *J Bone Joint Surg* 1995;77B:67-72.

Thirty-one of 36 patients (86%) treated by elbow replacement for distal humeral nonunion and available for long-term review had excellent or good results (average follow-up, 50.4 months). Five patients required reoperation: two for deep infections, two for particulate synovitis, and one for worn bushings. Two of these underwent resection arthroplasty. Two additional patients had deterioration in ulnar nerve function.

Papaioannou N, Babis GC, Kalavritinos J, et al: Operative treatment of type C intra-articular fractures of the distal humerus: The role of stability achieved at surgery on final outcome. *Injury* 1995;26:169-173.

Eighty-seven patients with type C fractures of the distal humerus were treated surgically between 1979 and 1992. In the early 1980s, a gradual transition in surgical tactic from limited internal fixation with postoperative cast immobilization to stable plate fixation by the AO technique with early mobilization occurred. Only 38% of patients with limited fixation compared to 77.8% of patients with stable fixation were satisfactory. In a subgroup of patients treated by the AO method in which stable fixation was achieved and postoperative cast immobilization was thereby avoided, the proportion of good results was 88%.

Sanders RA, Raney EM, Pipkin S: Operative treatment of bicondylar intraarticular fractures of the distal humerus. *Orthopedics* 1992;15:159-163.

This article documents a single surgeon's experience treating 17 fractures of the distal humerus with a lateral 3.5-mm DC plate and a posteromedial reconstruction plate. There were five excellent, eight good, two fair, and two poor results. All four of the fair or poor results occurred in patients with grade III open wounds. Three of these four patients had combination external and internal fixation.

Schemitsch EH, Tencer AF, Henley MB: Biomechanical evaluation of methods of internal fixation of the distal humerus. *J Orthop Trauma* 1994;8:468-475.

This study presents the biomechanics of distal humeral fracture fixation using a precontoured Dupont J-plate. They found maximum rigidity to anteroposterior and varus-valgus bending, axial compression and torsion with two plates, one each on the medial and lateral columns, placed parallel to one another. This rigidity was superior to that achieved by the traditional 90° configuration with reconstruction plates.

Self J, Viegas SF, Buford WL Jr, et al: A comparison of double-plate fixation methods for complex distal humerus fractures. *J Shoulder Elbow Surg* 1995;4:10-16.

A fixation method using 180° dual plate fixation with the additional use of bolts represented the focus of these biomechanical comparisons. Only axial compression was tested and a four-part fracture model was used. These tests found that 180° medial and lateral plates are more rigid and resist fatigue failure in axial compression testing better than a 90° medial and posterolateral plate combination, and that this effect is enhanced by the use of bolts.

Södergård J, Sandelin J, Böstman O: Mechanical failures of internal fixation in T and Y fractures of the distal humerus. *J Trauma* 1992;33:687-690.

Of 61 consecutive patients with T- or Y-type distal humeral fractures treated with surgical fixation, 18 (30%) had early failure of fixation. The authors related these failures to osteoporosis and inadequate fixation. Twelve of these 18 patients ultimately attained a good functional result following either repeat fixation or later treatment with plate fixation and autogenous bone graft for established nonunion.

Stricker SJ, Thomson JD, Kelly RA: Coronal-plane transcondylar fracture of the humerus in a child. *Clin Orthop* 1993;294:308-311.

Coronal shear fractures may also occur in children. There was no growth disturbance in this case.

Wang KC, Shih HN, Hsu KY, et al: Intercondylar fractures of the distal humerus: Routine anterior subcutaneous transposition of the ulnar nerve in a posterior operative approach. *J Trauma* 1994;36:770-773.

Seventy-five percent excellent or good results were achieved in the surgical treatment of 20 bicolumnar distal humerus fractures (three Group C1, 11 Group C2, and six Group 3 according to the AO classification). They related the fact that no patient complained of ulnar nerve symptoms postoperatively to their routine use of anterior subcutaneous transposition of the ulnar nerve. Of further interest, all of the patients with closed fractures had delayed surgery (5 to 10 days) without apparent disadvantage, indicating that the delay in definitive treatment inherent in referral to a more experienced surgeon is justified.

44

Olecranon and Coronoid Fractures

Shawn W. O'Driscoll, MD, PhD, FRCSC

Olecranon Fractures

Etiology

Olecranon fractures usually occur as a result of a fall and are caused by either a direct blow or eccentric contraction of the triceps during resisted flexion of the elbow to break the fall. These fractures are usually displaced and retracted proximally, with occasional rupture of the thin overlying skin. One consistent observation is the frequency with which patients describe a direct blow to the posterior elbow, even in the absence of any skin marks. Fracturing the bone results in sudden, severe pain that feels indistinguishable from a direct blow. A Scandinavian study of 4,012 adult patients with extremity fractures found that increased body mass index was descriptive of patients with displaced fractures at the elbow, and that obesity is a predisposing factor.

Classification

Several classification systems have been proposed, but the one by Morrey is perhaps most useful in guiding treatment (Fig. 1). Fractures are classified according to displacement, comminution, and elbow stability. Type I fractures are undisplaced (IA, noncomminuted; IB, comminuted but still undisplaced). Type II fractures are displaced (IIA, displaced but not noncomminuted; IIB, displaced and comminuted). Type III fractures are displaced with elbow joint instability (IIIA, noncomminuted; IIIB, comminuted). This classification not only influences treatment, but also correlates with injury severity.

Evaluation

The diagnosis is usually quite obvious from the clinical examination, which reveals tenderness and swelling over the olecranon. If the fracture is displaced, a gap can be felt at the fracture site and weakness of extension is noted. The ability to actively extend the elbow indicates that the anconeus and/or triceps fascial expansion is intact around the olecranon.

Appropriate radiographic examination includes anteroposterior and lateral radiographs of the elbow. Careful inspection for concentric articulation of the ulna with the trochlea is essential, especially for comminuted fractures and those entering the joint distally toward the coronoid. Instability, evidenced by anterior subluxation of the ulna with respect to the humerus, is more likely in those fractures.

In every case of an olecranon fracture, the radiographs should be carefully studied to determine whether or not the coronoid has also been fractured. Fractures, especially if they are comminuted, of both the coronoid and olecranon in combination can be particularly ominous and difficult to treat.

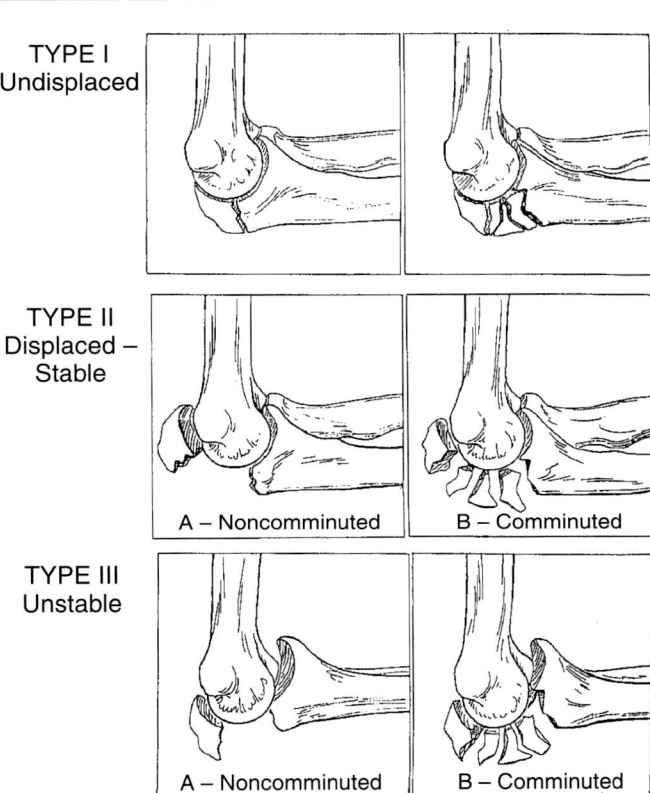

Fig. 1 Morrey classification of olecranon fractures. See text for details. (Reproduced with permission from Morrey BF (ed): *The Elbow and Its Disorders*, ed 2. Philadelphia, PA, WB Saunders, 1993.)

Treatment

As is the case for all articular fractures, obtaining and maintaining fracture reduction and joint stability so that early motion can be commenced is the treatment that most predictably assures preservation of function of both the joint and the limb. Thus, except for stable undisplaced fractures, the treatment is almost always surgical.

Treatment of these fractures is based on a sound understanding of the biomechanics and functional anatomy. Deforming forces primarily relate to the unbalanced pull of the triceps, causing distraction of the fracture, and of the biceps/brachialis, causing anterior subluxation of the ulna on the trochlea.

Type I: Undisplaced Fractures The balance of these two potentially deforming forces is maintained in undisplaced fractures by the intact soft tissues, thus no specific treatment is required. These patients can be protected briefly in a splint or sling and gentle motion permitted as is comfortable. The patient should be reexamined with radiographs after 7 to 10 days to confirm that no displacement has occurred. Flexion beyond 90° is generally avoided for the first 3 weeks.

Type II: Displaced Fractures The principle of treating this most common fracture pattern is based on the tension band concept. The deforming forces can be neutralized in this manner by using a posterior figure-of-8 wire with intramedullary Kirschner wires (K-wires). A posterior plate is an alternative, but a posterior figure-of-8 wire with two intramedullary K-wires is recommended and used by most. The K-wires should be bent, advanced into the canal, retracted 1 cm, bent 180°, and then, after placing the tension band wire, the K-wires are impacted into the olecranon through little vertical slits in the triceps tendon, which are then sewn over the K-wires to prevent backing out. Some surgeons prefer an intramedullary screw to K-wires.

For type IIB (comminuted) fractures, compression at the fracture site is not always possible, and if not, the tension band principle cannot be applied. Failure to recognize this limitation will result in one of two avoidable complications (Fig. 2). If too much tension is applied to the figure-of-8 wire, overcompression and narrowing of the semilunar notch of the ulna will occur and lead to premature arthritis. Alternately, if

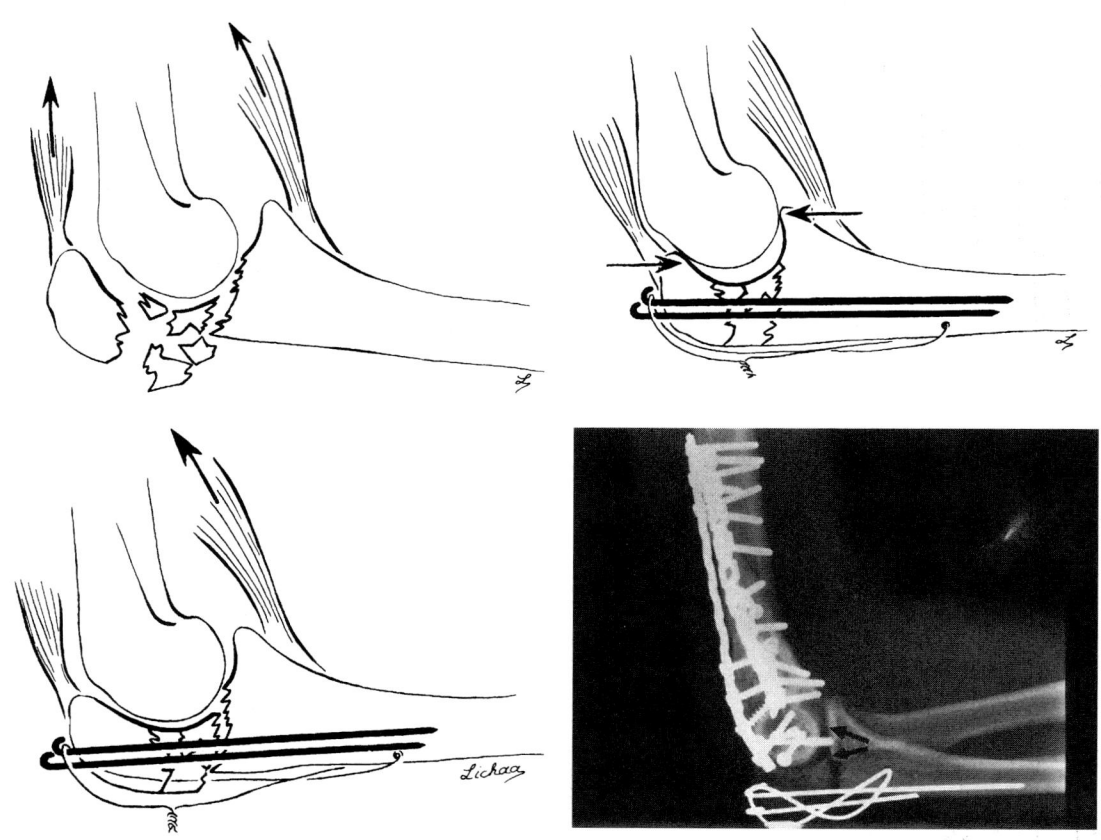

Fig. 2 Top left, Fractures of the olecranon can be unstable due to extension of the fracture toward the coronoid. Comminution increases this instability. The proximal ulna typically subluxates anteriorly because of the unopposed pull of the elbow flexors (brachialis, etc). These fractures behave quite differently from the usual olecranon fractures, are difficult to treat, and are associated with a poorer prognosis.
Top right, The traditional AO/ASIF method for internal fixation of olecranon fractures with intramedullary K-wires and tension banding relies on compression at the fracture site, which is not possible in comminuted fractures. If compression is applied the semilunar notch of the ulna will be narrowed (*arrows*), resulting in joint incongruity. **Bottom left,** If compression is not applied, the reduction is unstable and the fracture can displace. Anterior ulnohumeral subluxation occurs because of the unopposed pull of the anterior elbow flexors. **Bottom right,** Radiograph of a patient who had been treated by K-wires and tension band technique for an unstable olecranon fracture-subluxation. Stability was not possible because of the comminution and distal fracture line; thus, subluxation recurred. Careful inspection of the radiograph reveals that the ulna is still subluxated anteriorly, as indicated by the gap between the coronoid and the trochlea anteriorly (*arrows*). (Reproduced with permission from O'Driscoll SW: Technique for unstable olecranon fracture-subluxations. *Op Tech Orthop* 1994;4:49-53.)

one does not tension the wire, the reduction will not be stable, permitting fracture displacement joint subluxation, which also leads to arthritis. These problems can be avoided by application of a contoured plate posteriorly as described for type III fractures (Figs. 3, 4, and 5).

Plate fixation is an option for all olecranon fractures, and if the plate is placed posteriorly it functions not only as a tension band but also as a buttress. However, it is only necessary in unstable fracture-subluxations (type III) and some comminuted fractures (type IIB), and because hardware prominence sometimes causes irritation, most surgeons reserve plates for those situations. One biomechanical study compared lateral plating with a 3.5-mm reconstruction plate to placing the plate posteriorly for comminuted olecranon fractures. The two techniques yielded similar results in the test model.

In an attempt to prevent the problems associated with prominent hardware, biodegradable screws and pins have been tested. Two Finnish studies documented the use of these implants in 41 olecranon fractures. Two fractures displaced from failure of fixation and required reoperation. Three developed sinuses from tissue reaction to the polyglycolide, but healed. This technique has some potential advantage related to decreasing the need for hardware removal. Concerns relating to foreign body granulomatous reaction and failure of fixation need to be addressed before these techniques are recommended for routine use.

Excision of small comminuted fragments with triceps reattachment is recommended for elderly patients if internal fixation is expected to be unsuccessful or contraindicated. Keeping in mind that loss of stability has been shown in a biomechanical study by An and associates to be proportional to the amount of olecranon excised, no more than half of the olecranon should be removed. More importantly, this treatment is not acceptable for distal fractures entering the joint close to the coronoid, because the risk of instability is too high in such cases.

The surgical approach is posterior, but it is wise to avoid placing the incision directly over the tip of the olecranon, in the presence of the hardware and bursa. Wound breakdown in that area is more likely and more problematic to manage than a wound slightly off to the lateral or medial side. The scar will also be less prone to irritation or injury, especially if a plate is used. In all cases, the triceps expansion is repaired as well.

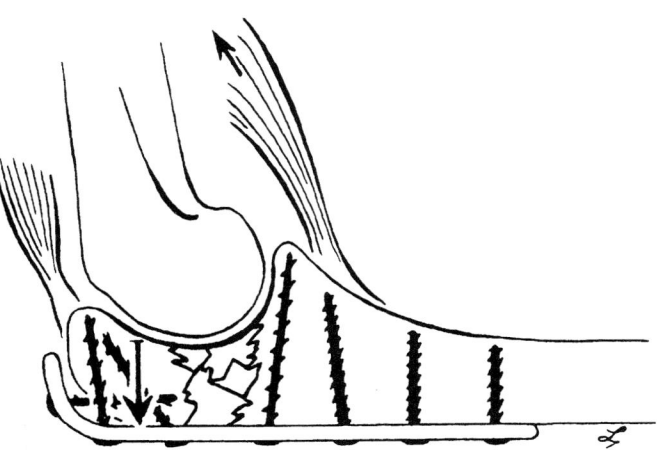

Fig. 3 Treatment of unstable comminuted fracture-subluxations is best accomplished using a posterior 3.5 mm dynamic compression plate that has been contoured around the proximal olecranon. Plate breakage is extremely unlikely. Three screws can be inserted into the small proximal fragment. Arrow shows resistance to the deforming pull of the anterior elbow flexors. (Reproduced with permission from O'Driscoll SW: Technique for unstable olecranon fracture-subluxations. *Op Tech Orthop* 1994;4:49-53.)

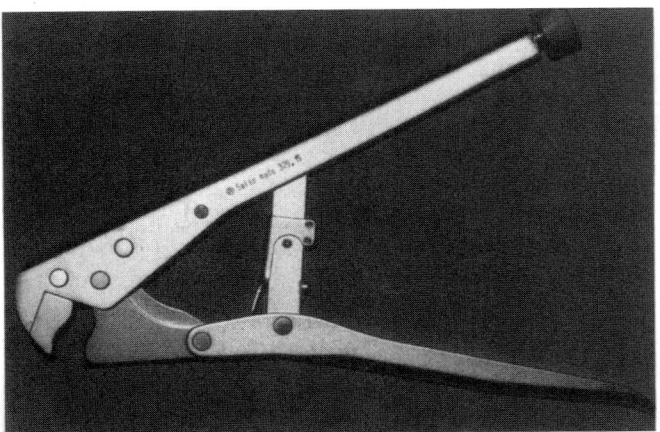 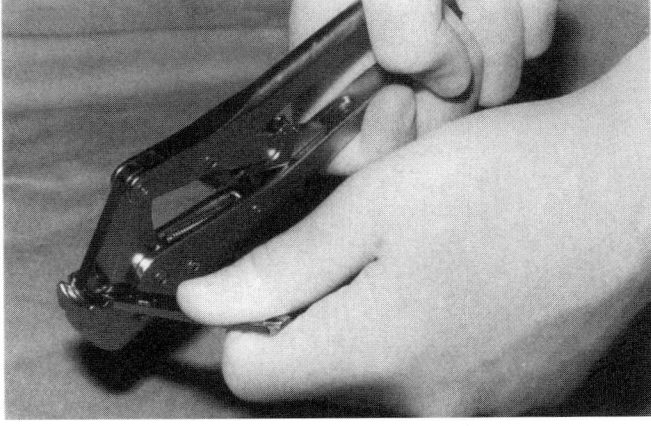

Fig. 4 Contouring the 3.5-mm dynamic compression plate. **Left,** The bending pliers that are used are supplied with the AO/ASIF small fragment set. **Right,** The proximal end of the plate is bent with the pliers to an 80° angle. A low contact dynamic compression or reconstruction plate can also be used, but the dynamic compression is preferable. (Reproduced with permission from O'Driscoll SW: Technique for unstable olecranon fracture-subluxations. *Op Tech Orthop* 1994;4:49-53.)

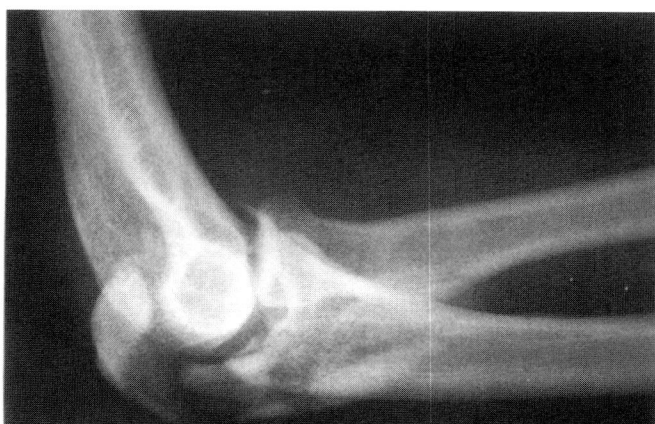 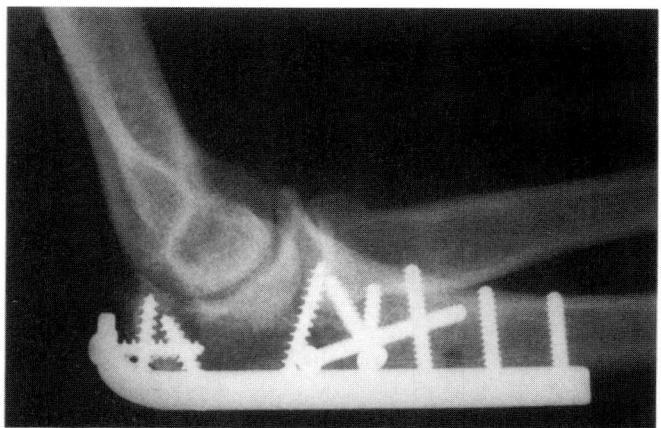

Fig. 5 **Left,** Lateral radiograph of a patient with an open comminuted olecranon fracture-subluxation. The ulna is subluxated anteriorly. The coronoid is also displaced, which is best seen on the anteroposterior (postoperative) view. **Right,** Postoperative radiograph. The wound was debrided and the fracture treated immediately with a contoured 3.5-mm dynamic compression plate and interfragmentary compression screws. Stable anatomic reduction was possible despite the comminution. Active motion was initiated when the wound was closed 3 days after debridement and open reduction and internal fixation. The fracture healed in 6 weeks. (Reproduced with permission from O'Driscoll SW: Technique for unstable olecranon fracture-subluxations. *Op Tech Orthop* 1994;4:49-53.)

Type III: Displaced Fractures With Joint Instability This is the category of fractures that creates challenges for the surgeon and problems for the patient. The distinguishing component of this injury is the instability of the elbow joint. Usually the ulna and radius subluxate anteriorly on the distal humerus because of the unbalanced pull of the biceps and brachialis. This instability might not be present on the initial films. Risk factors predicting joint instability include distal fractures entering the joint near the coronoid, severely comminuted fractures, and associated fractures of the coronoid. These unstable fracture-subluxations cannot be treated by the tension band technique and require plate fixation. A reliable method is the application of a contoured 3.5-mm dynamic compression (DC) plate to the flat posterior cortex of the proximal ulna. This plate configuration allows placement of three screws in the small proximal fragment, posterior buttressing against anterior subluxation, buttressing of the intercalary fragments, and, if the fracture can be converted to essentially a two-part fracture, interfragmentary compression and use of the tension band principle (Fig. 5). Some have tried plating along the medial or lateral borders of the ulna. This method is not as reliable because it is only possible to place one or two short screws in the proximal fragment. Another reason that plating medially or laterally is less desirable is that the plate must be contoured exactly to meet the curvature of the proximal ulna or it will cause displacement. The posterior surface of the ulna is flat and requires no contouring except around the tip of the olecranon (Fig. 4).

The principles of treating these unstable comminuted fracture-subluxations are to: (1) obtain stable fixation of the small proximal fragment; (2) buttress the ulnar shaft against the proximal fragment to resist the deforming pull of the anterior elbow flexors; (3) buttress the comminuted fragments within the fracture site; (4) obtain stable fixation of the ulnar shaft; and (5) secure fixation of the coronoid if fractured. This is best accomplished using a posterior 3.5-mm DC plate that has been contoured around the proximal olecranon. Plate breakage is extremely unlikely. Three screws can be inserted into the small proximal fragment. The plate must be contoured around the tip of the olecranon and be strong enough to resist bending and breaking. The DC, low contact dynamic compression (LCDC), or reconstruction plates suffice. This method of plating comminuted proximal ulnar fractures with elbow subluxation has the advantages of stable fracture fixation, excellent purchase on even small proximal fragments, and buttressing against elbow subluxation, all of which permit immediate motion.

Associated coronoid fractures should be carefully sought, identified, and fixed. Ligament injuries are repaired acutely.

If the fractures cannot be rigidly fixed and joint stability achieved, a hinged external fixation device is used to maintain joint alignment while the soft periarticular tissues heal sufficiently to maintain reduction.

Postoperative treatment in all cases consists of brief splinting for a day or two, then early motion. If the posterior tension band has been restored and is secure, full active motion is permitted. When the security of fixation is in question, motion is limited to an arc from 30° to 110° for the first 3 to 6 weeks.

Results

In a study of 45 displaced olecranon fractures treated by tension band wiring, 97% had good or excellent results when the fracture was isolated to the olecranon. Hardware complications were largely prevented by proper technique.

In one randomized study of 25 olecranon fractures, 15 were fixed with bioabsorbable wires and screws or pins and ten with metal tension bands (intramedullary K-wires and a tension band). The authors did not find a significant difference in outcomes except that secondary operations for hardware removal were not necessary in the group treated with the absorbable devices. Another study reported 41 patients treated with bioabsorbable implants. Implant fixation occurred in two, requiring revision. A sinus tract developed from tissue reaction in three, but did not affect fracture healing.

In a review of six patients with comminuted unstable fracture-subluxations of the olecranon treated by a posteriorly placed contoured DC plate, a functional arc of motion was achieved in five of six patients. The results were excellent (functional arc, no or minimal pain, excellent strength) in four cases. There were three reoperations: one for plate removal, one for ulnar nerve transposition (related to an open distal humerus fracture with soft tissue loss), and one for ligament repair and open reduction and internal fixation of a displaced coronoid fracture. The unsatisfactory outcome resulted from inadequate fixation and displacement of a comminuted type III coronoid fracture.

Fragment excision and triceps tendon reattachment should only be considered for small olecranon fractures in the elderly. The loss of elbow joint stability is proportional to the amount of the olecranon excised. In a recent series of patients treated by olecranon fragment excision, results were excellent in seven patients, good in four, and poor in one.

Few studies report the results of treatment of olecranon nonunions. In one study, 20 olecranon nonunions were treated surgically. The olecranon fragment was excised in one, fixed and grafted in 16, and the joint replaced in three. Four patients also had distraction arthroplasty. At a mean follow-up of 18 months, motion averaged 98° (improvement of 11°). Results were excellent in 12 patients, good in four, fair in six, and poor in two. Union was achieved in 15 of the 16 patients treated by osteosynthesis.

Complications

The most common complication of olecranon fractures is the need for hardware removal. In one series, this complication was reportedly as high as 80% of patients. This complication is usually caused by irritation from the tips of the K-wires protruding at the posterior aspect of the olecranon, or the twists in the tension band wiring. Protruding K-wires can be largely avoided by bending the K-wire tips around 180° and advancing them fully into the bone, then suturing the triceps over the buried wire. Prominence of the wire twists can be almost eliminated by using a Harris wire-tier, and rather than twisting the wire, a low profile, flat square knot is tied distally and laterally where there is muscle protecting it.

The second most common complication is loss of motion, particularly extension. This is caused by failure to initiate early postoperative motion and adequate efforts to rehabilitate the elbow. Starting motion in the first day or two postoperatively, and using splints if necessary, will assist in regaining motion starting 3 to 6 weeks after surgery, or later if the need was not recognized.

The remaining cartilage on the ulna and trochlea is also prone to damage from the severity of the blunt trauma, raising the possibility for chronic posttraumatic pain and/or arthritis.

Ulnar neuritis or neuropathy can occur either as a result of the injury itself or the surgical intervention. Hardware should be placed such that it does it compromise the ulnar nerve.

Instability and incongruity resulting from inappropriate application of the tension band technique were discussed previously.

Coronoid Fractures

Etiology

Isolated fractures of the coronoid are rare. Coronoid fractures are usually seen in association with elbow instability, either as part of a complex fracture dislocation or as a minimally displaced fracture indicative of subluxation and reduction of the elbow. Nothing usually attaches to the very tip of the coronoid. A cadaveric study of 20 elbows revealed that the capsule attaches 6 mm distally on average. This confirms that small flake fractures are not avulsion fractures, but are shear fractures caused by instability as previously postulated. Often they are accompanied by radial head fractures. Type III coronoid fractures, which involve more than 50% of the coronoid, often occur in association with comminuted fractures of the proximal ulna including the olecranon. Biomechanically, the coronoid is most vulnerable to fracture under axial load with the elbow flexed 80°.

Classification

Coronoid fractures have been classified by Regan and Morrey into three types. A type I fracture is a small shear fracture of just the tip of the coronoid. It has been erroneously referred to as an avulsion fracture. The capsule inserts 4 to 6 mm distal to the tip of the coronoid and the brachialis further down. These small fractures are usually caused by a traumatic elbow subluxation as the coronoid passes beneath the trochlea, a mechanism that has been reproduced in cadaver elbows (Fig. 6, *top*). It indicates that the elbow has been unstable, just as a bony Bankart lesion of the glenoid indicates anterior shoulder instability. Type II fractures involve up to 50% of the coronoid, and almost always are seen in association with fractures of the radial head and elbow dislocation (Fig. 6, *center*), known as the terrible triad of the elbow. Type III fractures involve more than 50% of the coronoid and are usually comminuted, often involving the olecranon (Fig. 6, *bottom*). These fractures are difficult to approach or fix, render the elbow unstable if left unfixed, and carry a grave prognosis. Indeed, in a complex fracture-dislocation of the elbow, the presence of a coronoid fracture is the most important concern.

Evaluation

The diagnosis should be suspected following an elbow dislocation or olecranon fracture. Plain anteroposterior and lateral radiographs usually suffice but oblique views can be helpful. Lateral tomograms are highly reliable if the diagnosis is in doubt.

Fractures of both the coronoid and olecranon in combination can be particularly ominous and difficult to treat, especially when they are comminuted.

Treatment

Type I Fractures Type I coronoid fractures only require fixation if the radial head has been fractured or if there is severe

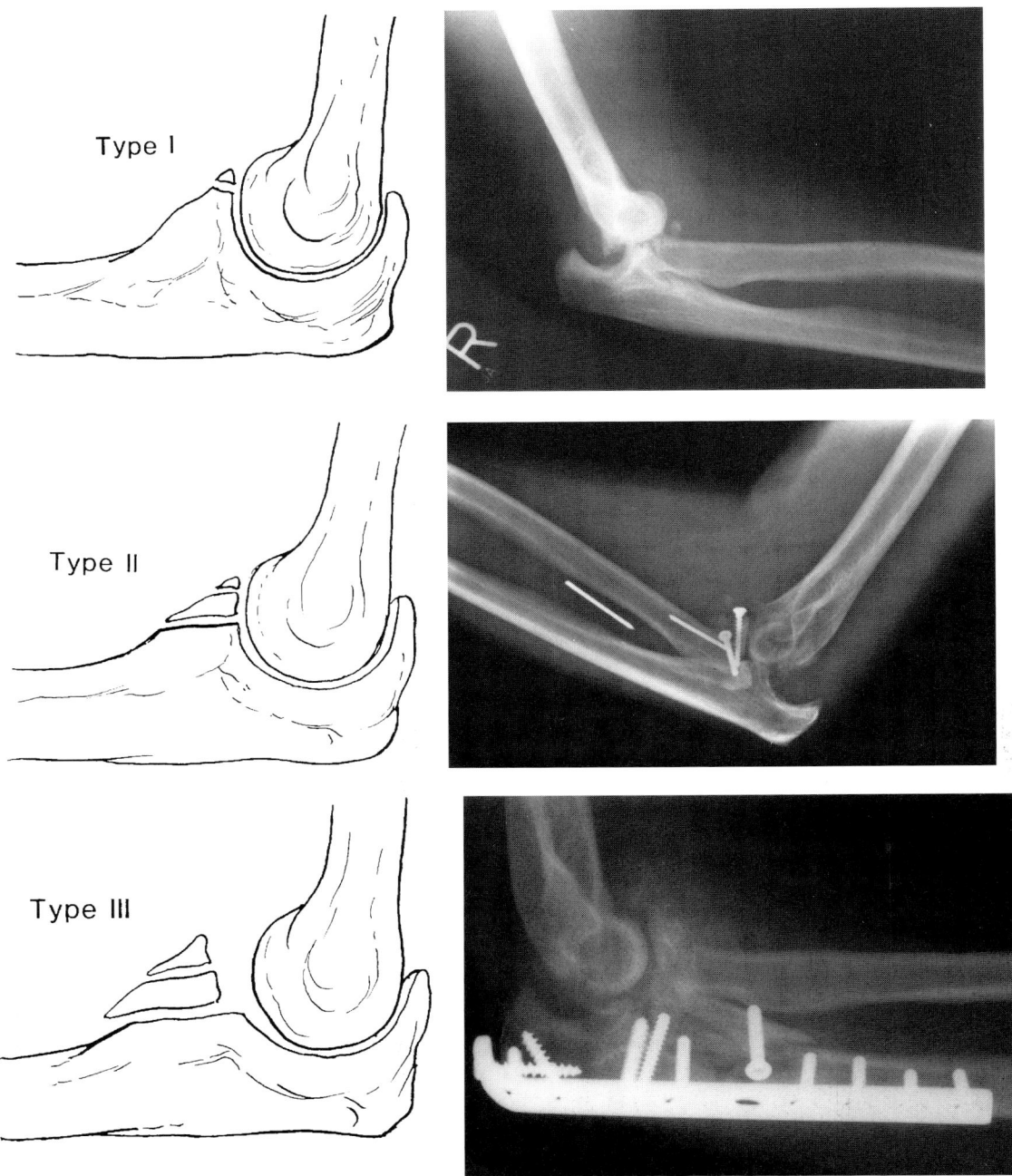

Fig. 6 Classification of coronoid fractures. See text for details. (Top left, center left, bottom left reproduced with permission from Morrey BF (ed): *The Elbow and Its Disorders*, ed 2. Philadelphia, PA, WB Saunders, 1993.)

instability such as when the entire distal humerus is stripped of its soft tissues. Screws cannot be used in the small fragment, so wires or sutures are placed over it and pulled through the ulna as described for type II fractures.

Type II Fractures A reliable method of fixation is to pass two heavy (No. 5) nonabsorbable sutures or wires through the ulna from the subcutaneous border emerging at the proximal (articular) edge of the fracture. These are then passed over the coronoid fragment, through the attached capsule, and back down through two separate holes in the ulna just proximal to the distal edge of the fracture and tied tightly (Fig. 7). Perfect anatomic reduction of these smaller fragments is not as important as restoration of the anterior buttress. The technique is based on principles similar to a volar plate advancement arthroplasty for proximal interphalangeal fracture-

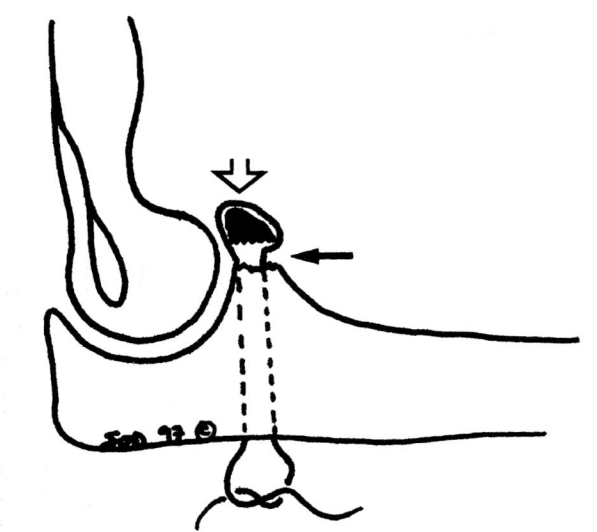

Fig 7 Technique for suture (or wire) fixation of small coronoid fractures. This technique is recommended whenever there is a type I or II coronoid fracture in the presence of a dislocated elbow unless the elbow is stable following closed reduction (which is rarely the case in these injuries).(© 1997 Shawn O'Driscoll, MD, Mayo Clinic, Rochester, MN.)

dislocations. The surgical approach is through the soft-tissue disruption laterally. Often the radial head is fractured and displaced, which facilitates the exposure.

Type III Fractures This ominous fracture pattern is one for which reliable and practical treatment has not been determined, which is one of the reasons it bears such a poor prognosis. Open reduction and stable internal fixation is the goal, but if this cannot be accomplished, a hinged external fixator is used to maintain the joint in the reduced position while the fragments heal.

The surgical approach depends on the fracture type and need for other surgery such as ligament reconstruction. A posterior skin incision just off the midline permits deep access laterally and medially. Type I and II fractures can be reduced and fixed through a lateral arthrotomy, as the soft-tissue dissection has already been performed by the traumatic dislocation. Access is facilitated if the radial head is fractured. Type III fractures can sometimes be fixed through the displaced olecranon fracture gap, but if there is no olecranon fracture, they require exposure from either the medial or lateral side. The optimum approach is not yet known. A direct anterior approach is difficult because of the brachialis insertion.

Chronic fracture-dislocations can be approached with a Bryan-Morrey posterior approach, reflecting the triceps laterally and dislocating the elbow to permit access to the entire joint, including the anterior structures. This permits placement of hardware from anterior to posterior through the reduced coronoid fragment.

If the fractures cannot be rigidly fixed and joint stability achieved, a hinged external fixation device is used to maintain joint alignment while the soft periarticular tissues heal sufficiently to maintain reduction. One study reported success in six of seven patients with complex unstable fracture-dislocations treated in this manner.

As with olecranon fractures, postoperative treatment consists of brief splinting for a day or two, then early motion. Full active motion is allowed if the posterior tension band has been restored and is secure. If security of fixation is in question, motion is limited to an arc from 30° to 110° for the first 3 to 6 weeks.

Nonunions There are no reports dealing with coronoid nonunions. Anecdotal experience indicates that these require treatment if the elbow is unstable. Open reduction and internal fixation with bone grafting, or structural bone grafting is recommended (Fig. 6). Displaced radial head fracture fragments that are removed can be sculpted and used to recreate the coronoid. The shape must be correctly restored.

Results

Little has been written regarding coronoid fractures. Regan and Morrey reviewed 35 cases and found that the likelihood of success was inversely related to the amount of coronoid involvement. Whereas over 80% of the small type I fractures had satisfactory outcomes, about 80% of the large comminuted type III fractures had unsatisfactory results. Type II fractures fell between the two extremes and were successfully managed in about 50% of the cases. The results are usually related to the success in controlling elbow instability.

Complications

The most common complication following coronoid fractures is elbow instability. The joint resultant force vector, which is posterior and superior, requires the coronoid to resist posterior displacement of the ulna under the humerus. Thus, the likelihood and severity of such instability is directly related to how much coronoid is lost or displaced.

Nonunions of small fragments do not seem to affect the outcome provided that elbow stability has been maintained.

Rapidly progressive posttraumatic arthritis usually is seen in patients with joint incongruity caused by displaced type II or III coronoid fractures that permit posterior subluxation.

Selected Bibliography

Olecranon

An K-N, Morrey BF, Chao EY: The effect of partial removal of proximal ulna on elbow constraint. *Clin Orthop* 1986;209:270-279.

The loss of elbow joint stability is proportional to the amount of the olecranon excised.

Bostman OM: Body mass index of patients with elbow and ankle fractures requiring surgical treatment. *J Trauma* 1994;37:62-65.

Obesity was a predisposing factor for patients with displaced elbow fractures.

Cobb TK, Morrey BF: Use of distraction arthroplasty in unstable fracture dislocations of the elbow. *Clin Orthop* 1995;312:201-210.

A hinged external fixator is a salvage option for unstable fracture-dislocations that cannot be repaired. Though not a problem in this series, deep sepsis from the pin across the distal humerus is a serious risk.

Helm RH, Hornby R, Miller SW: The complications of surgical treatment of displaced fractures of the olecranon. *Injury* 1987;18:48-50.

Forty-eight patients treated by either tension band wiring (34) or screw fixation (14) were reviewed. There was a higher rate of fracture distraction with screw fixation alone.

Inhofe PD, Howard TC: The treatment of olecranon fractures by excision of fragments and repair of the extensor mechanism: Historical review and report of 12 fractures. *Orthopedics* 1993;16:1313-1317.

Of 12 patients treated by olecranon fragment excision, results were excellent in seven, good in four, and poor in one.

Juutilainen T, Patiala H, Rokkanen P, et al: Biodegradable wire fixation in olecranon and patella fractures combined with biodegradable screws or plugs and compared with metallic fixation. *Arch Orthop Trauma Surg* 1995;114:319-323.

In this randomized study of 25 olecranon fractures, 15 were fixed with bioabsorbable wires and screws or pins and ten with metal tension bands (intramedullary K-wires and a tension band). The authors did not find a significant difference in outcomes except that secondary operations for hardware removal were not necessary in the group treated with the absorbable devices.

King GJ, Lammens PN, Milne AD, et al: Plate fixation of comminuted olecranon fractures: An in vitro biomechanical study. *J Shoulder Elbow Surg* 1996;5:437-441.

Lateral plating with a 3.5-mm dynamic compression reconstruction plate was found biomechanically to be similar to placing the plate posteriorly for comminuted olecranon fractures. Either technique should be satisfactory if there is adequate fixation in the small proximal fragment.

Cabanela ME, Morrey BF: Fractures of the proximal ulna and olecranon, in Morrey BF (ed): *The Elbow and Its Disorders,* ed 2. Philadelphia, PA, WB Saunders, 1993, pp 405-428.

Murphy DF, Greene WB, Dameron TB Jr: Displaced olecranon fractures in adults: Clinical evaluation. *Clin Orthop* 1987;224:215-223.

Thirty-eight patients were treated by a variety of surgical techniques. Hardware problems occurred in 80% of those who used the AO/ASIF tension band technique, and instability occurred in one of seven in whom the fragment was excised.

ODriscoll SW: Technique for unstable olecranon fracture-subluxations. *Op Tech Orthop* 1994;4:49-53.

Unstable fracture-subluxations cannot be treated by the tension band technique and require plate fixation. A reliable method is the application of a contoured 3.5-mm dynamic compression plate to the flat posterior cortex of the proximal ulna. This plate configuration allows placement of three screws in the small proximal fragment, posterior buttressing against anterior subluxation, buttressing of the intercalary fragments, and, if the fracture can be converted to essentially a two-part fracture, interfragmentary compression and use of the tension band principle. The posterior surface of the ulna is flat and requires no contouring except around the tip of the olecranon.

Papagelopoulos PJ, Morrey BF: Treatment of nonunion of olecranon fractures. *J Bone Joint Surg* 1994;76B:627-635.

Of 24 patients with olecranon nonunions, 20 were operated on. The olecranon fragment was excised in one, fixed and grafted in 16, and the joint replaced in three. Four patients also had distraction arthroplasty. At a mean follow-up of 18 months motion averaged 98° (improvement of 11°). Results were excellent in 12 patients, good in four, fair in six, and poor in two. Union had been achieved in 15 of the 16 patients treated by osteosynthesis.

Partio EK, Hirvensalo E, Bostman O, et al: Absorbable rods and screws: A new method of fixation for fractures of the olecranon. *Int Orthop* 1992;16:250-254.

Forty-one patients were treated with bioabsorbable implants. Implant fixation occurred in two, and revision was required. A sinus tract developed from tissue reaction in three, but did not affect fracture healing.

Wolfgang G, Burke F, Bush D, et al: Surgical treatment of displaced olecranon fractures by tension band wiring technique. *Clin Orthop* 1987;224:192-204.

Forty-five displaced olecranon fractures treated by tension band wiring had 97% good or excellent results when the fracture was isolated to the olecranon. Proper technique prevented most hardware complications.

Coronoid

Amis AA, Miller JH: The mechanisms of elbow fractures: An investigation using impact tests in vitro. *Injury* 1995;26:163-168.

Cage DJ, Abrams RA, Callahan JJ, et al: Soft tissue attachments of the ulnar coronoid process: An anatomic study with radiographic correlation. *Clin Orthop* 1995;320:154-158.

A cadaveric study of 20 elbows revealed that nothing usually attaches to the very tip of the coronoid. The capsule attaches 6 mm distally on average. This confirms that small flake fractures are not avulsion fractures, but are shear fractures due to instability as previously postulated. Type III coronoid fractures, which involve more than 50% of the coronoid, destabilize the medial collateral ligament.

Hanks GA, Kottmeier SA: Isolated fracture of the coronoid process of the ulna: A case report and review of the literature. *J Orthop Trauma* 1990;4:193-196.

Cabanela ME, Morrey BF: Fractures of the proximal ulna and olecranon, in Morrey BF (ed): *The Elbow and Its Disorders,* ed 2. Philadelphia, PA, WB Saunders, 1993, pp 405-428.

O'Driscoll SW: Classification and spectrum of elbow instability: Recurrent instability, in Morrey BF (ed): *The Elbow and Its Disorders,* ed 2. Philadelphia, PA, WB Saunders, 1993, pp 453-463.

A classification that unifies the clinical, radiographic and pathologic features along with implications for treatment of elbow instability is presented based on scientific laboratory data and clinical experience. Shear fractures at the tip of the coronoid occur as the ulna dislocates under the trochlea, creating a lesion analogous to the bony Bankart lesion of traumatic anterior shoulder instability.

O'Driscoll SW: Elbow instability. *Hand Clin* 1994;10: 405-415.

An important feature to recognize is that the small (type I) flake fractures of the coronoid are not avulsion fractures, but are shear fractures caused by impaction of the coronoid against the trochlea as the ulna dislocates under the humerus.

Regan W, Morrey B: Fractures of the coronoid process of the ulna. *J Bone Joint Surg* 1989;71A:1348-1354.

Coronoid fractures are classified.

Index

Page numbers in italics refer to figures; page numbers with t refer to tables

A
Abduction, painful arc of, 136
Ablation surgery, 248
Achievement of 90° of abduction, 293
Acromial fracture, 159, *159*
Acromioclavicular joint, 6–7, 31, 105. *See also* Shoulder
    arthritis in, 157, 217
    injuries to, 104–106, *105*
    resection of, 151
Acromionectomy, 158
    lateral, 158
Acromioplasty, 151, 159, 187, 218, *219*, 220
Activity level and acute dislocations, 69
Adhesive capsulitis, 255, 257
Age, as factor in
    acute dislocations, 69
    cuff tendon degeneration, 277
    rotator cuff injury, 135
Allograft interposition, 161
American Shoulder and Elbow Surgeons (ASES)
  Standardized Shoulder Assessment and Shoulder
  Score Index, 49, *50, 51*, 51–53, *52, 53*
Amyloidosis, 234
Analgesics in management of rheumatoid arthritis, 217
Anchor technique, 273, *273*
Anterior capsule of elbow, 306
    tear of, 319
Anterior capsulolabral reconstruction, 104
Anterior instability, recurrent, 104, 114–115
Anterior interosseous neuropathy, 373–374
Anterior medial collateral ligament (AMCL) and elbow
  instability, 345, 346, 347
Anterior shoulder pain
    classification of, 102–103
    diagnosis of, 101–102
Anterior stability tests, 61
Anterosuperior instability, 223
AO classification systems, 44
Arthritis. *See also* Degenerative arthritis; Elbow
  arthritis; Osteoarthritis; Posttraumatic arthritis;
  Rheumatoid arthritis
    in acromioclavicular joint, 157, 217
    arthroscopy in managing primary degenerative, 360
    glenohumeral, 157, 201
    inflammatory, of shoulder, 215, 223–224
      clinical presentation, 217
      complications, 222–223
      nonsurgical management, 217–218
      pathophysiology, 215–*216*, 217
      results/outcome, 221–222
      surgical management, 218, *218, 219,* 220–221
    posttraumatic, 195
Arthrodesis, 228
    in surgical repair of rotator cuff tears, 168–169
    in treating osteoarthritis, 229
Arthrography, in evaluating
    frozen shoulder, 256
    rotator cuff, *140*, 140–141, *141*
Arthrokatadysis in hip, 215
Arthropathy. *See also* Cuff tear arthropathy
    capsulorrhaphy, 227
Arthroplasty, 220–221, 237. *See also* Bipolar arthroplasty; Glenohumeral arthroplasty; Hemiarthroplasty
    Coonrad-Morrey total elbow, 380
    interposition, 380

    joint replacement, 380–381, *381*
    nonconstrained total joint, 229
    Outerbridge-Kashiwagi, 358
    prosthetic replacement, 228, 229
    resection, 174, 228
    results of, 233
    in surgical repair of rotator cuff tears, 168–169, 174–175
    in treating rheumatoid arthritis, 215, 217
    ulnohumeral, 383
Arthroscopic anterior glenohumeral reconstruction, 95, 99
    lesion identification, 96, *96*
    patient selection, 95–96
    surgical reconstruction
      labrum repair, 97–98
      ligament repair, *96*, 98, *99*
      midsubstance ligamentous laxity, *96*, 98–99, *99*
      postoperative rehabilitation, 99
      technique, 97
Arthroscopic capsular release, 327
Arthroscopic evaluation of anterior shoulder instability, 78–79
Arthroscopic stabilizations, intraoperative complications of, 112
Arthroscopic staple capsulorrhaphy, 113
Arthroscopic subacromial decompression, 103, 159
Arthroscopic synovectomy, 218, 229
Arthroscopy, 269
    of elbow, 319–320, *320, 321*
    for frozen shoulder, 260–261, *261*
    for primary degenerative arthritis, 360
Arthrosis, radiocapitellar, 393
Articular surface fractures, *186,* 186–187
Articulation
    glenohumeral, 42
    scapulothoracic, 7
    ulnohumeral, 387
Athletes
    anterior instability in throwing, 77
    elbow injuries in, 311, 321
      anterior, 319
      biomechanics, 311–313, *312*
      lateral, 317
      medial, 313–317, *315*
    shoulder pain in, 101–108, *105, 106, 107, 108*
Athletic Shoulder Outcome Rating Scale, 53
Atraumatic osteolysis of distal clavicle, 105–106
Atraumatic subluxation, exercise program for, 87
Avascular necrosis, 233
Axillary artery occlusion, 107–108
Axonotmesis, 245, 369
Axon reflex testing in evaluating brachial plexus injuries, 245

B
Bankart lesions, 59, 78, 79, 102
Bankart repairs, 111–112
    failure of, 116
Baseball pitching, *34,* 34–35
Biceps, 304
    rupture of, 163
Biceps tendinitis, 319
Biceps tendon, 15–16, *16. See also* Distal biceps tendon injury
    long head of, 5, *5*
Biochemical abnormalities, role in development of multidirectional instability, 86
Biodegradable fixation devices, 116
Biodegradable tacks, 113
Biomechanics
    of glenohumeral stability, *11,* 11–17, *12, 13, 14, 16*
    of total elbow arthroplasty, 306–308, *307*
Bipolar arthroplasty, 228. *See also* Arthroplasty
    of rotator cuff tear, 175

Bone block procedures, 113
Bone trough, 152
Bony stabilization procedure, 91
Brachial artery, risk for injury, 208
Brachialis, 304
Brachialis tendinitis, 319
Brachial plexopathy, 249
    metastatic, 251
    prognosis of radiation-induced, 251
Brachial plexus, 245
    anatomy of, 243, *243, 244*
    relationship of clavicle to, 192
Brachial plexus injuries, 106, 243
    closed, *245,* 245–246, 246t
        nonsurgical treatment of, 246–247
        obstetric, 249–250
        palliative treatment, 248
        reconstructive procedures, 247–248
        surgical treatment of, 247, *248*
    methods of evaluation, 243–245, *244*
    oncologic and radiation-induced, 251
    open wounds, 250–251
    postanesthetic palsy, 250
    sports-related, 251–252
Brachioradialis, 304
Bristow procedure, 79, 104, 113
    complications associated with, 113, *115*
Bryan-Morrey posterior approach, 411
Burners, 251–252
Burner syndrome, 106
Bursa
    subacromial, 6, 218
    subdeltoid, 218

C

C8 radiculopathy, 371
Caisson disease, 227
Calcification
    degenerative, 277
    reactive, 277–278, *278*
Calcifying tendinitis, 277
    diagnostic techniques, 280–281, *281, 282*
    management, 281–282
    pathoanatomy, *278,* 278–280, *279, 280*
    pathogenesis, 277–278, *278*
    surgical management, 282
Calcium pyrophosphate dihydrate (CPPD)
    deposition of crystals, 283
    intra-articular deposition of, 282–283
Capsular ligaments, biomechanical analysis of, 59
Capsular staples, loosening and migration of, 113, *113*
Capsulectomy, 401–402
Capsulitis, adhesive, 255, 257
Capsuloligamentous tissues, *302,* 302–304, *303*
Capsulorrhaphy, 91
    medial, 88
    staple, 112
Capsulorrhaphy arthropathy, 227
Cardiac disease, relationship between frozen shoulder and, 256
Carrying angle, 304–305
Caspari technique, 95, 272–273, *273*
Cervical disk disease, referred pain related to, 157
Cervical spine evaluation, 138
Cervical spine radiographs in evaluating brachial plexus injuries, 244
Checkrein shoulder, 255
Cheilectomy, open, 228–229
Chloroquine in management of rheumatoid arthritis, 217
Chondrocalcinosis (pseudogout), 227, 282–283
    diagnosis, 283, *283*
    pathology, 283
    therapy, 283

Chondromalacia, 317–318
Chondrosarcoma, 238
Chronic impingement syndrome, indications for surgery, 151
Chronic low grade traction, 369–370
Chronic refractory tennis elbow following failed surgical intervention, 338, *339*
Chronic valgus instability, 394
Clarke pectoralis major transfer, 250
Clavicle
    anatomy of, 191, *191*
    motion of, 191
Clavicle fractures
    classification, *192,* 192–193
    clinical evaluation, 192
    complications
        malunion, 195
        neurovascular injuries, 195
        nonunion, 195
        posttraumatic arthritis, 195
    etiology, 191–192
    radiologic evaluation, 192
    treatment
        closed management of middle third, 193
        lateral type, 194–195
        medial third, 195
        open management of middle third, *193,* 193–194
Clavicular instability, 160–161
Climber's elbow, 319
Closed chain rehabilitation, 293, *293, 294, 295*
Coaptation splint, 205
Codman exercises, 69
Codman's paradox, 31
Cold vasodilation test in evaluating brachial plexus injuries, 245
Colles' fracture and frozen shoulder, 256
Compass elbow hinge, 330–331, *332*
Compass Hinge™, 382
Compression plating, 209
Computed tomography (CT), in assessing
    brachial plexus injuries, 244
    clavicle fractures, 192
    elbow, 326
    proximal humerus fractures, *182,* 182–183
    rheumatoid arthritis, 217
    rotator cuff tears, 167
Computed tomographic (CT) arthrography, in assessing glenohumeral joint stability, 63
Conoid ligament, 6
Constant Score, 49
Constrained total shoulder arthroplasty of rotator cuff tear, 175
Coonrad-Morrey total elbow arthroplasty, 380, 381, 382
Coracoacromial arch, 22, *22,* 125–127, *126*
    abnormalities of, 130
    mechanical forces about, 126–127
Coracoacromial ligament, 6, 160, 259
    excision, 151
    repair of, 152, 223
    resection, 159
Coracohumeral ligament, 5, *13,* 13–14, 19
    anatomy and function of, 123
    and frozen shoulder, 258–259
    in frozen shoulder, 257
Coracoid bone block, fracture of, 113
Coracoid fractures, 201
Core decompression, 234, 235
Coronoid fractures, 350–351
    classification, 409, *410*
    complications, 411
    etiology, 409
    evaluation, 409
    results, 411
    treatment, 409–411, *411*

Coronoid impingement syndrome, 319
Corticosteroids. *See also* Steroids
   in managing rheumatoid arthritis, 217, 379
   in managing rotator cuff tear, 145
Cortisone injections for epicondylitis, 338
Crepitus, 135
Cubital tunnel syndrome, 370, 371
   treatment of, 372
Cubitus valgus, 370–371
Cubitus varus, 370–371
Cuff-capsule complex, 19, 20
Cuff tear arthropathy, 238. *See also* Rotator cuff
   complications, 175–176
   etiology, *173*, 173–174
   evaluation, 174, *174*
   results, 176
   treatment, 174
      bipolar arthroplasty, 175
      constrained total shoulder arthroplasty, 175
      glenohumeral arthrodesis and resection arthroplasty, 174–175
      hemiarthroplasty, 175
      nonsurgical, 174
      semiconstrained total shoulder arthroplasty, 175
      surgical debridement and acromioplasty, 174
      unconstrained total shoulder arthroplasty, 175

D
Darrach procedure, 394
Dead arm sensation, 86
Dead arm syndrome, 60
Debridement
   in managing humeral shaft fractures, 205, 229
   in managing osteoarthritis of the shoulder, 229
   in managing rotator cuff tears, 167–168
Decompression
   complications related to, *158*, 158–161, *159, 160, 161*
   in managing rotator cuff tears, 167–168
Decompression sickness, 227
Degeneration, 317
Degenerative arthritis. *See also* Arthritis
   arthroscopic treatment of primary, 360
   of glenohumeral joint, 92
Degenerative calcification, 277
Deltoid detachment, *158*, 158–159
Deltoid dysfunction, 169
Deltopectoral approach, 111
Diabetes
   and compressive neuropathy, 369
   relationship between frozen shoulder and, 256
Directed imaging studies of elbow, 326
Displaced glenoid fractures, 201–202
Distal biceps tendon injury
   classification, 339
   partial detachment, 339
   partial rupture, *339*, 339–340
   strain, 339
   treatment, 339
Distal humerus, 301, *301*, 305–306. *See also* Humerus
   fractures of, 397
      complications, 401–402
      epidemiology/etiology, 397
      evaluation, 397–398, *398*
      results/outcome, 400–401
      treatment, 398–400, *399, 400*
Distant muscle transfer in surgical repair of rotator cuff tears, 168
Dorsal scapular nerve, 243
Double crush syndrome, 369
Drawer test, 61
DREZ ablation, 248
Dropped shoulder, 160–161

Dupuytren's contracture, 255, 256, 258, 259
   and frozen shoulder, 256
   steroid injections for, 259–260
Dynamic Joint Distractor™, 382

E
Edge effect, 369
Ehlers-Danlos syndrome, 347
Elbow
   arthroscopy, 319–320, *320, 321*
   athletic injuries of, 311, 321
      anterior, 319
      biomechanics, 311–313, *312*
      lateral, 317
      medial, 313–317, *315*
   biomechanics of total arthroplasty, *207*, 306–308
   contractures of, 325
   force transmission, 305
   functional anatomy
      capsuloligamentous tissues, *302*, 302–304, *303*
      muscles, 304
      osteology, *301*, 301–302
   instability
      classification of, 347–348, *348*
      complications, 352
      constraints, 347
      epidemiology, 345
      etiology, *345*, 345–347, *346*
      evaluation, 348–350, *349*
      results of treatment, 351–352
      treatment, 350–351, *351*
   kinematics, 304
      flexion-extension, *304*, 304–305
      prosupination, 305
   loose bodies of
      classification, 355
      complications, 360
      etiology, 355
      evaluation, *355*, 355–356, *356*
      results, 360
      treatment, 356, *357, 358, 358, 359,* 360
   nerve injuries and neuropathies about
      anterior interosseous, 373–374
      median neuropathy at, 373
      pathophysiology, 369–370
      ulnar neuropathy, 370–373
   osteochondritis dissecans of, 363
      clinical presentation, *363*, 363–364, *364*
      complications, 366
      etiology, 363
      natural history and treatment, 364–365, *365*
      results, 365–366
   rehabilitation, 320
   restoration of function in, 248
   stability, 387–388, *388*
   stabilizers, 305–306
      capsuloligamentous tissues, 306, *306*
      muscles, 306
   stiffness and ankylosis of, 325
      classification, 325
      complications, 333
      etiology, 325
      evaluation, 325–326
      incidence, 325
      nonsurgical management, *326*, 326–327, *327*
      results, 332–333
      surgical management
         extrinsic contracture, 327–329, *329*
         intrinsic contracture, *330*, 330–332, *331, 332*

tendon injuries and tendinopathies of
  chronic refractory tennis elbow, following failed
    surgical intervention, 338, *339*
  distal biceps tendon injury, classification, 339
  epicondylitis, *337*, 337–338
  medial epicondylitis, 338–339
  triceps, 342
  treatment of floating, 206
Elbow arthritis, 379
  osteoarthritis, 382–384
    etiology and presentation, 382
    evaluation, 382
    results, 384
    treatment, 382–383
  posttraumatic, 381–382
    arthrodesis, 382
    complications, 382
  rheumatoid, 379
    evaluation, 379
    nonsurgical treatment, 379
    surgical treatment, 379–381
Elbow arthroplasty, 220
Elbow arthroscopy, 311
Elbow flexion
  with pressure over ulnar nerve test, 371
  treatment of loss of, 250
Elbow flexion test, 371
Electrical shock, osteonecrosis following, 234
Electrodiagnostic studies in evaluating brachial plexus injuries, 244
Electromyography, 34–35
  in evaluating brachial plexus injuries, 244
Endurance training, 70
Entrapment neuropathy of lateral antebrachial cutaneous nerve, 377
Epicondylectomy, medial, 372
Epicondylitis, 317, *337*, 337–338
  lateral, 317
  medial, 338–339
Epineural radial nerve repair, 208
L'Episcopo procedure, 248, 250
Erb-Duchenne-Klumpke palsy, 249, 250
  surgical treatment for, 249
Erb's point, 243
Essex-Lopresti lesion, 394
Essex-Lopresti prosthetic replacement, 393
Ethanol, 234
Eulerian system, 31–32, *32*
Exercise. *See also* Isometric exercises
  in managing rheumatoid arthritis, 217
  in managing rotator cuff tear, 145–147, *146, 147*
  pendulum
    in managing rheumatoid arthritis, 217
    in managing shoulder dislocations, 69
  plyometric, 70–71
Extensor carpi radialis brevis (ECRB), 337
  and posterior interosseous neuropathy, 375
Extensor carpi radialis longus (ECRL) and posterior interosseous neuropathy, 375
External rotation lag sign (ERLS), 137–138
Extracorporeal shock wave therapy, 282

F
Familial hyperlipidemia, 227
Fibromatosis, 257–258
  Peyronie's penile, 258
Fisk view, 140, *140*
Fixation device, overimpaction of, 112–113
Flexible nails, 207, *207*
Flexion-extension of elbow, *304*, 304–305
Flexor-pronator strain, 316
Floating elbow, treatment of, 206
Forearm rotation, 387
Forearm stability after radial head fracture, 389, *390*
Four-part fractures and fracture-dislocations, 185–186

Fractures. *See also* Clavicle fractures; Humeral shaft fractures; Proximal humerus fractures; Scapula fractures
  acromial, 159, *159*
  coracoid, 201
  of coronoid, 350–351
    classification, 409, *410*
    complications, 411
    etiology, 409
    evaluation, 409
    results, 411
    treatment, 409–411, *411*
  of distal humerus, 397
    complications, 401–402
    epidemiology/etiology, 397
    evaluation, 397–398, *398*
    results/outcome, 400–401
    treatment, 398–400, *399, 400*
  of olecranon, 350
    classification, 405, *405*
    complications, 409
    etiology, 405
    evaluation, 405
    results, 408–409
    treatment, 405–408, *406, 407, 408*
  of radial head, 387
    biomechanics, 387–388, *388, 389, 390*
    complications following, 393–394
    evaluation, 388–389, *390*
    prosthetic replacement of, 392–393, *393*
    treatment based on modified Mason classification, 389–392, *391, 392*
Free muscle grafts, in restoring elbow and hand function, 247
Free tissue grafts, in repair of rotator cuff tears, 168
Frozen shoulder, 255, 261
  arthroscopic surgical release, 260–261, *261*
  associated conditions, 256
  clinical presentation, 255–256
  definition, 255
  diagnostic tests, 256, *256*, 256–257, *257*
  functional anatomy of rotator interval, 258–259
  incidence, 255
  natural history of, 259
  pathology, 257–258, *258*
  surgical exploration, 257
  terminology, 255
  treatment
    conservative, 259
    manipulation under anesthesia, 260
    steroid injection, 259–260
    surgical release, for frozen shoulder, 260
Fulcrum maneuver, 270, *271*
Full-thickness rotator cuff tears
  results of open repair, 153
  surgical technique for repair of, 152

G
Garrod's knuckle pads, 258
Gaucher's disease, 227, 233, 235, 237
Gerber's classification scheme, 167
Geyser sign, 141, *141*
Glenohumeral arthritis, 157, 201
Glenohumeral arthrodesis, 174, 235
  and resection arthroplasty of rotator cuff tear, 174–175
Glenohumeral arthroplasty
  glenoid component, *39t*, 40
    conformity of articulation, 42
    fixation, 42, *43*
    radiolucent lines and failure, 40–41
    rotator cuff considerations, 42
    thickness, *41*, 41–42
  humeral component
    fixation, 38–39, *39t*
    offset and soft-tissue reconstruction, *38*, 39

modular components, 39–40
prosthetic design considerations of, 38
Glenohumeral articulation, conformity of, 42
Glenohumeral degeneration from rheumatoid arthritis, 217
Glenohumeral fulcrum, 215
Glenohumeral instability
　complications stemming from treatment of, 111
　　intraoperative, 111–113, *112, 113*
　　postoperative, 113–114
　failed repairs, 114–116
　and misdiagnosis, 157
　pathophysiology of, 95
　revision surgery, 116–117
Glenohumeral joint, 31, 37–38. *See also* Arthroscopic anterior glenohumeral reconstruction; Shoulder
　capsule, *4*, 4–5
　degeneration of, 173
　labrum, 3–4
　long head of biceps tendon, 5, *5*
　multidirectional instability, 85
　　complications, 89
　　diagnosis, 86–87, *87*
　　etiology, 85–86
　　results, 88–89
　　treatment, 87–88, *88*
　osseous structures, 3
　posterior instability, 89
　　complications, 92
　　diagnosis, 89–90, *90*
　　etiology, 89
　　results, 91–92
　　treatment, 90–91, *91*
　rotator cuff interval, 5
　stability
　　biomechanical analysis of, 59
　　and classification systems, 64
　　clinical evaluation, 59–62, *61*
　　pathophysiology of instability, 59, *59, 60*
　　radiographic evaluation, 62, *63*
　　　magnetic resonance imaging and computed tomographic imaging, *63*, 63–64
Glenohumeral ligaments and capsule, *13*, 13–15, *14*
Glenohumeral motion, normal, 37
Glenohumeral stability
　dynamic contributors to
　　biceps tendon, 15–16, *16*
　　individual components of rotator cuff, 15
　　joint compression, 15
　　preloading ligaments, 15
　　proprioception, 15
　　scapular rotators, 16
　　relative importance of various components to, *16*, 16–17
　static contributors to
　　glenoid labrum, 12
　　glenoid version, 11–12, *12*
　　humeral version, 11, *11*
　　intra-articular pressure, 12–13
　　ligaments and capsule, *13*, 13–15, *14*
　　surface area and articular conformity, 12
Glenohumeral synovectomy, 220
Glenohumeral synovitis, 215
Glenoid articular cartilage, aberrant drilling through, 112
Glenoid bone
　fractures of, 201–202, 227
　intraoperative fracture of, 227
　preoperative diagnosis of involvement, 235
　in rheumatoid shoulders, 221
Glenoid component, presence of radiolucent lines about, 223
Glenoid labral compression test, 102
Glenoid labrum, 12
Glenoid loosening, 223
Glenoid osteotomy, 92
　for posterior instability, 227

Glenoid reamers, 223
Glenoid resurfacing, 221, 222
Glenoid rim fractures, 202
Glenoplasty, 91
Glucocerebroside, 235, 237
Glycosaminoglycans (GAG), 26
Gold salts in management of rheumatoid arthritis, 217
Golf, 35, 312
Golgi tendon organs, desensitizing, 71
Gout, 227
Gunshot wounds, 251
Gymnastics, 312–313

H
Hawkins sign, 136, *136*
Hawkins test, 62
Health Status Questionnaire Short Form 36 (SF 36), 176
Hemiarthroplasty
　for chronic posterior dislocation, 74
　for cuff tear arthropathy, 174, 176
　for inflammatory arthritis of shoulder, 220, 221
　for osteoarthritis of the shoulder, 228
　for rotator cuff tear, 175
Hemochromatosis, 237–238
Hereditary epiphyseal dysplasia. *See* Osteochondritis dissecans
Heterotopic bone formation, 187
Heterotopic ossification, 160, *160*, 284, *284*
　postoperative, 229
Hill-Sachs lesions, 59, 102
Histamine sensitivity testing in evaluating brachial plexus injuries, 245
Holstein-Lewis fracture, 208
Home stretching in treating frozen shoulder, 259
Horii circle, 346
Horizontal subscapularis muscle-splitting approach, 111
Horner's syndrome in evaluating brachial plexus injuries, 244
Hospital for Special Surgery System for Assessing Shoulder Function, 49
Humeral functional brace, 205
Humeral head
　blood supply of, 44t, 44–45
　replacement of, 185–186, 228, 234–235
Humeral hemiarthroplasty, 221
Humeral shaft fractures, 205
　complications
　　nonunion, 208–209
　　radial nerve injury, 208
　　vascular injury, 208
　etiology, 205
　evaluation, 205
　imaging, 205
　nonsurgical management, 205, *206*, 209
　periprosthetic, 229
　of rheumatoid bone, 222–223
　surgical treatment, 205–206, *206*, 209
　　fixation using plates and screws, 206, *207*
　　intramedullary fixation, 206–208, *207, 208*
Humeral site anterior inferior glenohumeral ligament avulsion, 95
Humerus. *See also* Distal humerus
　distal, 301, *301*, 305–306
　rotational osteotomy of, 91
　rotation of, *31*, 31–32, *32*
Hyperlipidemia, fibromatosis, 227
Hyperuricemia, 227

I
Imatani Scoring System, 48, 54
Impingement, 60
　diagnosis of, 157
　internal, 101, 103
　outside, 101
　pain in, 382–383
　posteromedial, 317–318, *318*

postoperative, 229
and rotator cuff lesions, 103–104
signs of, 102
symptomatic, of humeral head, 92
Impingement syndrome, 128–129
coronoid, 319
indications for surgery in chronic, 151
surgical management for, 158
Impingement tests, 61–62
Inadequate decompression, 159
Infection
postoperative, in rheumatoid arthritis, 222
Yersinia enterocolitica, 238
Inferior capsular shift procedure, 87–88, 89, 104
Inferior glenohumeral ligament (IGHL), 3, 4, *4, 14,* 14–15
Inferior stability tests, 61
Inflammatory process, 257–258
Infraclavicular injuries to brachial plexus, 245–246
Infraspinatus fossa, 265
Infraspinatus muscle, 19–20, 123
weakness, 291
Infraspinatus-splitting approach, 112
Instability. *See also* Glenohumeral instability; Multidirectional instability
anterior
recurrence rate of, 114–115
recurrent, 104
anterosuperior, 223
chronic valgus, 394
clavicular, 160–161
posterolateral rotatory, 317, 348
recurrent anterior, 104
after shoulder arthroplasty for rheumatoid arthritis, 223
superior glenohumeral, 160
valgus, 347, 350, 351, 379, 394
varus, 347–348
Instability complex, 101
Intact rotator cuff with subacromial decompression, 152–153
Interlocked nails, 207–208, *208*
Internal fixation, techniques of, 183, *184*
Internal impingement, 101, 103
Internal rotation lag sign (IRLS), 137, 138
Interposition arthroplasty, 380
Intra-articular fracture
of distal humerus, 351
of glenoid, 92
Intramedullary fixation, 206–208, *207, 208*
Intrinsic contracture, surgical management of, *330,* 330–332, *331, 332*
In vitro glenohumeral kinematics, 33
Iontophoresis in managing rotator cuff tear, 145
Ischemic necrosis, 233
Isokinetic training, 69, *70*
Isolated glenohumeral synovitis, synovectomy for, 218, *218*
Isolated greater tuberosity fractures, 184
Isometric exercises
in managing rheumatoid arthritis, 217
in managing shoulder dislocation, 69

J
Jobe's augmentation and relocation tests, 270
Jobe sign, 138
Joint Active System (JAS), 327
Joint replacement arthroplasty, 380–381, *381*
Joint stiffness, 187
Jones procedure to resect humeral head for fractures, 228

K
Klumpke's palsy, 249

L
Labrum, 3–4
detachment, 97
fraying, 97
repair, 97–98
tears, 157
Lateral acromionectomy, 158
Lateral antebrachial cutaneous nerve, 376–377
Lateral collateral ligament (LCL), *302,* 302–303, 306, *306*
and elbow instability, 345, 346, 347, 349, 351
Lateral epicondylitis. *See* Epicondylitis
Lateral humeral offset, 37, *38*
Lateral pivot-shift apprehension test, 345, 349–350
Lateral tomograms in diagnosing loose bodies, 356
Latissimus dorsi muscle transfer, 170, 248, 250
Lift-off test, 137
Ligament augmentation device (LAD™), 340, 341
Little Leaguer's elbow, 363
Load and shift maneuver, 270, *271*
Local muscle repairs or transfer in surgical repair of rotator cuff tears, 168
Long thoracic nerve palsy, 252
Loose bodies of elbow, 317–318
classification, 355
complications, 360
etiology, 355
evaluation, *355,* 355–356, *356*
removal, 358, *358, 359,* 360
results, 360
treatment, 356, *357,* 358, *358, 359,* 360
Loss of motion, 135

M
Magnetic resonance imaging (MRI), in assessing
brachial plexus injuries, 244–245
clavicle fractures, 192
complete rupture from tuberosity, *340,* 340–342, *341*
distal biceps tendon injury, 340
elbow injuries, 311, 326
frozen shoulder, 256
glenohumeral joint stability, 63
rheumatoid arthritis, 217
rotator cuff, 142–144, *143, 144*
rotator cuff tears, 167
shoulder lesions, 271
Magnetic resonance imaging (MRI) arthrography, in assessing glenohumeral joint stability, 63
Magnusen-Stack procedure, 79, 104, 113, 116, 117
Malunion
of clavical fractures, 195
of proximal humerus fractures, 187
of scapular neck fractures, 201
Mason-Allen technique, 152
Matrix of direction cosines, 31
Mayo device, 330, 331, *331*
Mayo Elbow Performance Score (MEPS), 381
Mayo-modified Coonrad device, 306
McLaughlin procedure, 74
Medial capsulorrhaphy, 88
Medial collateral ligament (MCL), 303, *303,* 305, 306
and elbow instability, 345, 346, 347, 349, 350, 351
Medial epicondylectomy, 372
Medial epicondyle fractures, 316
Medial epicondylitis, 316, 338–339
Medial triceps subluxation, 371
Median neuropathy at elbow, 373
Metallic staples, 95
Metastatic brachial plexopathy, 251
Methotrexate in management of rheumatoid arthritis, 217
Methylmethacrylate, prosthetic glenoid fixation with, 228–229

Microspheroliths, 277
Middle glenohumeral ligament (MGHL), 3, 4, *4*, 14
Milwaukee shoulder, 173
Misdiagnosis, complications of rotator cuff surgery related to, 157–158
Mononeuritis of suprascapular nerve, 265
Motion/strength testing, 138
Multidirectional instability, 85
    complications, 89
    diagnosis, 86–87, *87*
    etiology, 85–86
    results, 88–89
    treatment of, 87–88, *88,* 115
Muscle repair or transfer, 168
Myelography in evaluating brachial plexus injuries, 244

N

Necrosis
    avascular, 233
    ischemic, 233
Neer classification of proximal humeral fractures, 44, 181–182, 183
Neer impingement sign, 136, *136*, 270
Neer impingement test, 61–62
Neer modification of McLaughlin procedure, 186
Nerve conduction velocity studies in evaluating brachial plexus injuries, 244
Nerve grafting, 247
Nerve injuries to elbow, 316–317
    anterior interosseous, 373–374
    median neuropathy at, 373
    pathophysiology, 369–370
    ulnar neuropathy, 370–373
Nerve transfer, 247, *248*
Neurapraxias, 245, 369
Neurologic entrapment syndromes, diagnosis and treatment of, 265–267, *266*
Neurologic injury, *162*, 162–163
Neuropathy, 409
Neurotization, 247, *248*
Neurotmesis, 245, 369
Neurovascular injuries
    to athlete's shoulder, 106
        long thoracic nerve, 106
        quadrilateral space syndrome, 107, *108*
        suprascapular nerve entrapment, 106–107, *107*
    and clavicle fractures, 195
Nonanatomic stabilization procedures, 113
Nonconstrained total joint arthroplasty, 229
Nonsteroidal anti-inflammatory drugs (NSAIDs)
    and formation of heterotopic bone, 402
    in managing rheumatoid arthritis, 217
    in managing rotator cuff tear, 145
Nonsurgical management
    of acute anterior dislocation of shoulder, 69–71, *70, 71*
    of arthritis, 217–218
    of brachial plexus injuries, 246–247
    of cuff tear arthropathy, 174
    of humeral shaft fractures, 205, *206,* 209
    of osteoarthritis of glenohumeral joint, 228
    of rheumatoid arthritis, 217–218, 379
    of rotator cuff tear, 174
    of rotator cuff tears, 144–147, *146, 147,* 174
    of scapular fractures, 201–202
    of stiffness and ankylosis of the elbow, *326,* 326–327, *327*
Nonunion
    of clavicle fracture, 195
    of humeral shaft fractures, 208–209
    of proximal humerus fracture, 187

O

O'Brien test, 102
    for superior labrum anterior and posterior (SLAP) lesions, 270, *270*
Obstetric injuries to brachial plexus, 249–250
Ochronosis, 227
Olecranon, fractures of, 350
    classification, 405, *405*
    complications, 409
    etiology, 405
    evaluation, 405
    results, 408–409
    treatment, 405–408, *406, 407, 408*
Olecranon osteotomy, 400
Oncologic-induced injuries, 251
Open capsular release, 327–328
Opening wedge osteotomy, 91
Open reduction and internal fixation, 184, 185
Orthotherapy, 146
Osgood-Schlatter disease, 318
Osseous structures, 3
Ossification
    of clavicle, 191
    heterotopic, 284, *284*
Osteoarthritis, 355. *See also* Arthritis
    etiology and presentation, 382
    evaluation, 382
    of glenohumeral joint
        clinical evaluation of, 227–228
        complications, 229
        etiology of, 227
        nonsurgical treatment of, 228
        radiographic features of, 228
        results/outcomes, 229
        surgical intervention, 228
    results, 384
    secondary, 227
    treatment, 382–383
Osteochondral fractures, 317. *See also* Osteochondritis dissecans
Osteochondritis dissecans, 360
    in children, 364
    of elbow, 363
        clinical presentation, *363,* 363–364, *364*
        complications, 366
        etiology, 363
        natural history and treatment, 364–365, *365*
        results, 365–366
Osteochondrosis. *See* Osteochondritis dissecans
Osteology, *301,* 301–302, *302*
Osteonecrosis, 45, 187. *See also* Osteochondritis dissecans
    of glenoid, 92
    nontraumatic, 233–234
        evaluation, 234
        of proximal humerus, 227
        treatment and results, 234–235, *236*
    posttraumatic, 233, *234*
        evaluation, 233, *235*
        surgical treatment, 233
    of shoulder, 237
Osteophytes, 317–318
    removal of, 358, *358, 359,* 360
Osteotomy, 113, 187
    olecranon, 400
    periarticular, 228
Outerbridge-Kashiwagi arthroplasty, 358
Outside impingement, 101

P

Paget's disease, 227
Pain
    anterior shoulder, 101–103
    in cervical disk disease, 157
    in cuff tear arthropathy, 174, 176
    impingement, 382–383
    in rotator cuff tears, 135

shoulder, in athletes, 101–108, *105, 106, 107, 108,* 129
suprascapular nerve in entrapment, 265
Palsy
    Erb-Duchenne-Klumpke, 249, 250
    Klumpke's, 249
    long thoracic nerve, 252
    suprascapular, 252
Pancreatitis, 227
Panner's disease. *See* Osteochondritis dissecans
Paravertebral nerve blocks, 251
Partial-thickness tears, surgical management of rotator cuff disease, 151–152
Particulate synovitis, 392
Pectoralis transfer, 248, 250
Pediatric supracondylar elbow fractures, 377
Pendulum exercises
    in managing rheumatoid arthritis, 217
    in managing shoulder dislocations, 69
D-penicillamine in managing rheumatoid arthritis, 217
Periarthritis, 255
Periarticular osteotomy, 228
Periprosthetic humeral shaft fractures, 229
Perthes disease of hip, 364
Peyronie's penile fibromatosis, 258
Phenobarbitone, 256
Phenytoin, 256
Phlebotomy, 238
Phonophoresis in managing rotator cuff tear, 145
Physical therapy in managing rheumatoid arthritis, 217
Physiotherapy in treating frozen shoulder, 259
Pigmented villonodular synovitis, 284
Plantar fibromatosis, 258, 259
Plates, fixation using, 206, *207, 208*
Plica band syndrome, 317
Plyometric exercise, 70–71, 295, *295*
Postanesthetic brachial plexus palsy, 250
Posterior apprehension test, 102
Posterior bone block, 91, *91*
Posterior elbow injuries, 317–319
Posterior glenoid bone loss, 228
Posterior interosseous nerve and lateral epicondylitis, 337, 338
Posterior interosseous neuropathy, 375–376
Posterior medial impingement, *318*
Posterior stability tests, 61
Posterior stabilization surgery, 112
Posterior stress test, 90
Posterolateral rotatory apprehension test, *349,* 349–350
Posterolateral rotatory instability, 317, 348
Posteromedial impingement, 317–318
Postoperative impingement, 229
Postoperative rehabilitation, 163
Postoperative stiffness, 163
Posttraumatic arthritis, 195, 381–382
    arthrodesis, 382
    complications, 382
Progressive abduction of shoulder, 85
Pronator syndrome, *374,* 374–375
Proprioception, 15
Prosthetic arthroplasty, 228–229
Prosthetic glenoid fixation with methylmethacrylate, 228–229
Prosthetic replacement of radial head, 392–393, *393*
Proximal humerus, blood supply of, 233
Proximal humerus fractures, 42, 227
    classification of, 44
    complications, 187
    etiology, 181
    evaluation, 181–183, *182*
    general considerations for open reduction and internal fixation, 44
    treatment/results, 183–187, *184, 185, 186*
Proximal radioulnar joint, 347
Proximal radius, 305
Proximal ulna, 301, *302,* 305

Psammomas, 277
Pseudodislocation, 192
Pseudogout. *See* Chondrocalcinosis (pseudogout)
Putti-Platt procedure, 79, 104, 113, 117
    development of osteoarthrosis following, *114*
    reverse, 91

Q
Quadrilateral space syndrome, 107, *108*
Quality Adjusted Life Years (QALY) analysis, 47–48
Quality of Life Index, 47

R
Racquet sports, 312
Radial head, fractures of, 351, 387
    biomechanics, 387–388, *388, 389, 390*
    complications following, 393–394
    evaluation, 388–389, *390*
    prosthetic replacement of, 392–393, *393*
    treatment based on modified Mason classification, 389–392, *391, 392*
Radial nerve
    entrapment of, 317
    injury to, 208
Radial nerve neuropathy at elbow, 375
Radial nerve palsy, 342
    managing, 208
Radial tunnel syndrome, 376, *376*
Radiation-induced injuries, 251
Radiocapitellar arthrosis, 393
Radiocapitellar chondromalacia, 317
Radiocapitellar overload syndrome, 317
Radiographs, in assessing
    brachial plexus injuries, 244
    clavicle fractures, 192
    proximal humerus fractures, *182,* 182–183
    rotator cuff, *138,* 138–140, *139, 140*
    rotator cuff tears, 167
Radius, proximal, 305
Range-of-motion testing of cervical spine, 62
Reactive calcification, 277–278, *278*
Reaming, 207
Recurrent anterior instability, 104
Recurrent tear, 161–162
Referred pain related to cervical disk disease, 157
Reflex sympathetic dystrophy, 163
Rehabilitation
    of elbow, 320
    of shoulder, 289
        constraint systems around, 289–290
        force couples around, 290, 290t
        guidelines for implementing, 291–292
        kinematic chain, 290, 290t
        organization of progression, *292,* 292–295, *293, 294, 295*
        pathophysiology accompanying injury, 290–291
        physiologic and biomechanical basis for, 289, 289t
        postoperative protocol, 295–297
Renal transplantation, 227
Repetitive hyperangulation, 101
Repetitive microtrauma, 103
Resection arthroplasty, 174, 228
Resorption phenomenon, 279
Reverse Putti-Platt repair, 91
Rheumatoid arthritis, 215, 379. *See also* Arthritis
    clinical presentation, 217
    evaluation, 379
    nonsurgical management, 217–218, 379
    pathophysiology, 215, *216,* 217
    surgical treatment, 379–381
Rheumatoid bone, fracture of, 222–223
Rheumatoid foot deformities, 220
Rheumatologist in managing rheumatoid arthritis, 217
Rocking horse glenoid, 175, 220

Rotational osteotomy of humerus, 91
Rotation matrix, 31
Rotationplasty of subscapularis muscle, 168
Rotator cable, 23
Rotator cuff, 38. *See also* Cuff tear arthropathy
   anatomy of
      abnormal, 125
      arterial supply of, 123
      coracoacromial arch, 22, *22*
      infraspinatus muscle, 19–20
      microstructure, 21, *21, 22*
      normal, 123, *124*
      subscapularis muscle, *20*, 20–21
      supraspinatus muscle, 19, *19, 20*
      teres minor, 20
      vascularity, 21
   biochemistry, 26
   biomechanics, 22–26, *23, 24, 25*
   as critical factor in outcome of glenohumeral arthroplasty, 42
   dysfunctional, 69
   exercises for, 294
   function of, 127–128
   imaging of
      arthrography, *140*, 140–141, *141*
      magnetic resonance imaging, 141–144, *143, 144*
      plain radiographs, *138*, 138–140, *139, 140*
      ultrasound, *141*, 141–142
   intact, with subacromial decompression, 152–153
Rotator cuff diseases, 123
   etiology, 129–130
   natural history, *130*, 130–131
   pathogenesis, 128–129
      vascular factors, 128
   as source of impingement, 129
Rotator cuff injury, 26, 291
   etiology of diseases, *27*, 27–28, *28*
   pathology, *26*, 26–27
   tendinosis, 26–27
Rotator cuff repair
   complications related to, 161–163, *162*
   for rheumatoid arthritis, 220
Rotator cuff surgery, complications of
   related to decompression, *158*, 158–161, *159, 160, 161*
   related to misdiagnosis, 157–158
   related to postoperative rehabilitation, 163
   related to repair, 161–163, *162*
   related to wound healing, 163
Rotator cuff tears, 125, 167, 170
   full-thickness
      results of open repair, 153
      surgical technique for repair of, 152
   history of, 135
   massive
      clinical evaluation of, 167
      failed, 169, *169, 170*
      surgical management of, 167
         arthrodesis and arthroplasty, 168–169
         debridement and decompression, 167–168
         distant muscle transfers, 168
         free tissue grafts, 168
         local muscle repairs or transfer, 168
         synthetic grafts, 168
   nonsurgical management of, 144, 174
      corticosteroid injection, 145
      exercise, 145–147, *146, 147*
      iontophoresis, 145
      nonsteroidal anti-inflammatory medication, 145
      phonophoresis, 145
      ultrasound, 145
   pain in, 135
   physical examination, 135–138, *136, 137*
   and rheumatoid arthritis, 215
   surgical management of partial-thickness, 151–152
   surgical techniques for patients with intact, 151
Rotator interval, 19
   functional anatomy of, 258–259
Rowe score, 54
Rush pin technique, 184

S

Salicylates in management of rheumatoid arthritis, 217
Sarcoidosis, 234
Scapula, anatomy of, *199*, 199–200
Scapular fractures, 199
   classification, 200–201
   complications, 201
   evaluation, 201
   nonsurgical treatment and results, 201–202
   prevalence and associated injuries, 200, *200*
   surgical approaches and technique, 202
   surgical treatment and results, 202, *202*
Scapular inclination as factor in inferior instability of shoulder, 85
Scapular muscle failure, 291
Scapular neck fractures, 200
Scapular rotators, 16
Scapular stabilization, 293
Scapulothoracic articulation, 7. *See also* Shoulder
Scapulothoracic crepitus, 201
Scapulothoracic dissociation, 201
Scapulothoracic joint, 31
Screw, fixation using, 206, *207, 208*
Screw-displacement axis system, 32
Secondary osteoarthritis, 227
Segmental shortening, 394
Semiconstrained total shoulder arthroplasty of rotator cuff tear, 175
Semmes Weinstein monofilaments, 370
Severity Index for Chronically Painful Shoulders, 49
SF-36 assessment, 48
Shock wave therapy for epicondylitis, 338
Shoulder. *See also* Acromioclavicular joint;
   Glenohumeral joint; Scapulothoracic articulation;
   Sternoclavicular joint; Subacromial space
   acute anterior dislocation, 67
      initial treatment, 67–69, *68*
      natural history, 69
      nonsurgical treatment, 69–71, *70, 71*
      presentation and examination, 67
      radiographic evaluation, 67, *67, 68*
      surgical treatment of initial anterior dislocation, *71*, 71–72
   acute posterior dislocation, 72
      initial treatment of, 73
      presentation and examination of, 72
   chronic anterior dislocations, 73–74
   chronic posterior dislocations (locked), 74–75
   frozen (*See* Frozen shoulder)
   inflammatory arthritis of, 215, 223–224
      clinical presentation, 217
      complications, 222–223
      nonsurgical management, 217–218
      pathophysiology, 215–*216*, 217
      results/outcome, 221–222
      surgical management, 218, *218, 219*, 220–221
   kinematics and kinesiology, *31*, 31–35, *32, 34*
   primary role of, 31
   recurrent anterior instability, 77
      complications, 80–81
      evaluation, 77–79, *78*
      treatment, 79–80, *80, 81*
   relevant anatomy and biomechanics of, *37*, 37t, 37–38, *38*
Shoulder arthrodesis, 247–248
Shoulder disorders
   evaluating outcomes in treatment of, 47, *47*
      quality of life and general health assessments, 47–48, 48t

global or universal shoulder assessments, 48t, 48–53
  assessments for specific diseases, 53–54
  evaluating outcomes, 54
Shoulder girdle
  acromioclavicular joint, 6–7
  glenohumeral joint, 3–5, *4, 5*
  scapulothoracic articulation, 7
  subacromial space, 5–6
Shoulder joint capsule, *4*, 4–5
Shoulder motion
  descriptions of, *31*, 31–32, *32*
  electromyography, 34–35
  mathematical models, 33–34
  radiographic techniques, 32
  in vitro and in vivo studies, 32–33
Shoulder Pain and Disability Index, 53
Shoulder replacement surgery for osteonecrosis, 237
Sickle cell disease, 233, 237
Silicone synovitis, 392
Simple Shoulder Test, 53, 176
SLAP. *See* Superior labrum anterior and posterior (SLAP) lesions
Smoking and risk of osteonecrosis, 234
Snow cap subarticular sclerosis, 174
Soft-tissue injury, 201
Soft-tissue repairs for posterior instability, 91
Somatosensory-evoked potentials in evaluating brachial plexus injuries, 244
Sonography in postoperative shoulder, 142
Speed tests, 137
Spinoglenoid notch, 265
  entrapment, 266–267
Spiral tomography of elbow, 326
Splinting of elbow, *326*, 326–327, *327*
Sports-related injuries to brachial plexus, 251
Spurling's test, 138
Spur removal, 229
Staple capsulorrhaphy, 112
Staples, 161
  loosening and migration of capsular, 113, *113*
  metallic, 95
Static progressive splinting, *326*, 326–327
Steindler flexorplasty, 248, 250
Stereophotogrammetry, 3, 127
Sternoclavicular joint, 7, 31. *See also* Shoulder
Sternocleidomastoid transfer, 248
Steroids. *See also* Corticosteroids
  in osteonecrosis, 234
  in treating frozen shoulder, 259–260
Stimson maneuver, 67
Stingers, 251–252
Stinger syndrome, 106
Stress fractures, 317–318
Stryker notch view, 78
Subacromial bursa, 6, 218
Subacromial bursectomy, 218, *219*, 220
Subacromial space, 5–6
  decompression of, 161
Subdeltoid bursa, 218
Subscapularis, *20*, 20–21
  postoperative ruptures of, 111
  recession or lengthening, 228
Subscapular recess, 258
Sulcus sign, 86, *87*, 102
Sulfasalazine in management of rheumatoid arthritis, 217
Superior capsule-cuff complex, 23
Superior glenohumeral instability, 160
Superior glenohumeral ligament (SGHL), 4, 5, *13*, 13–14
Superior labrum anterior and posterior (SLAP) lesions, 96, 97, 102, 269
  surgical management of, 271
  test for, 269, 270, *270*
Superior shoulder suspensory complex (SSSC), 199, *199*
  double disruption of, 202
Supraclavicular traction injuries, 245
Supracondylar elbow fractures, pediatric, 377
Supracondylar fracture of distal humerus, 351
Suprascapular nerve, 157, 265
  entrapment, 106–107, *107*, 265
    anatomy, 265
    complications, 267
    etiology, 265
    evaluation, 265–266, *266*
    results, 267
    treatment, 266–267
  palsy, 252
Suprascapular notch, 265
Supraspinatus fossa, 265
Supraspinatus muscle, 19, *19, 20*
  selective strengthening of, 69, *70*
Supraspinatus outlet, 19
Supraspinatus tendon, 19
Supraspinatus test, 137
Suretac absorbable anchor, 95
Suretac technique, 272, *272*
Surgical management. *See also specific surgeries*
  of calcifying tendinitis, 282
  debridement and acromioplasty of rotator cuff tear, 174
  for frozen shoulder, 260
  of shoulder lesions, 271–274, *272, 273, 274*
Suture anchors, 95, 152
Swanson Hospital for Special Surgery, 53
Swanson Scoring System, 48–59
Swimming
  breaststroke, 35
  butterfly stroke, 35
Symptomatic impingement of humeral head, 92
Synovectomy
  in managing elbow arthritis, 379–380, *380*
  in managing isolated glenohumeral synovitis, 218, *218*
Synovial fluid deficiencies, 173
Synovial osteochondromatosis, 238
Synovitis
  particulate, 392
  pigmented villonodular, 284
  silicone, 392
Synthetic grafts in surgical repair of rotator cuff tears, 168
Systemic lupus erythematosus, 227

T
Tadpole lesion, 369
Tendinitis
  biceps, 319
  brachialis, 319
  calcifying, 277–282, *278, 279, 280, 281, 282*
  triceps, 318–319
Tendinosis, rotator cuff, 26–27
Tendon injuries and tendinopathies about the elbow
  chronic refractory tennis elbow following failed surgical intervention, 338, *339*
  distal biceps tendon injury
    classification, 339
    complete rupture from the tuberosity, 340–342, *340, 341*
    partial rupture, *339*, 339–340
    strain, 339
  epicondylitis, *337*, 337–338
    medial, 338–339
  triceps tendon injury, 342
    diagnosis, 342
    treatment, 342
Tendon transfers, 248
Tennis elbow. *See also* Epicondylitis
  chronic refractory, following failed surgical intervention, 338
Tennis swing, 35
Tension band wiring, 185

Teres minor weakness, 291
Teres muscle, 20
Thoracic outlet syndrome, 106, 157, 371
Three-part fractures and fracture-dislocations, 185
Throwing
    anterior instability in athlete, 77
    injuries to elbow, 311–312, 313
    phases of, *34*, 34–35
Tinel's sign, 370, 371, 374
Total elbow arthroplasty, 402
    biomechanics of, 306–308, *307*
Total shoulder arthroplasty, 174
T-plasty modification of Bankart procedure, 88
T plate fixation, 185
Traction apophysitis, 318
Traction neurapraxia, 111
Transosseous suture technique, 152
Triceps tendinitis and rupture, 318–319
Triceps tendon
    injury
        diagnosis, 342
        treatment, 342
    transfer, 248, 250
Tuberosity fractures, 222–223
Turnbuckle splint, 327, *327*
Two-part tuberosity fractures, 184
Two-point discrimination, 370

U
UCLA scores, 49, 53, 54
Ulna, proximal, 301, *302*, 305
Ulnar collateral ligament (UCL)
    acute rupture of anterior band of, 315–316
    injury, 313–316, *315*
    stress test, 315
Ulnar nerve
    anatomy of, 370
    dysfunction, 402
    etiology, 370–371, *371*
    transposition, 317
    and neurolysis, 401–402
Ulnar neuritis, 372, 409
Ulnar neuropathy at elbow, 370–373
Ulnohumeral arthroplasty, 383
Ulnohumeral articulation, 387
Ultrasound, in assessing
    rotator cuff, *141*, 141–142
    rotator cuff tear, 145
Unconstrained total shoulder arthroplasty of rotator cuff tear, 175

V
Valgus extension overload syndrome, 314t, 316
Valgus instability, 347, 350, 351, 379
    chronic, 394
Valgus moment, 345
Varus instability, 347–348
Vascular injury, 208
Vascular synovitis, 259

W
Walch-Duplay Score, 54
Wallerian degeneration, 245
Wartenberg sign, 371
Watertight closure, 162
Weight lifting, 312–313
West Point axillary view, 78
Whipple test, 271, *271*
Wound healing, complications of rotator cuff surgery related to, 163

Y
Yergason test, 137
Yersinia enterocolitica, infections with, 238